Register Now for Online Access to Your Book!

SPRINGER PUBLISHING
CONNECT™

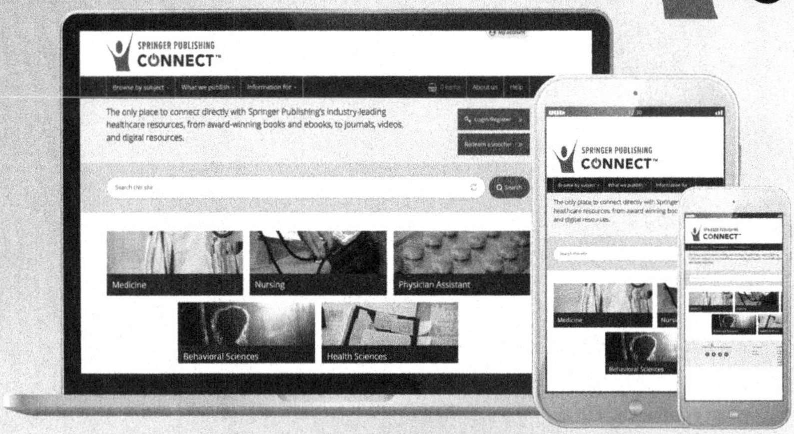

AF676617

Your print purchase of *Clinical Neurophysiology Board Review Q&A, Second Edition* **includes online access to the contents of your book**—increasing accessibility, portability, and searchability!

Access today at:
http://connect.springerpub.com/content/book/978-0-8261-8188-6
or scan the QR code at the right with your smartphone
and enter the access code below.

KJ0JNUWK

Scan here for quick access.

If you are experiencing problems accessing the digital component of this product, please contact our customer service department at cs@springerpub.com

The online access with your print purchase is available at the publisher's discretion and may be removed at any time without notice.

Publisher's Note: New and used products purchased from third-party sellers are not guaranteed for quality, authenticity, or access to any included digital components.

Clinical Neurophysiology Board Review Q&A

Second Edition

Puneet K. Gupta, MD, MSE, FACNS
Epileptologist and Neurohospitalist
Neurology Consultants of Dallas, P.A.
Director, Neurodiagnostics and Epilepsy
Medical City Dallas
Adjunct Assistant Professor
Department of Neurology and Neurotherapeutics
University of Texas Southwestern Medical Center
Dallas, Texas

Pradeep N. Modur, MD, MS
Director
Ascension Comprehensive Epilepsy Program
Professor
Department of Neurology
Dell Medical School at the University of Texas at Austin
Austin, Texas

Srikanth Muppidi, MD
Clinical Associate Professor
Neuromuscular Section
Department of Neurology and Neurological Sciences
Stanford School of Medicine
Stanford, California

demosMEDICAL
An Imprint of Springer Publishing

First Springer Publishing edition 2015.

Springer Publishing Company, LLC
11 West 42nd Street, New York, NY 10036
www.springerpub.com
connect.springerpub.com/

Acquisitions Editor: Beth Barry
Compositor: diacriTech

ISBN: 9780826181879
ebook ISBN: 9780826181886
DOI: 10.1891/9780826181886

22 23/ 5

Medicine is an ever-changing science. Research and clinical experience are continually expanding our knowledge, in particular our understanding of proper treatment and drug therapy. The authors, editors, and publisher have made every effort to ensure that all information in this book is in accordance with the state of knowledge at the time of production of the book. Nevertheless, the authors, editors, and publisher are not responsible for any errors or omissions or for any consequence from application of the information in this book and make no warranty, expressed or implied, with respect to the content of this publication. Every reader should examine carefully the package inserts accompanying each drug and should carefully check whether the dosage schedules therein or the contraindications stated by the manufacturer differ from the statements made in this book. Such examination is particularly important with drugs that are either rarely used or have been newly released on the market.

Library of Congress Cataloging-in-Publication Data
Library of Congress Control Number: 2020907804

Publisher's Note: **New and used products purchased from third-party sellers are not guaranteed for quality, authenticity, or access to any included digital components.**

Printed in the United States of America by Gasch Printing.

To our children—Nayan and Sonali; Sara, Maya, and Ross; and Medha—who are old enough to now understand the sacrifices we make for our patients' well-being. Their innocent and unrelenting inquisitiveness regarding the purpose of Board Review books is a true inspiration to revise and make this edition more meaningful. We are ever grateful to our children for their unconditional love, inspiration, and encouragement.

Contents

Preface

Five years have passed since publishing the first edition of *Clinical Neurophysiology Board Review Q&A*. This revision has provided us with an opportunity to include updates and advancements in neurodiagnostics that have occurred during this time. For example, invasive EEG monitoring has seen an increase in the use of stereo-EEG (SEEG), allowing for better assessment of the epileptic network for presurgical evaluations in a minimally invasive way; quantitative EEG (QEEG) has helped to expand the use and meaning of prolonged bedside critical care monitoring; and there is an increasing use of imaging for neuromuscular disorders (e.g., ultrasound for compressive neuropathies).

The objective of this second edition is the same as the first edition, which is to help solidify concepts, identify knowledge gaps, and, more importantly, provide the confidence to not only pass but also to perform well in various testing environments, from attending rounds to board examinations. Although this text was initially aimed for physicians, we were happy to hear positive reviews from technologists who stated that it helped them pass their respective boards as well. The digital platform has also been a great resource to many readers, and we hope that it continues to be so.

In this second edition, we continued to strive to make this resource more valuable. We revised and added a fifth answer choice to all (more than 800) the questions to better mimic the testing environment. In addition, more than 80 new questions and answers have been added to further expand the breadth and depth of knowledge.

We continue to be determined to make this book as comprehensive, user-friendly, and error-free as possible. We hope the book continues to help you reach your goals.

Good luck! As always, we welcome constructive feedback to help with future editions.

Puneet K. Gupta, MD, MSE, FACNS
Pradeep N. Modur, MD, MS
Srikanth Muppidi, MD

Acknowledgments

We would like to express our gratitude to the many people who continue to support us through this project:

To our editors and publishers—Beth Barry, Jaclyn Shultz, and Demos Medical Publishing—whose guidance and accountability helped us to complete this revision in a timely manner.

To our spouses—Paula, Lisa, and Kavitha—whose love and tolerance of our shenanigans knows no bounds.

To our children—Nayan and Sonali; Sara, Maya, and Ross; and Medha—who love to question everything in life but for our love of them.

To our teachers, mentors, and colleagues—past and current—for providing us the education.

To our patients—past, current, and future—for providing the motivation.

Puneet K. Gupta, MD, MSE, FACNS
Pradeep N. Modur, MD, MS
Srikanth Muppidi, MD

1

Anatomy and Physiology

QUESTIONS

1. Which of the following is an example of a near-field potential?
   A. P100
   B. Wave I recorded at Cz
   C. P13/14 recorded at the scalp
   D. N34
   E. P31

2. Which of the following results in a slower nerve conduction velocity?
   A. Larger nerve diameter
   B. Smaller nerve fiber diameter
   C. Shorter nerve length
   D. Low transmembrane capacitance
   E. High transmembrane resistance

3. The membrane permeability of which of the following ions contributes the most during depolarization, repolarization, and in maintaining the resting membrane potential, respectively?
   A. Calcium; chloride; potassium
   B. Sodium; potassium; chloride
   C. Sodium; potassium; potassium
   D. Sodium; chloride; potassium
   E. Calcium; potassium; chloride

4. Which of the following determines the flow of ions across a channel?
   A. Chemical gradient
   B. Electrical gradient
   C. Membrane conductance
   D. A and B
   E. A, B, and C

ANSWERS TO THIS SECTION CAN BE FOUND ON PAGE 12

5. In addition to voltage-gating, what is the other main gating mechanism for the neuronal ion channels?
   A. Light-gating
   B. Temperature-gating
   C. Ligand-gating
   D. Mechanosensitivity
   E. Intracellular second messenger gating

6. Which of the following types of nerve fibers within a given nerve contribute to the conduction velocity measured with nerve conduction studies?
   A. Fastest conducting nerve fibers
   B. Slowest conducting nerve fibers
   C. Unmyelinated fibers
   D. A and B
   E. A, B, and C

7. All of the following statements regarding the neuronal potentials are true *except:*
   A. Intracellular potential of a neuron is about −60 mV
   B. Action potentials contribute to the generation of the extracellular field potentials
   C. Postsynaptic potentials contribute to the generation of the extracellular field potentials
   D. There is net influx of cations into the neuron with an excitatory postsynaptic potential
   E. There is net outflow of cations from the nerve cell with an inhibitory postsynaptic potential

8. Which of the following is likely during repetitive nerve stimulation in a patient with myasthenia gravis?
   A. Decrease in limb temperature increases compound muscle action potential (CMAP) decrement
   B. Decrease in limb temperature decreases CMAP decrement
   C. Increase in limb temperature increases CMAP decrement
   D. Increase in limb temperature decreases CMAP decrement
   E. Limb temperature has no effect on CMAP decrement

9. Which of the following muscles is innervated by the peroneal nerve above the level of the fibular head?
   A. Semimembranous
   B. Semitendinosus
   C. Long head of biceps femoris
   D. Short head of biceps femoris
   E. None of the above

10. All of the following statements about the generation of EEG waveforms are true *except:*
    A. A negative field potential develops at the surface with activation of a superficial excitatory synapse
    B. A positive field potential develops at the surface with activation of a deep inhibitory synapse
    C. Excitatory postsynaptic potentials (EPSPs) in the upper dendrites of the neurons summate to produce depolarization

D. Postsynaptic potentials contribute to the generation of the EEG waveforms
E. Thalamocortical feedback loops modulate the amplitude of EEG waveforms

11. Which of the following ions has a higher concentration inside the cell than outside?
A. Sodium
B. Potassium
C. Calcium
D. Chloride
E. C and D

12. Which of the following statements is correct regarding the effect of limb temperature on nerve conduction velocity and latency?
A. Conduction velocity increases and latency increases with drop in temperature
B. Conduction velocity decreases and latency increases with drop in temperature
C. Conduction velocity increases and latency decreases with drop in temperature
D. Conduction velocity decreases and latency decreases with drop in temperature
E. Effect of temperature can be ignored as long as the limb is rewarmed to at least 29°C

13. Abductor pollicis brevis is innervated by the median nerve. The motor fibers for this innervation come from which of the following roots?
A. C6, C7, C8
B. C7, C8
C. C5, C6, C7
D. C8
E. C8, T1

14. Which of the following is most readily recorded as EEG activity with scalp electrodes?
A. Excitatory activity in the sulcal cortex
B. Excitatory activity in the apical dendrites in cortical layer 2
C. Inhibitory activity in the soma in cortical layer 5
D. B and C
E. A, B, and C

15. Which of the following defines the absolute refractory period?
A. Inactivation of the sodium (Na)+ channels
B. Activation of the sodium (Na)+ channels
C. Activation of the potassium (K)+ channels
D. Inactivation of the chloride (Cl)– channels
E. Activation of the calcium (Ca)+ channels

16. While performing the tibial H reflex, the H wave amplitude decreases with increasing stimulus intensity because:
A. At higher stimulus intensity, Ia afferent fibers are inhibited
B. At higher stimulus intensity, Ia afferent fibers are excessively activated
C. At higher stimulus intensity, there is increased collision between antidromic motor stimulus and orthodromic H reflex potentials
D. At higher stimulus intensity, the M response suppresses H waves
E. At higher stimulus intensity, there is synergy between antidromic motor stimulus and orthodromic H reflex potentials

17. Which of the following statements best describes the paroxysmal depolarization shifts (PDSs)?
A. They refer to fluctuations of postsynaptic potentials
B. They are characterized by rapid depolarization–repolarization sequences lasting less than 40 ms
C. They correlate with surface negative direct current (DC) fluctuations at the beginning of a seizure
D. They reflect the resting activity of the normal hippocampal neurons
E. They reflect the resting activity of the normal cortical pyramidal neurons

18. Which of the following fibers have the slowest conduction velocity?
A. Aα
B. Aβ
C. Aγ
D. Aδ
E. C

19. Which of the following receptor types exerts its effects through the calcium (Ca++) ions?
A. Alpha-amino-3-hydroxy-5-methyl-4-isoxazolepropionic acid (AMPA)
B. Kainic acid (KA)
C. N-methyl-D-aspartate (NMDA)
D. Glycine
E. All of the above

20. Which of the following statements is true about the myelinated nerves?
A. Sodium and potassium channels are evenly distributed in the myelinated nerves
B. Increased potassium conductance leads to repolarization in myelinated nerves
C. Myelin reduces membrane capacitance
D. Myelin reduces transmembrane resistance
E. Myelin promotes fast conduction uniformly along the nerve fibers

21. Which of the following statements is true regarding the transmission of action potentials along myelinated nerves?
A. Transmission is enhanced by increasing the internodal transmembrane capacitance
B. Transmission may fail if the internodal distance is too great
C. Transmission may fail if the internodal myelin thickness is increased
D. Transmission relies on opening of potassium channels in the internodal membrane
E. Transmission is enhanced by decreasing the internodal transmembrane resistance

22. Which of the following is true regarding the sodium–potassium pump?
A. It helps to neutralize the membrane potential
B. It enhances transport of sodium and potassium ions along their concentration gradients
C. It actively transports two sodium ions out of the cell and one potassium ion into the cell
D. It allows for secondary active transporters to function via the use of the sodium gradient
E. Its function is to remove net negative charge from the intracellular space

23. Which of the following is true regarding volume conductors?
A. They have conductivity but no capacitative properties
B. Different body regions have the same volume conduction
C. Volume conductor models have no effect on source analysis for magnetoencephalography (MEG)
D. Volume conduction is mainly based on conductivity in EEG
E. The morphology of motor unit potentials seen during needle electromyography (EMG) is independent of volume conduction

24. How does the compound muscle action potential morphology change as the recording electrode is moved farther away from the generator?
A. Latency remains the same
B. Amplitude increases
C. Rise time becomes sharper
D. Polarity tends to become positive
E. There is no change in morphology

25. Abnormal somatosensory evoked potential can be expected after damage to which of the following structures?
A. Spinothalamic tract
B. Tractus gracilis
C. Superior olivary nucleus
D. Lateral lemniscus
E. Medial geniculate body

26. All of the following statements regarding the neuronal membrane potential are true *except:*
A. It is dependent on the differential ionic concentrations across the membrane
B. It is dependent on the permeability of ions across the membrane
C. It is calculated using the Hodgkin–Huxley model
D. It is calculated using the Goldman equation
E. It is close to the Nernst potential for chloride (Cl) ions

27. Which of the following nerve pairs originates directly from the cervical nerve roots?
A. Suprascapular and dorsal scapular nerves
B. Long thoracic and dorsal scapular nerves
C. Suprascapular and subscapular nerves
D. Subscapular and thoracodorsal nerves
E. Long thoracic and thoracodorsal nerves

28. Which of the following is the generator of physiological theta waves?
A. White matter
B. Suprachiasmatic nucleus
C. Hippocampus
D. Thalamic pacemaker cells
E. Temporal neocortex

29. Safety factor at the neuromuscular junction refers to which of the following?
A. Separation of acetylcholine into primary, secondary, and tertiary presynaptic quanta
B. Amplitude of end-plate potential above the threshold value needed to generate muscle fiber action potential
C. Amplitude of end-plate potential below the threshold value needed to generate muscle fiber action potential
D. Minimum amplitude of the nerve action potential needed to open presynaptic calcium channels
E. The minimum number of acetylcholine receptors needed to generate the muscle fiber action potential

30. Which of the following statements is true regarding the interface between the EEG electrode and the electrolyte paste?
A. It acts as an electrical double layer that impedes current flow
B. It is potentially unstable, causing "pop" artifacts with new electrodes
C. It acts as a half-cell potential that remains stable despite movement of the electrode
D. It prevents development of electrical polarization
E. It becomes highly polarized when a silver–silver chloride interface is used

31. Which of the following waveform morphologies is likely to be seen when there is no volume conduction?
A. Symmetric monophasic negative potential
B. Asymmetric monophasic negative potential
C. Biphasic potential with an initial positive peak
D. Biphasic potential with a trailing positive peak
E. Triphasic potential with both initial and trailing positive peaks

32. Which thalamic nucleus helps in synchronization of EEG?
A. Reticular nucleus
B. Anterior nucleus
C. Pulvinar
D. Medial geniculate nucleus
E. Centromedian nucleus

33. Stimulation of the median nerve at the wrist with recording from the scalp to obtain somatosensory evoked potential causes activation in all of the following structures *except:*
A. Medial and lateral cords of brachial plexus
B. Nucleus cuneatus
C. Lateral lemniscus
D. Medial lemniscus
E. Ventral posterolateral nucleus of thalamus

34. Alpha rhythm is:
A. Restricted to the visual cortex
B. Can be seen in visual, somatosensory, and temporal cortices
C. Neither facilitatory nor inhibitory during attentional processes
D. Generated in the thalamus
E. Generated by the pyramidal neurons in layer VI of the visual cortex

35. Which of the following potentials is considered a standing wave?

A. The motor response seen when stimulating the peroneal nerve above the knee
B. The popliteal fossa potential seen with tibial nerve stimulation at the ankle
C. The sensory response in standard bipolar digit sensory nerve conduction
D. The P37 potential seen when stimulating the posterior tibial nerve
E. The P9 potential seen when stimulating the median nerve

36. Which of the following statements is true about a synapse generating excitatory postsynaptic potentials (EPSPs)?

A. There is inward flow of negative ions into the cell
B. There is a current source at the synapse
C. There is a current sink at the synapse
D. A positive potential is recorded by an electrode in the extracellular space at the synapse
E. A negative potential is recorded by an electrode in the extracellular space away from the synapse

37. Which of the following is primarily responsible for the rising phase of the action potential?

A. Gap junctions
B. Voltage-gated sodium channels
C. Voltage-gated potassium channels
D. Voltage-gated calcium channels
E. Sodium–potassium pump

38. Magnetoencephalography (MEG) is a measure of the magnetic fields generated by:

A. Tangential current dipoles
B. Radial current dipoles
C. Tangential and radial current dipoles
D. Cortical current dipoles on the convexity of gyri
E. Summated volume currents

39. Which of the following statements best describes the EEG signal?

A. The action potential contributes to the signal because the spike amplitude decays rapidly
B. The action potential contributes to the signal because the spike duration is long (3–4 ms)
C. Postsynaptic potentials are likely to contribute to the signal because they have longer durations (10–250 ms)
D. The signal recorded at the cortex tends to be of longer duration than the signal recorded simultaneously at the scalp
E. The signal is unaffected by the characteristics of the moving dipole

40. Delta waves are characterized by all of the following *except:*

A. They arise from interplay between transient calcium currents and rectifier sodium and potassium currents in the thalamus
B. They disappear in the cat thalamocortical neurons after decortication
C. They are synchronized by direct intracortical linkages
D. They are synchronized by cortico-thalamo-cortical projections
E. They are synchronized by networks of gap junctions

41. Which of the following is true regarding the relative difference between the intracellular and extracellular potentials across the membrane?
   A. Intracellular polarity is negative during maximal sodium influx
   B. Extracellular polarity is more positive during hyperpolarization
   C. Intracellular polarity is positive during the resting state
   D. Extracellular polarity is negative during the resting state
   E. The intracellular and extracellular potentials are isoelectric during the resting state

42. What is the most caudal point where the auditory information is represented bilaterally?
   A. Cochlear nucleus
   B. Rostral medulla
   C. Superior olivary nucleus
   D. Inferior colliculus
   E. Medial geniculate body

43. Which of the following is not a determinant of ion flow?
   A. Concentration gradient
   B. Channel conductance
   C. Electrical potential
   D. Transmembrane resistance
   E. Selective permeability

44. All of the following statements about theta activity in the EEG are true *except:*
   A. It is prominently seen in the CA1 hippocampal neurons
   B. It is more prominent during spatial navigation tasks
   C. It is more frequent during memory processing
   D. It is modulated by supramammillary nucleus of the hypothalamus
   E. It is felt to be caused by the GABA-mediated inhibitory postsynaptic potentials

45. Which of the following statements is true regarding the chloride ion?
   A. Its concentration is similar in both extracellular and intracellular compartments
   B. Its equilibrium potential is much lower than the resting membrane potential
   C. It is passively transported across the cell membrane
   D. It contributes as much as potassium to the resting membrane potential
   E. It contributes to excitatory postsynaptic potentials

46. Which of the following muscles is supplied by the accessory peroneal nerve?
   A. Peroneus brevis
   B. Peroneus tertius
   C. Tibialis anterior
   D. Tibialis posterior
   E. Extensor digitorum brevis

47. Which of the following statements is true regarding glial cells?
   A. Their intracellular potential is close to that of sodium (Na) ions
   B. They generate postsynaptic potentials
   C. They generate small action potentials
   D. They depolarize in response to an increase in extracellular potassium concentration
   E. They generally dampen extracellular field potentials

48. Which of the following statements is true regarding the voltage-gated sodium channels?
A. They are insensitive to changes in membrane potential
B. They alternate between the resting and active states
C. They close due to changes in calcium conductance
D. They function in a feedforward manner to promote sodium influx
E. They are responsible for the rising phase of the action potential

49. Paroxysmal depolarization shift (PDS) refers to:
A. The rising phase of the action potential
B. A period of time when neurons are hyperpolarized
C. A phenomena that helps to disrupt seizure propagation
D. A wave of cortical depolarization, leading to synchronized neuronal spiking
E. Occurrence of successive action potentials without intervening refractory periods

50. The resting membrane potential of a neuron is typically:
A. –90 mV
B. –70 mV
C. 0
D. +55 mV
E. +70 mV

51. Which of the following statements is true regarding the waveform potential recorded by an electrode located near the site of depolarization/repolarization sequence in a nerve situated inside a volume conductor?
A. The site of depolarization acts as a current source
B. The current lines fan away from the site of depolarization
C. The recorded waveform potential is asymmetric
D. The recorded waveform potential is usually monophasic and negative
E. The waveform duration remains the same regardless of the distance between the electrode and the site of depolarization

52. Which of the following statements is true regarding fast beta–gamma rhythms?
A. They are generated in the subcortical nuclei
B. Gamma oscillations reflect spatial synchronization of cortical areas for information processing
C. They are mainly associated with decreased levels of alertness
D. There is an increase in beta activity before movement with an increase in gamma activity after movement
E. They are associated with activity in the pyramidal cells

53. Which of the following statements best describes the EEG activity during sleep?
A. K-complexes become irregular and less frequent with deepening of sleep
B. Spindles are generated by the dorsal nucleus of the thalamus
C. Gamma-aminobutyric acid (GABA)ergic neurons underlie generation of sleep spindles
D. Sleep spindles facilitate transmission of afferent stimuli to the cortex
E. Increased brainstem cholinergic activity underlies the bursting feature of the spindles

54. The primary contributor for the extracellular potential measured in EEG is:
   A. Calcium action potential
   B. Depolarizing afterpotential
   C. Hyperpolarizing afterpotential
   D. Postsynaptic potential
   E. None of the above

55. Which of the following serves as the main mechanism to help move sodium ions into the cell during depolarization?
   A. Passive transport
   B. Active transport
   C. Facilitated diffusion
   D. Transcellular transport
   E. Carrier-mediated transport

56. Which of the following is true regarding the neurophysiology of nerve conduction studies (NCS)?
   A. Stimulators used in NCS are typically monopolar
   B. The depolarization of the axon occurs under the anode
   C. The stimulation current needs to be high to overcome the high resistance of the extracellular space
   D. The cross-sectional resistance of an axon is inversely proportional to the diameter of the axon
   E. Smaller nerves depolarize with a lower stimulus intensity than larger nerves

57. Which of the following is a near-field potential?
   A. N18
   B. P100
   C. Wave V
   D. P14
   E. Compound motor action potential

58. A 45-year-old man is referred to the electrodiagnostic laboratory for evaluation of brachial plexopathy. On examination, he is noted to have severe atrophy in the first dorsal interosseus muscle. This most likely localizes to which part of the brachial plexus?
   A. Lateral cord
   B. Posterior cord
   C. Upper trunk
   D. Middle trunk
   E. Lower trunk

59. Which of the following electrodiagnostic findings is least likely to occur as a result of cold limb temperature?
   A. Increased motor amplitude
   B. Prolonged distal latency
   C. Slowed nerve conduction velocity
   D. Decreased motor amplitude
   E. Increased sensory amplitude

60. What is the typical morphology of an end-plate spike?
   A. Monophasic negative deflection
   B. Monophasic positive deflection
   C. Biphasic with an initial negative followed by a final positive deflection
   D. Biphasic with an initial positive followed by a final negative deflection
   E. Triphasic with an initial positive, a middle negative, and a final positive deflection

61. Which of the following is a characteristic of the postsynaptic potentials (PSPs)?
   A. They are all-or-none phenomena
   B. They summate temporally but not spatially
   C. An action potential is generated when an excitatory PSP (EPSP) reaches −50 mV
   D. Acetylcholine generates inhibitory PSPs (IPSPs)
   E. Only inhibitory PSPs contribute to the generation of EEG waveforms

62. Resting membrane potential (RMP):
   A. Is close to the equilibrium potential of the potassium ions
   B. Is close to the equilibrium potential of the chloride ions
   C. Is around −60 mV
   D. Keeps the cell in a nonpolarized state
   E. Is depolarized by the sodium–potassium pump

63. Which of the following is NOT part of the Papez circuit?
   A. Hippocampus
   B. Fornix
   C. Mammillary bodies
   D. Centromedian nucleus of the thalamus
   E. Cingulate

64. Which of the following statements is true regarding the EEG activity recorded at the scalp?
   A. Alpha rhythm has the same amplitude regardless of whether it is recorded on the cortical surface or scalp
   B. About 2 cm^2 of the cortical surface needs to be involved for a given activity to be seen at the scalp
   C. Horizontally oriented dipoles are more likely to be seen at the scalp
   D. Widespread activity is more likely to be attenuated at the scalp
   E. Faster frequency activity is more likely to be attenuated at the scalp

65. Which of the following statements best describes the experimental evidence regarding the brainstem control of sleep and wakefulness?
   A. Stimulation of brainstem in anesthetized cats enhanced synchronized activity in the EEG
   B. A large lesion placed in the midbrain tegmentum produced desynchronized EEG resembling wakefulness
   C. Midpontine pretegmental transection in cat produced a permanent state resembling coma
   D. Midpontine pretegmental hemisection in cat produced synchronization resembling sleep in the ipsilateral hemisphere
   E. Midpontine hemisection combined with an ipsilateral midbrain hemisection in cat produced synchronization resembling sleep/coma in the ipsilateral hemisphere

ANSWERS

1. **A.** The P100 is a near-field response because it is recorded over the occipital lobe, not from widely separated electrodes over the scalp. Certain dipole potentials can be recorded as near-field and far-field potentials. Wave I, for instance, recorded at Cz, is a far-field potential, but Wave I, recorded at the ear, is a near-field potential. In another example, P13/14 of the median nerve somatosensory evoked potential (SSEP) measured at the scalp is felt to be a far-field rostral response, whereas the N13 measured from the dorsal neck is felt to be a near-field cervical cord response. N34 is a subcortical far-field potential reflecting activity in the brainstem and thalamus. P31 is a far-field potential reflecting activity in the caudal medial lemniscus.

2. **B.** Larger fiber diameter allows more ions to flow into the nerve, making it easier for the current to travel along the nerve. Myelin allows for low transmembrane capacitance and high transmembrane resistance, both of which lead to faster velocities. Shorter nerve length does not typically lead to slower conduction velocity.

3. **B.** Sodium contributes the most to neuronal depolarization and potassium to neuronal hyperpolarization. Although potassium helps to maintain the resting membrane potential, the resting membrane is most permeable to chloride. Therefore, the resting membrane potential, typically −60 to −70 mV, is nearest to the Nernst potential for chloride (around −65 mV), rather than potassium (around −90 mV).

4. **E.** All of them affect ionic flow across channels. The chemical driving force is defined by concentration gradients. The electrical driving force is determined by the membrane potential. The membrane conductance is a measure of how ions permeate through the channel pore. In general, medications alter the membrane conductance in order to achieve their clinical effect.

5. **C.** The two main gating mechanisms are voltage-gating and ligand-gating. However, there are a number of other types of channel gating: intracellular second messenger gating (e.g., inward-rectifier potassium channels); light-gating (e.g., rhodopsin channel); mechanosensitive ion channels (e.g., stretch receptors); cyclic nucleotide-gating (channels that are activated by cAMP or cGMP); and temperature-gating (e.g., transient receptor potential ion channel).

6. **A.** Only the fastest fibers contribute to the conduction velocity and latency measurements with nerve conduction studies. Slow and intermediate fibers do not contribute to those measurements. On the other hand, all the stimulated fibers contribute to amplitude and duration measurements on nerve conduction studies.

7. **B.** Postsynaptic potentials, not action potentials, are thought to contribute primarily to the generation of the extracellular field potentials. Other statements are true.

8. **B.** Decrease in limb temperature causes a decrease in CMAP decrement and may lead to false negative repetitive stimulation study in patients with myasthenia gravis. Therefore, it is important to warm the extremity before doing repetitive stimulation.

9. **D.** Short head of biceps femoris is innervated by a branch of the peroneal nerve above the fibular head. Other muscles described above are supplied by the tibial part of the sciatic nerve. EMG of the short head of biceps femoris helps distinguish between selective peroneal nerve pathology at or below the fibular head versus peroneal pathology at the knee or proximally.

10. **B.** A negative field potential develops at the surface with the activation of either a superficial excitatory synapse or a deep inhibitory synapse. The ascending action potentials elicit individual excitatory postsynaptic potentials in the upper dendrites of the neurons, which summate to cause depolarization in accordance with the discharge frequency. EEG waveforms are generated by grouped and synchronous influx in the afferent fiber systems toward the superficial generator structures; this activity is believed to be modulated by the thalamocortical feedback loops.

11. **B.** Sodium, chloride, and calcium are more concentrated outside the cell than inside. Potassium and organic anions (such as amino acids and proteins) are more concentrated inside the cell than outside. Sodium and chloride ions tend to flow into the cell along the concentration gradient, whereas potassium ions tend to flow outward. Because of their large size, organic anions are unable to move out of the intracellular compartment.

12. **B.** Conduction velocity decreases by 1.5 to 2 m/sec and latency increases by 0.2 ms with every 1°C drop in temperature. This information can be used to correct for cold limb temperature. Ideally, the limb should be rewarmed but this may not be possible in certain situations. The acceptable limb temperature is greater than 32°C for upper limb and greater than 30°C for lower limb.

13. **E.** Although the median nerve has fibers from multiple roots (C5–T1), the motor fibers that innervate abductor pollicis brevis come from C8 and T1 roots. Median sensory fibers that innervate the hand come from the C6 root.

14. **D.** Because of the columnar organization of the pyramidal neurons along with their sheetlike organization parallel to the scalp, any activity in the superficial or deep cortical layers leads to the generation of radial (vertical) dipoles, which can be readily detected by the scalp EEG electrodes. Furthermore, because of the location of the current sinks, both superficial excitatory activity (in layers 2 and 3) and deep inhibitory activity in (layer 5) result in surface negative extracellular potential at the scalp. On the other hand, activity in the sulcal cortex may lead to the generation of tangential dipoles, which may cancel each other out, and therefore, not readily recorded on the scalp. Such tangential dipoles, however, may be more conducive for recording by magnetoencephalography (MEG).

15. **A.** Inactivation of Na+ channels defines the absolute refractory period. Activation of K+ channels leads to hyperpolarization. Activation of Cl− channel helps to stabilize the hyperpolarized membrane potential. Activation of calcium (Ca)+ channels helps depolarization in some dendrites.

16. **C.** As the stimulus intensity is increased, there is increased collision between antidromic motor stimulus and orthodromic H reflex potentials, resulting in decreased H wave amplitude. Ia afferent fibers continue to be stimulated at a higher intensity but this also results in increased stimulation of motor fibers, ultimately resulting in collision.

17. **C.** Paroxysmal depolarization shifts refer to oscillations of the membrane potential. They begin with a steep depolarization that, on exceeding the membrane threshold, triggers a series of action potentials. This is followed by a plateau and then a steep repolarization and hyperpolarization after 80 to 100 ms. PDSs are characteristic of the epileptiform activity of individual neurons. With the DC recording, it can be noticed that the PDSs in pyramidal neurons are coupled at the beginning of the convulsive seizure with surface negative DC potentials and at the end of the seizure with positive DC potentials.

18. **E.** Type C nerve fibers have the slowest conduction velocity, generally in the range of 1 to 2 m / sec. Aα fibers have the fastest conduction velocity, in the range of 80 to 120 m / sec; these fibers are usually not assessed during motor and sensory studies as they are only involved in muscle stretch reflexes.

19. **C.** AMPA, KA, and NMDA receptors are subtypes of glutamate receptors. NMDA receptors affect Ca++ movement across the membrane. AMPA and KA receptors are ligand-gated ionic channels that are permeable to sodium Na+ and potassium K+. In general, KA receptors have slower kinetics and differential binding properties with specific agonists. NMDA receptors have both ionotropic and metabotropic properties and are important in synaptic plasticity. Glycine receptors exert their effects via chloride (Cl^-) ions.

20. **C.** In myelinated nerves, the sodium and potassium channels are unevenly distributed; the sodium channels are concentrated at the junction of Schwann cells (called nodes of Ranvier), whereas the potassium channels are concentrated underneath the myelin. Increased potassium conductance contributes to repolarization in unmyelinated nerves, not myelinated nerves. The myelin reduces the membrane capacitance and increases the transmembrane resistance, which allows the action potential to jump from node to node, known as saltatory conduction.

21. **B.** Transmission of action potentials along a myelinated nerve is referred to as saltatory conduction. This process relies on opening of sodium channels at the nodes of Ranvier. Although greater internodal distance leads to faster conduction velocities, there is an internodal length that, when reached, will lead to signal transmission failure. Transmission is enhanced by increasing the internodal myelin thickness, increasing the internodal transmembrane resistance, and decreasing the transmembrane capacitance.

22. **D.** The sodium–potassium pump helps to create a sodium gradient that provides the driving force for several secondary active transport systems, which import glucose, amino acids, and other nutrients into the cell. The pump helps to maintain, not neutralize, the membrane potential. It actively transports three sodium ions out of the cell and two potassium ions into the cell against their concentration gradients, resulting in net removal of one positive charge from the intracellular space.

23. **D.** Volume conduction is mainly based on conductivity in EEG. Volume conduction is the transmission of electric or magnetic fields from an electric current source through the intervening tissue toward a sensor. Overall, volume conductors have both conductivity as well as capacitative properties; these properties are variable, resulting in differing levels of volume conduction in different body regions. Volume conductor models are the basis for source analysis for EEG and MEG. In EEG, the transmission can be modeled mainly by conductivity (or resistivity), ignoring the tissue impedances from capacitors, inductors, and electromagnetic propagation. All motor and sensory nerve conduction waveforms as well as waveforms seen during needle EMG (e.g., spontaneous discharges and motor unit potentials) are substantially affected by volume conductor properties.

24. **D.** Compound muscle action potentials recorded at a distance from the generator are positive. Increasing the distance between the recording electrode and the generator can lead to changes in waveform morphology depending on the volume conduction in that body region. In general, nerve conduction latencies become erroneous at some distance from the generator, action potential amplitudes decrease quickly with increasing distance from the generator, and the waveform rise time slows or increases with increasing distance from the generator.

25. **B.** Somatosensory evoked potentials (SSEPs) test the integrity of dorsal columns that include gracile and cuneate tracts. The spinothalamic tract carries pain and temperature sensations, lies laterally in the spinal cord, and is not tested by SSEPs. Superior olivary nucleus, lateral lemniscus, and medial geniculate body are tested by the brainstem auditory evoked potentials.

26. **C.** The resting membrane potential is calculated using the Goldman equation, which takes into account the different concentrations of ions across the membrane as well as the permeability to ionic flow across the membrane. On the other hand, the Hodgkin–Huxley model is a set of nonlinear differential equations that approximates the electrical characteristics of excitable cells and describes how action potentials in neurons are initiated and propagated. The neuronal resting membrane potential (around −70 mV) is closest to the Nernst potential for chloride ions (around −65 mV).

27. **B.** Only long thoracic and dorsal scapular nerves originate from the cervical roots. Suprascapular nerve originates from the upper trunk. Subscapular and thoracodorsal nerves originate from the posterior cord.

28. C. The hippocampus is felt to be a generator for physiological theta waves. The higher amplitude theta waves are felt to be generated near the fissure that separates the CA1 molecular layer from the dentate gyrus. Physiological delta waves (e.g., N3 sleep stage) can originate in the thalamus (in coordination with the reticular formation) or in the cortex (in coordination with the suprachiasmatic nucleus). Thalamic pacemaker cells are felt to mediate the alpha range rhythms, including the posterior dominant rhythm, which are felt to be generated in the cortex. Dysfunction of white matter typically leads to pathological medium to high amplitude polymorphic delta slowing.

29. B. Safety factor refers to the amplitude of the end-plate potential above the threshold value needed to generate the muscle fiber action potential. In neuromuscular junction disorders, the safety factor is reduced. In myasthenia gravis, during slow repetitive stimulation, the end-plate potential falls below the threshold to produce muscle fiber action potential, resulting in the decrement pattern.

30. B. The interface between the EEG electrode and the electrolyte paste constitutes an "electrical double layer" that contributes to the stability of the interface and also represents a capacitance that augments current flow. The electrical double layer undergoes sudden transitions that produce electrode "pops," especially with new electrodes. The junction between the metal electrode and the ionic electrolyte develops a half-cell potential similar to half of an electrical battery. These half-cell potentials can be altered in various ways (e.g., drying of the paste, dilution by sweat or other fluids, relative differences in temperature, wear and tear, movement of the electrode against the electrolyte and the skin) causing disruption of the electrical double layer. Passage of direct current through the double layer causes chemical changes at the metal surface, including electrical polarization, which impedes the free flow of current in one direction more than the other and increases the impedance for low frequencies. However, a silver–silver chloride interface is resistant to polarization and is suitable for recording low-frequency and direct current recordings.

31. B. Without volume conduction, there will be no fanning out of the current lines from the generator. Therefore, there will be no approaching or trailing wave fronts and no initial or trailing positive peaks. Only a monophasic negative potential will be seen when the depolarization is just under the recording electrode. The morphology will be asymmetric given that repolarization takes more time than depolarization.

32. A. The reticular nucleus, part of the reticular activating system (RAS) that modulates the thalamocortical pathways, helps to synchronize and desynchronize the EEG. Typically, the EEG is synchronized when the thalamic relay neurons are in the burst mode and desynchronized when they are in the tonic mode. Stimulation of the RAS suppresses slower activity (e.g., delta) and stimulates faster activity (e.g., gamma). This modulation leads to distinct changes in cerebral electrical activity during wakefulness and sleep. The anterior nucleus of the thalamus (part of the Papez circuit) and the centromedian nucleus have been shown as sites for neurostimulation for seizure control. The pulvinar is the largest nucleus in the human thalamus, and lesions of the pulvinar can result in neglect and attentional deficit syndromes. The medial geniculate nucleus is the thalamic relay between the inferior colliculus and the auditory cortex.

33. C. Impulses after stimulation of median nerve are carried through medial and lateral cords of brachial plexus, C5–T1 roots, nucleus cuneatus, medial lemniscus, and ventral posterolateral (VPL) nucleus of thalamus to the parietal cortex. Lateral lemniscus carries auditory information.

34. B. Rhythmic activity in the alpha frequency range can be recorded from the visual cortex, somatosensory cortex (mu rhythm), and temporal cortex (tau rhythm). Alpha rhythm has both facilitatory and inhibitory roles during attentional processes. More recent studies performed in monkeys suggest a cortical generator for alpha rhythms. Horizontal intracortical linkages are essential for the spread of alpha activity. In the visual cortex, alpha waves are generated by an equivalent dipole layer centered at the level of the somata and basal dendrites of pyramidal neurons in layers IV and V.

35. E. The P9 potential generated by stimulating the median nerve is the best known standing wave, also known as a virtual dipole, which is felt to result from the waveform traveling from the arm into the trunk. It is also known as the junctional or boundary potential because it is felt to occur when the waveform moves from one body region into another. Other such potentials can be seen traveling from the arm to the hand.

36. C. At the site of the synapses generating EPSPs, a current sink occurs because of inward flow of positive ions into cell with a corresponding current source at a distance from the synapse from where the positive ions come out of the cell. The current flows from the source to the sink. Therefore, an extracellular electrode records a negative potential at the synapse generating an EPSP, but it records a positive potential away from the synapse. The opposite situation occurs with inhibitory postsynaptic potentials (IPSPs), creating a current source at the synapse and a current sink away from the synapse.

37. B. The voltage-gated sodium channels are primarily responsible for the rising phase of the action potential through a positive feedback mechanism. The voltage-gated calcium channels allow for stronger and longer depolarization, whereas the voltage-gated potassium channels facilitate repolarization. The sodium–potassium pump, via the use of ATP, reestablishes the concentration gradient as it moves sodium out of the cell and potassium into the cell. Gap junctions allow for direct electrical communication between cells; although they are not directly involved in the rising phase of the action potential, they allow free flow of ions between cells, enabling rapid nonchemical-mediated transmission between cells as well as enhancing synchronous firing among coupled cells.

38. A. MEG is a measure of the magnetic fields perpendicular to the skull generated by the tangential current dipoles. The radial current dipoles do not generate magnetic fields outside a sphere-shaped volume conductor, and therefore, do not contribute to the MEG. In contrast, EEG is a measure of both tangential and radial components. The main intracortical dipolar current sources are perpendicular to the cortical surface. Therefore, MEG mainly measures the cortical current dipoles lying within the sulci (which mainly produce tangential dipoles) and not on the convexity of the gyri (which mainly produce radial dipoles). Unlike EEG, MEG is not affected by the volume currents and, therefore, the MEG signal tends to be more focal in distribution than the corresponding EEG signal.

39. C. The action potential does not contribute to the EEG signal because its spike amplitude decays with distance depending on dendritic morphology and drops quickly away from the dendritic tree. Furthermore, the action potential does not contribute to EEG signal due to its short duration (1–2 ms). On the other hand, the postsynaptic potentials that have longer durations (10–250 ms) contribute to the EEG signal. The propagation of electrical activity in the cortex results in the phenomenon of time dilation in which an EEG signal (e.g., epileptiform spike) recorded at the cortex tends to be of shorter duration than the signal recorded simultaneously at the scalp. This is because a moving dipole from a longer distance can be observed over a longer time period than the one from a shorter distance.

40. B. Delta oscillations in the thalamus arise from interplay between the transient calcium current underlying the low threshold spike and a hyperpolarization-activated cation current, a noninactivating inward (anomalous) rectifier carried by sodium and potassium. Delta oscillations are found *in vivo* in the thalamocortical neurons of the cat after decortications. Delta oscillations are synchronized by direct intracortical linkages, cortico-thalamo-cortical projections, and networks of gap junctions.

41. B. The extracellular space is relatively positive and the intracellular space is relatively negative at rest; this difference becomes more pronounced during membrane hyperpolarization. During depolarization, the relative potentials of the intracellular and extracellular spaces begin to equalize and ultimately reverse during maximal sodium influx.

42. C. Vibrations produced by the sound waves are sensed by the hair cells in the organ of Corti. Hair cells contact with the afferent fibers originating from the spiral ganglion cells. The central processes of the spiral ganglion cells form the cochlear nerve, which terminates in the ipsilateral cochlear nucleus located in the rostral medulla (ventral portion for low-frequency tones and dorsal portion for high-frequency tones). From the cochlear nuclei, the neurons project to both ipsilateral and contralateral superior olivary nuclei; in other words, the auditory information is bilaterally represented at this point. Neurons in the superior olive then project through the lateral lemniscus in the pontine tegmentum to the inferior colliculus, which in turn projects to the medial geniculate nucleus of the thalamus. Fibers from the medial geniculate in turn project to the Heschl's gyrus (superior temporal gyrus), the primary auditory cortex.

43. D. Ion flow is determined by ionic concentration gradients, selective permeability of ion channels (often referred to as the channel conductance), and electrical forces that arise from the membrane potential. Action potential transmission, not ion flow, is determined by transmembrane resistance.

44. E. Theta activity is felt to represent a dynamic state emerging from the hippocampal networks engaged in spatial navigation and memory processes. More prominent theta activity has been reported in the left anterior hippocampus and parahippocampal cortex during goal-directed navigation relative to aimless movements. Theta oscillations are also frequent during memory processing, and even more evident during recall than learning tasks. Recent studies have shown that the supramammillary nucleus of the hypothalamus, strongly connected to the medial septum, brainstem, and diencephalon, may play a role in modulating hippocampal theta activity. According to some investigators, the hippocampal CA1 pyramidal cells receive rhythmic inputs in the theta frequency range from other sources that consist of atropine-sensitive and atropine-resistant inputs; the former would drive the somata and the latter the distal dendrites. The atropine-sensitive theta rhythm is felt to be mainly caused by chloride (Cl)-mediated, not GABA-mediated, inhibitory postsynaptic potentials on the pyramidal cells.

45. C. Chloride ions are passively transported across the membrane via the chloride channels, which are open during the resting state. The extracellular concentration of chloride (about 150 mM) is more than 10 times the intracellular concentration (about 13 mM). The resting membrane potential most closely resembles the equilibrium (Nernst) potential for chloride. Chloride does not contribute significantly to the resting membrane potential. Inward flow of negative ions (such as chloride) into the cells can contribute to inhibitory, not excitatory, postsynaptic potentials.

46. E. The accessory peroneal nerve is a normal anatomical variant that supplies the extensor digitorum brevis muscle. Its presence should be suspected when the peroneal motor amplitude is higher with stimulation at the fibular head compared to the ankle. More than 25% of normal healthy adults may have an accessory peroneal nerve. Peroneus brevis, peroneus tertius, and tibialis anterior are supplied by the peroneal nerve and tibialis posterior is supplied by the tibial nerve.

47. D. Glial cells are depolarized by an increase in extracellular potassium concentration. Intracellular potential of a glial cell approximates the potassium equilibrium potential and hence somewhat exceeds the neuronal membrane potential. Glial cells do not exhibit action potentials or postsynaptic potentials. Glial cells are believed to amplify extracellular field potentials.

48. E. The voltage-gated sodium channels open in response to changes in the membrane potential. They are responsible for the rising phase of the action potential. The increase in sodium influx is due to a positive feedback loop. The sodium channels exist in one of three distinct states: resting, active, or inactive. The sodium channels close (become inactive) at the peak of the action potential because of their intrinsic channel properties but not due to changes in calcium conductance or membrane potential.

49. D. The PDS is a wave of cortical depolarization, leading to synchronized spiking of a group of neurons. This burst of action potentials can be detected by EEG as epileptiform activity as it serves as the cellular manifestation of epilepsy. It is thought that there is a calcium (Ca)-mediated depolarization, which causes voltage-gated sodium (Na) channels to open, resulting in action potentials. This depolarization is followed by a period of hyperpolarization mediated by Ca-dependent potassium (K) channels or gamma-aminobutyric acid (GABA)-activated chloride (Cl) influx.

50. B. The outside of the cell is by convention defined as zero and the resting membrane potential is, therefore, equal to the voltage inside the cell. In neurons, the usual range of the resting membrane is −60 mV to −70 mV, close to the equilibrium potential of chloride ions. In muscle, it is typically closer to −90 mV. The typical equilibrium potentials for potassium and sodium are −90 mV and +55 mV, respectively.

51. C. A depolarization/repolarization sequence occurring in a nerve located inside a volume conductor produces characteristic changes. The actual site of depolarization acts as a current "sink," with the current lines fanning into it from the adjacent current "source." The recorded waveform potential is usually triphasic, consisting of an initial, small positive (downward) deflection, a large, negative (upward) deflection, and a trailing, small positive (downward) deflection. The waveform is asymmetric because repolarization is slower and has less dense current lines than depolarization.

52. B. Gamma (30–70 Hz) rhythms are felt to be generated in the superficial somatosensory cortical layers II/III, while beta rhythms (20–30 Hz) are felt to be generated in deep layer V mainly in association with activity in the fast-spiking interneurons. Gamma oscillations reflect a general mechanism that synchronizes neuronal networks in spatially separate cortical areas to enable fast routing and processing of information in the cortex. Despite their presence during sleep and under anesthesia, fast oscillations are mainly associated with increased levels of alertness, thus closely following the onset of activity in cholinergic neurons of the brainstem and basal forebrain. Increase of beta activity has been demonstrated after finger or foot movement when the muscles relax (postmovement beta rebound). Related to this postmovement beta rebound, there is an increase of gamma activity (greater than 30 Hz) immediately preceding the finger movement, which is felt to be associated with activation of cortical motor neurons.

53. C. K-complex is a recurrent depolarizing–hyperpolarizing sequence within an oscillatory cycle. With deepening of sleep, the K-complexes become more rhythmic, regular, and faster (approaching 1 Hz). During late stages of sleep, most of the K-complexes may be confounded with delta waves. Spindles are generated within the thalamus because they persist in the thalamus after decortication and high brainstem transection. In particular, the reticular nucleus, consisting of GABAergic neurons, is felt to generate the spindle oscillations because spindles are abolished in the dorsal thalamus after disconnection from the reticular nucleus but are preserved in the rostral part of the reticular nucleus severed from the dorsal thalamus. The decreased activity of brainstem cholinergic neurons at the onset of sleep contributes to the hyperpolarization of thalamocortical cells, facilitating the occurrence of bursting discharges. Such clusters of high-frequency action potentials excite the dendrites of neurons in the reticular nucleus, and trigger the dendrodendritic avalanche leading to synchronization of the entire reticular nucleus. Bursting of reticular neurons causes powerful GABAergic inhibitory postsynaptic potentials in thalamocortical neurons. The end of this inhibition triggers a rebound low threshold spike (LTS), crowned by a high-frequency burst of action potentials, which in turn excites the target reticular cells. The main functional correlate of sleep spindles is to block incoming stimuli to the cortex at the thalamic level, which promotes cortical deafferentation.

54. D. Although the postsynaptic potentials primarily contribute to the extracellularly measurable potentials, other relatively slow variations of membrane potential, such as those associated with depolarizing or hyperpolarizing afterpotentials and dendritic events as calcium action potentials, can also be contributory.

55. A. Sodium ions move passively (i.e., without expenditure of energy) along their concentration gradient into the cell via voltage-gated sodium channels during depolarization. Facilitated diffusion, which is also energy-independent, is a process by which substances, such as glucose and chloride, move across the cell membrane and down the concentration gradient with the help of carrier molecules. Although sodium ions can be transported by this mechanism, the movement of ions during depolarization is mainly through passive transport. Active transport uses energy, typically ATP, to move ions usually against the normal gradients; the sodium–potassium pump is an example.

56. D. The cross-sectional resistance of an axon is inversely proportional to the diameter of the axon. Therefore, larger axons depolarize with lower stimulus intensities compared to smaller axons. The stimulators used in NCS are typically bipolar, with a cathode and an anode. The depolarization of the axon occurs below the cathode. On the other hand, hyperpolarization of the axon occurs below the anode. The extracellular space has low resistance, allowing for current to flow easily to the axon. Therefore, the intensity of the stimulation current needed for depolarization is dependent mainly on the size of the desired nerve to be stimulated rather than the resistance characteristics of the extracellular space.

57. B. The P100, a long latency visual evoked potential response generated by the striate (visual) cortex, is considered a near-field potential. Far-field potentials are waveforms recorded by electrodes far from the current source having a low spatial gradient (i.e., rate of change in potential with respect to distance). Examples of far-field potentials include Wave V, P14, and N18 as well as other subcortically generated potentials measured at the scalp. Of note, the compound motor action potential is a composite of both near- and far-field potentials.

58. E. Severe atrophy of the first dorsal interosseus muscle suggests involvement of C8/T1 nerve roots. The differential diagnosis of that would be ulnar neuropathy, medial cord/lower trunk brachial plexopathy, or C8/T1 radiculopathy.

59. D. Cold temperature affects both sensory and motor nerve conduction studies. With decreased limb temperature, conduction velocity is slowed and distal latency is prolonged. Sensory and motor amplitudes are higher with cold limb temperature compared to normal body temperature.

60. C. End-plate spikes typically start with depolarization of the end-plate stimulated directly by the needle tip resulting in an initial negativity. This is followed by a final positivity as the depolarization travels away from the end plate.

61. C. PSPs are graded responses that can vary depending on sodium influx. In contrast, action potentials are all-or-none phenomena that cannot be stopped once started. When an EPSP reaches a threshold of −50 mV, an action potential is generated. In contrast, when an IPSP occurs, the membrane becomes hyperpolarized. PSPs occurring simultaneously in multiple synapses summate spatially. Similarly, PSPs that overlap in time summate temporally. Acetylcholine generates an EPSP, whereas GABA generates an IPSP. Both EPSPs and IPSPs contribute to the generation of EEG waveforms.

62. B. RMP is close to the equilibrium potential of the chloride ions, which is usually around −70 to −80 mV. At this potential, the cell is said to be in a polarized state. At the resting state, the concentration of potassium ions is 20 times higher inside the cell than outside, whereas the concentration of sodium ions is 10 times higher outside the cell than inside.

This concentration gradient is maintained by the sodium–potassium pump. An excitatory postsynaptic potential depolarizes the cell as a result of influx of sodium ions such that the RMP becomes less negative. When the RMP reaches −50 to −60 mV, an action potential is generated.

63. D. Papez circuit consists of hippocampus, fornix, mammillary bodies, anterior nucleus of the thalamus, and cingulate cortex. It was originally felt to underlie the processing of emotional expression, but more recent evidence suggests that it is involved spatial and episodic memory processing. Stimulation of the anterior nucleus of the thalamus, which is part of the Papez circuit, modulates activity in the hippocampus and cortex. This is the basis for deep brain stimulation for epilepsy.

64. E. Cortical activity gets attenuated by cerebrospinal fluid (CSF), dura, skull, and scalp. As a result, the amplitude of alpha rhythm is 300 μV or greater over the cortex, but <100 μV at the scalp. It has been shown that approximately 6 cm^2 of the cortical surface needs to be involved for a given activity to be seen at the scalp electrode. Radially oriented dipoles contribute to the EEG activity detected at the scalp, whereas the horizontally oriented diploes, running parallel to the cortical surface, contribute to the magnetoencephalographic (MEG) activity at the scalp. Focal activity tends to be more attenuated (as high as 5,000:1) than widespread activity (as low as 2:1). Faster frequency activity is more attenuated than the slower frequency activity by intervening tissues between the cortex and the scalp.

65. E. In their stimulation experiments in anesthetized cats, Moruzzi and Magnoun showed that stimulation of brainstem resulted in cessation of synchronized slow activity in the ipsilateral hemisphere produced by anesthesia, which changed to a low-voltage desynchronized pattern resembling wakefulness. Further lesioning experiments by Lindsley et al. showed that a large lesion of the midbrain tegmentum resulted in the desynchronized EEG (resembling wakefulness) being replaced by synchronized EEG with recurring bursts of spindles and slow waves (resembling sleep). These findings led to the conclusion that the ascending reticular activating system, located in the midbrain and diencephalon, is critical for EEG activation and wakefulness.

Batini et al. showed that midpontine pretegmental transection in cat produced permanent desynchronization resembling wakefulness, suggesting the presence of a sleep-inducing center in the caudal part of the brainstem. Experiments by Cordeau and Mancia showed that midpontine pretegmental hemisection in cat produced desynchronization resembling wakefulness in the ipsilateral hemisphere while the synchronized activity resembling sleep was preserved on the contralateral side. In their second set of experiments, Cordeau and Mancia found that when a midpontine hemisection was combined with an ipsilateral midbrain hemisection, the ipsilateral desynchronization (wakefulness) pattern changed to permanent synchronization (sleep / coma) pattern. Furthermore, they found that an arousal stimulus changed the synchronized EEG to desynchronized pattern in the contralateral but not in the ipsilateral hemisphere. Results of midpontine hemisection suggested that ipsilateral permanent desynchronization is due to interruption of a synchronizing mechanism (sleep promoting center) located in lower brainstem, whereas the results of midbrain hemisection suggested that the ipsilateral permanent synchronization is due to interruption of afferent flow from the desynchronizing mechanism (ascending reticular activating system).

2

Electronics and Instrumentation

QUESTIONS

1. The impedance in a resistor–capacitor circuit decreases with:
   A. Increase in the amplifier gain
   B. Decrease in amplifier gain
   C. Decrease in signal frequency
   D. Increase in capacitance
   E. Decrease in capacitance

2. Which of the following is true regarding electrode impedance when performing an EEG?
   A. It should be more than 5 kΩ for scalp electrodes
   B. It is not critical because the electrode–electrolyte interface does not resemble a resistor–capacitor (RC) circuit
   C. Large electrode impedances can lead to large artifacts
   D. It is increased by removing the scalp oil
   E. It is important for it to be as high as possible

3. Impedances from the adjacent electrodes should be similar in order to:
   A. Increase the impedance mismatch
   B. Prevent "salt bridging" effects
   C. Prevent aliasing
   D. Ensure a pathway for current to flow from one electrode to another
   E. Maintain signal fidelity in the differential amplifier

ANSWERS TO THIS SECTION CAN BE FOUND ON PAGE 37

The figures in this chapter can be viewed in a larger size by accessing the digital version of this chapter found on Springer Publishing Company Connect™. Refer to the front of this book for access instructions.

4. Across a resistor in a resistor–capacitor (RC) circuit, the voltage drop is characterized by all of the following *except:*
A. It is maximal at the outset of an applied square wave pulse
B. It is very sensitive to sudden changes in applied voltage
C. It acts like a high-frequency filter
D. It acts like a high-pass filter
E. It decreases over time to zero dependent on the time constant.

5. In a resistor–capacitor (RC) circuit, a larger resistor will cause the time constant to be:
A. Longer
B. Shorter
C. Unchanged
D. More dependent on the capacitor size
E. Less dependent on the capacitor size

6. Which of the following factors may introduce artifacts in the repetitive nerve stimulation study with recording from the abductor pollicis brevis (APB) muscle with median stimulation at the wrist, compared to recording from the abductor digiti minimi (ADM) muscle with ulnar stimulation at the wrist?
A. Simultaneous ulnar nerve stimulation at the wrist
B. Movement of recording electrode
C. Cold thumb temperature
D. 60 Hz artifact, which is more likely in distal muscles
E. Inability to relax APB muscle between stimulations

7. Current by convention
A. Flows from the negative pole to positive pole
B. Flows from the positive pole to the negative pole
C. Refers to the rate of flow of electrons summated over a period of time
D. Refers to the movement of the negative charge
E. Refers to flow in the same direction as the flow of electrons

8. During a motor nerve conduction study, the sensitivity of the display was changed from 5 mV per division to 1 mV per division. How can this change affect the compound muscle action potential (CMAP)?
A. Increases the CMAP duration
B. Increases the CMAP amplitude
C. Decreases the CMAP amplitude
D. Increases the measured CMAP latency
E. Decreases the measured CMAP latency

9. In the sural antidromic sensory study shown below, what is the sweep speed likely to be?

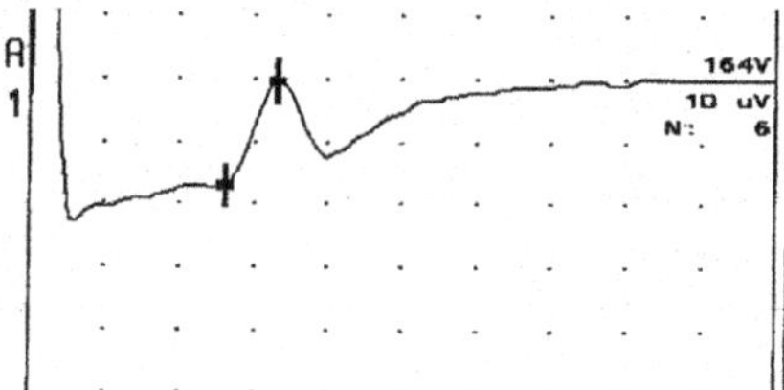

Recording Site :Lat Mal

STIMULUS SITE	LAT1 ms	LAT2 ms	AMP uV	TEMP °C
A1: Lower leg(14cm)	2.6	3.3	16.74	33.7
A2:				

A. 0.1 ms/division
B. 0.5 ms/division
C. 1 ms/division
D. 2 ms/division
E. Cannot be determined from the information provided

10. Which of the following is true regarding cathode?
A. It is the positively charged terminal of a galvanic cell
B. It is the neutral charged terminal of a galvanic cell
C. It is the negatively charged terminal of a galvanic cell
D. It repels electrons
E. It represents the terminal into which the current flows

11. Which of the following situations will lead to a phase shift to the left?
A. Decreasing the low-frequency filter; decreasing the high-frequency filter
B. Decreasing the low-frequency filter; increasing the high-frequency filter
C. Increasing the low-frequency filter; decreasing the high-frequency filter
D. Increasing the low-frequency filter; increasing the high-frequency filter
E. None, because filter changes do not affect phase shifts

12. While performing an electrodiagnostic study in an ICU setting, excess electrical artifact can be removed by undertaking all of the following steps *except:*
A. Turning off all devices that do not need to be "on" during the study
B. Using adequate electrode gel
C. Using coaxial cables
D. Using submaximal stimulation for nerve conduction studies
E. Preparing the skin

13. While performing antidromic sensory studies, the technologist decreases the distance between the active and reference electrodes without making any changes to the distance between the stimulation point and active electrodes. This will likely result in which of the following changes to the sensory nerve action potential (SNAP)?
A. Increased duration
B. Increased peak latency
C. Increased onset latency
D. Decreased onset latency
E. Decreased amplitude

14. Decreasing the time constant will cause the waveform to appear:
A. Sharper
B. Smoother
C. Phase shift to the right
D. Larger
E. Unchanged

15. Which of the following outcomes is likely if the high-frequency filter cutoff is reduced from 10,000 Hz to 500 Hz during needle EMG?
A. No change in motor unit action potential (MUAP) amplitude
B. Reduction in MUAP amplitude
C. Increase in MUAP amplitude
D. Increases the number of phases in the MUAP
E. Any of the above, depending on the type of needle used

16. What happens to the P100 latency of the visual evoked potential if the high-frequency filter cutoff is lowered?
A. There may be an apparent increase in the P100 latency
B. There may be an apparent decrease in the P100 latency
C. There may be a bifid pattern of the peak latency
D. The P100 waveform will merge with the N75 waveform
E. There will be no change in the apparent P100 latency

17. Silver chloride electrodes are used for routine neurophysiological studies because:
A. They develop the necessary amount of capacitance
B. They behave like a built-in low-frequency filter
C. They are not susceptible to "pops"
D. The chloride ions prevent polarization
E. They are nonreversible

18. All of the following statements about sensitivity are true *except:*
A. It is typically expressed as microvolts/millimeter
B. Increase in gain increases the sensitivity
C. It alters the dynamic range of the amplifier
D. It represents the size of the deflection seen on the paper or display
E. The typical sensitivity for scalp EEG is 7 μsec/mm

19. Undersampling during analog-to-digital conversion can lead to which of the following?
A. Artificial reduction of low-frequency components
B. Artificial increase of high-frequency components
C. Decrease in amplitude resolution
D. Decreased ability to analyze direct current (DC) potentials
E. Aliasing

20. Which of the following strategies can be used to minimize analog-to-digital converter (ADC) sampling artifact?
A. Increase the sampling rate to equal the maximum desired resolvable frequency
B. Apply a high-frequency filter to the input data
C. Apply a low-frequency filter to the input data
D. Open the dynamic range beyond the extremes of the desired input voltages
E. Use an ADC with a small bit rate

21. In a resistor–capacitor (RC) circuit, the voltage output across a capacitor:
A. Behaves like a high-frequency filter
B. Behaves like a high-pass filter
C. Is sensitive to high frequencies

D. Is linear
E. Is independent of the time constant

22. During needle EMG recording in a patient, the electrodiagnostic fellow notices that a single motor unit has started to appear once per sweep on the screen (sweep speed set at 10 ms/division; 20 divisions on the screen). This particular motor unit seems to move rightward on the screen. The firing frequency of this potential is likely to be
A. 4 Hz
B. 5 Hz
C. 6 Hz
D. 10 Hz
E. Directly proportional to the sweep speed

23. Temporal resolution of the raw data is limited by which of the following?
A. Amplifier sampling frequency
B. Bit rate of analog-to-digital converter (ADC)
C. Input range of the amplifier
D. Screen resolution
E. Recording electrode

24. What is the maximum recommended electrode impedance for recording EEG?
A. 1 ohm
B. 500 ohms
C. 1,000 ohms
D. 5,000 ohms
E. 50,000 ohms

25. In a resistor–capacitor (RC) circuit, impedance is equal to:
A. Resistance only
B. Capacitive reactance only
C. Capacitive reactance and inductive reactance
D. Resistance and capacitive reactance
E. Resistance, capacitive reactance, and inductive reactance

26. How does the number of bits in the analog-to-digital converter (ADC) affect the sampling rate?
A. It reduces it
B. It increases it
C. It depends on the bit rate
D. It depends on the filter settings
E. It does not affect the sample rate

27. In calculating impedance, the inductive reactance is subtracted from the capacitive reactance because:
A. They have the same phase
B. They are 45 degrees out of phase
C. They have opposite phases
D. The capacitive reactance already includes the inductive reactance
E. The inductive reactance is not part of the overall impedance

28. Capacitors have all of the following characteristics *except:*
A. They permit and restrict flow of ions through the lipid bilayer
B. They indirectly produce neurophysiological potentials
C. They contribute to impedance
D. They can store potential energy
E. Their capacitive reactance is directly proportional to frequency

29. Which of the following correctly lists the order in which the analog signals are converted to digital signals?
A. Analog signal is sensed, amplified, filtered, and sampled at discrete time intervals
B. Analog signal is sensed, filtered, amplified, and sampled at discrete time intervals
C. Analog signal is sensed, amplified, sampled at discrete time intervals, and filtered
D. Analog signal is sensed, sampled at discrete time intervals, filtered, and amplified
E. Analog signal is sensed, sampled at discrete time intervals, amplified, and filtered

30. Increasing the high-frequency filter cutoff will cause the waveform to appear:
A. Sharper
B. Smoother
C. Phase shifted to the right
D. Smaller
E. Smoother and phase shifted to the right

31. What is the charge moving across a potential energy gradient?
A. Resistance
B. Current
C. Energy
D. Power
E. Impedance

32. Which of the following statements best describes the time constant in a resistor–capacitor (RC) circuit?
A. It is the time required for the capacitor to reach approximately 37% of its charge
B. It is directly proportional to the applied voltage
C. It is inversely proportional to the resistance
D. It is inversely proportional to the capacitance
E. It is prolonged by higher capacitance

33. The effective alternating current (AC) equivalent to the direct current (DC) across a resistor is obtained by applying which of the following mathematical operations to the maximum current amplitude?
A. Division
B. Integral
C. Root mean square
D. Square
E. Derivative

34. What is the rate of transfer of energy?
A. Charge
B. Current
C. Capacitance

D. Power
E. Inductance

35. An infinitely large resistance between the anode and cathode causes:
A. An infinitely large current and open circuit
B. An infinitely small current and open circuit
C. An infinitely large current and short circuit
D. An infinitely small current and short circuit
E. No effect on the current between the anode and cathode

36. Which of the following statements is NOT a characteristic of an amplifier?
A. Its gain is given by the ratio V_{out}/V_{in} of the signal
B. Its gain is commonly expressed in decibels
C. Its dynamic range is the voltage range over which it behaves linearly
D. Its sensitivity is expressed as microvolts per millimeter
E. Its gain is directly proportional to sensitivity

37. A 47-year-old female has a history of chronic alcohol abuse and seizures. She was non-compliant with her antiepileptic drugs (AEDs) and had a seizure resulting in a right parietal scalp contusion. She subsequently had another generalized convulsion a few hours later. What is seen on her EEG (filter 1–70 Hz) below?

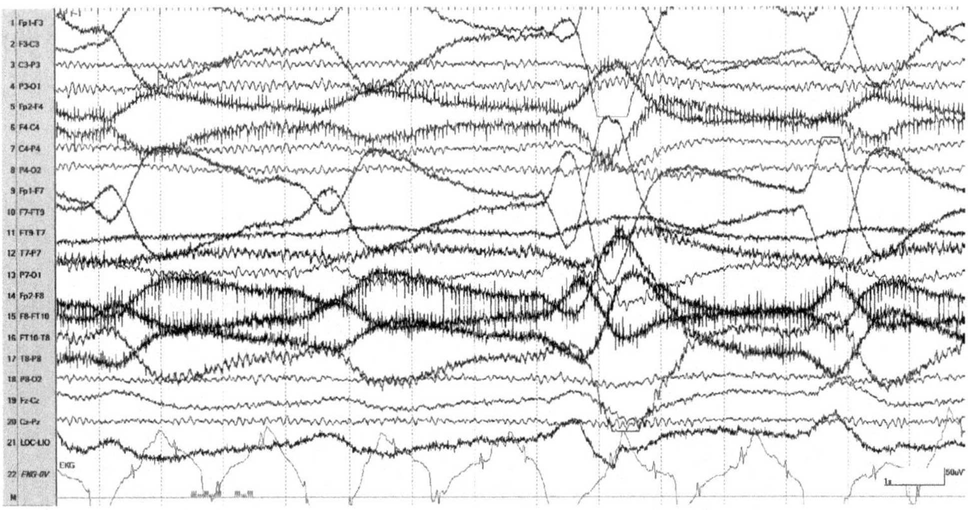

A. Sweat artifact
B. Eye movement artifact
C. Ventilator artifact
D. Cable artifact
E. Myogenic artifact related to photic stimulation

38. Which of the following situations will lead to a phase shift to the right?
A. Decreasing the low-frequency filter; decreasing the high-frequency filter
B. Decreasing the low-frequency filter; increasing the high-frequency filter
C. Increasing the low-frequency filter; decreasing the high-frequency filter
D. Increasing the low-frequency filter; increasing the high-frequency filter
E. Adjusting the filter settings has no effect on phase shifts.

39. What types of signals are used in the calibration process for EEG?
A. Square wave inputs
B. Sine wave inputs
C. Cosine wave inputs
D. Triangular wave inputs
E. Hyperbolic wave inputs

40. Which of the following does *not* increase the EEG impedance?
A. Interface between the scalp and the electrode
B. The wiring from the electrode to the amplifier
C. Display of the acquired EEG waveform on the computer screen
D. Skull thickness
E. Recording electrode

41. Ideally, where should the reference electrode be palced in relation to the recording electrode in order to get the most robust waveform?
A. On a well-defined anatomical landmark
B. Adjacent to
C. Far from
D. Anywhere
E. Depends on the electrode type used

42. Which of the following is closest to the percentage of the input amplitude that will pass at the cutoff frequency of a filter?
A. 0%
B. 25%
C. 50%
D. 75%
E. 100%

43. When multiple capacitors are placed in a circuit, they exhibit the behavior opposite to that of
A. Inductors
B. Resistors
C. Invertors
D. Operative amplifiers
E. Differential amplifiers

44. Which of the following statements regarding analog-to-digital conversion of the EEG is true?
A. Analog EEG measures the data at discrete time points
B. Digital EEG is made up of continuous nondiscrete data
C. The higher the sampling rate, the closer the digital signal resembles the analog signal
D. The less number of bits an analog-to-digital converter (ADC) has, the more the digital sample resembles the analog signal
E. The ideal sampling rate is 1.5 times the highest frequency in the analog signal

45. All of the following statements regarding inductors are true *except:*
A. Their currents are generated by the electrical field surrounding a wire that creates currents in other wires
B. They have a reactance similar to resistors
C. They pose an impediment to current generated by another source
D. The reactance is directly proportional to the inductance
E. Inductance is measured in henries

46. While performing a sensory nerve conduction study, the neurology resident in the electrodiagnostic laboratory notices a stimulus artifact before the sensory response. Which of the following techniques can help reduce the stimulus artifact?
A. Increase the stimulus intensity
B. Decrease the distance between the stimulator and recording electrode
C. Place the ground electrode on the contralateral extremity
D. Rotate the anode of the stimulator
E. Decrease the stimulus intensity to deliver a submaximal stimulus

47. All of the following statements about common mode signals are true *except:*
A. Common mode signals are dissimilar potentials at different electrode sites that should be ideally rejected
B. Amplifiers are designed to preferentially block common mode signals and to pass the differential-mode signals
C. Unequal impedances between electrodes can affect common mode signals
D. It is recommended that the common mode signals be rejected at a ratio of 80 dB
E. Ideally, the common mode gain is zero and the common mode rejection ratio (CMRR) is infinity

For Questions 48–51:

A 27″ computer screen has a resolution of 1,920 (horizontal) by 1,080 (vertical) pixels with vertical borders of 250 pixels each. An EEG sampled at 1,000 Hz is displayed at 15 seconds per page.

48. How many pixels per inch (PPI) are present on the computer screen?
A. 12.2
B. 40
C. 63.1
D. 71.1
E. 81.6

49. How many pixels are available to display 1 second of EEG?
A. 39
B. 95
C. 105
D. 128
E. 142

50. What is the maximum frequency of the EEG activity that can be displayed based on the specified parameters?
A. 47 Hz
B. 63 Hz
C. 96 Hz
D. 121 Hz
E. 635 Hz

51. What would be the maximum resolvable frequency if the margins of the screen are eliminated and the number of seconds per page is reduced from 15 seconds to 10 seconds?
A. 47 Hz
B. 96 Hz
C. 192 Hz
D. 500 Hz
E. 1000 Hz

For Questions 52–55:

Assume an EEG acquisition system has a 10-bit analog-to-digital converter (ADC) with a voltage range of −2 mV to +2 mV.

52. In how many discrete voltage bins can the digital signal be placed?
A. 4
B. 10
C. 512
D. 1,024
E. 2,000

53. The voltage resolution of the sampled data is closest to which value?
A. 0.2 μV
B. 2 μV
C. 0.4 μV
D. 4 μV
E. 8μV

54. What will happen to the voltage resolution if the voltage range of the EEG system is reduced to the −1 mV to +1 mV range?
A. It will remain the same because the number of bins has not changed
B. It will decrease by a factor of 2
C. It will increase by a factor of 2
D. It will decrease by a factor of 4
E. It will increase by a factor of 4

55. What will be the approximate voltage resolution if a 12-bit analog-to-digital converter (ADC) is used instead of the 10-bit ADC in the EEG system?
A. 1 μV
B. 2 μV
C. 4 μV
D. 8 μV
E. 16 μV

56. Which of the following statements regarding EEG artifacts is true?

A. Glossokinetic artifact resembles temporal delta activity
B. Electrocardiogram artifact most commonly appears in the bipolar montages
C. Pulse artifact on scalp EEG is synchronous with the QRS complex
D. Electrical 60 Hz artifact is usually not affected by the ground electrode
E. Electrode pop artifact may mimic a focal ictal discharge

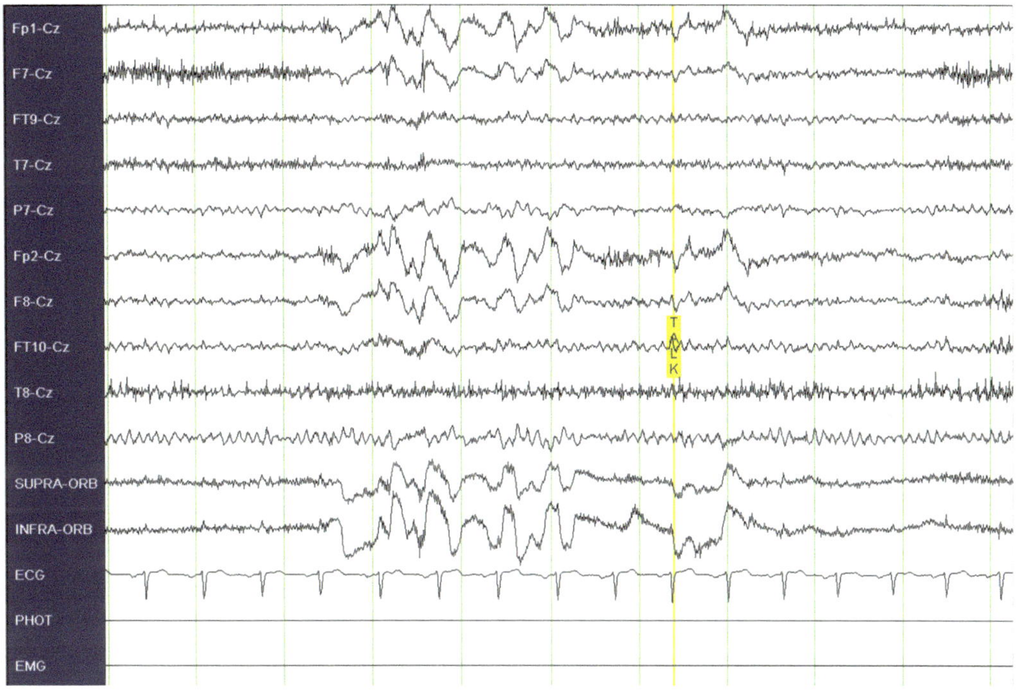

Figure A

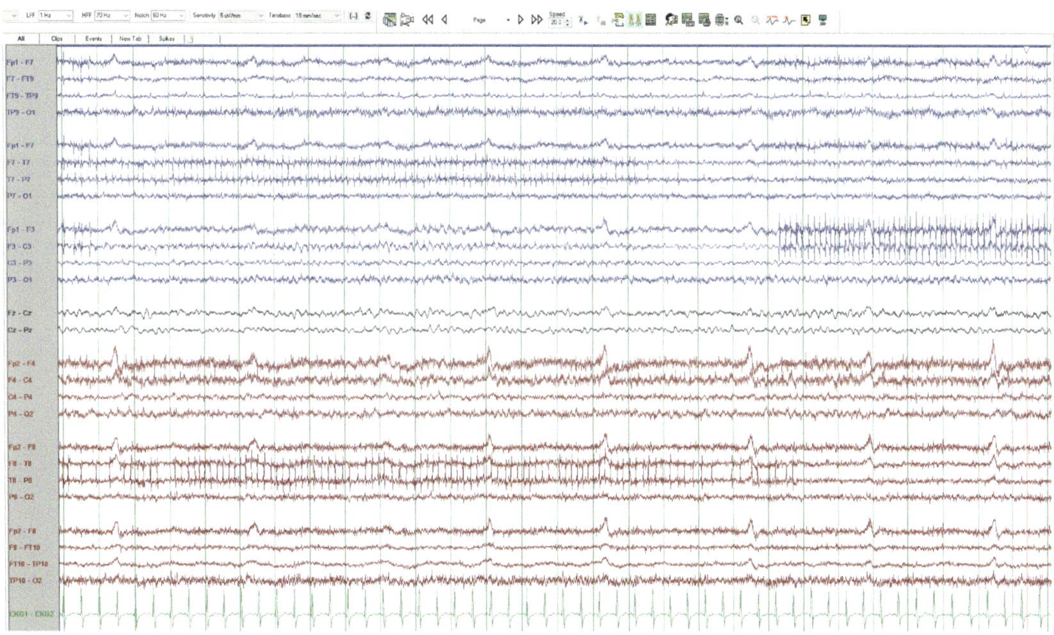

Figure B

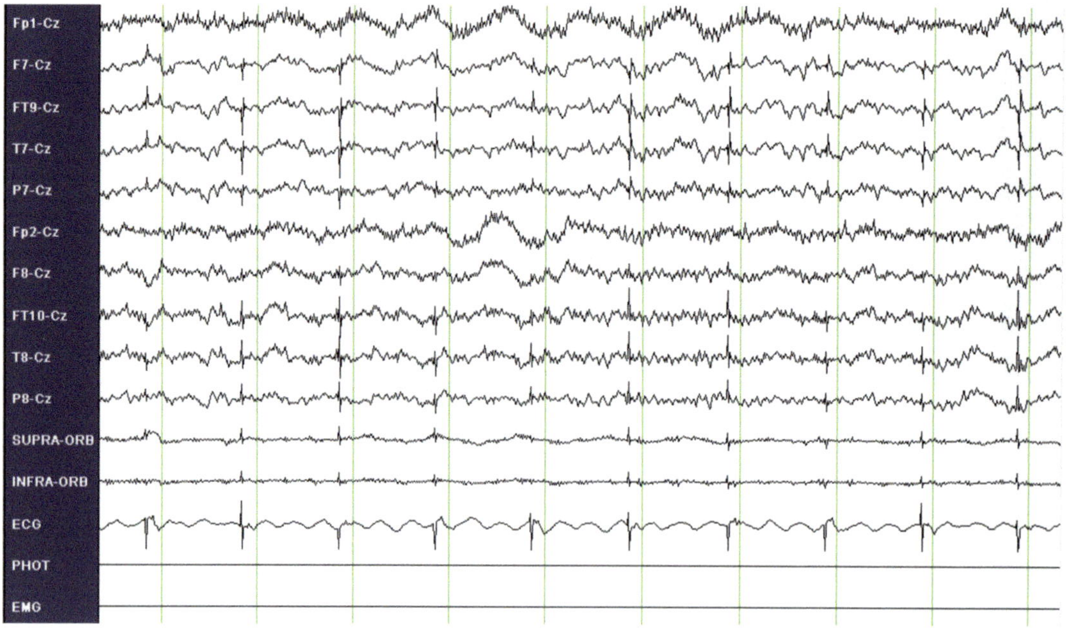

Figure C

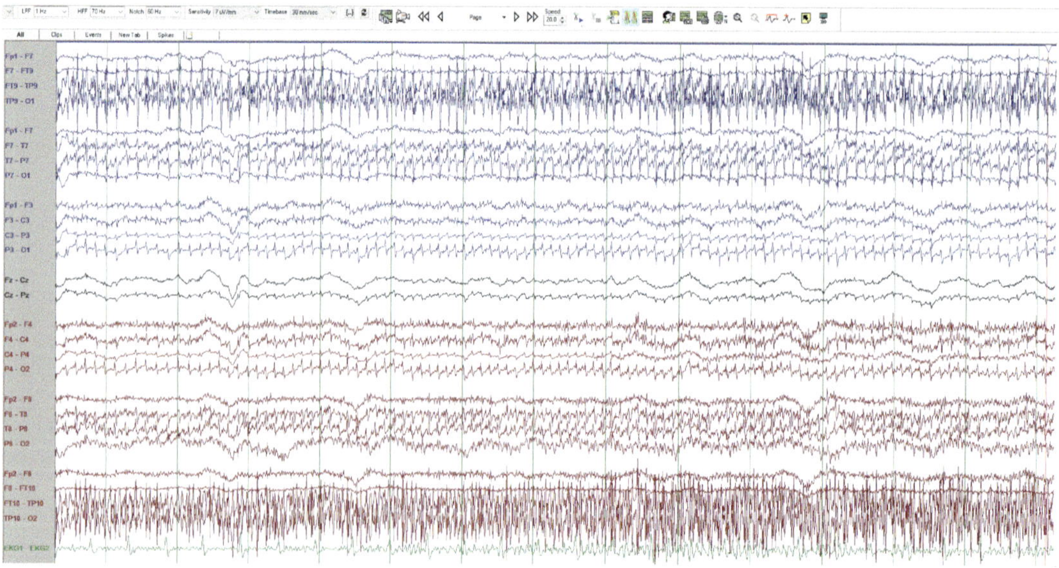

Figure D

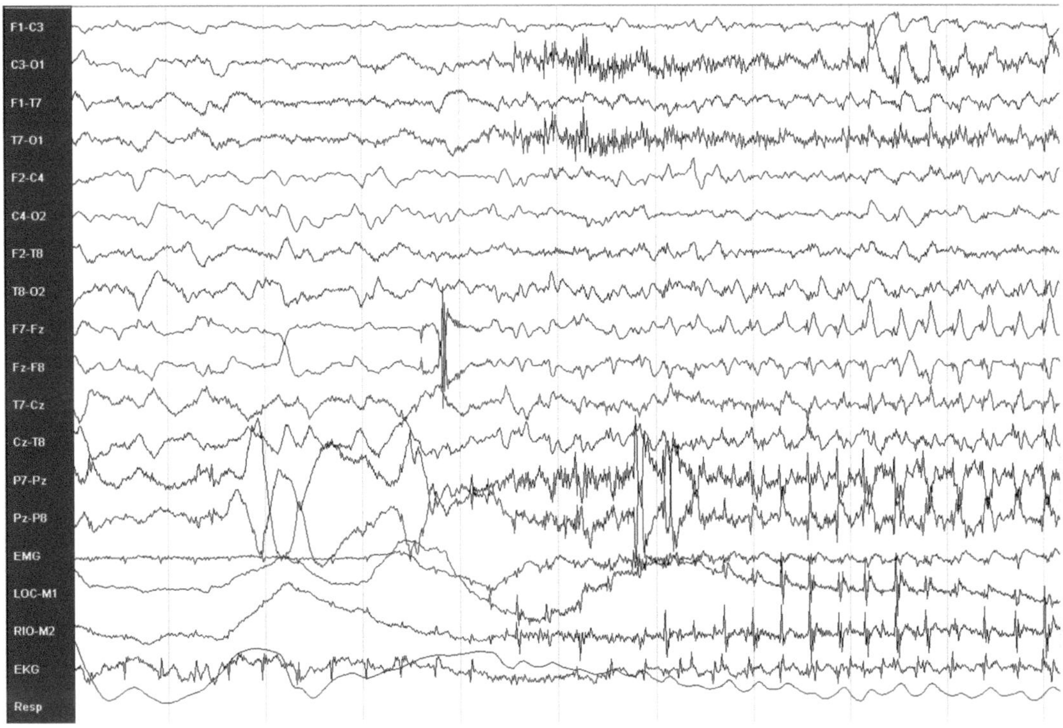

Figure E

For Questions 57–61:

Match Figures A, B, C, D, or E to one of the clinical scenarios listed below:

57. A 40-week CA neonate had spells of lip smacking and desaturations prompting an EEG evaluation. During the study, the baby started to scream and cry, prompting her mother to pick her up to console her.

A. Figure A
B. Figure B
C. Figure C
D. Figure D
E. Figure E

58. A 17-year-old had an asthma attack requiring intubation and sedation. The ventilator was on assist control set to 12 breaths per minute, but the patient was overbreathing the ventilator.

A. Figure A
B. Figure B
C. Figure C
D. Figure D
E. Figure E

59. A 56-year-old patient presents status post cardiac arrest in the setting of a seizure disorder and is being prepped for therapeutic hypothermia. The ED notes diffuse body tremors. The patient is noted to be febrile to 102°F and is on pressors for hypotension.
A. Figure A
B. Figure B
C. Figure C
D. Figure D
E. Figure E

60. A 12-year-old was getting an EEG for seizures. The patient loved candy and told the EEG technologist that her favorite type was "little licorice lollipops" which she repeated three times in a row.
A. Figure A
B. Figure B
C. Figure C
D. Figure D
E. Figure E

61. A 57-year-old presented with an episode of aphasia. A code stroke was activated and the patient had a CT head scan, which was unremarkable. An MRI brain scan could not be done due to the presence of incompatible metal in the body. An EEG was done to assess for seizures.
A. Figure A
B. Figure B
C. Figure C
D. Figure D
E. Figure E

62. Which of the following statements comparing subdural grids and stereoencephalography (SEEG) is most *true*?
A. SEEG is not ideal for bilateral explorations
B. Subdural grids are placed through multiple burr holes
C. SEEG requires angiography images as part of the planning process
D. Subdural grids are ideal for recording from sulcal areas, deep brain structures, and noncontiguous lobes
E. Robotic guidance has improved the safety and accuracy of placing subdural grids

ANSWERS

1. **D.** The impedance (Z), given by the equation $1/(2\pi FC)$, decreases as either frequency (F) or capacitance (C) increases. Gain refers to the ratio of the signal coming out of the amplifier to that going in, and it does not affect impedance.

2. **C.** Because the electrode–electrolyte interface resembles an RC circuit, it is important for the electrode impedance to be as low as possible, typically less than 5 kΩ for scalp electrodes. Large electrode impedances can cause large artifact potentials even by small local currents induced by ambient electric fields (Ohm's law: V = IR, V = IZ). Preparing the site (e.g., with alcohol) to remove oil helps to lower the impedance to desired levels.

3. **E.** Because inputs from neighboring contacts are compared using differential amplifiers, their input impedances must be comparable. If there is an impedance mismatch, the signal fidelity will be degraded because the common sources of artifact will not be effectively subtracted. Higher impedances lead to lower than true amplitudes and loss of lower frequencies. Excessively low impedances (e.g., a "salt bridge" caused by a smeared electrode gel between the contacts) can also cause erroneously low amplitudes. Impedance is not related to aliasing, which is caused by sampling the signal at a rate inadequate to represent the highest frequency present in the waveform.

4. **C.** When a square wave pulse is applied to an RC circuit, the voltage drop across the resistor is immediately equal to the input voltage. Hence, the voltage across the resistor is maximal at the outset but decreases in relation to the time constant and eventually equals zero. Thus, the voltage output across the resistor is very sensitive to sudden changes in input voltage (i.e., passes high frequencies) but very insensitive to relatively unchanging voltage (i.e., blocks low frequencies). Therefore, a resistor acts as a high-pass filter (i.e., low-frequency filter).

5. **A.** When voltage is applied to an RC circuit, the current immediately flows across the resistor and begins to accumulate on the capacitor. Over time, the capacitor charges and accrues voltage exponentially that opposes further current flow. If the power source is turned off, the capacitor discharges in the same exponential manner but in the opposite direction. This exponential change is described by the circuit's time constant, τ, which is the time required for the capacitor to reach approximately 63% of its charge. This time is independent of the applied voltage but depends on resistance and capacitance, and is given by the equation

$$\tau = R * C,$$

where τ is the time constant, R is the resistance, and C is the capacitance. A larger resistor permits less current to flow to charge the capacitor, resulting in a longer τ. Similarly, a larger capacitor takes longer to charge, resulting in a longer τ as well. Note that the resistor and capacitor equally affect the time constant.

6. **B.** Movement of the recording electrode changes the compound muscle action potential and may introduce errors in the calculation of the decrement. Other factors are no more likely to introduce errors when recording from the APB muscle with median stimulation compared to recording from the ADM muscle with ulnar repetitive stimulation.

7. **B.** Current can be the flow of positive and/or negative charges, but by convention, current refers to the movement of the positive charge and therefore is described as flowing from the positive pole to the negative pole. Conventional current flows in the opposite direction to the flow of electrons. Current is not a summated value over time.

8. **E.** When the sensitivity changes from 5 to 1 mV per division, the earliest deflection from the baseline also changes and occurs earlier, and this leads to a decrease in the measured latency. Decreasing the sensitivity does not affect the amplitude or the duration of a compound muscle action potential.

9. **C.** From the table, the peak latency (LAT2) is 3.3 ms and the peak can be seen after three divisions. Similarly, the onset latency (LAT1) is 2.6 ms and this is seen after two divisions. Based on this, each division has to be 1 ms.

10. **A.** Cathode is the positively charged terminal of a galvanic cell, whereas anode is the negatively charged terminal. There is no neutral charged terminal in a galvanic cell. In a circuit, the electrons flow into the cathode and, by convention, the current flows out of the cathode.

11. **D.** Increasing both the low-frequency and high-frequency filter settings will lead to a phase shift to the left.

12. **D.** Excessive electrical artifact is not uncommon while performing studies in ICU and various precautions will help minimize this artifact. Turning off unnecessary devices, preparing the skin, using electrode gel, and using appropriate cables will help minimize electrical artifact. Submaximal stimulation will not affect the electrical artifact and is not recommended.

13. **E.** When the distance between the active and reference electrodes is decreased, there will be excess phase cancellation, which can result in decreased SNAP amplitude, duration, and peak latency. Onset latency will not change because the difference between the stimulation point and active electrode is unchanged.

14. **A.** Decreasing the time constant will result in a sharper waveform. A shorter time constant results in a higher cutoff frequency for the low-frequency filter based on the equation

$$F_c = 1/(2\pi\tau) \approx 0.16/\tau,$$

where F_c is the cutoff frequency and τ is the time constant. Note that F_c is the frequency above which greater than 70% of the input amplitude will pass. A higher cutoff frequency will result in attenuation of higher amplitude slow activity. This will result in smaller and sharper waveforms with a phase shift to the left.

15. **B.** When the high-frequency filter cutoff is reduced, it reduces the rapidly changing waveforms and, in turn, results in reduction in MUAP amplitude. It may also decrease the number of phases in the motor unit potential.

16. **A.** Decreasing the high-frequency cutoff will exclude higher frequencies that contribute to the peak of the waveform. As a result, the peak will appear artificially later, resulting in an apparent increase in the P100 latency. The P100 waveform will not merge with the N75 waveform. The N75 waveform is a smaller, negative peak, which is often seen and occurs prior to the P100 waveform.

17. **D.** Electrodes are made of metallic materials, allowing them to detect electrical potentials from the patient and to conduct them to the recording device. Electrodes may be polarized (nonreversible) or nonpolarized (reversible). Polarized electrodes tend to develop significant capacitance and behave like low-frequency filters that can interfere with transmission of underlying biological signals, so they are commonly avoided. For intracranial recordings, gold or platinum can be used but they are expensive. Silver chloride electrodes are nonpolarized (reversible) electrodes in which polarization is avoided because the chloride ion is common to both the electrode and the electrolyte. The silver chloride electrodes are commonly used for routine neurophysiological studies. However, they are still susceptible to "pops," especially when new, because the electrode–electrolyte interface undergoes sudden transitions.

18. **B.** Sensitivity is expressed as microvolts per millimeter and refers to the size of the vertical deflection seen on the paper or screen that represents the voltage. Typical sensitivity settings for scalp EEG are 7 μV/mm Changing the sensitivity of the EEG changes the dynamic range of the amplifier. The gain and sensitivity are inversely proportional. Therefore, an increase in the amplifier gain causes a decrease in the sensitivity.

19. **E.** Undersampling refers to fewer discrete digital time samples obtained during analog-to-digital conversion; this is not related to amplitude resolution. Undersampling causes distortion of high-frequency components by artificially converting them to lower frequencies, a phenomenon called aliasing. To avoid distortion, the sampling rate should be greater than twice the highest input frequency component of interest to be recorded (the Nyquist frequency). The alias frequency is mathematically defined as the sampling frequency minus the Nyquist frequency.

20. **B.** ADC sampling artifact can be minimized by applying a high-frequency, not low-frequency, filter to the input data to cut off undesirable high-frequency elements. The desired sampling rate should be at least two times the maximum desired resolvable frequency. The dynamic range should closely encompass the extremes of the desired input voltages. An ADC with the highest bit rate possible will allow for voltages to resemble the analog values as closely as possible.

21. **A.** When a square wave pulse is applied to an RC circuit, there is a lag in the appearance of the voltage across the capacitor, and the initial voltage drop across the capacitor is zero. However, the voltage across the capacitor increases in relation to the time constant

and eventually equals the pulse voltage. Thus, the voltage output across the capacitor is very insensitive to sudden changes in input voltage (i.e., blocks high frequencies) but very sensitive to relatively unchanging voltage (i.e., passes low frequencies). Therefore, a capacitor acts like a high-frequency filter (or low-pass filter).

22. **A.** The whole screen sweep duration is 200 ms (20 multiplied by 10 ms). This means if the motor unit potential appears at the same spot after each sweep screen, its firing frequency is 5 Hz. If it appears to move to the left, then it should be firing slightly faster than 5 Hz, and if it appears to move to the right, then it should be firing slightly slower than 5 Hz. In this case, because the potential is moving to the right, a firing frequency of 4 Hz appears more likely. The firing frequency is not 10 Hz because the motor unit would have to fire twice during this sweep to achieve this frequency. The firing frequency is a property of the motor unit and independent of the display screen characteristics. Therefore, the motor unit firing frequency is independent of the sweep speed.

23. **A.** Temporal resolution refers to the resolution of discrete measurements with respect to time. The amplifier sampling frequency, or the frequency at which the amplifier measures the voltage (i.e., number of data points per second), determines the temporal resolution of the data. Although the screen resolution can impact the resolution of what can be displayed on the screen (e.g., decreasing the number of seconds displayed increases the temporal resolution displayed), it does not impact the resolution of the raw data. The bit rate of the ADC and the amplifier input range determine the voltage resolution of the raw data. Temporal resolution is not limited by the recording electrode, which senses the data continuously.

24. **D.** The recommended electrode impedance is 5,000 ohms or less to minimize electrode-related artifact.

25. **D.** In a circuit, only the individual components present (resistor, R; inductor, L; capacitor, C) contribute to the impedance. Therefore, in a RC circuit, impedance is equal to resistance and capacitive reactance. In a resistor–inductor–capacitor (RLC) circuit, all three components would contribute to the impedance.

26. **E.** The sampling rate is the number of measurements per second expressed as Hz. It is independent of the number of bits in the ADC. The latter affects the voltage resolution of the acquired data, not the sampling rate. The sample rate is also independent of the filter settings.

27. **C.** Inductive and capacitive reactance have opposite phases (i.e., 90 degrees out of phase). Therefore, when inductive reactance is smaller than capacitive reactance, inductive reactance is subtracted from capacitive reactance in calculating impedance. The opposite is true when capacitive reactance is smaller than inductive reactance.

28. **E.** Capacitors can maintain separated charge and store potential energy. In biological systems, the lipid bilayer membrane of nerve tissue acts as a capacitor, permitting and restricting the flow of ionic currents. The intermittent fluctuations in current ultimately lead to the potentials studied in clinical neurophysiology. The amount of capacitive reactance, which contributes to impedance, is inversely proportional to the frequency of the activity and is given by the equation

$$Xc = 1/(2 * \pi * f * C),$$

where Xc is the capacitive reactance in ohms, *f* is the frequency of the current in hertz (Hz), and C is the capacitance in farads. For example, 4 Hz theta activity will lead to higher capacitive reactance than 16 Hz beta activity. Of note, other sources of biological capacitance, such as the cerebrospinal fluid, skull, and scalp, can interfere with these signals.

29. **A.** Analog signals are first sensed by electrodes. They are then amplified, filtered, and sampled at discrete time intervals as dictated by the sampling frequency. The resolution of the voltage steps is determined by the number of bits in the analog-to-digital converter (ADC).

30. **A.** Increasing the high-frequency components will make the waveform appear sharper. In general, a higher cutoff frequency will result in inclusion of higher frequency components that tend to be sharper and smaller in amplitude. Due to the presence of higher amplitude lower frequencies, the overall waveform size may not change much. However, the superimposed faster frequencies may make the waveform sharper (more spiky) along with a phase shift to the left. Decreasing the high-frequency filter cutoff will result in a smoother waveform with a phase shift to the right.

31. **C.** Energy is the charge moving across a potential gradient and is measured in joules (J). Power is the rate of transfer of energy and is measured in watts (W) or J/sec. Current refers to the rate of flow of charge in response to an applied electrical potential or voltage and is measured in amperes (A). Resistance is the impediment to the flow of charge and is measured in ohms (Ω) and is typically the measurement in direct current (DC) circuits. Impedance (also measured in ohms (Ω)), on the other hand, is used in alternating current (AC) circuits and includes the effects of the inductors (inductance) and capacitors (capacitance). The impedance caused by these two effects is collectively referred to as reactance. Of note, impedance forms the imaginary part of complex impedance whereas resistance forms the real part of impedance.

32. **E.** The time constant of a circuit, τ, is the time required for the capacitor to reach approximately 63% of its charge. This time is independent of the applied voltage but depends proportionally on both resistance and capacitance and is given by the equation

$$\tau = R * C,$$

where τ is the time constant, *R* is the resistance, and C is the capacitance. Thus, the time constant can be prolonged by higher capacitance or resistance.

33. **C.** The effective current in an AC circuit across a resistor is given by the root mean square (RMS) value, which is equal to 0.707 * the maximum AC amplitude. Due to the sinusoidal nature of AC, the average current over any given complete cycle is zero. This means that the amount of charge delivered at the end of a cycle of stimulation is near zero. Also, because AC is only at its maximum amplitude for an instant, it will not produce the same heating effect as an equivalent DC. These are some of the reasons for using AC instead of DC for brain mapping.

34. **D.** Power is the rate of transfer of energy and is measured in watts (W) or joules per second (J/sec). Current refers to the rate of flow of charge in response to an applied electrical

potential or voltage and is measured in amperes (A). Charge is the physical property of matter that causes it to experience a force when close to other electrically charged matter and is measured in coulombs (C). Capacitance is the ability of a substance to store an electric charge and is measured in farads (f). Inductance poses an impediment to current flow in inductors and contributes to a circuit's overall impedance.

35. **B.** If the resistance between the anode and cathode is infinitely large, then the current becomes infinitely small (close to zero) and the circuit acts like an open circuit. On the other hand, if the resistance is infinitely small, then the current is infinitely large and the circuit acts like a short circuit. Any resistance in between these two extremes allows current to flow and is considered a closed circuit.

36. **E.** Amplifiers multiply the input signal by a factor called gain that is given by the ratio, V_{out}/V_{in}. The gain is commonly expressed in decibels (20 * log10). The dynamic range is the voltage range over which the amplifier behaves linearly. The sensitivity, expressed as microvolts per millimeter, alters the dynamic range of an amplifier. The gain and sensitivity are inversely proportional. Thus, increasing the sensitivity will reduce the amplifier gain.

37. **D.** The EEG shows cable artifact caused by someone stepping on the cable between the jack box and the amplifier. Sweat artifact can present with very slow activity (usually 0.25–0.5 Hz) due to the sodium chloride and lactic acid from the sweat reacting with the electrodes producing the swaying. Such an artifact would have been attenuated in this example because the low-frequency filter setting was 1 Hz. Occasionally, sweating can be misinterpreted as slow roving eye movements when the sweat artifact is in the anterior channels. Eye movement artifact is produced because the eyeball acts as a dipole with the cornea being relatively positive compared to the retina. With eye closure, the eyeball rotates about its horizontal and vertical axes as it moves superior and lateral, respectively (referred to as the Bell phenomenon). This phenomenon typically lasts less than 0.5 seconds, which is faster than what is seen on the EEG shown in this example. Ventilator artifacts have highly variable morphology (made up of single or multiple waveforms) and amplitude, but they recur with each respiration. Myogenic artifact during photic stimulation presents as lower amplitude speculated activity over the frontal electrodes at various flash frequencies, not seen here.

38. **A.** Decreasing both the low-frequency and high-frequency filter settings will lead to a phase shift to the right. On the other hand, increasing both the low-frequency and high-frequency filter settings will lead to a phase shift to the left.

39. **A.** Calibration maneuvers use square wave inputs and are done to assess the fidelity of the recording system.

40. **C.** Display of the acquired EEG signal on the computer screen does not add to the EEG impedance. EEG impedance is a measure of the resistance along with the capacitive and inductive reactance. Impedance derives from any material through which the EEG signal passes from its generator to the analog-to-digital converter (ADC).

41. **C.** The reference electrode ideally should be far from the recording electrodes, regardless of the type of electrodes used, to subtract artifacts and noise that may be contaminating

both input electrodes (i.e., common mode rejection) and to enhance the underlying waveform because the reference electrode will likely be less involved in the particular electric field, contributing to the recording electrode waveform. Placing the reference electrode adjacent to the recording electrode will result in a small signal because both electrodes would still be exposed to similar electrical fields, resulting in cancellation of common fields, which is not ideal. Therefore, the location of the reference electrode is relevant and cannot be placed anywhere.

42. **D.** The cutoff frequency or corner frequency is the frequency either above or below which the power output of a circuit (e.g., an electronic filter) has fallen to a given proportion of the power in the passband (i.e., the band of frequencies that the filter lets through). Most frequently, this proportion is one-half the passband power, also referred to as the 3 dB point because a fall of 3 dB corresponds approximately to one-half power. Because power is the square of voltage, the resulting voltage value in relation to the passband voltage is

$$\upsilon = \sqrt[2]{\frac{1}{2}} = 0.707, \text{ or } 70\%.$$

43. **B.** Multiple capacitors in a circuit interact in a manner that is opposite to the behavior of resistors. When capacitors are placed in parallel, there is an additive effect. On the contrary, when capacitors are placed in series, they add in a reciprocal manner.

44. **C.** Analog EEG measures continuous (not discrete) data with respect to time and value. Digital EEG, on the other hand, intermittently samples data at discrete moments, and the corresponding amplitudes at that moment are assigned to the nearest discrete values. The degree of fidelity with which the digitally sampled data resembles the original analog data depends on how finely it is sampled, that is, how many discrete steps there are with respect to time (i.e., sampling rate) and the amplitude (i.e., number of bits in the analog-to-digital converter or ADC). For a particular ADC, the number of bits tends to be fixed while the sampling rate can be altered. To prevent aliasing, the ideal sampling rate should be greater than 2 times the highest frequency present in the analog signal.

45. **A.** The inductive current is generated by the magnetic field, not the electrical field, surrounding a wire that creates currents in other wires. Inductance is similar to resistance in that it poses an impediment to current flow. In terms of inductors, the reactance is to the current generated by another source, which is directly proportional to the inductance, L (given in henries).

46. **D.** Increasing the stimulus intensity will only worsen the stimulus artifact. Multiple techniques are recommended to decrease the stimulus artifact. These include decreasing the stimulator intensity, increasing the distance between the stimulator and recording electrodes, placing the ground between the stimulator and recording electrode, and rotating the anode of the stimulator electrode. Additionally, one can reduce the stimulus intensity while making sure it is still supramaximal.

47. **A.** Common mode signals are potentials that are similar at different electrode sites. The ability of an amplifier to block common mode signals and to pass differential-mode

signals is called CMRR and is usually expressed in decibels (dB). Ideally, the common mode gain is zero, while the CMRR is infinity. Unequal impedances between electrodes can affect common mode rejection and can cause artifacts. It is recommended that the CMRR should be at least 80 dB (10,000:1) at the highest sensitivity of the amplifier.

48. **E.** The PPI of a display is related to the size of the display in inches and the total number of pixels in the horizontal and vertical directions. Note that the size of a display typically refers to the diagonal measurement across the screen. Therefore, if given the horizontal and vertical number of pixels, the number of pixels along the diagonal can be calculated in two steps:

(a) Calculate diagonal resolution in pixels using the Pythagorean theorem:

$$d_p = \sqrt{\omega_p^2 + h_p^2}$$

(b) Calculate PPI:

$$PPI = \frac{d_p}{d_i}$$

where

- d_p is diagonal resolution in pixels
- w_p is width resolution in pixels
- h_p is height resolution in pixels
- d_i is diagonal size in inches (this is the number advertised as the size of the display).

For example, for a 27–inch screen with a 1,920 × 1,080 resolution (in which w_p = 1,920, h_p = 1,080, and d_i = 27), we get 2,203 pixels along the diagonal and a PPI of 81.6.

49. **B.** The number of pixels displayed in the EEG is a reflection of the total number of horizontal pixels of the display subtracting the number of pixels in the border. To obtain the number of pixels per second of EEG, the number of pixels displayed in the EEG is divided by the number of seconds displayed.
In the stated case,

$$1920 \text{ horizontal pixels} - (250 \text{ border pixels} \times 2) = 1420 \text{ pixels per EEG page}$$

and

$$\frac{(1420 \text{ pixels / EEG page})}{(15 \text{ sec/ EEG page})} = 95 \text{ pixels per sec}$$

50. **A.** The maximum frequency that can be clearly displayed given the screen resolution and number of seconds of EEG per screen is 47 Hz. In general, the maximum frequency faithfully representable on a pixel display is one-half the number of pixels per second, which is 95 in this case. The maximum resolvable frequency of EEG, in this case, based

on the sampling rate of 1,000 Hz is 500 Hz (Nyquist frequency). However, this question is specifically referring to the maximum frequency of the EEG activity that can be displayed on the screen with the specified parameters. In this case, there are only 95 pixels available to be displayed per second of EEG. Therefore, this could be considered to be equivalent to a sampling rate of 95 Hz. Based on the Nyquist theorem, the maximum resolvable frequency is one-half of the sampling rate or 47.5 Hz. The maximum frequency displayed could be increased by decreasing the number of seconds displayed per page, thus increasing the number of pixels per second. Note that when a signal contains not just one but many different frequencies added together, the minimum sampling rate needed to avoid aliasing is twice the highest frequency present irrespective of how many other frequency components there are.

51. **B.** In the proposed scenario, the maximum resolvable frequency will be 96 Hz. After making the noted adjustments, there will be

$$\frac{(1920 \text{ horizontal pixels / EEG page})}{(10\text{s / EEG page})} = 192 \text{ pixels per sec,}$$

which would correlate to a sampling rate of 192 Hz. Based on the Nyquist theorem, the maximum resolvable frequency is one-half of the sampling rate, or 96 Hz in this case. Although digital EEG recording systems typically have very good resolution and dynamic range, the ability to display the data depends on the screen resolution of the monitors. The displayed resolvable frequency can be increased by increasing the screen resolution or decreasing the number of seconds displayed, both of which would increase the number of pixels per second. Thus, when evaluating for gamma activity or high-frequency oscillations, the number of seconds displayed on the screen is typically around 1 to 2 seconds.

52. **D.** The digital signal can be placed in 2^{10} or 1,024 bins or digitally assignable increments. The number of discrete voltage bins or divisions is determined by the number of bits an analog-to-digital converter (ADC) has, that is, 2^n, where *n* is the number of bits an ADC has.

53. **D.** The magnitude of the voltage step or resolution is equal to the dynamic range (i.e., the range of measurable voltage values) divided by the number of discrete bins (determined by the number of bits the analog-to-digital converter [ADC] has). In this case, the dynamic range is 4 mV (–2 mV to +2 mv), and the number of bins is 1,024. Thus, the voltage resolution is roughly 4 ∝V, which is calculated as follows:

$$4 \text{ mV} / 1024 \text{ bins} = 4000\ \mu\text{V} / 1024 \text{ bins} = 3.9\ \mu\text{V} \sim 4\ \mu\text{V}.$$

54. **C.** In the new scenario, the dynamic range has been reduced from the original −2 mV to +2 mV to the new −1 to +1 mV, that is, by a factor of 2 (from 4 mV to 2 mV). This will increase the voltage resolution by a factor of 2. In other words, the voltage resolution will be higher at 2 mV instead of the original 4 mV. This is calculated as follows:

$$2 \text{ mV} / 1024 \text{ bins} = 2000\ \mu\text{V} / 1024 \text{ bins} = 1.96\ \mu\text{V} \sim 2\ \mu\text{V}.$$

55. **A.** By increasing the bit depth of the ADC, the voltage resolution will increase by a factor of $2^{\Delta n}$, where Δn is the change in the number of bits. In this case, the new resolution will increase by a factor of 2^2 (= 4). So the new resolution will be 1 μV, which is calculated as follows:

$$\text{Original } 2^{10} \text{ bit depth} : 4 \text{ mV} / 1024 \text{ bins} = 4000\ \mu\text{V} / 1024 \text{ bins} = 3.9\ \mu\text{V} \sim 4\ \mu\text{V}$$

$$\text{New } 2^{12} \text{ bit depth} : 4 \text{ mV} / 4096 \text{ bins} = 4000\ \mu\text{V} / 4096 \text{ bins} = 0.97\ \mu\text{V} \sim 1\ \mu\text{V}$$

56. **E.** Electrode pop artifacts can mimic spike or sharp waves or even a calibration signal. They occur due to the changing properties of electrode paste and skin conductance. Sometimes, the pops may occur in a repetitive fashion and may mimic a focal ictal discharge presenting as evolving morphology and frequency. Glossokinetic artifact, produced by tongue movement, resembles frontal delta activity or eye movement. The tongue is electrically charged, with a negative tip and positive base or root. EKG artifact most commonly appears in the ear reference montages. The vector direction of the QRS complex results in both ears, and resulting electrodes A1 and A2, with opposite polarities. Connecting A1 and A2 electrodes will reduce ECG artifact. Pulse artifact on scalp EEG is seen when an electrode is near an artery. The pulse artifact typically lags behind the QRS complex by 200 to 300 ms due to the time required for the pulse wave to travel from the heart to the scalp. Note that pulse artifact is separate from ballistocardiographic artifact which is due to subtle body movements related that occur in conjunction with a systolic pulse wave. These appear as low voltage rhythmic delta activity. The ground electrode is used to eliminate 60 Hz artifact.

57. **E.** The clinical scenario best matches Figure E, which has an abundance of movement artifact, which is produced in this case by the mother patting her baby. Although, the rhythmic EEG changes could be mistaken for cerebral rhythmic delta activity or an ictal discharge, the multiple (double or sometimes triple) phase reversals can support a noncerebral etiology. In addition, the EEG technologist's annotations and viewing the associated video can help to identify certain artifacts.

58. **B.** The clinical scenario best matches Figure B, which has artifact that resembles respirator artifact. The artifact can resemble periodic complexes and can be differentiated from cerebral activity by correlating the complexes with the ventilator settings or the chest movements on the associated video. Of note, high-frequency ventilator artifact can produce diffuse sinusoidal artifact.

59. **D.** The clinical scenario best matches Figure D, which has artifact that resembles diffuse movement/muscle artifact, which in this case is due to shivering. Reviewing the phenomenology on the associated video could help to distinguish movement disorders from epileptic seizures.

60. **A.** The clinical scenario best matches Figure A, which has artifact that resembles glossokinetic artifact. Glossokinetic artifact, produced by tongue movement, resembles frontal delta activity or vertical eye movement, most prominently seen in Fp1 and Fp2. The tongue is electrically charged, with a negative tip and positive base or root. The artifact can be reproduced by asking the patient to say words or sound that have the letter "L."

61. C. The clinical scenario best matches Figure C, which has artifact that resembles pacemaker artifact. The artifact appears as needle-like spikes of variable amplitudes occurring prior to the QRS complex, best seen on the EKG channel. Note that even though a patient may have a paced rhythm, the EEG does not capture all the pacemaker artifacts due to the short duration of the pacer pulse and thus may occur in between time samples.

62. C. Extra-operative invasive EEG monitoring has allowed for increased ability to localize EEG abnormalities. Two techniques used are subdural electrodes and depth electrodes. One approach using depth electrodes is SEEG, which allows for bilateral recording from deep cortical areas as well as noncontiguous lobes. SEEG is based on anatomo-electro-clinical (AEC) correlations of the three-dimensional spatiotemporal organization of the ictal discharge. The anatomo-electrical correlation is dependent on accurate ictal EEG recordings to occur in the epileptogenic zone, thereby allowing for a secondary evaluation of the electro-clinical relationship as the ictal discharge spreads. SEEG has multiple advantages over subdural grid evaluation including avoidance of large craniotomies, reduced surgical morbidity, and broader coverage area. One limitation SEEG has is poor functional mapping. The other answer choices are false.

3

Nerve Conduction Studies and Electromyography

QUESTIONS

1. Compared to concentric electromyography (EMG) needles, monopolar needles have which of the following features?
   A. Smaller motor unit potential amplitude
   B. Increased pain
   C. Increased variability of motor unit potentials
   D. Recording smaller area of muscle
   E. Requires shorter duration to complete needle EMG

2. After a motor vehicle accident, a 40-year-old man develops weakness in the right arm and wrist drop. Evaluation in the emergency department (ED) reveals a fracture near the spiral groove. A radial motor study performed approximately 12 days after the accident reveals normal distal compound muscle action potential (CMAP) amplitude and absent response with stimulation above the spiral groove. These findings are most consistent with
   A. Radial nerve transection at the spiral groove
   B. Radial nerve neuropraxia at the spiral groove
   C. Radial nerve neuropraxia in the forearm from the cast
   D. Radial nerve neurotmesis at the spiral groove
   E. Poor technique leading to absent response on proximal stimulation

ANSWERS TO THIS SECTION CAN BE FOUND ON PAGE 131

The figures in this chapter can be viewed in a larger size by accessing the digital version of this chapter found on Springer Publishing Company Connect™. Refer to the front of this book for access instructions.

3. A 4-month-old boy is admitted to the hospital with weakness, difficulty breathing, and decrease in overall activity level. After an initial evaluation, a neuromuscular disease is suspected. A fast (20 Hz) repetitive stimulation revealed 60% increment. This boy likely has
   A. Congenital myasthenic syndrome
   B. Congenital myopathy
   C. Botulism
   D. Acquired Lambert-Eaton Myasthenic syndrome (LEMS)
   E. Congenital muscular dystrophy

4. Needle electromyography (EMG) in a patient with severe deltoid weakness revealed the following motor unit firing pattern on full activation. What does this finding suggest?

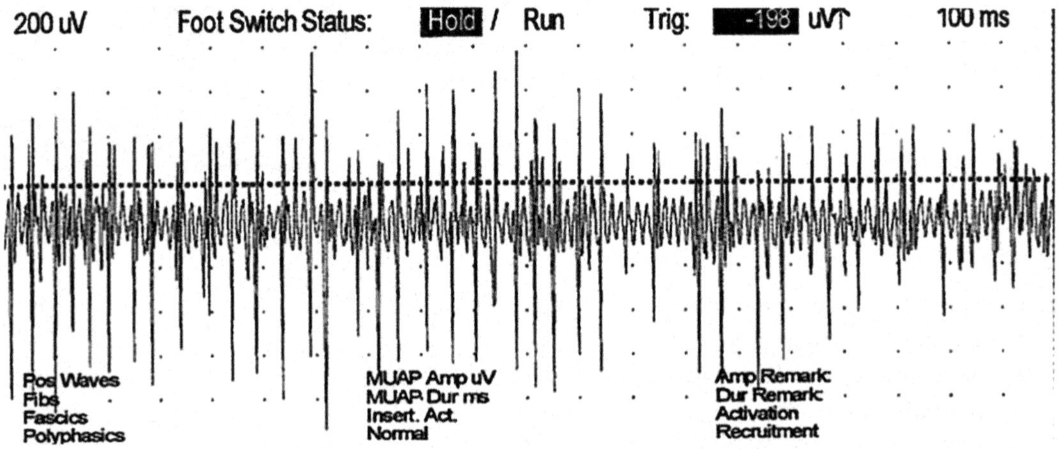

   A. An underlying myopathy
   B. An underlying neuromuscular junction dysfunction
   C. An underlying neurogenic process
   D. No motor unit activity
   E. This is a normal interference pattern

5. A 15-year-old boy presents to his neurologist with slowly worsening gait and weakness that he has had for many years. He underwent a peroneal motor study, as shown below. The findings suggest which of the following conditions?

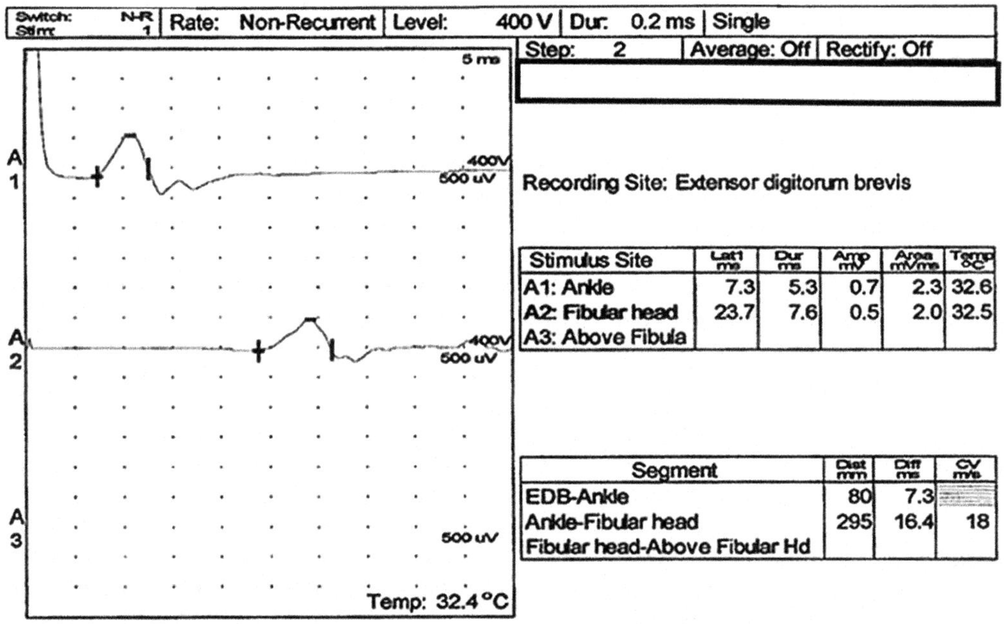

A. Charcot–Marie–Tooth (CMT) type 2A
B. CMT type 1
C. Normal nerve conduction for a 15-year-old
D. Spinal muscular atrophy
E. Distal myopathy

6. A 45-year-old man with type 1 diabetes for more than 15 years is admitted with right thigh pain. His overall glycemic control is poor. He noticed pain and swelling in the right thigh in the last 24 hours. On examination, he is not able to flex or extend his right knee because of severe pain. He also has mild distal weakness and symmetrical sensory loss in his lower limbs. Bilateral ankle reflexes are absent. Which of the following is the ideal initial diagnostic test?
   A. MRI of the right thigh
   B. MRI lumbar spine and lumbosacral plexus
   C. Nerve conduction study (NCS) and electromyography (EMG) study
   D. Muscle biopsy
   E. Spinal fluid analysis for elevated protein

7. Which of the following situations may lead to higher peroneal motor amplitude with stimulation at the fibular neck compared to ankle stimulation?
   A. Excessive stimulation at the fibular head
   B. Submaximal stimulation at the ankle
   C. Accessory peroneal nerve innervation
   D. All of the above
   E. None the above

8. All of the following are considered risk factors for developing acute quadriplegic myopathy in an ICU setting *except*

A. Liver transplant
B. Hemodialysis for end-stage renal disease
C. Prolonged high-dose oral corticosteroid therapy
D. High-dose intravenous (IV) corticosteroid therapy
E. Sedation with opiates

9. In an isolated posterior cord brachial plexopathy with associated weakness and sensory loss, which of the following abnormalities on deep tendon reflex testing is seen?

A. Absent triceps reflex only
B. Absent biceps and triceps reflexes
C. Absent biceps, brachioradialis, and triceps reflexes
D. Absent triceps and brachioradialis reflexes with normal biceps reflex
E. Normal deep tendon reflexes

10. On needle electromyography (EMG) of certain muscles, it is theoretically possible to injure the adjacent nerves. Among the options below, performing EMG of which muscle is *not* likely to injure the paired nerve?

A. Flexor pollicis longus and superficial radial nerve
B. Pronator teres and median nerve
C. First dorsal interosseous and ulnar nerve
D. Gluteus maximus and sciatic nerve
E. Iliopsoas and femoral nerve

11. Which of the following is the most sensitive test to detect myasthenia gravis (MG)?

A. Acetylcholine receptor (AChR) antibody titer
B. Repetitive stimulation of facial or spinal accessory nerves
C. Icepack test
D. Single-fiber electromyography (SFEMG) of the distal muscle in upper limbs
E. SFEMG of frontalis

12. A 55-year-old man noticed right leg weakness for a few weeks. On examination, he has weakness of his right toe extension and sensory loss on the dorsum of the foot. A peroneal motor study with recording from tibialis anterior is shown below. Which of the following is most likely to be the underlying etiology?

Switch: N-R Stim: 1	Rate:Non-Recurrent	Level: 400 V	Dur: 0.1 ms	Single

Step: 2	Average: Off	Rectify: Off

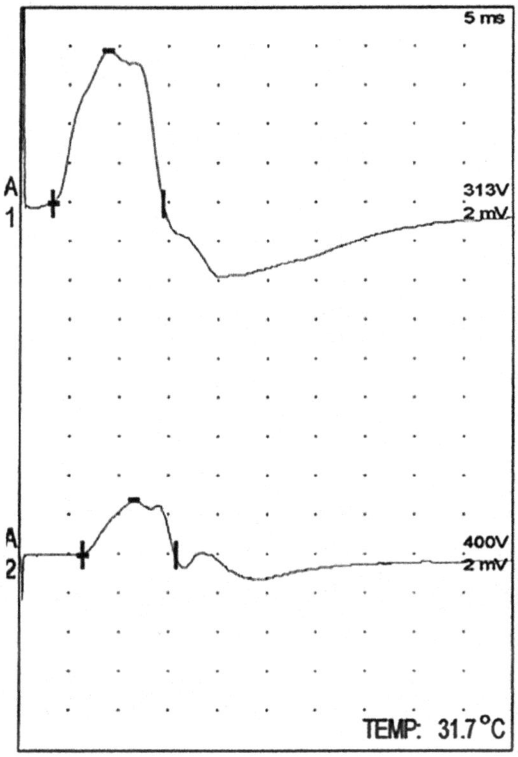

Recording Site : Tib. Ant.

Stimulus Site	Lat1 ms	Dur ms	Amp mV	Area mVms	Temp °C
A1: Fibular Hd.	3.2	11.2	7.8	57.8	31.8
A2: Popliteal fossa	6.3	9.4	2.8	16.8	31.8

Segment	Dist mm	Diff ms	CV m/s	Temp °C
Tib. Ant.-Fibular Hd.		3.2		31.8
Fibular Hd.-Popliteal fossa	95	3.1	31	31.8

A. Recent significant weight loss
B. Traumatic ankle fracture
C. Recent lumbosacral spine injury
D. Recent significant weight gain
E. Recent fracture of tibia

13. Which of the following features is highly suggestive of an acquired demyelinating polyneuropathy?
A. Prolonged distal latency
B. Severely reduced conduction velocity
C. Abnormal temporal dispersion
D. Severely reduced motor or sensory amplitude
E. Reduced recruitment patterns on needle electromyography (EMG)

14. A forearm exercise test was performed in a 25-year-old woman with fatigue and weakness. During the test, neither ammonia nor lactate levels are increased. This finding is compatible with which of the following?
A. Myophosphorylase deficiency
B. Phosphofructokinase deficiency
C. Myoadenylate deaminase deficiency
D. Insufficient effort from the patient
E. All of the above

15. A 30-year-old is suspected to have brachial plexus injury after trauma. He has weakness and sensory loss in the hands. Routine nerve conduction studies revealed mildly reduced median and ulnar motor amplitudes. The resident doing the procedure is unsure if F-wave studies of the median and ulnar nerve would be helpful. What is the correct response?
A. Median and ulnar F-wave responses will not help with localization in this case
B. F-wave responses will almost certainly be normal in this case
C. F-wave responses may help with localization in this case
D. F-wave responses are not useful because the amplitudes were mildly decreased
E. F-wave responses should be done in patients with trauma

16. While performing a nerve conduction study, the neurology resident notices that there is an initial positive deflection on a motor nerve study. He would like to repeat the study to eliminate the initial positive deflection. Which of the following is the best suggestion for him?
A. Move the G1 electrode to the belly of the recording muscle
B. Move the G2 electrode to increase the distance between the G1 and G2 electrodes
C. Move the stimulating electrode to increase the distance between the stimulating and G1 electrode
D. It is common to have an initial positive deflection in motor studies, so there is no need to repeat the study
E. If initial positive deflection is seen with proximal stimulation, then this can be ignored

17. In patients with neurogenic thoracic outlet syndrome, which of the following patterns of weakness and sensory loss is commonly seen?
A. Deltoid weakness and loss of sensation over the lateral aspect of shoulder
B. Finger extensor weakness and loss of sensation over the dorsum of the hand
C. First dorsal interosseous weakness and loss of sensation over the fifth digit
D. Abductor pollicis brevis muscle weakness and loss of sensation over the lateral forearm
E. Bicep weakness with sensory loss over the lateral aspect of forearm

18. Which electrodiagnostic feature on needle electromyography (EMG) is only seen in chronic neurogenic processes?
A. Reduced recruitment
B. Motor unit potentials with large duration and amplitude
C. Fasciculation potentials
D. Positive sharp waves
E. Fibrillation potentials

19. A 70-year-old man with multiple chronic comorbidities has been in the ICU for a few weeks for pneumonia and multiorgan failure. He required several weeks of sedation. After recovery from multiorgan failure, he was noted to have severe weakness in all his limbs. Which of the following techniques/studies may help differentiate critical illness neuropathy from critical illness myopathy?

A. Normal sensory responses
B. Motor unit morphology
C. Recruitment patterns on needle electromyography (EMG)
D. Direct muscle stimulation
E. All of the above

20. A very well-built 40-year-old guitar player presents with muscle stiffness that he has had most of his life, and also weakness in cold weather. On examination, he does not have any limb weakness. A routine electromyography (EMG) revealed repetitive discharges that wax and wane in frequency and amplitude. What does this patient most likely have?

A. Periodic paralysis
B. Myotonic dystrophy type I
C. Myotonic dystrophy type II
D. Myotonia congenita
E. Pompe disease

21. Which of the following findings is most likely to be abnormal in a patient with mild or early length-dependent axonal polyneuropathy?

A. Peroneal motor amplitude
B. Tibial motor amplitude
C. Peroneal F-wave response
D. Sural sensory response
E. Tibial F-wave response

22. Which of the following statements is *not* true about amyloid myopathy?

A. It is commonly seen in cases of secondary amyloidosis
B. It may cause hypertrophy of muscles
C. Peripheral neuropathy is seen in greater than 20% of cases
D. It is commonly seen with primary or hereditary amyloidosis
E. Needle electromyography (EMG) reveals myopathic changes

23. Calculation of the negative peak duration and area on the proximal and distal compound muscle action potential (CMAP) are most useful in assessing which of the following electrodiagnostic measures on motor nerve conduction studies?

A. Conduction velocity
B. Latency
C. Temporal dispersion
D. Stimulus intensity
E. Stimulus duration

24. A 65-year-old man has a history of difficulty walking for about a year. He recently noticed a tendency to drop objects. On examination, he was found to have weakness in both lower limbs, predominantly in his quadriceps muscles, along with weakness of finger flexion, which is worse on the left side. He had no significant sensory loss. Which of the following would most likely be found on needle electromyography (EMG)?

A. Short-duration, small-amplitude motor units with early recruitment
B. Long-duration, large-amplitude motor units with early recruitment
C. Long-duration, large-amplitude motor units with reduced recruitment
D. Normal EMG because his clinical presentation is consistent with an upper motor neuron disease
E. Only positive sharp waves and fibrillation in the weak muscles, but normal motor unit morphology

25. The low-frequency filter setting should be set at 0.5 Hz while performing which of the following tests?

A. Slow repetitive stimulation at 3 Hz
B. Fast repetitive stimulation at 50 Hz
C. Sympathetic skin response
D. Blink or facial studies
E. H-reflex studies

26. A 60-year-old man had extensive lumbar spine surgery for back pain and has a spinal stimulator. He recently complained of increasing weakness in his thoracic area. Needle electromyography (EMG) of the thoracic paraspinal muscles revealed the following spontaneous activity. What does this activity suggest?

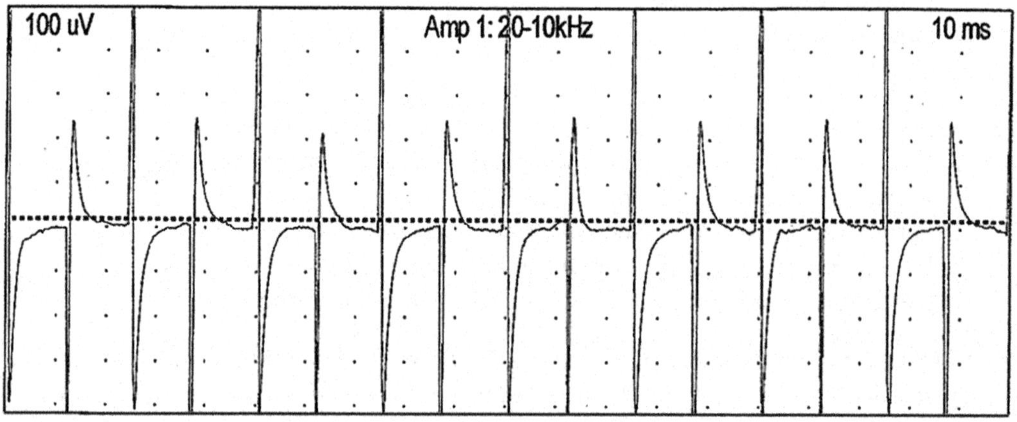

A. Regularly firing fibrillation potential
B. Fast-firing motor unit potential
C. Electrical artifact
D. Regularly firing positive sharp wave potentials
E. Myokymia

27. A 60-year-old man with weakness undergoes an ulnar motor study at baseline and after 15 seconds of exercise as shown below. What does it show?

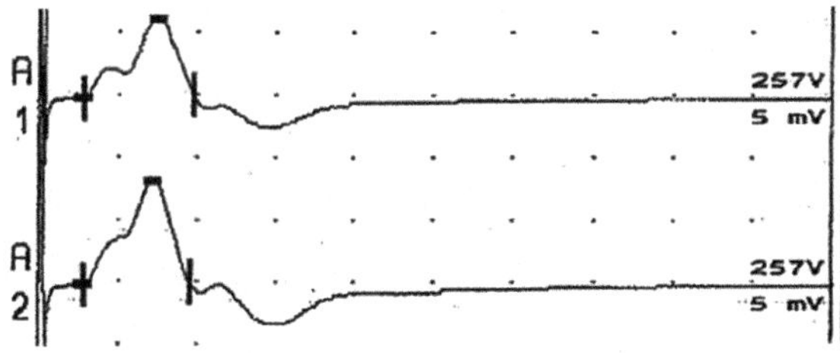

Recording Site : ADQ

STIMULUS SITE	LAT 1 ms	DUR ms	AMP mV	AREA mVms
A1: Wrist	2.7	7.0	6.458	22.13
A2: Wrist 15 s	2.7	6.8	8.476	28.39

A. Low compound muscle action potential (CMAP) amplitude at baseline and significant increment
B. Low-CMAP amplitude at baseline and nonsignificant increment
C. Normal CMAP amplitude at baseline and significant increment
D. Normal CMAP amplitude at baseline and nonsignificant increment
E. Normal CMAP amplitude at baseline and nonsignificant decrement

28. A median motor study from a 40-year-old man with painless weakness is shown below. This is most consistent with which of the following conditions?

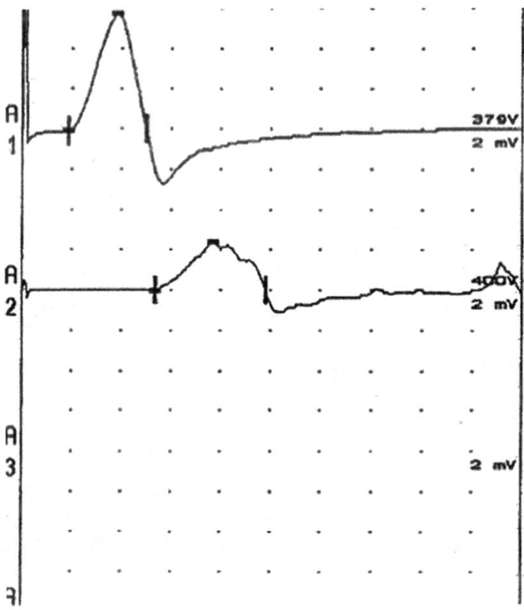

Exam.

Recording Site : APB

STIMULUS SITE	LAT 1 ms	AMP mV	AREA mVms	TEMP °C
A1: Wrist	4.6	5.906	24.15	34.8
A2: Elbow	13.3	2.396	14.81	34.8
A3: Axilla				
A4:				

SEGMENT	DIST mm	DIFF ms	CV m/s	CVco m/s
Wrist-Elbow	255	8.7	29	24

A. Amyotrophic lateral sclerosis
B. Multifocal motor neuropathy
C. Monomelic amyotrophy
D. Spinobulbar muscular atrophy (SBMA)
E. Neurogenic thoracic outlet syndrome

29. Which of the following findings on a nerve conduction study favors a diagnosis of acquired diffuse demyelinating polyneuropathy?

A. Reduced compound muscle action potential amplitude
B. Severely decreased conduction velocity
C. Severely prolonged distal latency
D. Abnormal temporal dispersion
E. Absent or prolonged F-wave

30. Motor nerve conduction study of the right radial nerve is shown below. What does this study show?

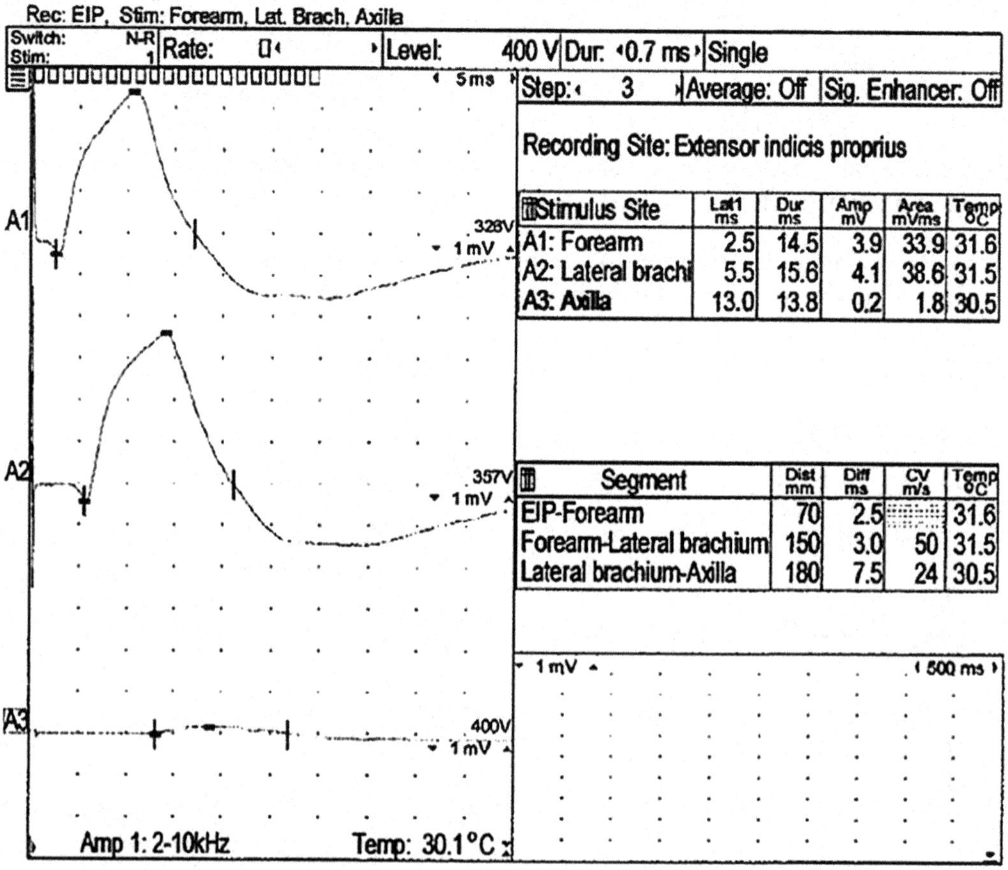

A. Severe diffuse distal demyelinating process
B. Conduction block in the arm
C. Severe temporal dispersion in the arm
D. Normal study
E. Submaximal distal stimulation

31. A 24-year-old administrator with hypothyroidism has noticed numbness in her hands. She frequently wakes up at night with tingling in her fingers and hands. Her primary care physician diagnosed her with carpal tunnel syndrome (CTS) and referred her for electrodiagnostic studies. Her median and ulnar motor studies were normal. Her median and ulnar antidromic sensory studies with recording from second and fifth digits were normal. Which of the following is the best step to find evidence of CTS in this patient?
A. Perform median and ulnar mixed palmar studies
B. Measure median and ulnar digit 4 sensory latencies
C. Median nerve study with inching across the wrist
D. Measure median and radial digit 1 sensory latencies
E. Any of the above

32. A patient is referred to the neuromuscular clinic for evaluation of brachial plexopathy. On examination, he was noted to have weakness in the deltoid and triceps; however, the pronator teres muscle and biceps brachii muscle strength was normal. Presuming that the pathology is in the brachial plexus, these findings are best localizable to which of the following structures?
A. Medial cord
B. Lateral cord
C. Posterior cord
D. C5–C6 roots
E. Upper trunk

33. Needle electromyography (EMG) of which of the following muscles can differentiate a medial cord brachial plexopathy from lower trunk brachial plexopathy?
A. First dorsal interosseous
B. Abductor pollicis brevis
C. Extensor indicis proprius
D. Flexor carpi ulnaris
E. Abductor digiti minimi

34. A 50-year-old man is admitted to the ICU with an unclear neurological disorder. He is sedated with propofol for severe agitation and is on ventilatory support. Electrodiagnostic study showed normal motor and sensory responses but absent F-wave responses. Which of the following is the most appropriate conclusion based on the available information?
A. He has Guillain–Barré syndrome (GBS) with agitation and needs spinal fluid analysis
B. Absent F-wave responses can be due to sedation with propofol
C. He will need somatosensory evoked potential (SSEP) studies to rule out peripheral nerve processes
D. Without repetitive nerve stimulation, it is not possible to come to a definitive conclusion
E. F-wave responses are always difficult to obtain in ICU setting because of other electrical noise

35. The waveforms shown below were acquired by repetitive nerve stimulation in the same patient at baseline (top) and immediately after exercise (bottom). The results are consistent with which of the following phenomena?

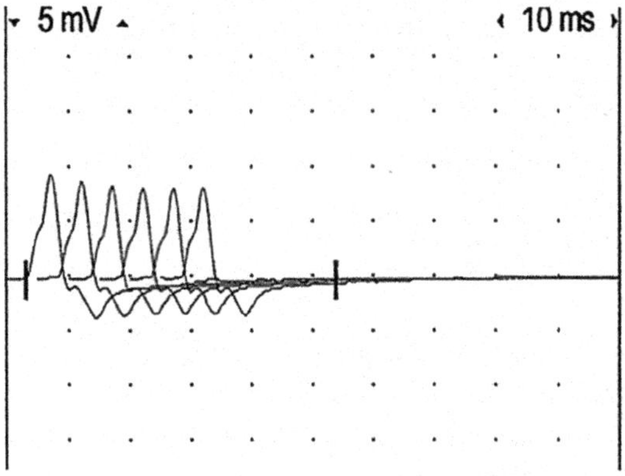

Stim Freq:	3 Hz	No. in Train:	6
Stim Dur:	0.1 ms	Stim Rjct:	0.5 ms
Stim Site: Wrist			
Time:	10:40:38		
Comment: baseline			

Pot No.	Peak Amp mV	Amp Decr %	Area mVms	Area Decr %	Stim Level
1	9.70	0	70.80	0	400V
2	8.99	7	65.40	8	400V
3	8.54	12	62.20	12	400V
4	8.41	13	60.70	14	400V
5	8.41	13	60.40	15	400V
6	8.51	12	62.00	12	400V

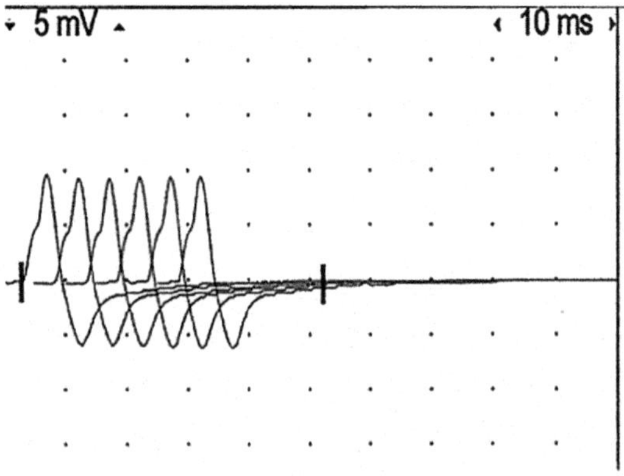

Foot Switch: Ready / Stimulate / Stop
Stim Mode: Train / Single

Stim Freq:	3 Hz	No. in Train:	6
Stim Dur:	0.1 ms	Stim Rjct:	0.5 ms
Stim Site: Wrist			
Time:	10:41:42	Stop Watch:	0:37
Comment: Imm after exer			

Pot No.	Peak Amp mV	Amp Decr %	Area mVms	Area Decr %	Stim Level
1	9.97	0	77.30	0	400V
2	9.83	1	74.30	4	400V
3	9.73	2	79.70	-3	400V
4	9.76	2	78.60	-2	400V
5	9.81	2	78.90	-2	400V
6	9.85	1	78.60	-2	400V

A. Facilitation but not repair
B. Repair but not facilitation
C. Both repair and facilitation
D. Neither repair nor facilitation
E. This is a fast repetitive stimulation, and so these phenomena cannot be assessed

36. A 45-year-old man with suspected myasthenia gravis had a 3-Hz repetitive stimulation (slow repetitive stimulation) of the left ulnar nerve with abductor digiti minimi (ADM) recording, which was normal. The next most appropriate step for evaluation of neuromuscular junction dysfunction would include:
A. Use a higher rate of stimulation such as 20 or 50 Hz
B. Make sure the limb is not cold, and warm the limb by 3°C to 4°C if needed
C. Administer pyridostigmine and repeat the test
D. Use a higher amplifier gain during the study
E. Administer Tensilon (edrophonium) and repeat the test

37. A median palmar mixed sensory study is shown below. Which part of the waveform is considered a far-field potential?

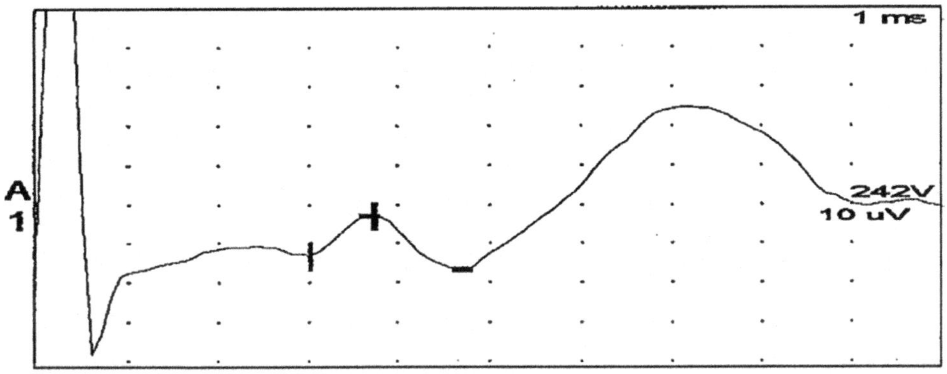

A. Stimulus artifact
B. Sensory response
C. Motor response
D. Only the sensory latency
E. Only the motor latency

38. A 60-year-old man presents with chronic history of difficulty walking and tendency to fall. On examination, he has mild distal weakness in the lower limbs, severe sensory loss in the lower limbs, and severe sensory ataxia. A motor nerve conduction study obtained from the right peroneal nerve with extensor digitorum brevis recording is shown below. Which of the following statements is true about this study?

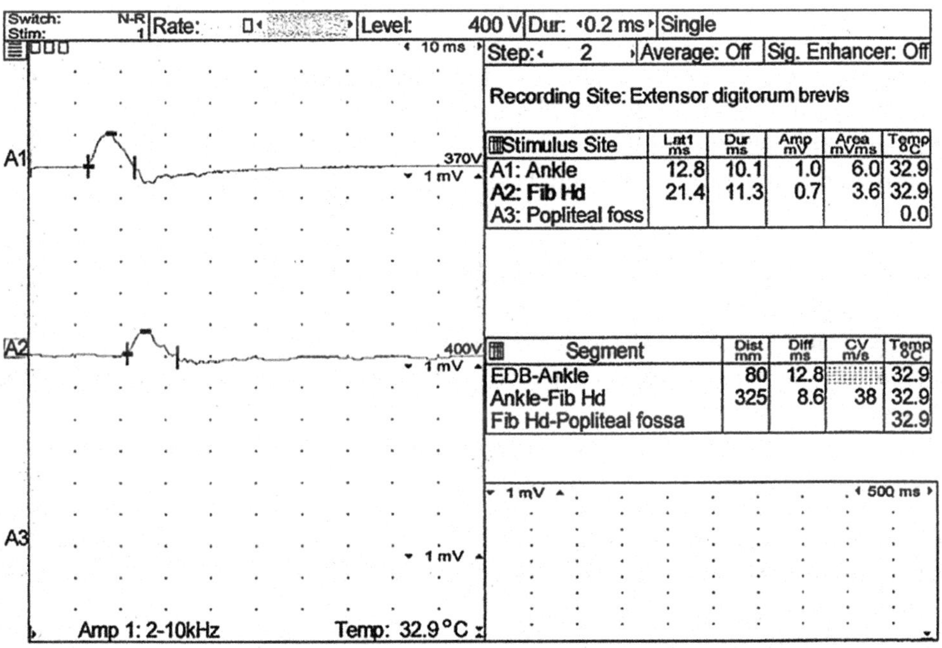

A. It suggests acquired demyelinating polyneuropathy
B. It suggests axonal polyneuropathy
C. It is a normal peroneal motor study for age
D. Because this is a motor study, it is not relevant to the severe sensory ataxia
E. Without needle electromyography (EMG), one should not interpret a motor nerve conduction study

39. Which of the following potentials on needle electromyography (EMG) has an irregular firing pattern?
A. Complex repetitive discharges
B. Positive sharp waves
C. Fibrillation potentials
D. Fasciculation potentials
E. Myokymic discharges

40. Short-duration motor unit potentials may be seen in all of the following conditions *except:*
A. Polymyositis
B. Lambert–Eaton myasthenic syndrome (LEMS)
C. During early reinnervation after severe denervation
D. Amyotrophic lateral sclerosis (ALS)
E. Critical illness myopathy

41. A 30-year-old South Asian man presented to the electrodiagnostic lab with slowly progressive weakness in the right hand over 18 months. He denies any sensory loss or pain. On examination, he has weakness in the right hand finger abductors, extensors, and flexors. Nerve conduction studies and electromyography (EMG) will likely reveal:
A. Decreased median and ulnar sensory amplitudes
B. Long-duration motor unit potentials with reduced recruitment patterns
C. More than 100% increment after 15-second exercise
D. Absent sural sensory response
E. Short-duration motor unit potentials with early recruitment patterns

42. Which of the following is true on a median motor study in patients with Martin–Gruber anastomosis (MGA) and carpal tunnel syndrome (CTS)?
A. Delayed distal latency only
B. Delayed distal latency and spuriously increased conduction velocity
C. Delayed distal latency, spuriously increased conduction velocity, and positive dip on proximal stimulation
D. MGA corrects for carpal tunnel compression, and so the median motor study is normal
E. Normal median sensory responses

43. Low compound muscle action potential (CMAP) amplitudes are seen in all of the following conditions *except:*
A. Adult-onset acid maltase deficiency
B. Severe critical illness myopathy
C. Lambert–Eaton myasthenic syndrome (LEMS)
D. During an episode of periodic paralysis
E. Hereditary distal myopathy

44. Which of the following features of the motor unit potential should be taken into consideration before analyzing individual motor units?
A. Duration of motor unit potential
B. Rise time
C. Number of phases or turns
D. Amplitude of motor unit potential
E. Number of motor unit potentials seen in one epoch

45. Which of the following studies can help differentiate a cervical root avulsion from brachial plexopathy?
A. Motor nerve amplitudes in upper limb
B. F-wave reflex testing in upper limb
C. Somatosensory evoked potential (SSEP) testing from the upper limb
D. Sensory nerve conduction study
E. Motor nerve conduction velocities in upper limb

46. Which of the following enzyme defects leading to a glycogen storage disorder (GSD) is not associated with neuromuscular manifestations?
A. Acid alpha-glucosidase deficiency
B. Beta enolase deficiency
C. Glucose 6-phosphate deficiency
D. Aldolase deficiency
E. None of the above

47. A 23-year-old woman presents to her neurologist with severe fatigue, generalized weakness, and occasional eye droop. To rule out myasthenia gravis (MG), repetitive stimulation of the spinal accessory nerve is done. The results of repetitive stimulation 2 minutes after exercise are shown below. What does it show?

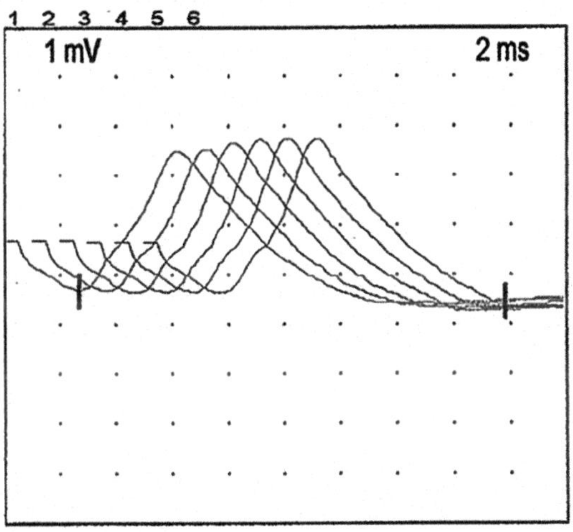

Foot Switch: Ready / Stimulate / Stop
Stim.Mode: Train / Single

Stim Freq: 3 Hz | No. in Train: 6
Stim Dur: 0.1 ms | Stim Rjct: 0.5 ms
Stim Site: Postauricular
Time: 08:08:50 | Stop Watch: 0:14
Comment:2 min post ex

Pot No.	P-P Amp mV	Amp. Decr %	Area mVms	Area Decr %	Stim. Level
1	3.12	0	12.60	0	178V
2	3.21	-3	12.60	0	178V
3	3.36	-8	13.10	-4	178V
4	3.48	-12	13.50	-7	178V
5	3.48	-12	13.40	-6	178V
6	3.46	-11	13.40	-6	178V

A. Significant decrement in compound muscle action potential (CMAP) amplitude
B. Mild increment in CMAP amplitude, which is normal
C. No change in CMAP amplitude
D. Repair suggestive of neuromuscular junction dysfunction
E. Patient unable to tolerate the study with poor baseline

48. The two waveforms below are from iliopsoas muscle during spontaneous activity recordings with different sweep speeds. What do these findings suggest?

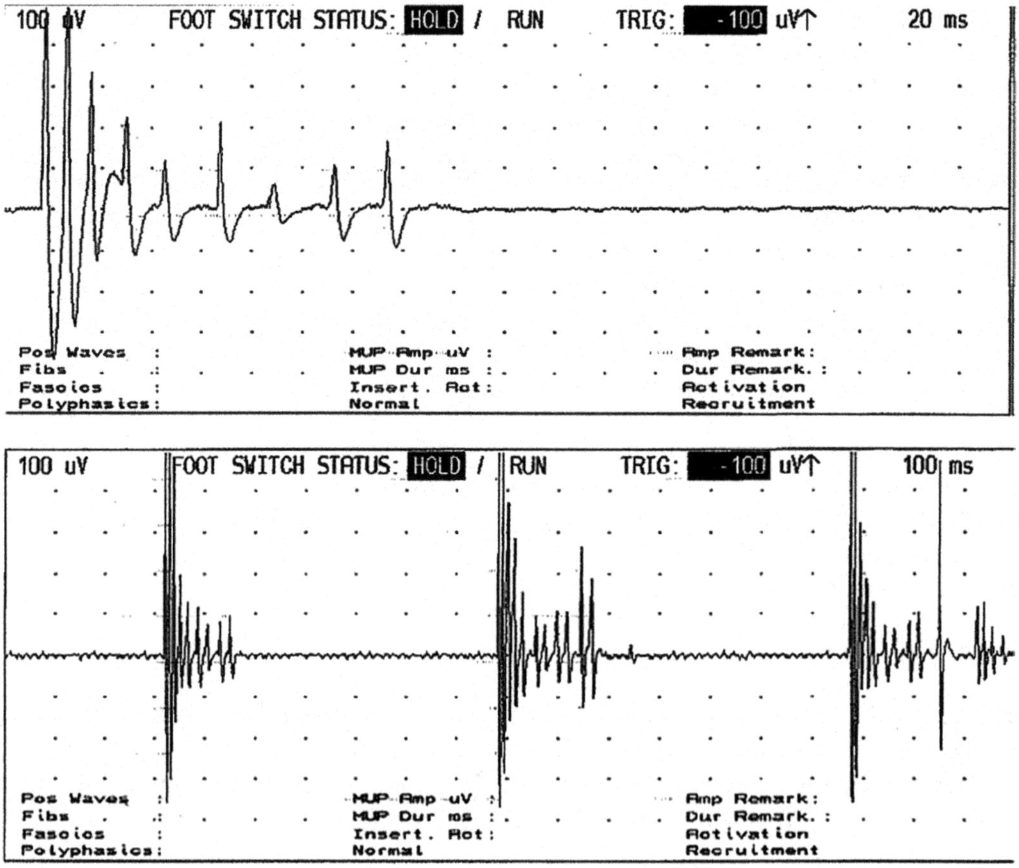

A. Fasciculation potentials
B. Fibrillation potentials
C. Tremor
D. Myokymia
E. Complex repetitive discharges

49. A 50-year-old man developed double vision and difficulty walking over 3 days. Initial examination in the emergency department (ED) revealed decreased eye movements. Strength in limbs was relatively preserved, all deep tendon reflexes were absent, and his gait was ataxic. What would the motor nerve conduction study in this patient likely reveal?

A. Normal motor amplitude and conduction velocity
B. Conduction block
C. Severely reduced motor amplitudes
D. Normal motor amplitudes but severely reduced conduction velocity
E. Prolonged distal latencies only

50. A 50-year-old woman noticed increasing tiredness and muscle pain over the last few months. On examination, she has symmetrical proximal limb weakness. On routine testing, she was noted to have elevated alanine aminotransferase (ALT) and aspartate aminotransferase (AST; five times above upper limit of normal). Which of the following is an appropriate next test in this patient?

A. Liver biopsy
B. Creatine phosphokinase (CPK) level and needle electromyography (EMG)
C. Muscle biopsy
D. Whole genome sequencing
E. Routine nerve conduction testing only

51. In the nerve conduction study shown below, which of the following statements is true regarding the change in stimulus intensity?

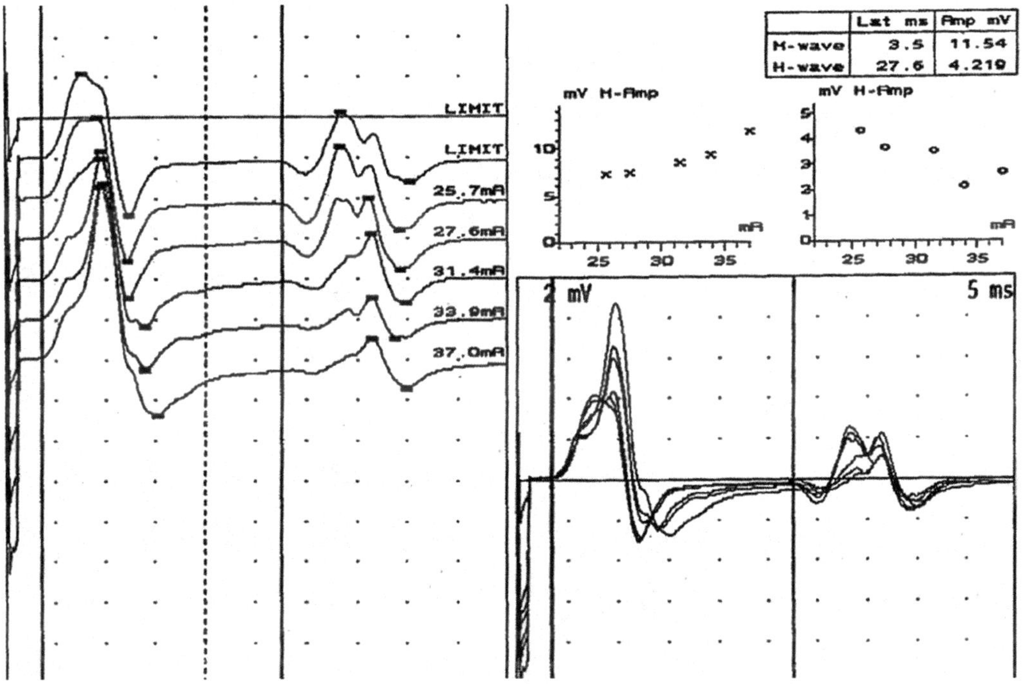

A. Fixed supramaximal stimulus
B. Fixed submaximal stimulus
C. Increasing submaximal stimulus
D. Decreasing supramaximal stimulus
E. Variable stimulus intensity to distract patient

52. The following waveforms show ulnar slow repetitive stimulation in a patient with suspected myasthenia gravis at baseline and after 1 minute of exercise. What is the best interpretation of this data?

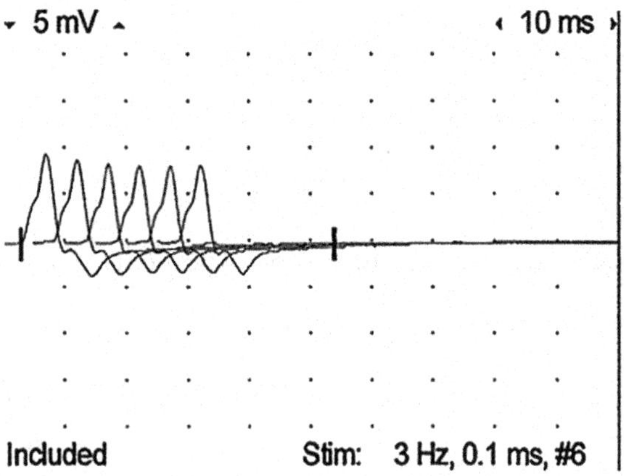

Stim Freq:	3 Hz	No. in Train:	6
Stim Dur:	0.1 ms	Stim Rjct:	0.5 ms
Stim Site: Wrist			
Time:	10:40:38		
Comment: baseline			

Pot No.	Peak Amp mV	Amp Decr %	Area mVms	Area Decr %	Stim Level
1	9.70	0	70.80	0	400V
2	8.99	7	65.40	8	400V
3	8.54	12	62.20	12	400V
4	8.41	13	60.70	14	400V
5	8.41	13	60.40	15	400V
6	8.51	12	62.00	12	400V

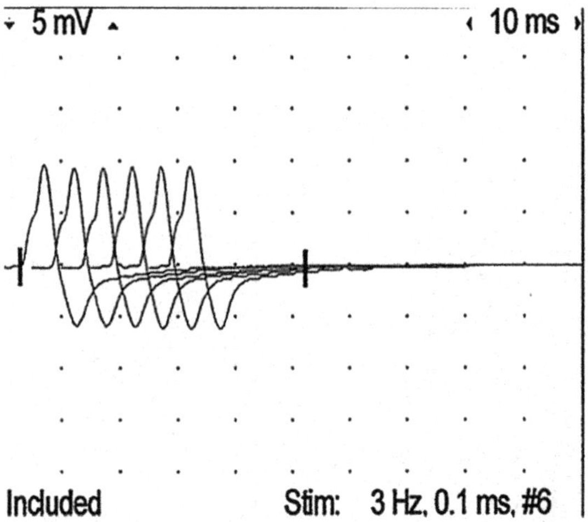

Foot Switch: Ready / Stimulate / Stop
Stim Mode: Train / Single

Stim Freq:	3 Hz	No. in Train:	6
Stim Dur:	0.1 ms	Stim Rjct:	0.5 ms
Stim Site: Wrist			
Time:	10:41:42	Stop Watch:	0:37
Comment: Imm after exer			

Pot No.	Peak Amp mV	Amp Decr %	Area mVms	Area Decr %	Stim Level
1	9.97	0	77.30	0	400V
2	9.83	1	74.30	4	400V
3	9.73	2	79.70	-3	400V
4	9.76	2	78.60	-2	400V
5	9.81	2	78.90	-2	400V
6	9.85	1	78.60	-2	400V

A. Repair of decrement
B. Both repair and facilitation
C. Only facilitation
D. This is a normal study
E. Normal study at baseline, but abnormal after exercise.

53. In the figure below, what is the firing rate of the most prominent motor unit potential?

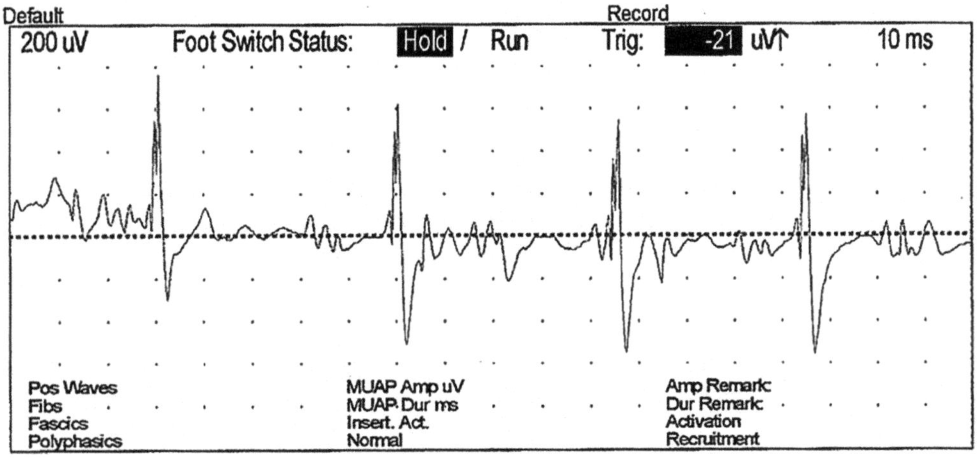

A. 20 Hz
B. 5 Hz
C. 50 Hz
D. 15 Hz
E. 4 Hz

54. A 40-year-old cyclist noticed recent onset sensory symptoms in his right hand. On examination, he has sensory loss in the right fifth digit but no weakness. His nerve conduction study is shown below. What is the most likely interpretation based on the clinical and nerve conduction data?

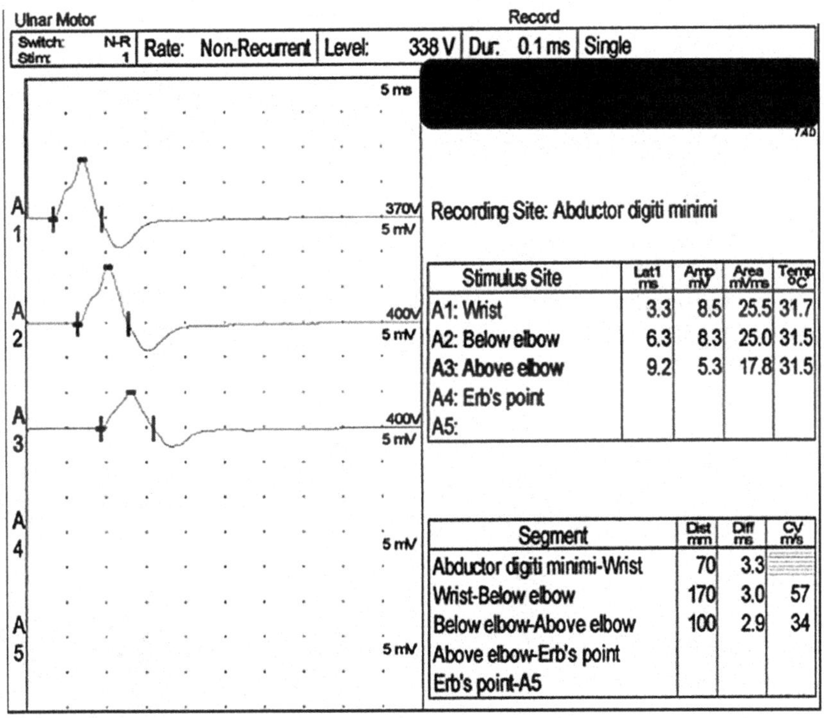

Stimulus Site	Lat1 ms	Amp mV	Area mVms	Temp °C
A1: Wrist	3.3	8.5	25.5	31.7
A2: Below elbow	6.3	8.3	25.0	31.5
A3: Above elbow	9.2	5.3	17.8	31.5
A4: Erb's point				
A5:				

Segment	Dist mm	Diff ms	CV m/s
Abductor digiti minimi-Wrist	70	3.3	
Wrist-Below elbow	170	3.0	57
Below elbow-Above elbow	100	2.9	34
Above elbow-Erb's point			
Erb's point-A5			

A. Ulnar neuropathy at the wrist
B. Ulnar neuropathy at the elbow
C. Medial cord or lower trunk plexopathy
D. Ulnar neuropathy in the forearm
E. Ulnar neuropathy in the palm

55. The blink reflex study shown below was performed in a patient with facial symptoms. Ipsilateral stimulation is shown in the left panel; contralateral stimulation is shown in the right panel; the top four traces are obtained after right-sided stimulation; the bottom four traces are obtained after left-sided stimulation. What does it suggest?

Stim Side	Ipsi R1-Lat ms	Ipsi R2-Lat ms	Contra R2-Lat ms	Diff R2-Lat ms
Right			42.0	
Left	10.8	32.2		

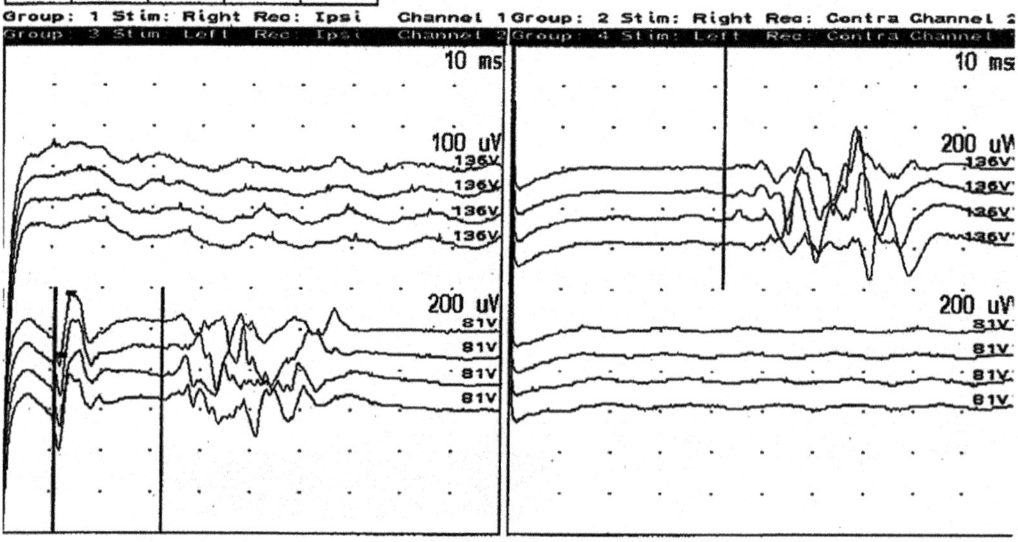

A. Right trigeminal neuropathy
B. Right facial neuropathy
C. Left trigeminal neuropathy
D. Right trigeminal neuropathy
E. Technically limited study as patient failed to relax right facial muscles

56. In a 25-year-old woman with hand numbness, a median antidromic sensory study was performed with stimulation at the wrist and then at the elbow as shown below. What does this study reveal?

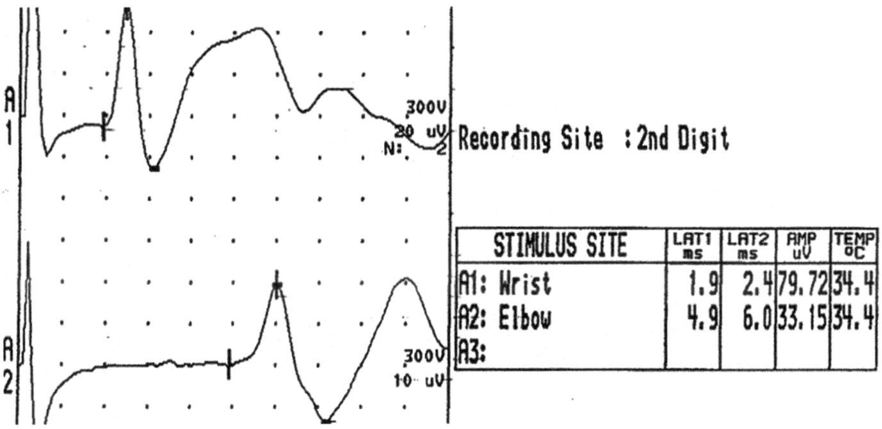

STIMULUS SITE	LAT1 ms	LAT2 ms	AMP uV	TEMP oC
A1: Wrist	1.9	2.4	79.72	34.4
A2: Elbow	4.9	6.0	33.15	34.4
A3:				

A. Conduction block in the forearm
B. Abnormal temporal dispersion in the forearm
C. Normal median sensory study
D. Carpal tunnel syndrome
E. Incorrect interpretation as latency and amplitude findings are from motor responses

57. With sciatic nerve compression, which of the following findings is relatively likely on electrodiagnostic testing?
A. Absent tibial response but normal peroneal and sural responses
B. Significantly decreased peroneal amplitude compared to tibial amplitude
C. Absent tibial and peroneal responses with preserved sural response
D. Normal tibial H-reflex
E. Decreased peroneal motor amplitude but normal peroneal F-wave responses

58. The conduction velocity of an action potential is *least* likely to be affected by which of the following?
A. Axon diameter
B. Axon temperature
C. Distance between nodes of Ranvier
D. Number of surrounding axons
E. Extent of myelination

59. A tibial motor study with abductor hallucis recording from a 45-year-old man with difficulty walking is shown below. A1 represents stimulation at the ankle and A2 represents stimulation at the popliteal fossa. The distance between the ankle and popliteal fossa stimulation is 40 cm. Sweep speed is 5 ms per division and gain is set at 5 mV. Which combination of the following latency, amplitude, and conduction velocity measurements is correct?

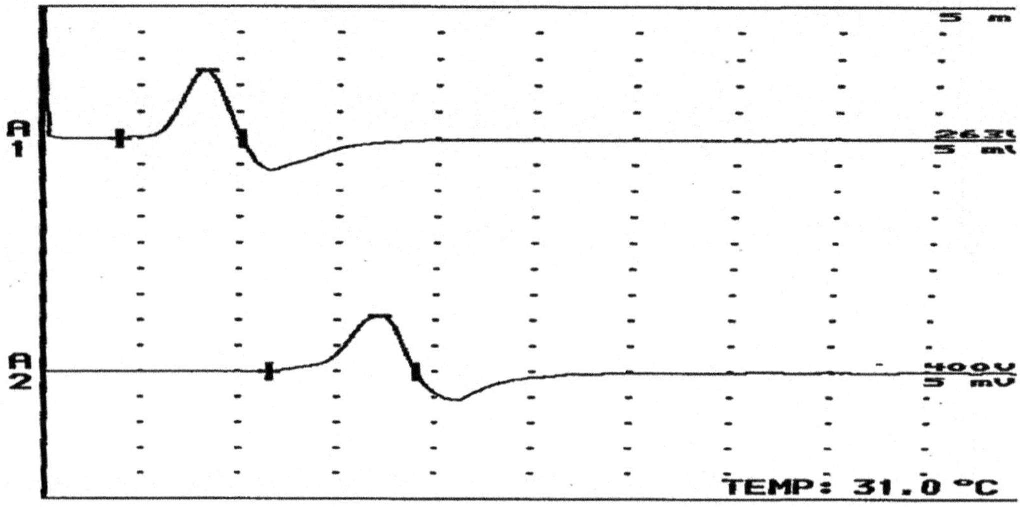

	Distal latency (ms)	Distal amplitude (mV)	Approximate conduction velocity (m/sec)
A	4	10	40
B	4	12	50
C	2	24	60
D	12	15	20
E	8	24	50

60. The normal recruitment frequencies in a limb and cranial muscle are

A. Around 16 Hz for cranial muscle and 7 to 10 Hz for limb muscle
B. Around 16 Hz for limb muscle and 7 to 10 Hz for cranial muscle
C. Around 25 Hz for cranial muscle and 50 Hz for limb muscle
D. Around 50 Hz for cranial muscle and 2 Hz for limb muscle
E. Around 5 Hz for cranial muscle and 10 Hz for limb muscle

61. A 35-year-old man noticed weakness in his right hand for the last few months and then recently developed painless left leg weakness with foot drop. He denies any pain in his limbs or sensory loss. His median motor study is shown below. Based on this nerve conduction study finding, what is the most likely diagnosis?

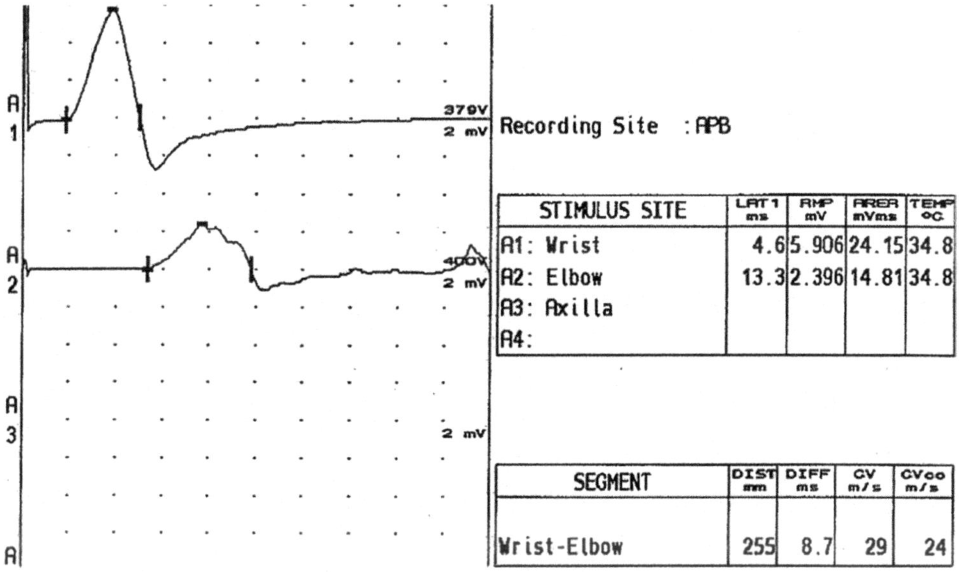

A. Carpal tunnel syndrome (CTS)
B. Multifocal motor neuropathy
C. Lower trunk brachial plexopathy
D. Hirayama's monomelic amyotrophy
E. Charcot–Marie–Tooth (CMT) with late manifestations

62. Nerve conduction and electromyography (EMG) studies are appropriate initial diagnostic procedures in all of the following conditions *except:*
A. A 5-year-old boy with high creatine phosphokinase (CPK), enlarged calf muscles, and positive Gower's sign
B. A 12-year-old boy with fatigue, weakness, and ptosis
C. A 15-year-old girl with slowly progressive distal weakness, atrophy, and sensory loss
D. A 22-year-old man with subacute onset of lower extremity numbness and weakness
E. A 65-year-old man with progressive painless weakness in multiple limbs

63. A forearm exercise test was performed in a man with suspected metabolic myopathy. Both ammonia and lactate levels were measured at regular intervals during the forearm exercise test. If the lactate level is elevated but not the ammonia level, it is suggestive of:
A. Myophosphorylase deficiency
B. Phosphofructokinase deficiency
C. Myoadenylate deaminase deficiency
D. Phosphoglycerate kinase deficiency
E. Mitochondrial myopathy

64. A 50-year-old woman presents with a 25-year history of bilateral ptosis and double vision. In addition, she has a history of cardiac arrhythmia for which she eventually needed a cardiac pacemaker. On examination, she has bilateral ptosis, limitation of the extraocular movement, and proximal weakness in limb muscles. Which of the following findings is likely to be seen on electrodiagnostic testing?
A. Greater than 10% decrement on slow repetitive stimulation
B. Greater than 100% on increment on fast repetitive stimulation
C. Short-duration motor unit potentials on needle electromyography (EMG)
D. Long-duration motor unit potentials on needle EMG
E. Normal needle EMG study in proximal limb muscles

65. A repeat electromyography (EMG) was performed in a patient diagnosed with acute motor axonal neuropathy after he noticed mild improvement in strength. The key finding was the presence of a few short-duration, small-amplitude polyphasic motor unit potentials. Which of the following helps in interpreting the clinical significance of these potentials?
A. Spontaneous activity
B. Degree of activation of muscle
C. Recruitment pattern
D. Findings on muscle biopsy
E. Creatine phosphokinase (CPK) level

66. After an extensive abdominal and pelvic surgery, a 40-year-old woman developed significant weakness in her left thigh. Needle electromyography (EMG) of the vastus lateralis performed a few months later revealed the following potentials during maximum activation. What is the firing frequency of the observed potential?

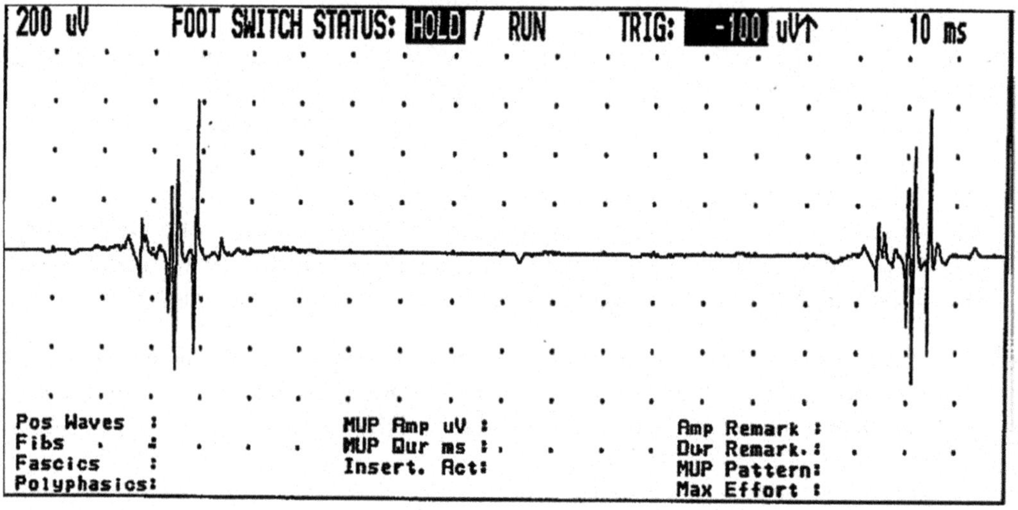

A. 5 Hz
B. 7 Hz
C. 10 Hz
D. 14 Hz
E. 2 Hz

67. A peroneal motor conduction study with three-point stimulation was performed. The distance between the ankle and fibular head stimulations is 350 mm, and between the fibular head and knee is 90 mm. What are the conduction velocities below and above the fibular head?

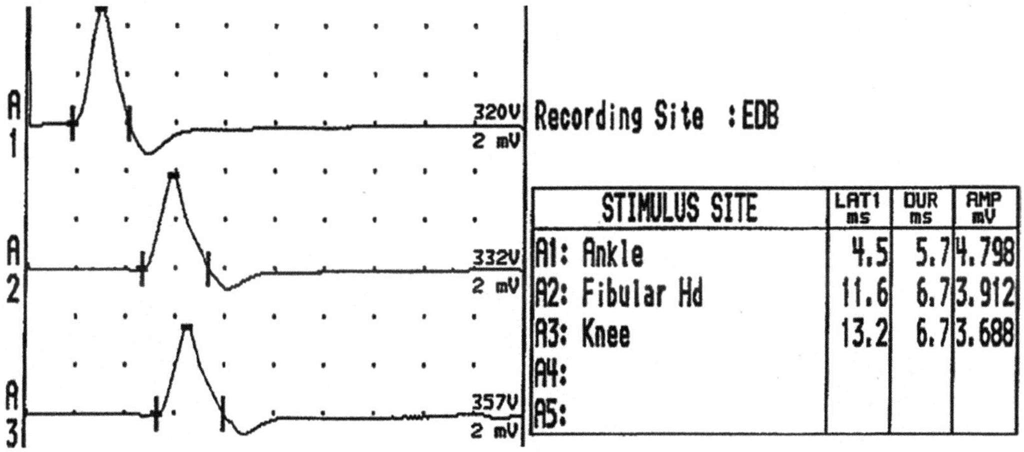

A. 60 and 69 m/sec
B. 49 and 56 m/sec
C. 49 and 29 m/sec
D. 49 and 49 m/sec
E. 56 and 49 m/sec

68. The electromyography (EMG) waveforms shown below were seen during maximum activation of the muscle in a 70-year-old man with weakness. This finding may be seen in which of the following conditions?

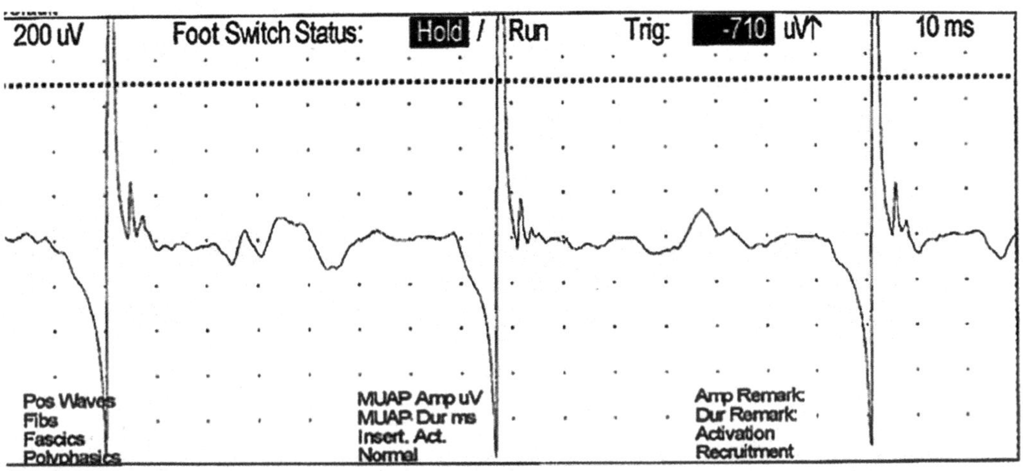

A. Polymyositis
B. Lambert–Eaton myasthenic syndrome (LEMS)
C. Chronic polyradiculopathy
D. Steroid-induced myopathy
E. Myasthenia gravis

69. On slow repetitive stimulation at 2 to 3 Hz, significant decrement may be seen in all of the following *except*
A. Botulism
B. Paramyotonia congenita
C. Neomycin toxicity
D. Becker muscular dystrophy
E. Lambert-Eaton myasthenic syndrome (LEMS)

70. When performing a three-point ulnar nerve stimulation (at the wrist, below elbow, and above elbow), it is important to perform the study with the elbow flexed as study performed with elbow extended will result in:
A. Erroneous increase in conduction velocity across the elbow
B. Erroneous decrease in conduction velocity across the elbow
C. Erroneous increase in ulnar compound muscle action potential (CMAP) amplitude
D. Erroneous decrease in ulnar CMAP amplitude
E. Erroneous increase in distal latency

71. Submaximal stimulation is used in which of the following nerve conduction studies?
A. Motor nerve conduction and F-wave responses
B. All sensory studies
C. H-reflex study
D. All nerve conduction studies are always performed with supramaximal stimulation, and submaximal stimulation should never be used.
E. Blink reflexes

72. During motor nerve conduction studies, it is important to measure the duration of the compound muscle action potential (CMAP) as this correlates with:
A. Duration of the electrical stimulus
B. Distal latency
C. Temporal dispersion
D. Conduction velocity
E. Patients ability to tolerate the study

73. Which of the following is shown in the figure below?

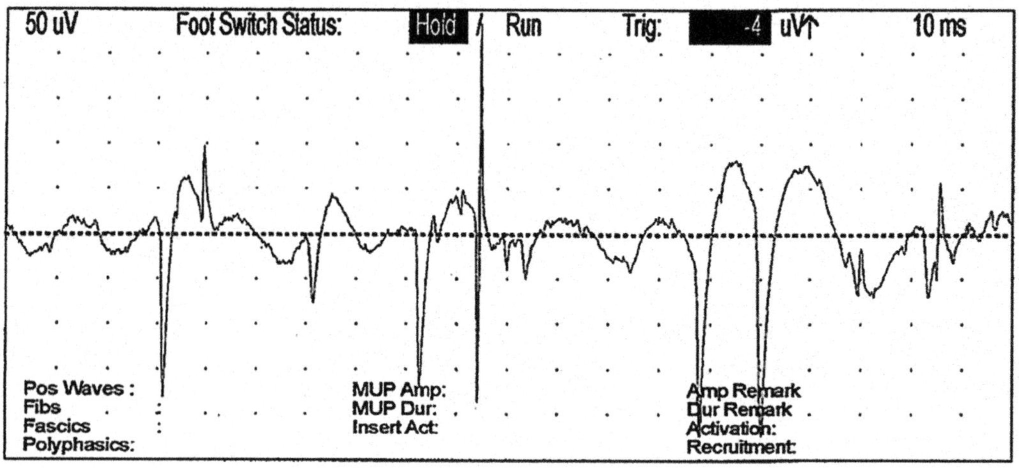

A. Many positive sharp waves and occasional fibrillation potentials
B. Many positive sharp waves and large-amplitude motor unit potentials
C. Complex repetitive discharges
D. Myokymia
E. Distant motor unit activity

74. While performing needle electromyography (EMG) and analyzing the motor unit potentials, all of the following factors directly affect the motor unit morphology *except:*
A. Age of the patient
B. Distance between the needle and the core of the muscle
C. Specific muscle being studied
D. Temperature
E. Concentric vs. monopolar needle used for needle EMG

75. A 60-year-old man developed Bell's palsy. He was treated with oral corticosteroids and antiviral agents but continued to have facial weakness. An ear–nose–throat physician requested facial electrodiagnostic studies before possible surgical intervention for the facial weakness. Electromyography (EMG) from the frontalis muscle during maximum activation is shown below. What does it reveal?

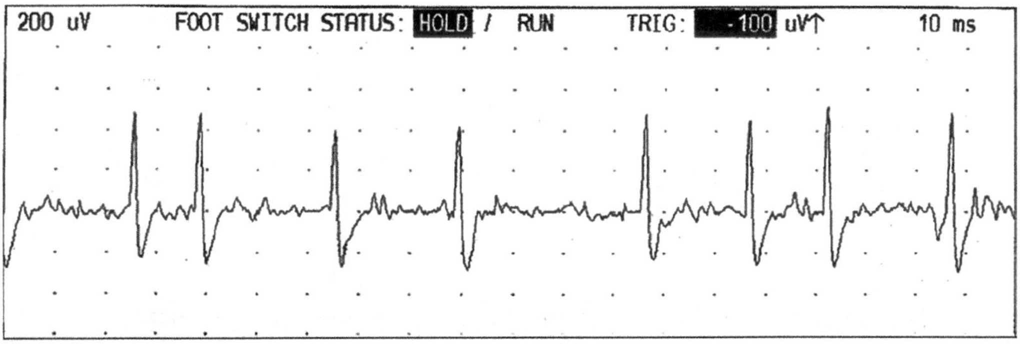

A. Early recruitment
B. Severely reduced recruitment
C. Normal recruitment for frontalis muscle
D. Synkinesis
E. Fasciculation potentials

76. A 60-year-old man has noticed difficulty over the past 2 months getting up from a chair, climbing steps at work, and lifting objects above his head. His primary care physician also noticed a rash on sun-exposed areas of the man's body. The patient was referred for electrodiagnostic testing. Needle electromyography (EMG) of weak proximal muscles in this patient would likely reveal
A. Decreased recruitment and large motor unit potentials
B. Early recruitment and large motor unit potentials
C. Early recruitment and small motor unit potentials
D. Decreased recruitment and small motor unit potentials
E. Normal recruitment and motor unit morphology

77. A 60-year-old male with sensory symptoms in his feet had routine nerve conduction studies. A tibial F-wave study is shown below. What do the additional waves seen between the M-waves and F-waves indicate?

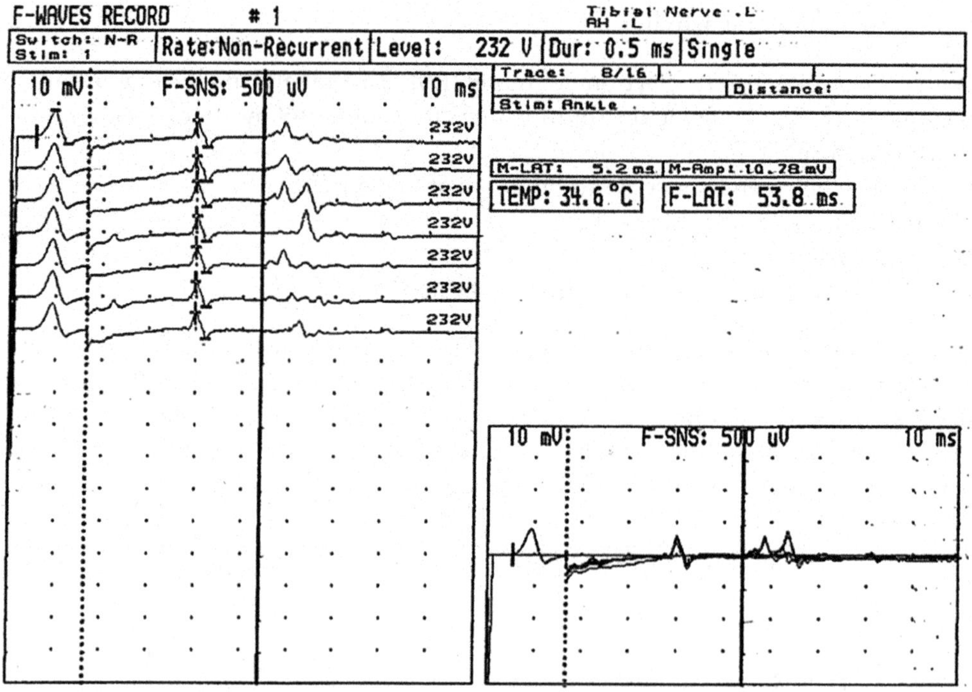

A. Electrical artifacts
B. A-waves
C. H-reflex waveforms
D. Waveforms related to excess patient movement with each stimulation
E. Artifact related to filter settings during F-wave studies

78. Which of the following statements is true regarding single-fiber needle electromyography (EMG)?
A. Normal patients have a jitter value of 100
B. Abnormal jitter is only seen with neuromuscular junction (NMJ) disorders
C. Blocking is always present in myasthenia gravis
D. Blocking may be seen in weak muscles in NMJ disorders
E. Normal upper limit of jitter does not change with muscles being tested

79. Myotonic discharges are most likely seen in which of the following disorders?
A. Duchenne muscular dystrophy
B. Acid maltase deficiency
C. Miyoshi myopathy
D. Hypokalemic periodic paralysis
E. Steroid myopathy

80. What does the waveform below show?

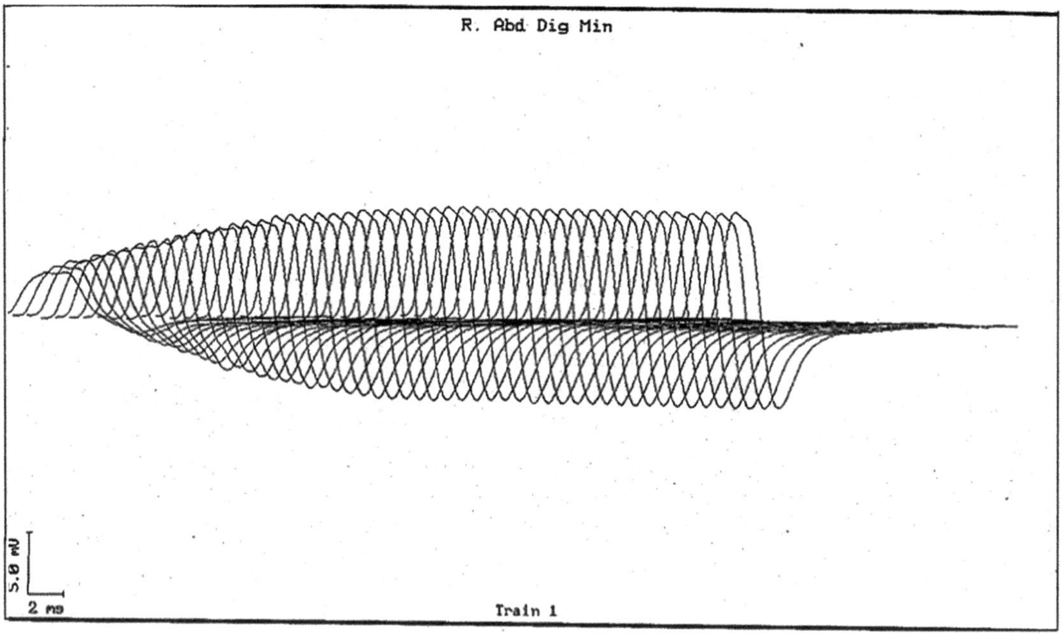

A. Slow repetitive stimulation and significant decrement
B. Fast repetitive stimulation and significant increment
C. Fast repetitive stimulation and significant decrement
D. Slow repetitive stimulation and significant increment
E. Normal fast repetitive stimulation

81. The commonly performed late response nerve conduction studies, F-wave and H-reflex, have certain unique differences. Which of the following statements is correct regarding these two late responses?

A. Both have fixed morphology with repeated stimulations
B. Both have shorter latencies with proximal stimulation
C. Both require supramaximal stimulation
D. The same nerve fibers carry afferent responses for both studies
E. Both require submaximal stimulation

82. A 25-year-old man was involved in a motor vehicle accident 3 weeks ago. He suffered a crush injury to his forearm and developed diffuse hand weakness. A few days after recovery from extensive surgery to his forearm, he continued to have weakness. An electromyography (EMG) of a distal weak muscle might reveal which of the following patterns?

Choices	Spontaneous activity	Motor unit duration	Motor unit amplitude	Recruitment pattern
A	Normal	Normal	Normal	Normal
B	Positive sharp waves and fibrillation potentials	Short duration	Small amplitude	Early recruitment
C	Positive sharp waves and fibrillation potentials	Normal	Normal	Decreased recruitment
D	Positive sharp waves and fibrillation potentials	Long duration	Large amplitude	Decreased recruitment
E	Normal	Long duration	Large amplitude	Normal

83. A 55-year-old with progressive gait difficulty and frequent falls was seen in clinic. On examination, he has severe large fiber distal sensory loss, mild distal weakness, ataxia, and mild intentional tremor. Peroneal motor study with extensor digitorum brevis recording was done as shown below. Which of the following tests might be most helpful to diagnose the underlying condition?

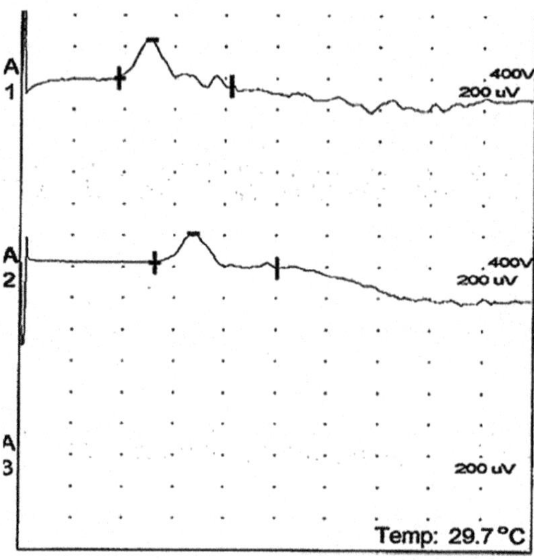

Recording Site: Extensor digitorum brevis

Stimulus Site	Lat1 ms	Dur ms	Amp mV	Temp °C
A1: Ankle	18.5	22.5	0.2	29.4
A2: Fibular head	26.0	23.9	0.2	29.4
A3: Popliteal fossa				

Segment	Dist mm	Diff ms	CV m/s
EDB-Ankle	80	18.5	
Ankle-Fibular head	310	7.5	41
Fibular head-Popliteal fossa			

A. Peripheral myelin protein (PMP) 22 duplication/deletion
B. Myelin-associated glycoprotein (MAG) antibodies
C. Antinuclear antibody (ANA), ds-deoxyribonucleic acid (ds-DNA) and complement levels
D. Paraneoplastic panel
E. Exome sequencing

84. Which of the following potentials is characterized by an irregular rhythm?
   A. Fasciculation potentials
   B. Positive sharp waves
   C. Complex repetitive discharges
   D. Fibrillation potentials
   E. Myokymia

85. An 80-year-old man has difficulty walking from an unclear neurodegenerative disease. Needle electromyography (EMG) recording from a distal upper limb muscle is shown below. What is the approximate firing frequency of the grouped motor unit activity below?

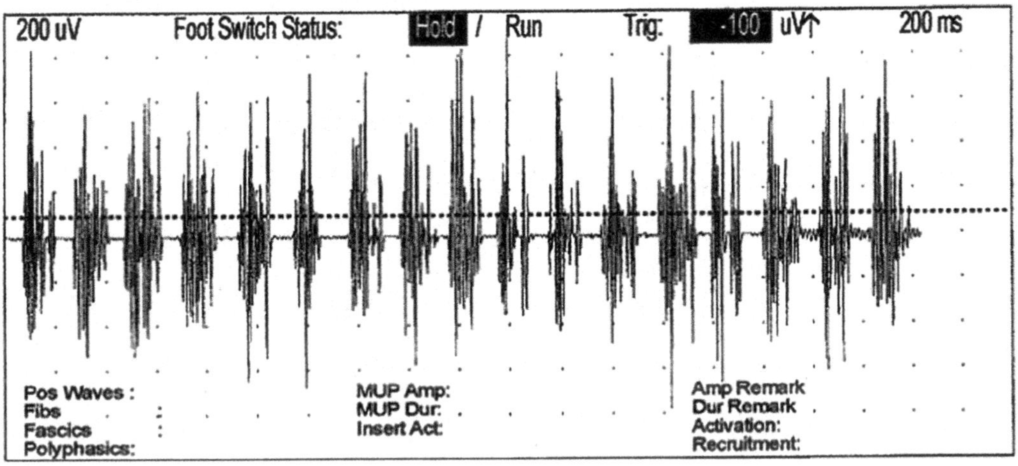

   A. 9 to 12 Hz
   B. 4 to 5 Hz
   C. 1 to 2 Hz
   D. 16 to 18 Hz
   E. 25 Hz

86. A 78-year-old man with chronic mild back pain presents with difficulty walking. On examination, he has sensory loss and mild distal weakness. Ankle reflexes are absent. Electrodiagnostic findings are shown below. What is the most appropriate interpretation?

Nerve conduction studies	Latency	Amplitude	Conduction velocity
Bilateral sural antidromic responses	No response	No response	
Bilateral peroneal motor responses	Normal	Mildly reduced amplitude	Mildly reduced conduction velocity
Bilateral tibial motor responses	Normal	Normal	Normal
Bilateral peroneal F-wave responses	Absent		

A. He has polyneuropathy because sural sensory responses are absent
B. He has polyneuropathy because peroneal motor conduction velocity is decreased
C. He has lumbosacral radiculopathy because peroneal motor amplitudes are decreased
D. He could either have polyneuropathy or lumbosacral radiculopathy; further differentiation is not possible based on the given data
E. These are normal findings in any 78-year-old, and so no further testing is required

87. A sural sensory study was performed in a 56-year-old man. This revealed a latency of 4.9 ms, amplitude of 12 μV, and conduction velocity of 36 m/sec. After the study, the electrodiagnostic technician noticed that the limb temperature was 27°C and repeated the study after rewarming the leg to above 30°C. Which of the following values are likely to be seen on the repeat sural study?

	Latency (ms)	Amplitude (μV)	Conduction velocity (m/sec)
A	5.0	12	42
B	5.0	8	36
C	4.2	14	33
D	4.2	8	42
E	5.5	16	30

88. The waveforms shown in the figure below may be found in all of the following conditions *except:*

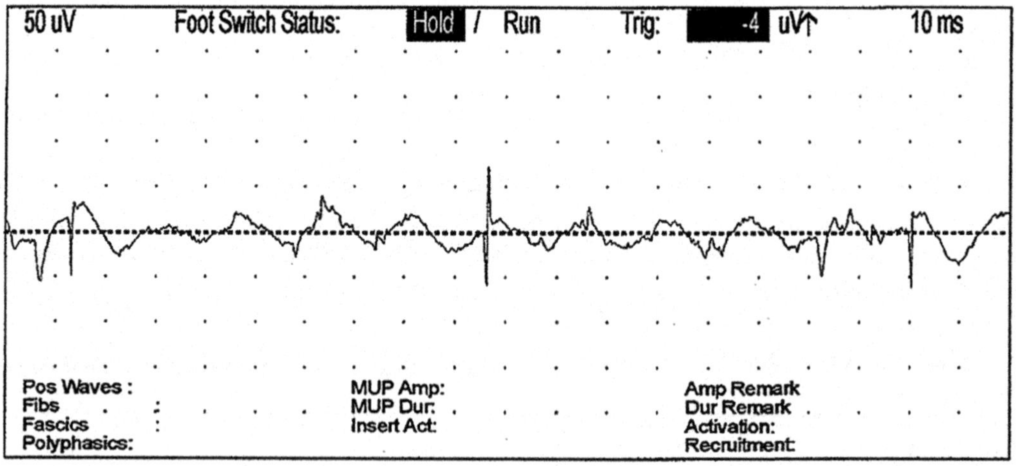

A. Steroid-induced myopathy
B. Toxic myopathies
C. Inflammatory myopathies
D. Glycogen storage disorders
E. Necrotizing myopathy

89. Which of the following factors increases the likelihood of neuropathy or myopathy related to colchicine toxicity?
A. Hepatic impairment
B. Renal failure
C. Cardiac failure
D. When used for nongouty conditions
E. If colchicine is taken intermittently

90. Which of the following patterns of electrodiagnostic abnormalities is likely in a patient with subacute nerve injury?

	Distal CMAP amplitude	Spontaneous activity on EMG	Motor unit morphology on EMG	Recruitment pattern
A	Normal	Normal	Normal	Normal
B	Decreased	Abnormal	Normal	Reduced
C	Decreased	Abnormal	Abnormal	Reduced
D	Normal	Normal	Normal	Reduced
E	Decreased	Normal	Normal	Normal

Note: CMAP, compound muscle action potential; EMG, electromyography.

91. Fibrillation potentials on the needle electromyography (EMG) are secondary to:
A. Irregular depolarization of all muscle fibers in a motor unit
B. Irregular depolarization of single muscle fiber
C. Regular depolarization of single muscle fiber
D. Regular depolarization of all muscle fibers in a motor unit
E. Regular depolarization of adjacent muscle fibers

92. A 50-year-old woman noticed weakness and pain in the right leg a few days after a cardiac angiogram. On examination, she has severe weakness in the right hip flexion and knee extension. Right knee reflex is absent. She has sensory loss in the medial aspect of the right leg. On a nerve conduction study (NCS)/ electromyography (EMG) performed about 2 weeks later, which of the following electrodiagnostic patterns is likely to be seen?
A. Absent peroneal and tibial motor responses and denervation in the tibialis anterior muscle
B. Absent femoral motor response only
C. Absent or reduced femoral motor response, absent saphenous and sural sensory responses
D. Absent or reduced femoral motor response, absent saphenous sensory response, and active denervation changes in the quadriceps muscle
E. Absent saphenous sensory response only

93. A 35-year-old man is undergoing surgery in the supraclavicular region to remove a tumor. The surgeon requests an intraoperative monitoring, specifically electromyography (EMG) of the abductor pollicis brevis (APB) muscle, to make sure there is no obvious lower trunk injury. Which of the following responses on needle EMG would indicate plexus injury during the surgery?

A. Positive sharp waves and fibrillation potentials
B. Myokymia
C. Neurotonic discharges
D. Fasciculation potential
E. Complex repetitive discharges

94. Routine nerve conduction and needle electromyography (EMG) studies are usually normal in which of the following conditions?

A. Lumbosacral radiculopathy
B. Mild large-fiber neuropathy
C. Small-fiber neuropathy
D. Lambert–Eaton myasthenic syndrome (LEMS)
E. Severe distal myopathy

95. Which of the following is true about F-wave latencies in children?

A. F-wave latency is similar to adult F-wave latency because slower conduction velocity and shorter limb length counteract each other
B. F-wave latencies are longer in children than adults because of lack of complete myelination
C. F-wave latencies are shorter as the limb length is shorter
D. F-waves are absent in children, so latency cannot be assessed
E. As repeated stimulation is not tolerated, F-wave studies should not be performed in children

96. A new neurology resident in the neuromuscular clinic starts to do a nerve conduction study and notices that when she stimulates the nerve, the resulting waveform has an initial positivity. Which of the following scenarios could explain this finding?

A. This is a normal response in all motor and sensory nerve conduction studies
B. This is due to a retreating wavefront
C. This is a bipolar digital sensory study
D. This is a motor response with the recording electrode far from the stimulated muscle
E. This is likely a result of submaximal stimulus

97. In a patient with suspected median mononeuropathy, a thorough electromyography (EMG) was performed after nerve conduction studies. The EMG findings are summarized below. What is the most likely diagnosis?

Muscle	Fibrillation/positive sharp waves	Motor unit morphology	Recruitment
Abductor pollicis brevis	2+	Increased duration and amplitude	Reduced
Flexor carpi radialis	1+	Increased duration and amplitude	Reduced
Pronator teres	1+	Increased duration and amplitude	Reduced
First dorsal interosseous	Normal	Normal	Normal
Extensor indices proprius	Normal	Normal	Normal

A. Median mononeuropathy at the wrist
B. Median mononeuropathy proximal to the nerve supply to pronator teres
C. Median mononeuropathy distal to the nerve supply to pronator teres
D. Lower trunk brachial plexopathy
E. Median cord brachial plexopathy

98. A 40-year-old man was admitted to the hospital with a 4-day history of progressive ascending weakness and currently has minimal distal limb movement. All of the testing including spinal fluid analysis is suggestive of Guillain–Barré syndrome (GBS). A needle electromyography (EMG) performed within 5 days of onset of symptoms will likely reveal:
A. Abundant positive sharp waves and fibrillation potentials
B. Fasciculation potentials
C. Normal needle EMG
D. Decreased motor unit recruitment patterns
E. Large duration and amplitude motor unit potentials with decreased recruitment patterns

99. A 75-year-old male with chronic back pain presents with recent onset right foot drop. He previously had right-sided foot drop a few years ago. He was diagnosed with lumbosacral radiculopathy at that time and had undergone a lumbar spine laminectomy surgery. Subsequently he regained most of the strength in the right leg until recently when he developed right foot drop again. After nerve conduction studies (NCS), an electromyography (EMG) of the right tibialis anterior was done. Which of the following is the most likely pattern of EMG findings?

Choices	Spontaneous activity	Motor unit duration	Motor unit amplitude	Recruitment pattern
A	Positive sharp waves and fibrillation potentials	Short duration	Small amplitude	Early recruitment
B	Positive sharp waves and fibrillation potentials	Normal	Normal	Normal
C	Positive sharp waves and fibrillation potentials	Long duration	Large amplitude	Decreased recruitment
D	Normal	Normal	Normal	Decreased recruitment
E	Normal	Long duration	Large amplitude	Normal

100. Which of the following electrodiagnostic findings in acute inflammatory demyelinating polyradiculoneuropathy (AIDP) is the most reliable predictor of poor prognosis?
A. Severely prolonged distal latency
B. Severely reduced compound muscle action potential (CMAP) amplitude
C. Severely reduced conduction velocity
D. Positive sharp waves and fibrillation potentials
E. Severely prolonged CMAP duration

101. In patients with shoulder girdle weakness, needle electromyography (EMG) abnormality in which of the following muscles localizes the lesion to cervical roots?
A. Deltoid
B. Infraspinatus
C. Biceps brachii
D. Serratus anterior
E. Pectoralis major

102. Decreased activation on needle electromyography (EMG) can be seen in which of the following conditions?
A. Pain limiting the effort by the patient
B. Upper motor neuron disease
C. Testing of a very strong muscle
D. Weakness in limb muscle after stroke
E. All of the above

103. Which of the following agents is *not* commonly known to cause necrotizing myopathy?
A. Cyclosporine
B. 3-hydroxy-3-methylglutaryl-CoA (HMG-CoA) reductase inhibitors
C. Amiodarone
D. Propofol
E. Alcohol

104. Needle electromyography (EMG) of the tibialis anterior muscle revealed the following motor unit potentials. What type of neuromuscular process does this suggest?

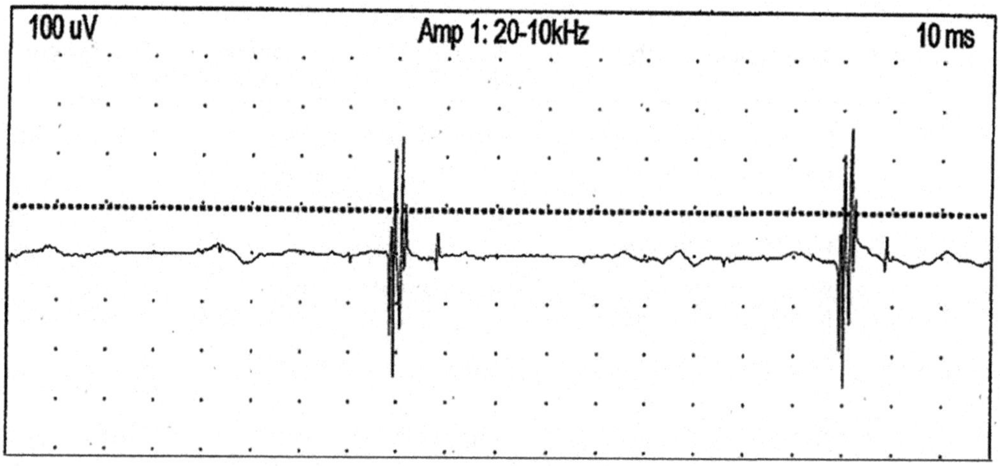

A. Acute neurogenic process
B. Acute myopathic process
C. Chronic reinnervation process
D. Acute neuromuscular junction dysfunction
E. Chronic neuromuscular junction dysfunction

105. Excess variability of motor unit potentials is seen in which of the following conditions?
A. Amyotrophic lateral sclerosis (ALS)
B. Chronic inflammatory demyelinating polyneuropathy (CIDP)
C. Polymyositis
D. Myasthenia gravis
E. Spinal muscular atrophy

106. A nerve entrapment at the Guyon's canal leads to abnormalities in which of the following nerve–muscle pairs on electrodiagnostic testing?
A. Median nerve and abductor pollicis brevis muscle
B. Ulnar nerve and first dorsal interosseous muscle
C. Radial nerve and extensor digitorum communis muscle
D. Ulnar nerve and flexor carpi ulnaris muscle
E. Posterior interosseous nerve and supinator muscle

107. A median motor nerve conduction study performed in a 15-year-old boy is shown below. This study is suggestive of which of the following?

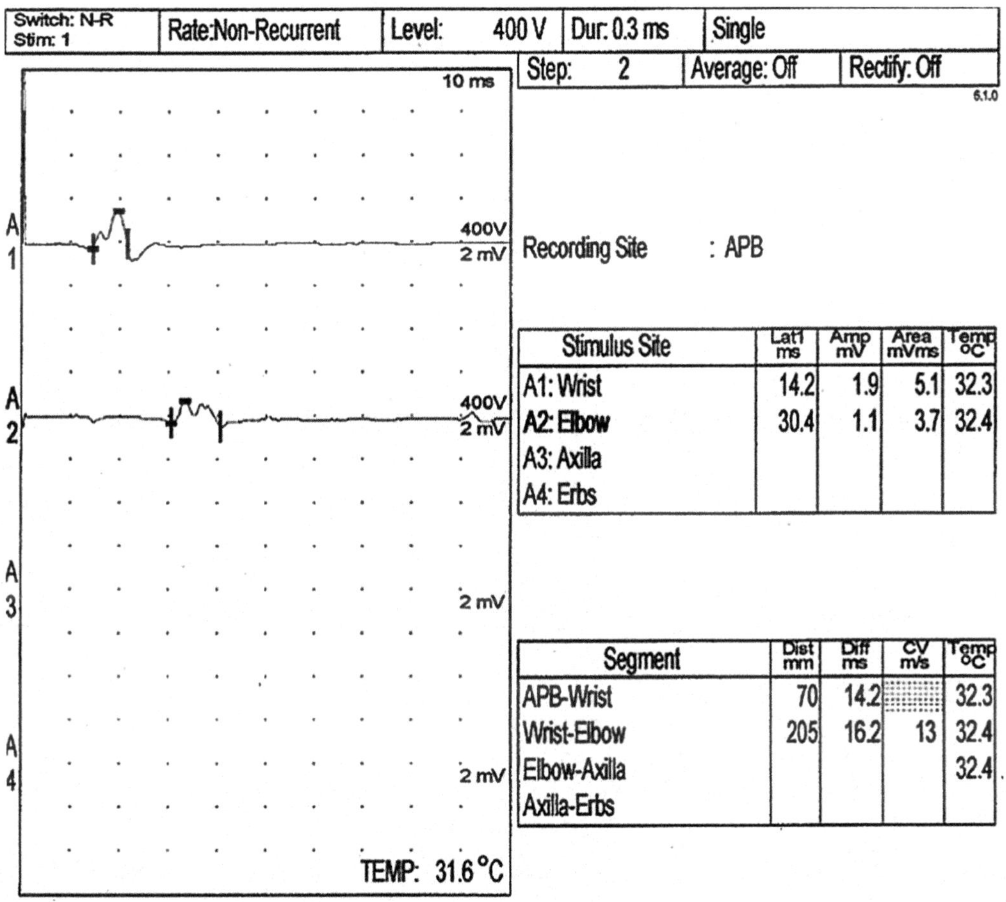

A. Severe carpal tunnel syndrome
B. Severe demyelinating neuropathy
C. Severe axonal neuropathy with carpal tunnel syndrome
D. Martin–Gruber anastomosis
E. Normal study as cold limb temperature caused to very slow velocities

108. Which of the following statements is true regarding F-wave and M-wave amplitudes?
A. F-wave amplitude is 50% of the M-wave amplitude
B. F-wave amplitude is 30% of the M-wave amplitude
C. F-wave amplitude is 3% to 5% of the M-wave amplitude
D. F-wave and M-wave amplitudes are the same
E. F-wave responses are 0.3% to 0.5% of M-wave amplitude

109. A 60-year-old man with low back pain has a tibial H-reflex testing performed. The afferent and efferent loops of the H-reflex are:
A. Antidromic sensory and orthodromic motor
B. Orthodromic sensory and orthodromic motor
C. Orthodromic sensory and antidromic motor
D. Antidromic sensory and antidromic motor
E. Afferent and efferent pathways vary by the nerve stimulated

110. The needle electromyography (EMG) waveforms shown below may be seen in all of the following conditions *except:*

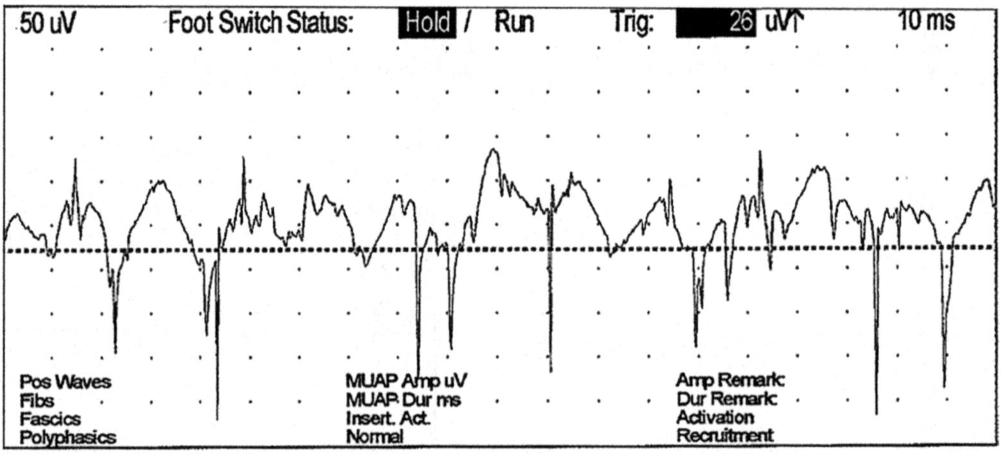

A. Motor neuron disease
B. Severe inflammatory polymyositis
C. Severe axonal polyneuropathy
D. Guillain–Barré syndrome (GBS) with demyelinating changes only
E. Traumatic neuropathy with severe weakness

111. A 35-year-old neurology resident noticed numbness over the dorsum of his left foot and weakness of the foot dorsiflexion for 6 months. Because his symptoms did not improve with rest, he ultimately had a nerve conduction study and needle electromyography (EMG) of the left leg muscles. EMG findings are tabulated below. What is the most likely localization for his weakness?

Muscle	Spontaneous activity	Motor unit morphology	Recruitment
Tibialis anterior	2+ positive sharp waves and fibrillations	Long-duration and large-amplitude motor unit potentials	Severely reduced
Medial gastrocnemius	1+ positive sharp waves and fibrillations	Mildly increased duration and amplitude motor unit potentials	Mildly reduced
Short head of biceps femoris	1+ positive sharp waves and fibrillations	Mildly increased duration and amplitude motor unit potentials	Mildly reduced
Gluteus medius	Normal	Normal	Normal

A. Peroneal nerve at fibular head
B. Peroneal nerve above the fibular head
C. L5 radiculopathy
D. Sciatic nerve
E. S1 radiculopathy

112. Which of the following features of the motor unit action potential is most suggestive of proximity of the needle electrode to the motor unit?
A. Duration
B. Rise time
C. Amplitude
D. Number of phases
E. Firing frequency

113. A 25-year-old woman noticed numbness in her left hand after she started wearing a new, tight-fitting bracelet. On examination, she has sensory loss over the dorsum of the left hand. There was no clear weakness on examination and deep tendon reflexes were normal. A nerve conduction study was requested. Apart from routine testing, which nerves should be tested to localize her neuropathy?
A. Bilateral lateral antebrachial cutaneous sensory studies
B. Bilateral median palmar sensory studies
C. Bilateral radial motor studies
D. Bilateral radial sensory studies
E. Bilateral medial antebrachial cutaneous sensory studies

114. Which of the following is the earliest abnormal feature seen in nerve conduction studies in a patient with acute demyelinating polyneuropathy?
A. Decreased conduction velocity
B. Absent sensory responses
C. Delayed or absent F-wave responses
D. Conduction block or abnormal temporal dispersion
E. Reduced motor amplitudes

115. Ulnar motor study performed in a woman with chronic distal weakness and sensory loss is shown below. What is this study consistent with?

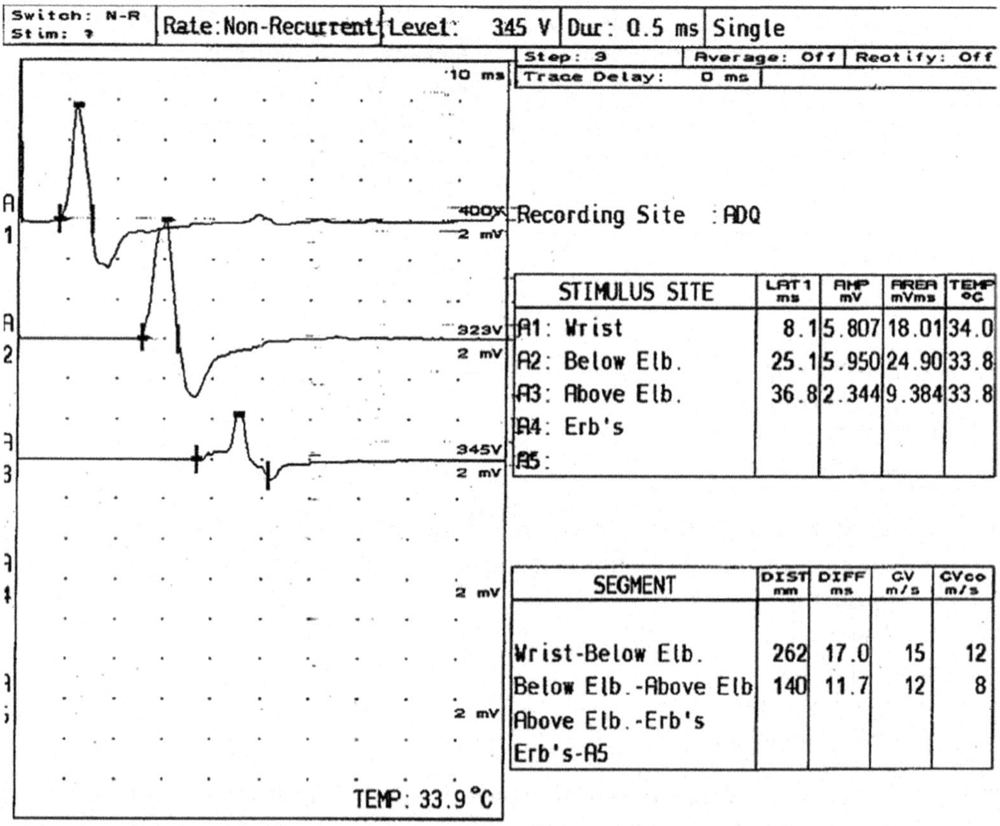

STIMULUS SITE	LAT 1 ms	AMP mV	AREA mVms	TEMP °C
A1: Wrist	8.1	5.807	18.01	34.0
A2: Below Elb.	25.1	5.950	24.90	33.8
A3: Above Elb.	36.8	2.344	9.384	33.8
A4: Erb's				
A5:				

SEGMENT	DIST mm	DIFF ms	CV m/s	CVco m/s
Wrist-Below Elb.	262	17.0	15	12
Below Elb.-Above Elb	140	11.7	12	8
Above Elb.-Erb's				
Erb's-A5				

A. Chronic inflammatory demyelinating neuropathy
B. Hereditary demyelinating neuropathy with partial conduction block
C. Hereditary axonal neuropathy with partial conduction block
D. Monomelic amyotrophy
E. Multifocal motor neuropathy (MMN)

116. Which of the following statements is *true* regarding motor unit potential morphology in infants as compared to normal healthy adults?
A. Infants and adults have similar motor unit morphology
B. Infants have significantly smaller motor unit amplitude than adults
C. Infants have larger motor unit amplitude than adults because of superior synchrony among muscle fibers within each motor unit potential
D. Only infants with myopathy have smaller motor unit amplitude than adults
E. Motor unit amplitude is larger in infants and reaches normal adult range after 5 years of age

117. A 20-year-old was stabbed with a long-blade knife in the neck during a fight. He noticed weakness and numbness in his right hand after the injury. Which of the following findings will differentiate brachial plexopathy from cervical root injury?
A. Ulnar sensory amplitude
B. Median H-reflex with flexor carpi radialis recording
C. Median somatosensory evoked potential study
D. Ulnar motor amplitude
E. Ulnar F-wave response

118. Which of the following electromyography (EMG) responses is generated from the motor unit?
A. Complex repetitive discharges
B. Fibrillation potentials
C. Myokymic discharges
D. Myotonic discharges
E. Positive sharp waves

119. A 60-year-old man has chronic low back pain. Previously, he had extensive lumbar spine surgery for disc disease and recently developed increasing back pain followed by right leg weakness. He undergoes nerve conduction studies in both legs and electromyography (EMG) of the right lower limb muscles. Which of the following statements best describes the need for needle EMG of the lumbar paraspinal muscles?
A. It is needed because active denervation in lumbar paraspinal muscle would indicate new lumbosacral radiculopathy
B. It is needed because active denervation in lumbar paraspinal muscle would indicate that his pain is not musculoskeletal
C. It is needed because active denervation in lumbar paraspinal muscle would indicate that he needs another surgery
D. It is not needed because active denervation can be secondary to postsurgical changes and therefore not helpful
E. It is not needed because active denervation in lumbar paraspinal muscles can be seen in normal individuals

120. A 25-year-old woman presents with chronic left shoulder pain and sensory symptoms in her hands. On examination, she has atrophy of the thenar and hypothenar muscle groups in the hand. A nerve conduction study was performed. This showed decreased median and ulnar motor amplitudes. Ulnar sensory response was absent whereas median sensory response was normal. Based on these findings, which of the following conditions is likely?
A. Carpal tunnel syndrome (CTS)
B. C7–C8 radiculopathy
C. Martin–Gruber anastomosis (MGA) and CTS
D. Neurogenic thoracic outlet syndrome
E. Ulnar neuropathy at elbow

121. Repetitive nerve stimulation was performed in a man with proximal limb weakness as shown below. Which of the following statements is correct?

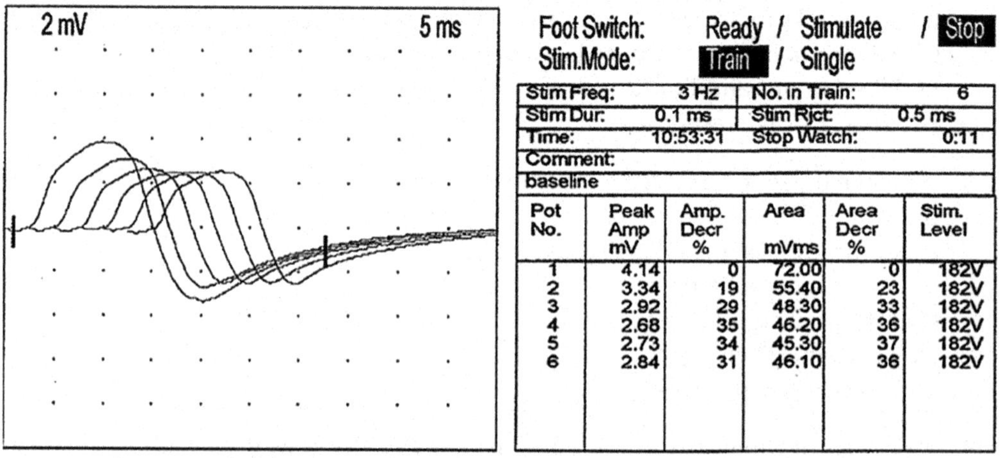

A. This is slow repetitive stimulation which reveals significant decrement
B. This is fast repetitive stimulation which reveals significant decrement
C. This is slow repetitive stimulation which reveals significant increment
D. This is fast repetitive stimulation which reveals significant increment
E. This is a slow repetitive stimulation with nonsignificant decrement

122. A 45-year-old woman had severe axillary neuropathy after trauma. Needle electromyography (EMG) of which of the following muscles is going to reveal denervation?
A. Teres major and teres minor
B. Deltoid and teres major
C. Deltoid and teres minor
D. Deltoid and triceps
E. Deltoid and anconeus

123. Significant decrement may be seen on slow repetitive stimulation in which of the following conditions?
A. Lambert–Eaton myasthenic syndrome (LEMS)
B. Myasthenia gravis
C. Botulism
D. Postsynaptic congenital myasthenic syndrome
E. All of the above

124. In a patient with muscle weakness, a muscle biopsy was completed. Muscle tissue was stained with adenosine triphosphatase at different pH values. On these stains, the patient was noted to have fiber-type grouping and loss of the usual checkerboard pattern of type 1 and type 2 fibers. Among the following, which type of electromyography (EMG) finding best correlates with fiber-type grouping on muscle biopsy?
A. Positive sharp waves and normal motor unit potentials
B. Motor unit potentials with large amplitude and long duration
C. Motor unit potentials with small amplitude and short duration
D. Fasciculation potentials
E. Fibrillation potentials and normal motor unit potentials

125. A 45-year-old man presents with weakness for more than 20 years. On examination, he has predominantly symmetrical, proximal more than distal, weakness with diminished reflexes and intact sensation. He was previously told that he had a form of muscular dystrophy. Needle electromyography (EMG) revealed few positive sharp waves and fibrillation potentials along with long-duration and large-amplitude motor unit potentials with severely reduced recruitment. If a muscle biopsy is performed in this patient, it will most likely reveal:
A. Rimmed vacuoles
B. Perifascicular atrophy
C. Fiber type grouping
D. Glycogen positive vacuoles
E. Necrotic fibers

126. A median motor study was performed in a 35-year-old woman with tingling paresthesias in her hands. Electrodiagnostic data is presented below. A small initial positive dip in the compound muscle action potential (CMAP) was seen with elbow stimulation only. Distance between the wrist and elbow stimulation is 250 mm. Distance between wrist stimulation and G1 electrode is 70 mm. What is the correct interpretation?

Median motor study with APB recording	Latency	Amplitude	Conduction velocity
Wrist stimulation	5.5 ms	5.0 mV	-
Elbow stimulation	8.0 ms	6.0 mV	100 m/sec

Note: APB, abductor pollicis brevis.

A. Median mononeuropathy at the wrist and Martin–Gruber anastomosis (MGA)
B. Median mononeuropathy in the forearm and MGA
C. Median mononeuropathy at the wrist only
D. Positive dip with elbow stimulation indicates a technical limitation and study should be repeated
E. Normal study as distal CMAP amplitude is normal

127. Which of the following combination of deep tendon reflex abnormalities is seen in an upper trunk brachial plexopathy?
A. Absent triceps reflex
B. Absent biceps reflex but preserved triceps and brachioradialis reflexes
C. Absent brachioradialis reflex but preserved biceps and triceps reflexes
D. Absent biceps and brachioradialis reflexes with preserved triceps reflex
E. All deep tendon reflexes are normal as middle and lower trunk function is preserved

128. A routine median motor study in a 50-year-old secretary with symptoms of hand numbness and weakness is shown below. What does this study reveal?

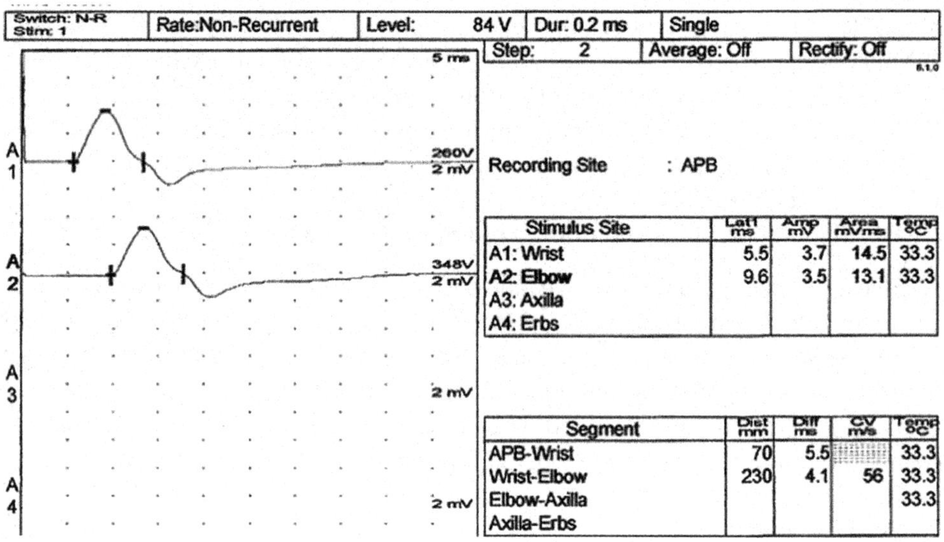

A. Normal median motor study
B. Evidence of median neuropathy in the wrist
C. Evidence of median neuropathy in the forearm
D. Conduction block in the forearm
E. No conclusions can be drawn without median sensory response

129. By what age do conduction velocities of motor nerves in a child reach the adult range?
A. 1 year
B. 2 years
C. 5 years
D. 7 years
E. 10 years

130. What is the firing frequency of the motor unit potential with the largest amplitude in the study shown below?

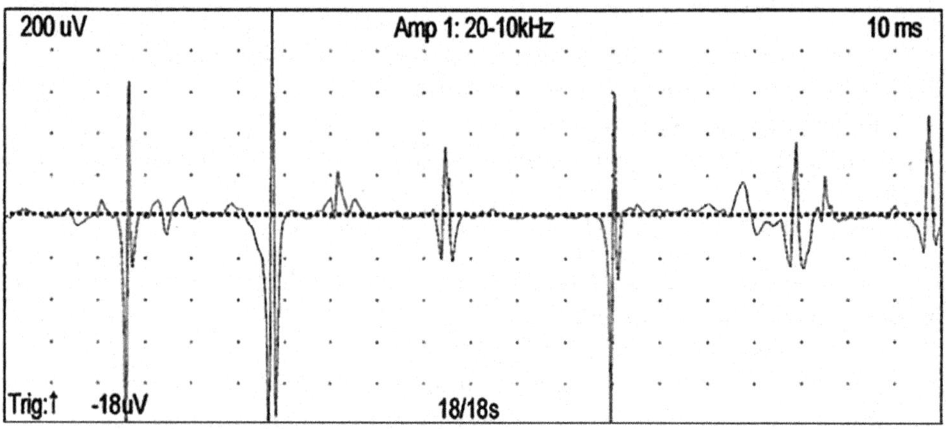

A. 20 Hz
B. 10 Hz
C. 5 Hz
D. 2.5 Hz
E. 40 Hz

131. A 70-year-old man is referred for evaluation of cervical radiculopathy. Needle electromyography (EMG) in a distal muscle shows the pattern below. This is most consistent with:

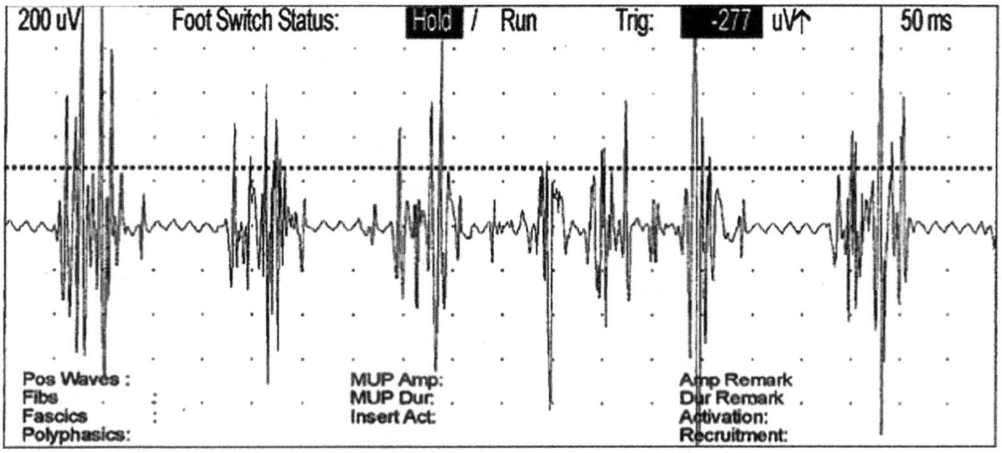

A. Myokymia
B. Diffuse fasciculation potentials
C. Complex repetitive discharges
D. Tremor
E. Normal motor unit firing pattern

132. Scapular winging may be seen in all the following conditions *except:*
A. Facioscapulohumeral muscular dystrophy
B. Spinal accessory nerve injury
C. Long thoracic nerve injury
D. Lower trunk brachial plexopathy
E. Dorsal scapular nerve injury

133. The time required for the appearance of fibrillation potentials or positive sharp waves after a peripheral nerve injury depends upon which of the following?
A. Distance between the site of the nerve injury and the muscle
B. Distance between the spinal cord and muscle
C. Extent of demyelination in the nerve
D. Distance between the spinal cord and the site of the nerve injury
E. Length of the limb

134. The ulnar motor nerve conduction response shown below is likely to be seen in which of the following conditions?

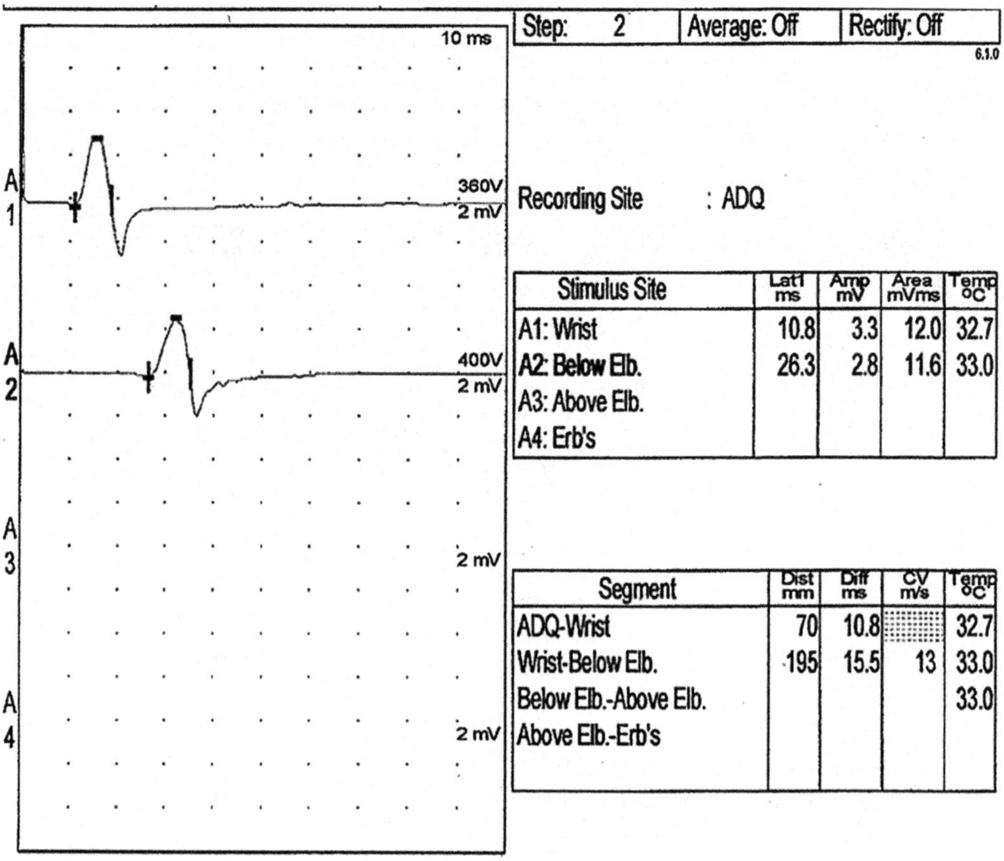

Stimulus Site	Lat1 ms	Amp mV	Area mVms	Temp ºC
A1: Wrist	10.8	3.3	12.0	32.7
A2: Below Elb.	26.3	2.8	11.6	33.0
A3: Above Elb.				
A4: Erb's				

Segment	Dist mm	Diff ms	CV m/s	Temp ºC
ADQ-Wrist	70	10.8		32.7
Wrist-Below Elb.	195	15.5	13	33.0
Below Elb.-Above Elb.				33.0
Above Elb.-Erb's				

A. Acute inflammatory demyelinating polyneuropathy
B. Chronic inflammatory demyelinating polyneuropathy
C. Hereditary demyelinating polyneuropathy
D. Lewis-Sumner syndrome
E. Multifocal motor neuropathy

135. A 35-year-old man presents with right arm weakness. On examination, he has weakness of the right elbow flexion but other muscle groups are strong. He also has sensory loss over the lateral forearm. Which of the following is the most likely cause for this clinical presentation?

A. C5–C6 radiculopathy
B. Medial cord brachial plexopathy
C. Lateral cord brachial plexopathy
D. Musculocutaneous neuropathy
E. Upper trunk brachial plexopathy

136. Which antidromic median sensory configuration would result in an initial positivity?
A. Recording from digit 3 with the reference electrode over digit 5
B. Recording from digit 3 with the reference electrode over digit 3
C. Recording from digit 5 with the reference electrode over digit 3
D. Recording from digit 2 with the reference electrode over digit 2
E. Any of the above configurations would result in an initial positivity if the stimulating anode and cathode were reversed with stimulation at the wrist.

137. All of the following drugs can cause neuromyopathy (combination of neuropathy and myopathy) *except:*
A. Disulfiram
B. Colchicine
C. Amiodarone
D. Chloroquine
E. Clofibrates

138. A 45-year-old man had extensive surgery in the right lower abdominal/groin area for retroperitoneal sarcoma. After surgery, he noticed significant weakness and sensory loss in the right lower limb. Because his symptoms did not improve after 8 weeks, bilateral nerve conduction studies were performed as shown below. What is the most likely localization?

Nerve	Latency	Amplitude	Conduction velocity
Bilateral peroneal motor study	Normal	Normal	Normal
Bilateral tibial motor study	Normal	Normal	Normal
Bilateral sural antidromic sensory study	Normal	Normal	Normal
Right saphenous sensory study	Absent	Absent	
Left saphenous sensory study	Normal	Normal	Normal

A. Sciatic nerve
B. Lower lumbosacral plexus
C. Femoral nerve
D. Lateral femoral cutaneous nerve of thigh
E. L2, L3, L4 nerve root injury

139. All of the following are features of Pompe disease *except:*
A. Myotonia in thoracic paraspinal muscles
B. Berry aneurysms
C. Cardiac abnormalities
D. Flexion contractures at the elbow
E. Reduced forced vital capacity

140. A 65-year-old man was referred for neuromuscular evaluation of head drop. Over the last 6 months, he noticed increasing weakness in his neck muscles and difficulty keeping his head up. On examination, he has severe neck extensor weakness (2/5) but strength in all other muscle groups is normal. Which of the following conditions is most likely?

A. Motor neuron disease presenting with head drop
B. Myasthenia gravis
C. Pompe disease
D. Isolated neck extensor myopathy
E. Inclusion body myositis

141. A 30-year-old woman presented with increasing fatigue, decreased exercise tolerance, and weakness over the last few years. On examination, she had proximal limb weakness with normal reflexes and sensation. Facial strength was normal. Her forced vital capacity was decreased. Routine motor and sensory nerve studies were normal. Needle electromyography (EMG) revealed short-duration, myopathic motor units in proximal muscles. What additional step during the electrodiagnostic testing would be helpful?

A. Facial EMG
B. Repetitive stimulation of the facial nerve
C. EMG of the thoracic paraspinal muscles
D. Diaphragmatic EMG
E. Long exercise test

142. One week after a pure neuropraxic injury in the forearm, a nerve conduction study may reveal all the following findings *except:*

A. Decreased distal compound muscle action potential (CMAP) amplitude
B. Decreased or absent proximal CMAP amplitude
C. Complete conduction block
D. No motor unit activity on needle electromyography (EMG)
E. Absent F-wave response

143. A 50-year-old male had an electromyography (EMG) for weakness in the upper limb. Below is the tracing from needle EMG. What is the amplitude and firing frequency of the largest motor unit shown? (Gain: 1 mV and sweep speed 10 ms)

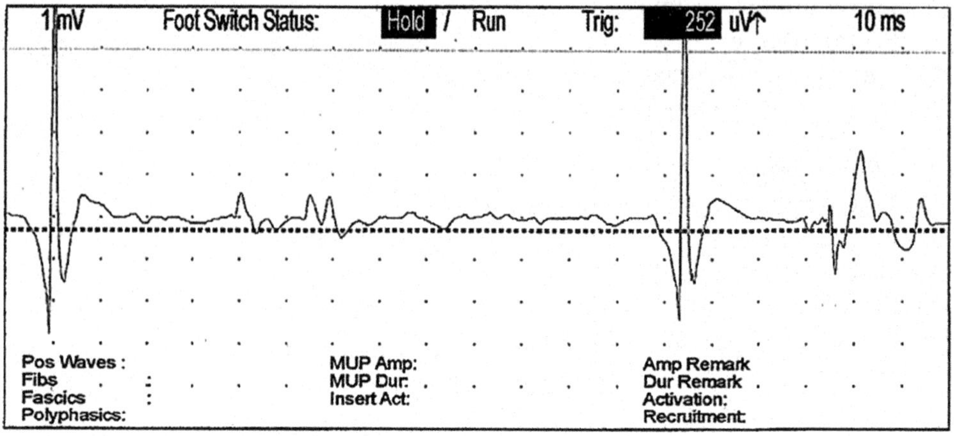

A. 7.5 mV and 5 Hz
B. 2 mV and 10 Hz
C. 7.5 mV and 10 Hz
D. 5 mV and 20 Hz
E. 10mV and 10 Hz

144. A nerve entrapment at the Arcade of Frohse can cause electrodiagnostic changes in which of the following nerve–muscle pairs?
A. Median nerve and abductor pollicis brevis
B. Ulnar nerve and first dorsal interosseous
C. Radial nerve and flexor carpi radialis
D. Median nerve and pronator teres
E. Ulnar nerve and abductor digiti minimi

145. A 70-year-old man developed complete right sciatic nerve injury after hip replacement surgery. On sensory examination, which part of the lower extremity is expected to be normal?
A. Dorsum of the foot
B. Lateral part of the calf
C. First web space between the great toe and second toe
D. Medial aspect of the leg (over the tibial bone)
E. Lateral aspect of the foot

146. A 30-year-old woman was admitted for ascending weakness and numbness for 36 hours. She also reports severe back pain. On examination, she has distal and proximal weakness, diffuse areflexia, and distal sensory loss. An urgent electrodiagnostic study was requested. Which of the following components of the electrodiagnostic study is most likely to be abnormal in this patient?
A. Sural sensory response
B. Peroneal motor response
C. H-reflexes
D. Blink responses
E. Slow repetitive stimulation testing

147. All of the following types of neuropathy may be associated with HIV infection *except:*
A. Symmetrical distal polyneuropathy
B. Acute inflammatory demyelinating polyradiculoneuropathy (AIDP)
C. Sensory neuronopathy
D. Multifocal motor neuropathy
E. Autonomic neuropathy

148. A neuromuscular fellow notices the findings shown below while performing an electromyography (EMG) of a weak muscle. What is the source of the waveforms shown?

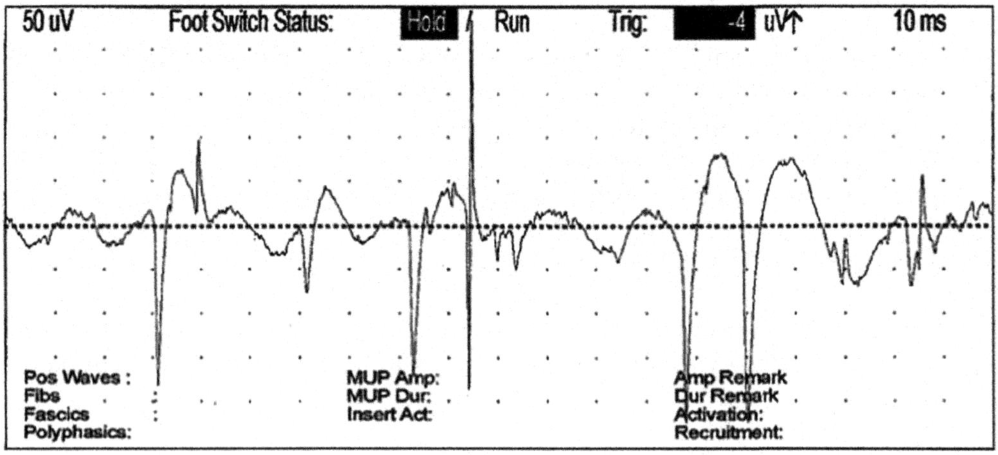

A. Anterior horn cells
B. Muscle fibers
C. Motor nerve axons
D. Ephaptic transmission in muscle fibers
E. Proximal nerve root

149. A 30-year-old man initially noticed difficulty walking and tendency to fall in his late teenage years, followed by gradual progression of his condition over the next decade. On examination, he has severe spasticity in his lower limbs and distal sensory loss and weakness. His 28-year-old brother also has similar manifestations. Electrodiagnostic study in this patient will most likely reveal:
A. Normal nerve conduction studies
B. Primarily low compound muscle action potential (CMAP) amplitude with mild slowing and reduced sensory amplitudes
C. Severe slowing of conduction velocity with mildly decreased amplitudes
D. Normal nerve conduction studies but severe denervation on needle electromyography (EMG) in proximal muscles
E. Normal nerve conduction studies but denervation on needle EMG in distal muscles

150. A 19-year-old man presents with difficulty walking for a few years and frequent falls. His peroneal nerve conduction study is shown below. Which of the following tests is most likely to be diagnostic in this patient?

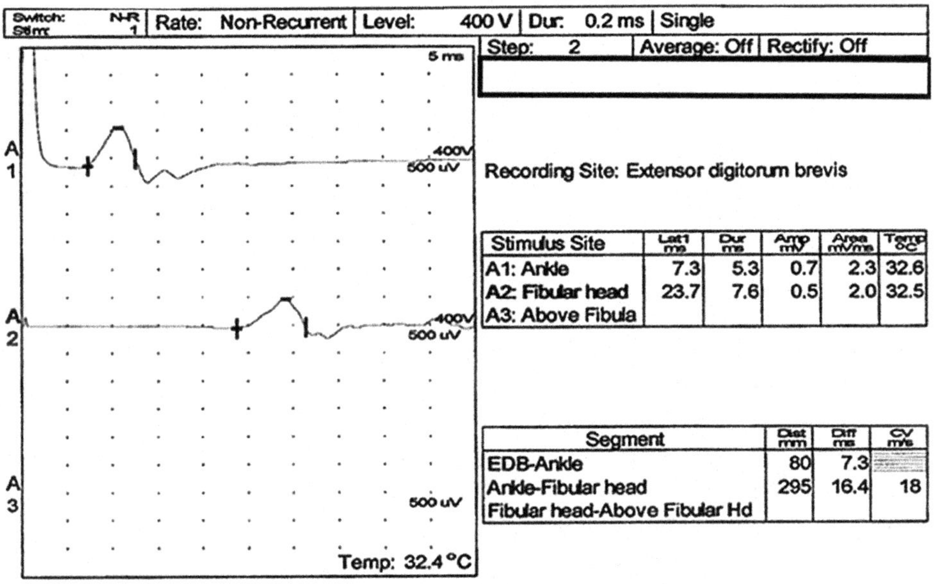

A. Mitofusin (MFN) mutation
B. Peripheral myelin protein (PMP) mutation analysis
C. Very long-chain fatty acids
D. Spinal fluid analysis
E. Fasting blood glucose levels

151. A 44-year-old man presented with increasing shortness of breath and orthopnea. Chest x-ray revealed elevated right hemi-diaphragm. Electromyography (EMG) tracing from right hemi-diaphragm below reveals:

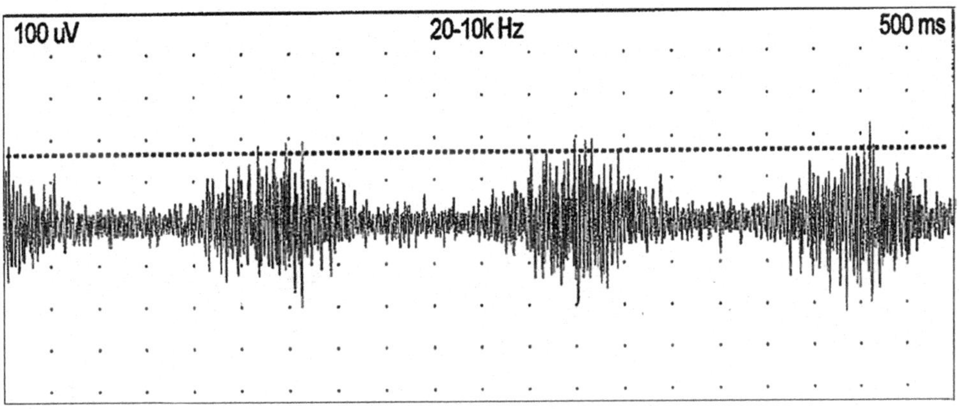

A. Active denervation and myopathic motor units with early recruitment
B. Normal changes with respiration
C. Myokymia
D. Neurogenic process with decreased recruitment
E. Myotonia

152. A 25-day-old infant was noted to have severely reduced tone. Her pediatrician would like to exclude an underlying neuromuscular cause for her decreased tone and requested an electrodiagnostic evaluation. Nerve conduction velocities of median and peroneal motor nerves were in the range of 25 to 26 m/sec. This finding suggests that the infant has
   A. Demyelinating polyneuropathy
   B. Axonal polyneuropathy
   C. Normal conduction velocity for age
   D. Myopathy
   E. Neuromuscular junction disease

153. Rapid or early recruitment on needle electromyography (EMG) is usually seen in which of the following conditions?
   A. Amyotrophic lateral sclerosis (ALS)
   B. Charcot–Marie–Tooth (CMT) disease
   C. Muscular dystrophy
   D. Hypokalemic period paralysis
   E. Hereditary spastic paraparesis

154. A 30-year-old woman presented with recent onset difficulty speaking and swallowing. In addition, she has ptosis and diplopia. She was given pyridostigmine but her symptoms worsened with this medication. Repetitive stimulation of the spinal accessory nerve revealed significant decrement. Acetylcholine receptor (AChR) antibody test was normal. What is the next best diagnostic step?
   A. Voltage-gated calcium channel antibody
   B. Muscle-specific kinase antibody
   C. Single-fiber electromyography (SFEMG)
   D. Muscle biopsy to evaluate mitochondrial diseases
   E. Genetic testing for congenital myasthenic syndrome

155. A 40-year-old man recently had a knee injury and noticed weakness in his right leg. The findings on peroneal motor study are shown below. What does this suggest?

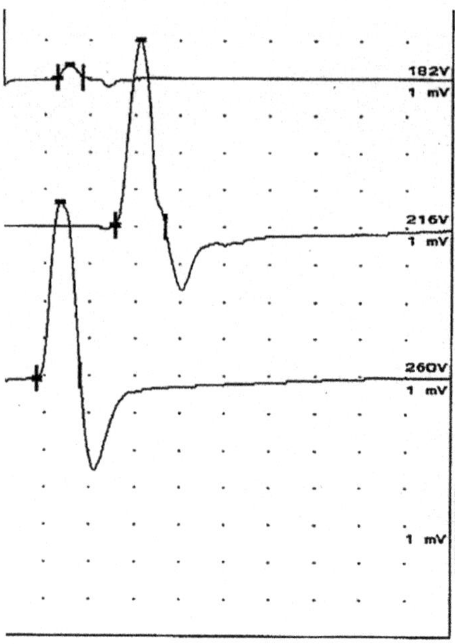

Recording Site : EDB

STIMULUS SITE	LAT1 ms	DUR ms	AMP mV	AREA mVms	TEMP °C
A1: Ankle	6.3	2.8	0.411	0.714	
A2: Fibular Hd	12.7	5.6	4.974	13.10	
A3: Accessary	4.1	4.8	4.789	12.92	
A4:					

SEGMENT	DIST mm	DIFF ms	CV m/s	CVoo m/s
Ankle-Fibular Hd	360	6.4	56	
Fibular Hd-Accessary		8.6		

A. Peroneal mononeuropathy at the fibular head
B. Peroneal mononeuropathy at the ankle
C. Normal variant
D. Peroneal mononeuropathy above the popliteal fossa
E. Normal peroneal study, but indirect evidence of tibial neuropathy as proximal compound muscle action potential (CMAP) is higher

156. A 20-year-old male was diagnosed with Guillain–Barré syndrome (GBS) in the emergency department (ED) based on acute onset of weakness 4 days ago, areflexia, and elevated cerebrospinal fluid protein. Nerve conduction study and electromyography (EMG) were performed on the day of admission when patient had severe limb weakness. EMG is most likely to reveal the following in the weak muscles

Choices	Spontaneous activity	Motor unit duration	Motor unit amplitude	Recruitment pattern
A	Positive sharp waves and fibrillation potentials	Short duration	Small amplitude	Early recruitment
B	Positive sharp waves and fibrillation potentials	Normal	Normal	Normal
C	Positive sharp waves and fibrillation potentials	Long duration	Large amplitude	Decreased recruitment
D	Normal	Normal	Normal	Decreased recruitment
E	Normal	Normal	Normal	Normal

157. A 40-year-old man is found to have diffuse myokymia on needle electromyography (EMG). Which of the following antibody testing is likely to be diagnostic?
A. Voltage-gated calcium channel antibody
B. Voltage-gated potassium channel antibody
C. Acetylcholine receptor (AChR) antibody
D. GM1 antibody
E. NT5C1A antibody

158. An ulnar nerve conduction study recording from the abductor digiti minimi is shown below. Needle electromyography (EMG) of the same muscle will likely reveal:

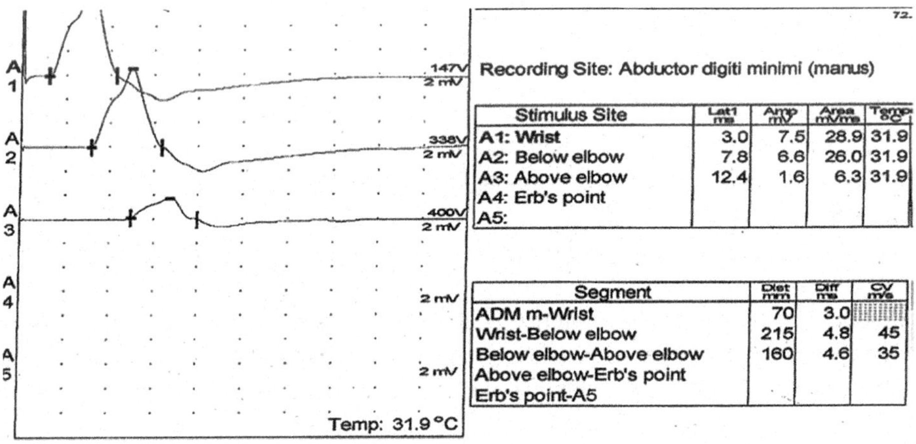

Stimulus Site	Lat1 ms	Amp mV	Area mVms	Temp °C
A1: Wrist	3.0	7.5	28.9	31.9
A2: Below elbow	7.8	6.6	26.0	31.9
A3: Above elbow	12.4	1.6	6.3	31.9
A4: Erb's point				
A5:				

Segment	Dist mm	Diff ms	CV m/s
ADM m-Wrist	70	3.0	
Wrist-Below elbow	215	4.8	45
Below elbow-Above elbow	160	4.6	35
Above elbow-Erb's point			
Erb's point-A5			

A. Positive sharp waves and fibrillation potentials
B. Large-amplitude and long-duration motor unit potentials
C. Reduced recruitment patterns
D. Increased insertional activity
E. Early recruitment patterns

159. A 34-year-old woman with chronic fatigue and various types of somatic pain is referred for evaluation of myasthenia gravis (MG). On examination, there is no clear weakness. Her slow repetitive stimulation studies performed at baseline and immediately after exercise are shown below. What is the appropriate interpretation?

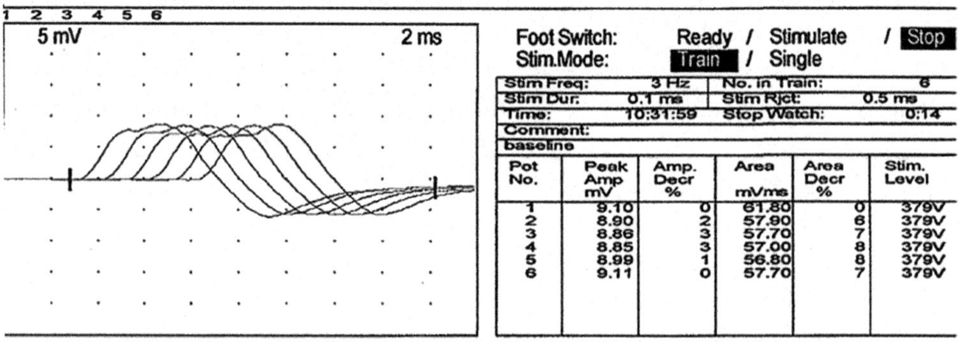

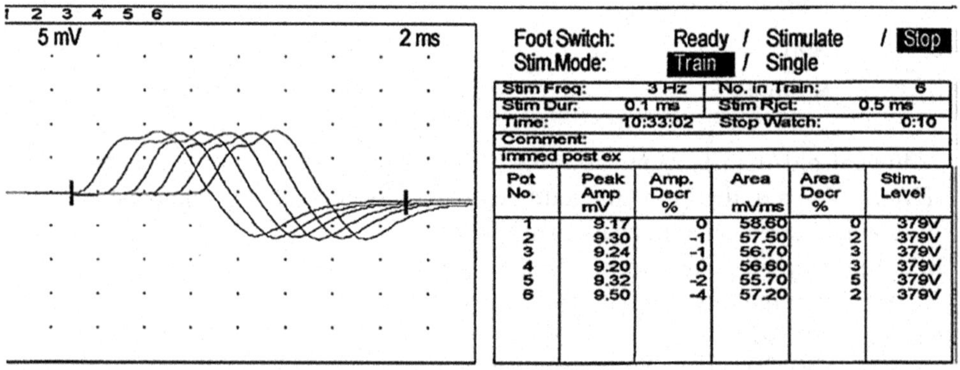

A. Significant decrement and repair
B. Significant decrement and facilitation
C. Normal repetitive stimulation
D. Significant decrement only
E. Significant decrement immediate postexercise and normal study at baseline

160. All of the following statements regarding the contribution of the reference electrode to the recorded waveform in the following motor nerve studies are true *except:*

A. In median nerve studies, the reference electrode does not contribute significantly to the waveform
B. In peroneal nerve studies, the reference electrode contributes significantly to the waveform
C. In tibial nerve studies, the reference electrode contributes significantly to the waveform
D. In ulnar nerve studies, the reference electrode contributes significantly to the waveform
E. In radial nerve studies, the reference electrode contributes significantly to the waveform

161. While performing needle electromyography (EMG), which of the following electrodiagnostic findings may be confused with fibrillation potentials?
A. Positive sharp waves
B. Fasciculation potentials
C. End-plate spikes
D. Tremor
E. Motor unit potentials

162. A needle electromyography (EMG) performed in a 60-year-old man with a history of weakness shows a recruitment frequency of 30 Hz. What is the most likely cause of his weakness?
A. Complete traumatic nerve injury with no reinnervation
B. Previous poliomyelitis
C. Lambert–Eaton myasthenic syndrome (LEMS)
D. Polymyositis
E. Myasthenia gravis (MG)

163. A neurology consultation was requested in a 40-year-old man in the hospital for evaluation of dysphagia. He recently had a motor vehicle accident and sustained extensive right leg injury that required right leg below-knee amputation. After surgery, he was noted to have severe dysarthria and dysphagia. On examination, he has mild facial weakness, ptosis, and mild distal limb weakness without any sensory loss. His wife reports a similar facial appearance for more than 10 years. She also reports similar but milder postanesthesia complication in the past. Electrodiagnostic study in this man will likely reveal
A. Myotonia on needle electromyography (EMG)
B. Decrement on repetitive stimulation
C. Significant increment on fast repetitive stimulation
D. Only myopathic motor unit potentials
E. Chronic neurogenic changes with reduced recruitment patterns

164. Which of the following parameters does not routinely effect the calculation of the F estimate?
A. Compound muscle action potential (CMAP) amplitude
B. CMAP distal latency
C. Conduction velocity
D. Distance between stimulator electrode to the spinal cord
E. Height of patient or limb length

165. Incomplete recovery from Guillain–Barré syndrome (GBS) can be characterized by all of the following pathological changes in the peripheral nerves or muscles *except*
A. Longer internodes
B. Shorter internodes
C. Onion bulb formation
D. Decrease in nerve fibers on skin biopsy
E. Loss of checkerboard pattern on muscle biopsy

166. Which of the following statements is true about steroid-induced myopathy?
- A. Type 1 muscle fiber atrophy is seen on muscle biopsy
- B. Type 2b muscle fiber atrophy is seen on muscle biopsy
- C. Irritative changes with positive sharp waves and fibrillation potentials are seen on electromyography (EMG)
- D. Nonflourinated corticosteroids are more likely to cause myopathy than flourinated corticosteroids
- E. Type 2a muscle fiber atrophy is seen on muscle biopsy

167. A 20-year-old man suffered an injury while riding his bike. He developed weakness, pain, and sensory loss in the left upper limb. Nerve conduction studies performed a few weeks later revealed normal median motor and ulnar motor and sensory responses. Left lateral antebrachial antidromic sensory response was absent. Findings on needle electromyography (EMG) of selected muscles in the left upper limb are shown below. What is the most likely localization?

Muscle	Spontaneous activity	Motor unit morphology	Recruitment
Left deltoid	3+ positive sharp waves and fibrillation potentials	No motor units seen	-
Left biceps brachii	3+ positive sharp waves and fibrillation potentials	No motor units seen	-
Left triceps	2+ positive sharp waves and fibrillation potentials	Mildly increased duration and amplitude	Mildly reduced
Left FDI	Normal	Normal	Normal
Left APB	Normal	Normal	Normal
Left serratus anterior	Normal	Normal	Normal

Note: APB, abductor pollicis brevis; FDI, first dorsal interosseous.

- A. C5, C6, and C7 roots
- B. Upper trunk of brachial plexus
- C. Posterior cord of brachial plexus
- D. Lower trunk of brachial plexus
- E. Medial cord of brachial plexus

168. A 25-year-old man developed a viral illness in the summer of 2012 followed by development of weakness in the left arm within a few weeks. On examination, he has severe weakness in the left hand and arm. A nerve conduction study performed 3 months later revealed the following findings. What is the most likely diagnosis?

Nerve conduction study	Latency	Amplitude	Conduction velocity
Left median sensory study (antidromic)	Normal	Normal	Normal
Left ulnar sensory study (antidromic)	Normal	Normal	Normal
Left radial sensory study (antidromic)	Normal	Normal	Normal
Left median motor study	No response	No response	-
Left ulnar motor study	No response	No response	-

A. Monomelic amyotrophy
B. West Nile-associated poliomyelitis type syndrome
C. Spinobulbar muscular atrophy (Kennedy's disease)
D. Early onset amyotrophic lateral sclerosis (ALS)
E. Multifocal motor neuropathy (MMN)

169. Which of the following drugs can cause a combination of toxic neuropathy and myopathy?
A. Metronidazole
B. Hydroxychloroquine
C. Isoniazid
D. Phenytoin
E. Cisplatin

170. A 25-year-old man was admitted to the intensive care unit (ICU) after a motor vehicle accident. He has a significant head injury and is not able to follow commands. His orthopedic surgeon would like to exclude radial neuropathy from a humerus fracture. A bedside radial nerve conduction study performed within 24 hours of the accident showed normal amplitude with stimulation at the elbow. What is the most appropriate conclusion?
A. Radial nerve is not injured
B. It is not possible to rule out radial nerve injury with the above information
C. Radial nerve is not injured below the elbow
D. Radial sensory response is needed to answer this question
E. Comparison with opposite limb distal radial compound muscle action potential (CMAP) amplitude is required

171. When requesting muscle biopsy in a patient with suspected myopathy, which of the following should be considered to increase the yield of the biopsy?
A. Biopsy a muscle with normal strength (5/5 on Medical Research Council [MRC] scale)
B. Biopsy a muscle with mild weakness (4/5 on MRC scale)
C. Biopsy a muscle with severe weakness (2–3/5 on MRC scale)
D. Obtain an MRI of the muscle before biopsy
E. Ideally select a muscle with no function so that larger portion can be obtained for biopsy

172. Which of the following neuromuscular manifestations may be seen in amiodarone toxicity?
A. Severe peripheral neuropathy only
B. Proximal myopathy only
C. Both peripheral neuropathy and myopathy
D. Neuromuscular junction dysfunction
E. Motor neuron disease

173. A 35-year-old man had extensive injuries in a motor vehicle accident. A few weeks after discharge from the intensive care unit (ICU), while underlying rehabilitative therapy, he was noted to have significant weakness in the right upper limb. Findings on needle electromyography (EMG) are shown in the table below. What is the best localization based on these findings?

Muscle	Spontaneous activity	Motor unit morphology	Recruitment
Right deltoid	2+ positive sharp and fibrillation potentials	Large duration motor unit potentials	Reduced
Right triceps	1+ positive sharp and fibrillation potentials	Large duration motor unit potentials	Reduced
Right biceps	Normal	Normal	Normal
Right first dorsal interosseous	Normal	Normal	Normal
Right abductor pollicis brevis	Normal	Normal	Normal

A. Lateral cord
B. Medial cord
C. Posterior cord
D. Lower trunk
E. Upper trunk

174. A 45-year-old man presents with a 5-year history of slowly progressive speech and swallowing difficulty. He recently noticed some limb weakness and this prompted a referral to a neuromuscular physician. On examination, he has dysarthria, flaccid limb weakness, decreased reflexes, and occasional fasciculations. Findings on sensory nerve conduction studies are shown below. Which of the following conditions does the patient most likely have?

Sensory nerve	Latency	Amplitude
Sural antidromic study	Absent response	Absent response
Median antidromic study	3.2	40
Ulnar antidromic study	3.1	25

A. Sporadic amyotrophic lateral sclerosis (ALS)
B. Primary lateral sclerosis (PLS)
C. Spinobulbar muscular atrophy
D. Spinal muscular atrophy (SMA)
E. Upper motor predominant ALS

175. A median motor study in a 60-year-old woman is shown below. A1 is with wrist stimulation and A2 is with elbow stimulation. The distance between the two stimulation points is 225 mm. Which of the following conclusions is correct?

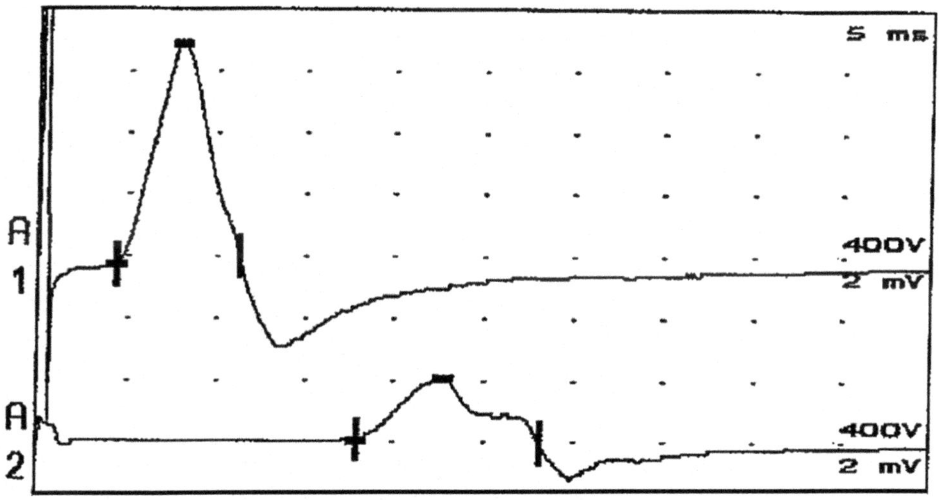

A. Conduction velocity is less than 20 m/sec and there is a partial conduction block
B. Conduction velocity is 30 m/sec and there is only an abnormal temporal dispersion
C. Conduction velocity is 50 m/sec and there is a partial conduction block
D. Conduction velocity is less than 20 m/sec and there is only an abnormal temporal dispersion
E. Conduction velocity is 50m/sec and there is abnormal temporal dispersion

176. A 20-year-old basketball player noticed painless shoulder weakness when a heavy dumbbell fell on his neck while lifting weights. He was able to play but has noticed difficulty performing push-ups. A sensory nerve conduction study revealed decreased median and radial sensory amplitudes. These findings best localize to:
A. C5 root injury
B. C6 root injury
C. Upper trunk brachial plexopathy
D. Spinal accessory nerve injury
E. Lower trunk brachial plexopathy

177. A 30-year-old woman presents with a 2-month history of ptosis, double vision, facial weakness, and mild proximal limb weakness. Myasthenia gravis (MG) is suspected and the patient is referred for electrodiagnostic studies. The technologist performs 3 Hz repetitive stimulation of the right ulnar nerve, which is normal. What is the next best step to do?
A. Give patient oral pyridostigmine and repeat the study
B. Repeat the study using 20 Hz stimulation
C. Perform repetitive stimulation of the facial nerve
D. Warm the hand by 2°C and repeat the ulnar repetitive study
E. Single-fiber electromyography (EMG) of the extensor digitorum communis muscle

178. While performing a sural sensory nerve conduction study, the examiner notices that the leg feels cold to the touch. Which of the following is the most appropriate step before continuing with the study?

A. Measure the temperature and proceed with nerve conduction study testing
B. Compare the response to motor studies in the lower limb
C. Measure the temperature and warm the lower limb
D. Measure the temperature and use formulas to correct for latency and velocity
E. Document colder foot temperature and let the referring physician decide the relevance of technical limitation

179. A 23-year-old man presented to the neurology clinic with a history of multiple episodes of weakness. Each episode usually lasts a few hours. He originally noticed these episodes during his teenage years. Episodes are often preceded by prolonged activity or large meals. On examination, he did not have any clinical myotonia. Nerve conduction studies (NCS) and electromyography (EMG) were done. Which of the following is most likely on EMG?

Choices	Spontaneous activity	Motor unit duration	Motor unit amplitude	Recruitment pattern
A	Normal	Normal	Normal	Normal
B	Positive sharp waves and fibrillation potentials	Normal	Normal	Normal
C	Positive sharp waves and fibrillation potentials	Normal	Normal	Decreased recruitment
D	Normal	Normal	Normal	Decreased recruitment
E	Normal	Increased	Increased	Early recruitment

180. Slow repetitive stimulations at baseline and immediately after exercise in a 40-year-old man with weakness are shown below. These studies are suggestive of:

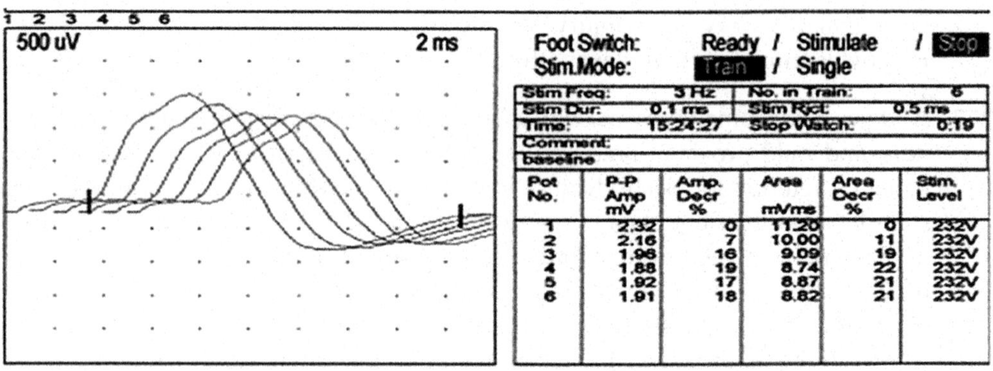

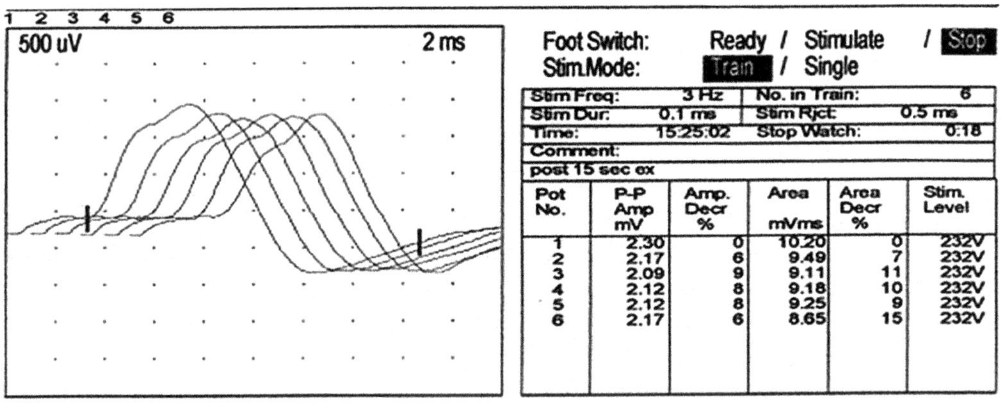

A. Significant decrement and repair
B. Significant decrement and facilitation
C. Normal repetitive stimulation
D. Significant decrement only
E. Technically very poor study, and so unable to interpret

181. In a patient with suspected myasthenia gravis (MG), needle electromyography (EMG) is most likely to reveal:
A. Positive sharp waves and fibrillation potentials
B. Large-amplitude polyphasic motor unit potentials
C. Variation in motor unit amplitude
D. Increased recruitment frequency if the muscle is weak
E. Positive sharp waves and fibrillation potentials with normal motor unit morphology

182. Motor unit potentials noted on needle electromyography (EMG) of the right tibialis anterior muscle are shown below. This type of motor unit morphology may be seen in which of the following conditions?

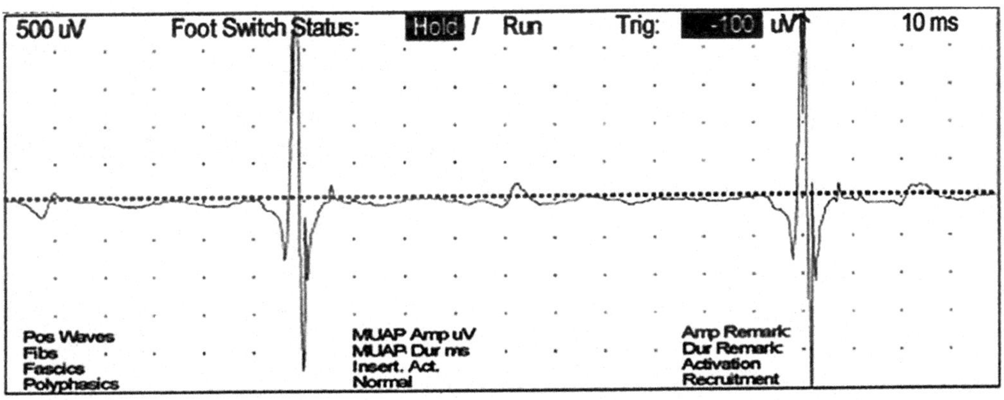

A. Toxic myopathies
B. Chronic polyradiculopathy
C. Chronic neuromuscular junction diseases such as myasthenia gravis
D. Acute inflammatory demyelinating polyradiculoneuropathy (AIDP)
E. Steroid myopathy

183. A 30-year-old female had isolated lower trunk brachial plexopathy with associated weakness and sensory loss. Deep tendon reflex testing would reveal which of the following?
A. Absent triceps reflex
B. Absent biceps and triceps reflexes
C. Absent biceps, brachioradialis, and triceps reflexes
D. Intact biceps, brachioradialis, and triceps reflexes
E. Absent brachioradialis reflex with normal biceps and triceps reflexes

184. A 25-year-old professional volleyball player developed recent right shoulder pain. Extensive workup for any shoulder joint pathology was negative. Routine nerve conduction studies in the right upper limb including Erb point stimulation were normal. Electromyography (EMG) of which of the following muscles might be most useful?
A. Triceps
B. Serratus anterior
C. Infraspinatus
D. Deltoid
E. Pectoralis major

185. A 45-year-old man has a few-month history of weight loss and low appetite. Extensive evaluation found an enlarged supraclavicular lymph node. He underwent biopsy of the lymph node. After the biopsy, he developed pain and weakness in his left shoulder area. Electromyography (EMG) of which of the following muscles is most likely to be abnormal?
A. Deltoid
B. Trapezius
C. Serratus anterior
D. Supraspinatus and infraspinatus
E. Biceps brachii

186. Needle electromyography (EMG) of which of the following muscles would help differentiate L5 radiculopathy from peroneal mononeuropathy *above* the popliteal fossa?
A. Short head of biceps femoris
B. Tibialis posterior
C. Medial gastrocnemius
D. Peroneus brevis
E. Tibialis anterior

187. Which of the following findings on a muscle biopsy is characteristic of dermatomyositis?
A. Rimmed vacuoles
B. Perifascicular atrophy
C. Endomysial inflammatory infiltrates
D. Myofiber necrosis
E. Cox negative fibers

188. Which of the following statements is true regarding the electrodiagnostic changes in patients with botulism?
A. Low compound muscle action potential (CMAP) amplitude and decrement on fast repetitive stimulation
B. Low-CMAP amplitude and increment with slow repetitive stimulation
C. Low-CMAP amplitude and normal findings on needle electromyography (EMG)
D. Low-CMAP amplitude, increment with fast repetitive stimulation, and active denervation potentials in weak muscles
E. Normal CMAP amplitude and increment with slow repetitive stimulation

189. Which of the following is the earliest needle electromyography (EMG) change seen in a patient with acute demyelinating polyneuropathy?
A. Abundant positive sharp waves and fibrillation potentials
B. Polyphasic motor unit potentials
C. Complex repetitive discharges
D. Decreased recruitment of motor units
E. Small duration motor unit potentials

190. In Martin–Gruber anastomosis (MGA), which of the following changes may be seen with median and ulnar motor studies with standard distal and proximal stimulations at wrist and elbow?
A. Less than 10% drop in ulnar amplitude on proximal stimulation
B. Less than 10% drop in median amplitude on proximal stimulation
C. More than 10% drop in ulnar amplitude on proximal stimulation
D. More than 10% drop in median amplitude on proximal stimulation
E. More than 10% drop in median and ulnar amplitudes on proximal stimulation

191. Continued insertional activity after moving a concentric electromyography (EMG) needle is considered normal if it lasts less than how many milliseconds?
A. 100 ms
B. 200 ms
C. 300 ms
D. 400 ms
E. 500 ms

192. A 60-year-old man presented with right foot drop that started a few months ago after significant weight loss. On examination, he has severe weakness in the right tibialis anterior and peroneal group of muscles. Needle electromyography (EMG) of the right tibialis anterior is shown below. In addition, he also has motor unit potentials with long duration and large amplitude and a decreased recruitment pattern. These findings in combination suggest which of the following?

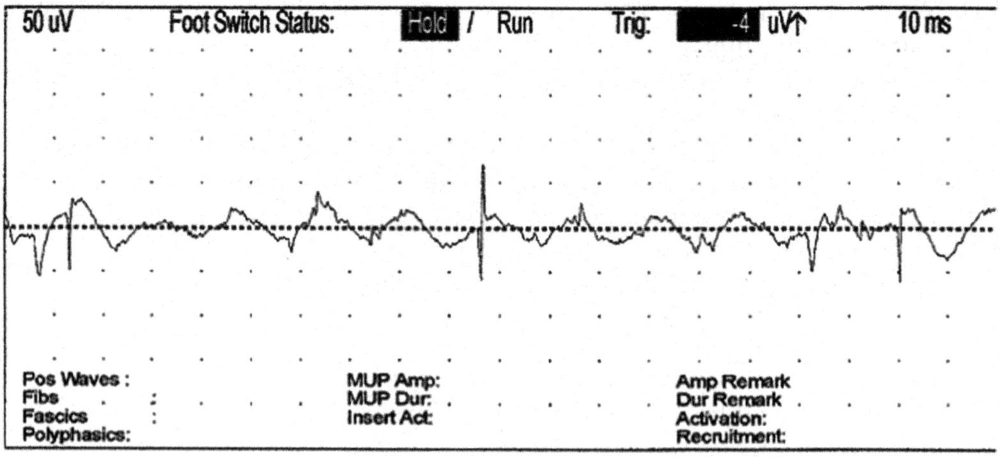

A. Only chronic reinnervation changes in the right tibias anterior muscle
B. Both active denervation and chronic reinnervation changes
C. Only active denervation changes
D. These findings are suggestive of focal myopathic process.
E. These findings can be normal in older patients.

193. A 20-year-old woman is admitted with progressive ascending weakness and sensory symptoms suggestive of Guillain–Barré syndrome (GBS). During the electrodiagnostic study, the technologist performs sural sensory response, which was normal. Before peroneal or tibial studies can be done, the patient requests that further studies be stopped as she cannot tolerate the testing. Based on the normal sural response, what would be the best conclusion or recommendation?
A. The patient does not have GBS
B. GBS cannot be ruled out because normal sural sensory response is not uncommon in GBS
C. Because sural sensory response is normal, the patient does not have any type of neuropathy
D. Repeat the study after the patient is sedated under anesthesia
E. Sural sensory response is always normal in GBS syndromes

194. Vitamin B6 toxicity typically leads to which of the following electrodiagnostic findings?
A. Absent motor responses
B. Absent motor responses and severe denervation in distal muscles
C. Absent sensory responses
D. Normal nerve conduction studies but denervation in proximal and distal muscles
E. "Myopathic motor unit potentials" on needle electromyography (EMG)

195. A 45-year-old woman presents with a few week history of weakness and difficulty climbing steps. On examination, she mostly has proximal weakness in her upper and lower limbs with normal distal examination. Reflexes and sensory function are preserved. She also noticed a new skin rash over her neck and chest. Which of the following combinations of findings is most likely to be found on the needle electromyography (EMG) of proximal muscles?

Choices	Spontaneous activity	Motor unit duration	Motor unit amplitude	Recruitment pattern
A	Normal	Normal	Normal	Normal
B	Positive sharp waves and fibrillation potentials	Short duration	Small amplitude	Early recruitment
C	Positive sharp waves and fibrillation potentials	Normal	Normal	Normal
D	Positive sharp waves and fibrillation potentials	Long duration	Large amplitude	Decreased recruitment
E	Normal	Short duration	Small amplitude	Normal

196. Bifid sensory nerve action potentials in children are seen because of which of the following?
A. Poor technique
B. Normal variant in children because of different degrees of myelination
C. Mild axonal neuropathy
D. Demyelinating neuropathy
E. Severe axonal neuropathy

197. A 70-year-old man, suspected to have brachial plexopathy based on history and examination, underwent nerve conduction studies. Motor and sensory responses of the median and ulnar nerves are summarized below. What is the most likely localization?

Nerve conduction study	Amplitude	Conduction velocity
Median motor response	Absent response	-
Median antidromic sensory response	Normal amplitude	Normal conduction velocity
Ulnar motor response	Absent response	-
Ulnar antidromic sensory response	Absent response	-

A. Upper trunk
B. Medial cord
C. Lateral cord
D. C8 and T1 roots
E. Posterior cord

198. Which of the following electromyography (EMG) findings is most likely in a patient with polymyositis?
A. Long-duration motor unit potentials with reduced recruitment patterns
B. Short-duration motor unit potentials with reduced recruitment patterns
C. Positive sharp waves/fibrillation potentials and short-duration motor unit potentials
D. Fasciculation potentials and short-duration motor unit potentials
E. Long-duration motor unit potentials with normal recruitment patterns

199. A 45-year-old man recently noticed weakness in his right hand. He works in the construction industry, and uses his palms and hands for manual labor. He does not report any sensory loss. His median motor and sensory studies were normal. Ulnar motor study with abductor digiti minimi recording and ulnar sensory study were also normal. Needle electromyography (EMG) revealed active denervation in the first dorsal interosseous muscle but not in the abductor digiti minimi or abductor pollicis brevis muscles. Which of the following is the most likely cause of his weakness?
A. Medial cord brachial plexopathy
B. Anterior interosseous neuropathy
C. Ulnar neuropathy in the forearm
D. Ulnar neuropathy in the palm
E. Ulnar neuropathy at the elbow

For Questions 200 to 204:

A 61-year-old African American man presented with recent onset eyelid droopiness and weakness over 4 weeks. He used to lift heavy weights but recently noticed difficulty lifting small objects above his head. A few days before coming to the hospital, he noticed a mild right eye droop. Initial examination was significant for right eye ptosis, facial weakness, mild weakness of neck flexion, and proximal limb weakness. The rest of the strength examination, reflexes, and sensation were normal.

200. Where does this presentation best localize to?
A. Peripheral nerve
B. Muscle
C. Neuromuscular junction (NMJ)
D. Anterior horn cells
E. Multiple cranial nerves and roots

201. Which of the following tests in the above patient is most likely to provide a quick confirmation of the diagnosis?
A. Creatine phosphokinase (CPK) level
B. Routine nerve conduction study to look for neuropathy
C. Repetitive nerve stimulation
D. Needle electromyography (EMG) testing
E. Spinal fluid analysis

202. What does the study obtained from the ulnar nerve shown below reveal in this patient?

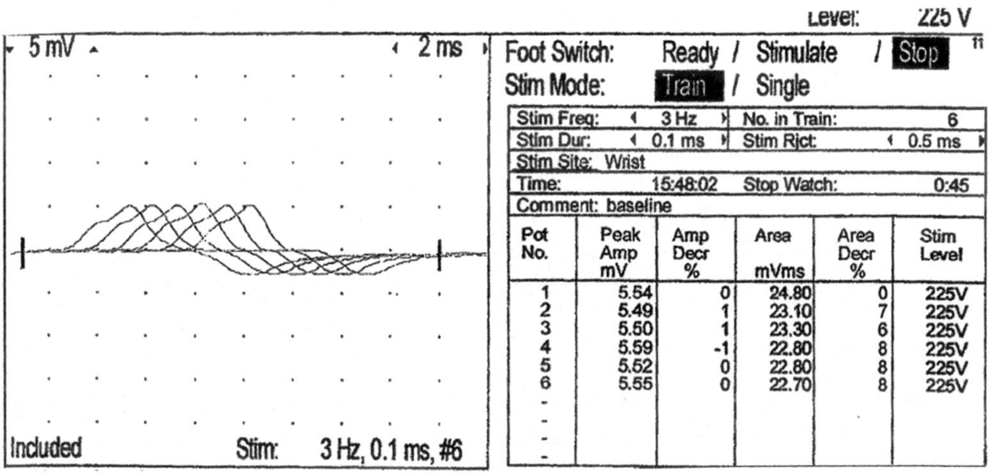

A. Abnormal decrement consistent with myasthenia gravis (MG)
B. Normal ulnar slow repetitive nerve stimulation
C. Abnormal increment consistent with Lambert–Eaton myasthenic syndrome (LEMS)
D. Normal ulnar fast repetitive stimulation
E. Abnormal ulnar fast repetitive stimulation

203. What does the study obtained from the right spinal accessory shown below reveal in this patient?

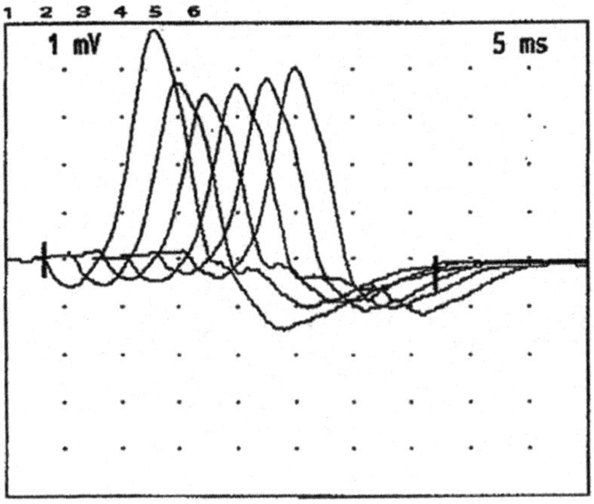

FOOT SWITCH: READY / STIMULATE / STOP
STIM.MODE: TRAIN / SINGLE

STIM FREQ: 3 Hz	NO. IN TRAIN 6
STIM DUR: 0.1 ms	STIM ADJST: 0.5 ms
TIME: 14:41:06	STOP WATCH: 0:31

COMMENT:
baseline

POT NO.	PEAK AMP mV	AMP. DECR %	AREA mVms	AREA DECR %	STIM. LEVEL
1	4.87	0	42.50	0	138V
2	3.67	25	30.10	29	138V
3	3.35	31	27.20	36	138V
4	3.73	23	30.00	29	138V
5	3.71	24	30.20	29	138V
6	3.94	19	32.40	24	138V
7					
8					
9					
10					

A. Abnormal decrement consistent with myasthenia gravis (MG)
B. Normal spinal accessory slow repetitive nerve stimulation
C. Abnormal increment consistent with Lambert–Eaton myasthenic syndrome
D. Normal spinal accessory fast repetitive stimulation
E. Abnormal increment of spinal accessory slow repetitive stimulation

204. Which of the following tests would be most appropriate to achieve diagnose in this patient?
A. Antibody testing for voltage-gated calcium channel
B. Acetylcholine receptor (AChR) antibodies and CT scan of chest
C. Muscle-specific kinase antibody (MuSK) and CT scan of chest
D. Paraneoplastic panel and positron emission tomography (PET) scan
E. Magnetic resonance (MR) brain and spine along with spinal fluid analysis

For Questions 205 to 209:

A 20-year-old college student presents with difficulty walking for 5 years but recently developed an increased tendency to trip and fall along with mild weakness in her hands. She also reports mild numbness in her feet. She denies any pain. Her birth and initial development were normal, but as a child she did not perform well in sports. On examination, cranial nerves are normal. Proximal limb strength is normal. She has distal weakness with bilateral foot drop and moderate finger extension and abduction weakness. She also has high-arched feet and atrophy of foot intrinsic muscles. Deep tendon reflexes are absent and there is length-dependent sensory loss.

205. What is the best neuroanatomical localization in the above patient?
A. Peripheral nerve and spinal cord
B. Peripheral nerve and muscle
C. Peripheral nerve only
D. Muscle only
E. Cervical and lumbosacral roots

206. What is the next best diagnostic step for this patient?
A. Nerve conduction studies
B. Repetitive nerve stimulation
C. Brain and spine MRI
D. Genetic testing
E. Spinal fluid analysis

207. Lower limb nerve conduction studies revealed absent motor and sensory responses. What does the upper limb study shown below reveal?

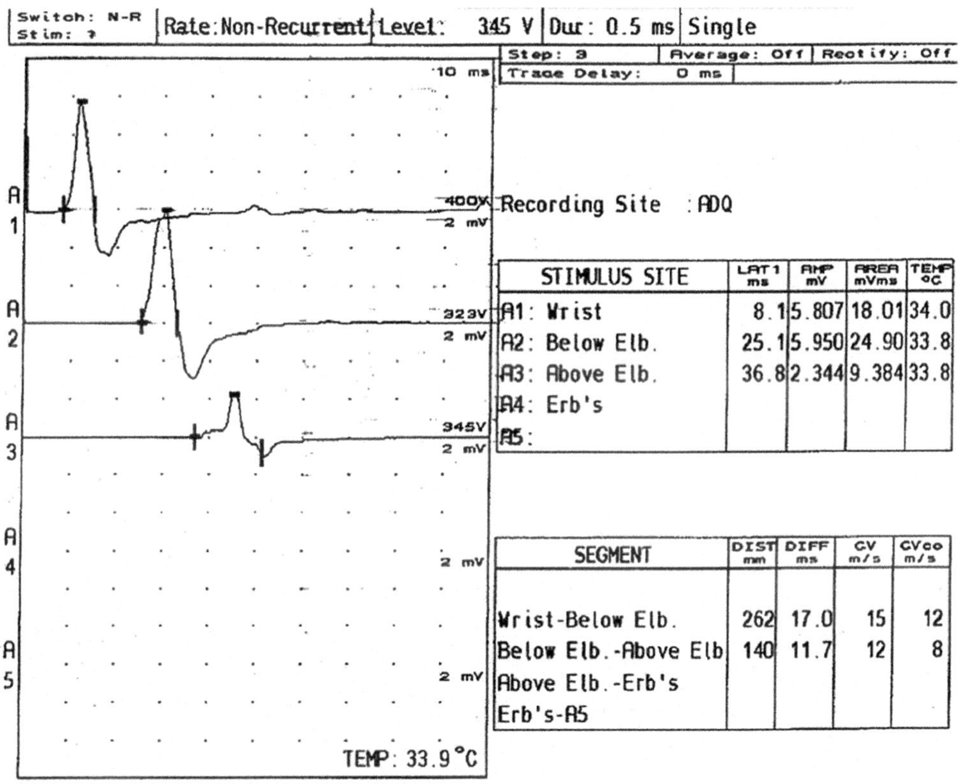

A. Demyelinating neuropathy with profoundly diminished conduction velocity and a partial conduction block
B. Demyelinating neuropathy with abnormal temporal dispersion
C. Demyelinating neuropathy with profoundly diminished conduction velocity
D. Axonal neuropathy
E. Mixed polyneuropathy

208. Based on the history, examination, and the above nerve conduction study, what is the most likely diagnosis in the above patient?
A. Acquired demyelinating polyneuropathy
B. Hereditary demyelinating polyneuropathy
C. Acquired axonal polyneuropathy
D. Distal myopathy
E. Hereditary axonal polyneuropathy

209. What is the next most appropriate test to perform in the above patient?
  A. Peripheral myelin protein (PMP) deletion/duplication genetic test
  B. Mitofusin (MFN) mutation test
  C. Spinal fluid analysis
  D. Muscle biopsy
  E. Sural nerve biopsy

For Questions 210 to 213:

A 55-year-old woman presented with progressive weakness over 4 months. Initially, she noticed increasing difficulty with climbing steps and getting up from the floor. She recently noticed difficulty lifting her arms when reaching above her head or brushing her hair. She reports a mild dull ache in her muscles. She does not have any skin rash. On examination, she has moderate proximal weakness in the upper and lower limbs with preserved distal limb strength. Deep tendon reflexes and sensory examination were normal. Cranial nerve examination revealed mild facial weakness. The rest of the neurological examination is normal.

210. The above clinical presentation best localizes to
  A. Peripheral nerve
  B. Skeletal muscle
  C. Neuromuscular junction
  D. Spinal cord
  E. Anterior horn cell

211. The above patient underwent a routine nerve conduction study as shown below. What does this tibial motor nerve reveal?

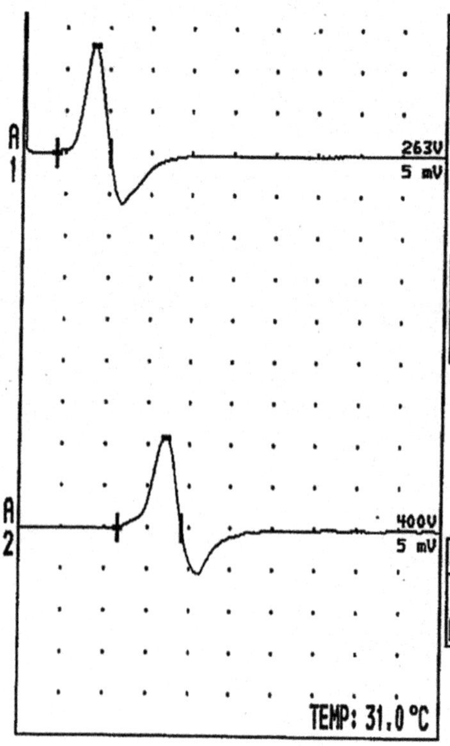

Recording Site :Abductor hallucis

STIMULUS SITE	LAT1 ms	DUR ms	AMP mV	AREA mVms
A1: Ankle	3.9	6.2	12.94	32.64
A2: Pop. fossa	11.5	7.5	10.81	34.33

SEGMENT	DIST mm	DIFF ms	CV m/s	CVco m/s
Ankle-Pop. fossa	405	7.6	53	55

A. Axonal neuropathy
B. Demyelinating neuropathy
C. Normal study
D. Decreased motor amplitude, but cause is unclear
E. Prolonged proximal motor latency

212. Needle electromyography (EMG) of the deltoid muscle from the above patient is shown below (trace A is at rest and trace B is on active muscle contraction). What do they reveal?

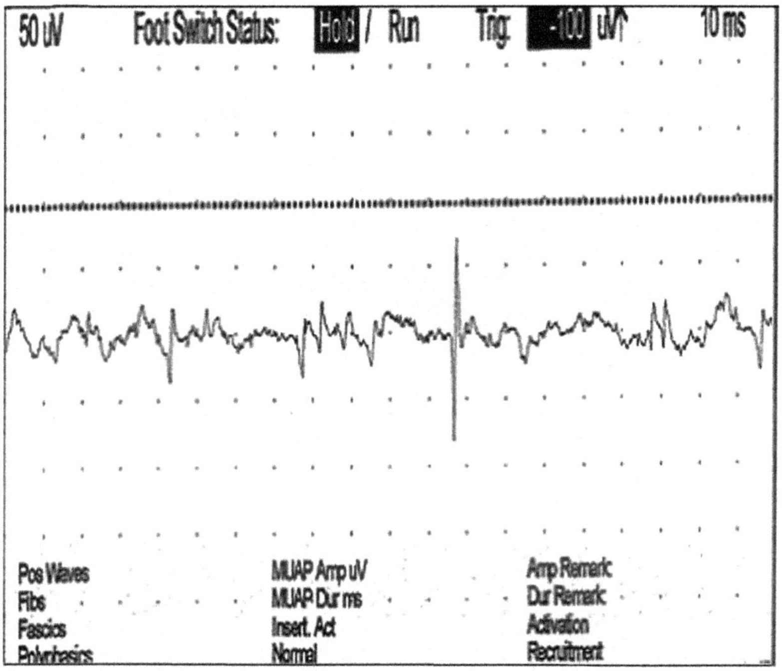

A

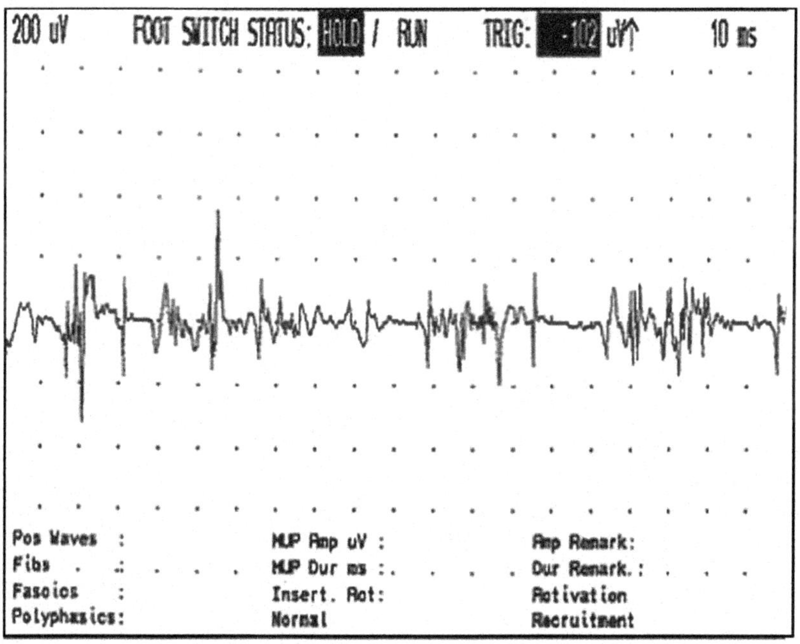

B

A. Positive sharp waves only at rest and normal motor unit potentials on contraction
B. Fibrillation potentials only at rest and normal motor unit potentials on contraction
C. Positive sharp waves and fibrillation potentials during rest and short-duration motor unit potentials on contraction
D. Positive sharp waves and fibrillation potentials at rest and long-duration motor unit potentials on contraction
E. Normal activity at rest and short-duration motor unit potentials on contraction

213. Needle electromyography (EMG) obtained from the deltoid in this patient with minimal effort against resistance is shown below. What does it show?

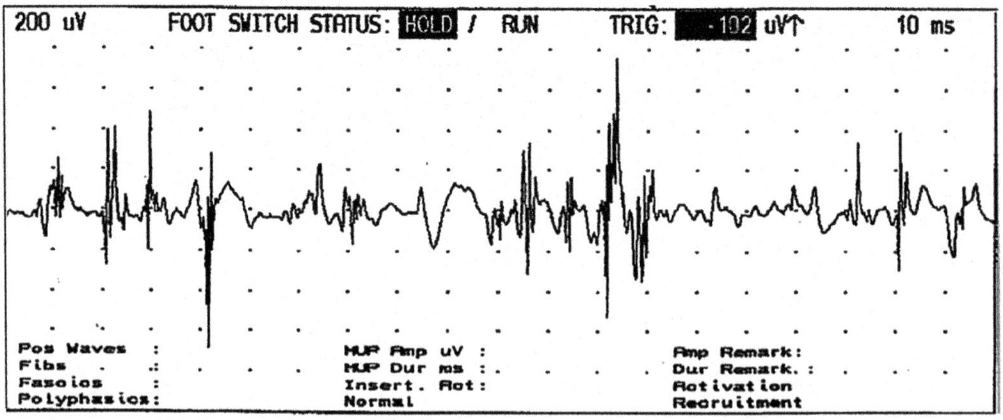

A. Decreased recruitment pattern
B. Normal recruitment pattern
C. Early recruitment pattern
D. Hyperexcitable recruitment pattern
E. Severely reduced recruitment patterns

For Questions 214 to 218:

A 55-year-old man presents with severe fatigue and weakness for over 4 months and recent onset of dry mouth. He does not report any obvious diplopia. He is a chronic smoker. On examination, he has mild facial weakness, mild to moderate weakness of neck flexion, and severe proximal limb weakness. Deep tendon reflexes are absent. Sensory examination is normal.

214. The most likely neuroanatomical localization for his symptoms is
A. Peripheral nerve
B. Neuromuscular junction (NMJ)
C. Muscle
D. Anterior horn cells
E. Cervical, thoracic, and lumbosacral roots

215. Routine nerve conduction study and needle electromyography (EMG) study in the above patient is expected to reveal which of the following?

A. Absent sensory responses
B. Decreased conduction velocity
C. Reduced motor amplitudes
D. Positive sharp waves and fibrillation potentials
E. Absent F-wave responses

216. Ulnar motor study done in this patient is shown below. Top trace is at baseline and the bottom trace is after 10 seconds of exercise. What does it reveal?

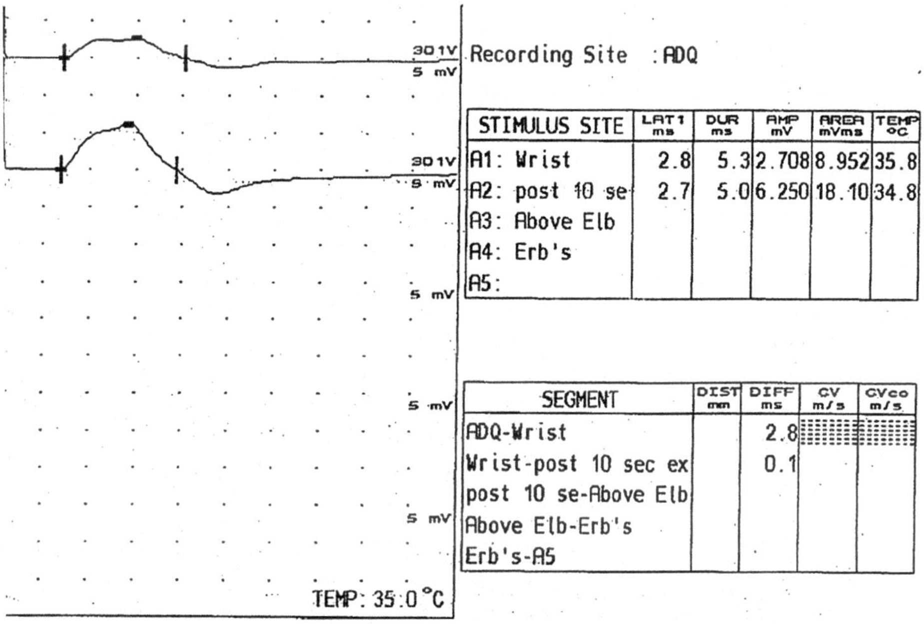

A. Normal increase in compound muscle action potential (CMAP) amplitude after 10 seconds of exercise
B. Decreased motor amplitude on repeat stimulation, suggestive of postsynaptic neuromuscular junction (NMJ) disorder
C. Increased motor amplitude on repeat stimulation, suggestive of presynaptic NMJ disorder
D. Technically limited study
E. This can study cannot be interpreted without proximal nerve stimulation

217. Which of the following tests will have the highest yield for diagnosis in the above patient?

A. Antibody testing for voltage-gated calcium channel antibody
B. Acetylcholine receptor (AChR) antibodies and CT scan of chest
C. Muscle-specific kinase antibody (MuSK) and CT scan of chest
D. Paraneoplastic panel and positron emission tomography (PET) scan
E. Spinal fluid analysis and magnetic resonance (MR) brain

218. Which of the following statements is true about the condition this patient has?

A. This is always a paraneoplastic syndrome
B. This can be either an autoimmune or paraneoplastic syndrome
C. The prognosis is very poor and life expectancy is always less than 1 year
D. Because this is a relatively common condition, there is generally no time lag between symptom onset and diagnosis
E. This condition responds dramatically well to treatment

219. A 35-year-old woman presented to the emergency department (ED) with progressive weakness over few months. What does the motor nerve conduction study waveform below reveal?

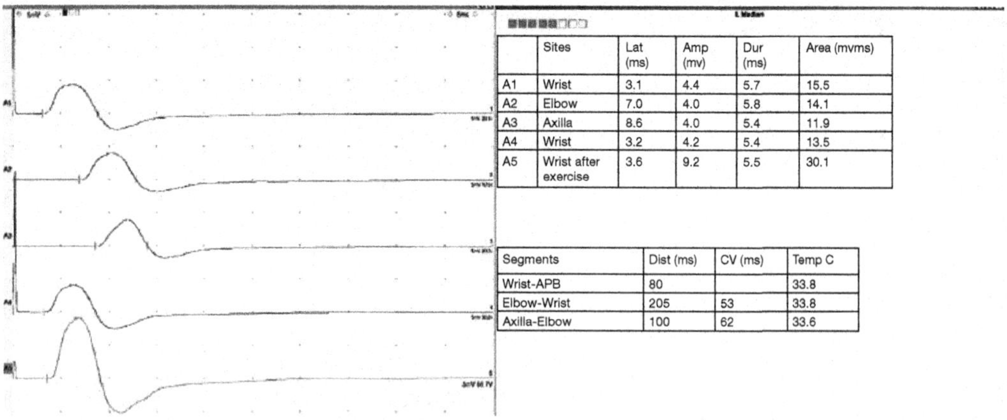

	Sites	Lat (ms)	Amp (mv)	Dur (ms)	Area (mvms)
A1	Wrist	3.1	4.4	5.7	15.5
A2	Elbow	7.0	4.0	5.8	14.1
A3	Axilla	8.6	4.0	5.4	11.9
A4	Wrist	3.2	4.2	5.4	13.5
A5	Wrist after exercise	3.6	9.2	5.5	30.1

Segments	Dist (ms)	CV (ms)	Temp C
Wrist-APB	80		33.8
Elbow-Wrist	205	53	33.8
Axilla-Elbow	100	62	33.6

A. Normal motor left median study
B. Normal median compound muscle action potential (CMAP) amplitude with normal postexercise increase in CMAP amplitude
C. Reduced CMAP amplitude at baseline and >100% increase in CMAP amplitude after brief exercise
D. Normal CMAP amplitude, but severely reduced velocity
E. Prolonged distal latency and reduced CMAP amplitude with preserved velocity.

220. A 48-year-old woman with progressive weakness is referred for nerve conduction and electromyography (EMG) studies. The following median motor study is most suggestive of?

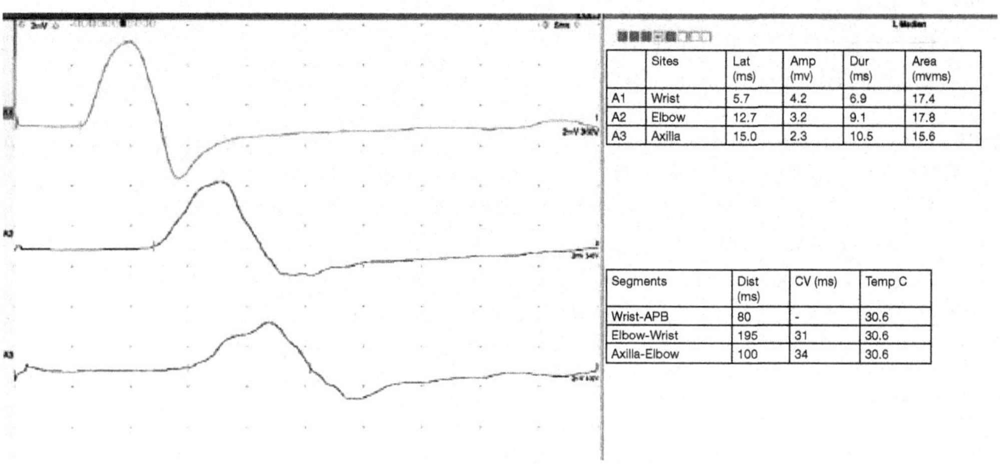

	Sites	Lat (ms)	Amp (mv)	Dur (ms)	Area (mvms)
A1	Wrist	5.7	4.2	6.9	17.4
A2	Elbow	12.7	3.2	9.1	17.8
A3	Axilla	15.0	2.3	10.5	15.6

Segments	Dist (ms)	CV (ms)	Temp C
Wrist-APB	80	-	30.6
Elbow-Wrist	195	31	30.6
Axilla-Elbow	100	34	30.6

A. Axonal polyneuropathy
B. Demyelinating polyneuropathy
C. Normal motor nerve conduction study
D. Distal myopathy
E. Motor neuron diseases such as amyotrophic lateral sclerosis (ALS)

221. A 50-year-old woman reports a history of diplopia and limb weakness in the past which improved with a short course of prednisone. She recently noticed similar limb weakness but without ocular symptoms. She was referred to a neurodiagnostic lab, and the following study was performed. What does it reveal?

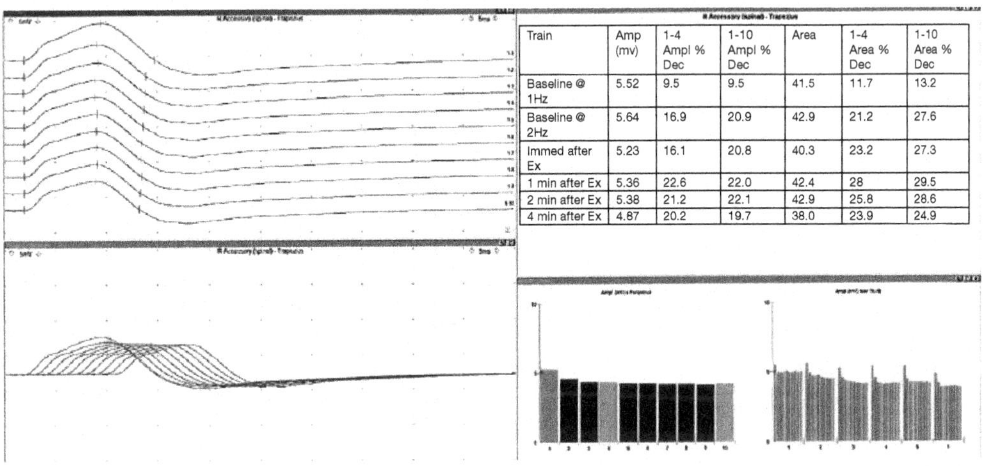

Train	Amp (mv)	1-4 Ampl % Dec	1-10 Ampl % Dec	Area	1-4 Area % Dec	1-10 Area % Dec
Baseline @ 1Hz	5.52	9.5	9.5	41.5	11.7	13.2
Baseline @ 2Hz	5.64	16.9	20.9	42.9	21.2	27.6
Immed after Ex	5.23	16.1	20.8	40.3	23.2	27.3
1 min after Ex	5.36	22.6	22.0	42.4	28	29.5
2 min after Ex	5.38	21.2	22.1	42.9	25.8	28.6
4 min after Ex	4.87	20.2	19.7	38.0	23.9	24.9

A. Normal slow repetitive stimulation
B. Abnormal slow repetitive stimulation with significant decrement
C. Abnormal slow repetitive stimulation with significant increment
D. Abnormal fast repetitive stimulation with significant decrement
E. Abnormal fast repetitive stimulation with significant decrement

222. Slow repetitive stimulation was performed in a 30-year-old with weakness. What does this study reveal?

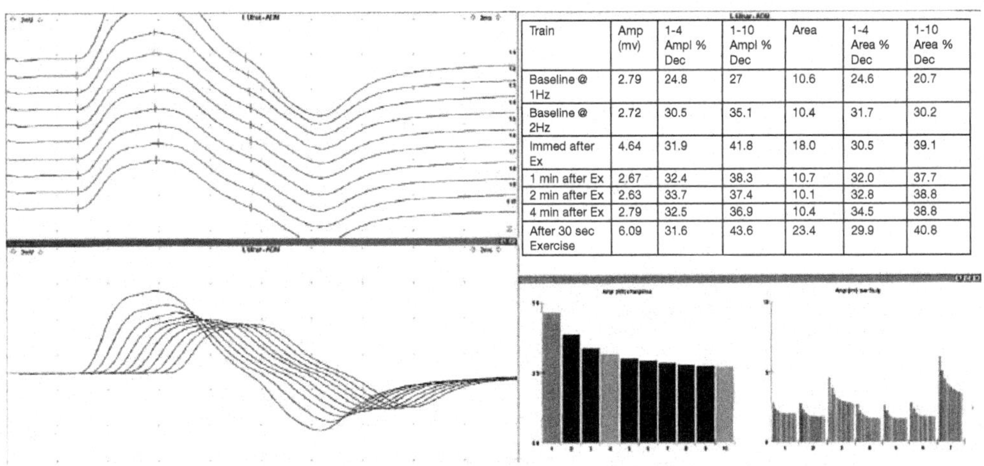

Train	Amp (mv)	1-4 Ampl % Dec	1-10 Ampl % Dec	Area	1-4 Area % Dec	1-10 Area % Dec
Baseline @ 1Hz	2.79	24.8	27	10.6	24.6	20.7
Baseline @ 2Hz	2.72	30.5	35.1	10.4	31.7	30.2
Immed after Ex	4.64	31.9	41.8	18.0	30.5	39.1
1 min after Ex	2.67	32.4	38.3	10.7	32.0	37.7
2 min after Ex	2.63	33.7	37.4	10.1	32.8	38.8
4 min after Ex	2.79	32.5	36.9	10.4	34.5	38.8
After 30 sec Exercise	6.09	31.6	43.6	23.4	29.9	40.8

A. Significant decrement on repetitive stimulation
B. Significant decrement on repetitive stimulation and facilitation
C. Significant increment on repetitive stimulation
D. Significant increment on repetitive stimulation and facilitation
E. Normal study

223. A 36-year-old man underwent left hip surgery under general anesthesia. Two to 3 days postoperatively he noticed severe pain over the left shoulder. Over the next 2 weeks, the pain gradually improved to a residual dull ache. However, as the pain improved, he noticed left shoulder weakness. On examination he has left elbow flexion weakness along with scapular winging. He thinks his left arm might have been positioned in an unusual way during the surgery. The most likely cause for his left arm weakness is:
A. Neuropraxic injury to brachial plexus from positioning
B. Inflammatory brachial plexopathy
C. C5/6 radiculopathy
D. Traumatic brachial plexopathy
E. Postsurgical inflammatory neuropathy associated with hip surgery

224. Performing needle electromyography (EMG) on which of the following muscles would help to differentiate a femoral neuropathy from a lumbosacral plexopathy in a 70-year-old man?
A. Iliopsoas muscles
B. Vastus lateralis muscles
C. Adductor longus
D. Lumbar (L2–L4) paraspinals
E. Gluteus medius or gluteus maximus muscles

225. Neuromuscular ultrasound has been shown to assist with the diagnosis of focal compressive neuropathies. Which of the following is likely to be seen when performing median nerve ultrasound in a patient with carpal tunnel syndrome?
A. Increased median nerve cross sectional area
B. Increased vascularity in the nerve
C. Hypoechogenicity
D. Reduced mobility of the nerve
E. All of the above

226. A 22-year-old reports intermittent episodes of weakness and falls. Which of the following electrodiagnostic tests is most helpful to diagnosis periodic paralysis?
A. Single-fiber electromyography (EMG)
B. Short exercise testing
C. Long exercise testing
D. Fast repetitive stimulation
E. Slow repetitive stimulation

227. A 60-year-old woman noticed slowly progressive right shoulder and arm weakness. She previously had radiation therapy over the right side of the neck for malignancy and was told she was in remission. She denies any pain with the recent weakness. Electromyography (EMG) study revealed myokymic discharges. Which of the following features makes radiation induced plexitis more likely compared to recurrence of malignancy?

A. Painless weakness
B. Upper trunk involvement with predominant shoulder muscle weakness
C. Myokymic discharges on needle electromyography (EMG)
D. Slow progression over many years
E. All of the above

228. In ammatory or autoimmune neuropathies may not be nonlength dependent unlike more common causes of peripheral neuropathy. Among the autoimmune neuropathies below, which type of neuropathy is distal predominant?

A. Myelin-associated glycoprotein (MAG) neuropathy
B. Acute inflammatory demyelinating polyradiculoneuropathy (AIDP)
C. Acute motor sensory axonal neuropathy (AMSAN)
D. Multifocal motor neuropathy (MMN)
E. Chronic inflammatory demyelinating polyneuropathy (CIDP)

229. While performing a motor nerve conduction study, a neurophysiology fellow notices abnormal temporal dispersion at a noncompressive site. This finding is most likely to be seen in which of the following conditions?

A. Charcot-Marie-Tooth hereditary neuropathy type 1A (CMT1A)
B. Charcot-Marie-Tooth hereditary neuropathy type 2 (CMT2)
C. Diabetic polyneuropathy
D. Neuropathy associated with chronic renal failure
E. Acute inflammatory demyelinating polyradiculoneuropathy (AIDP)

230. Which of the following best describes the findings in the single-fiber electromyography (EMG) of the orbicular oculi muscle?

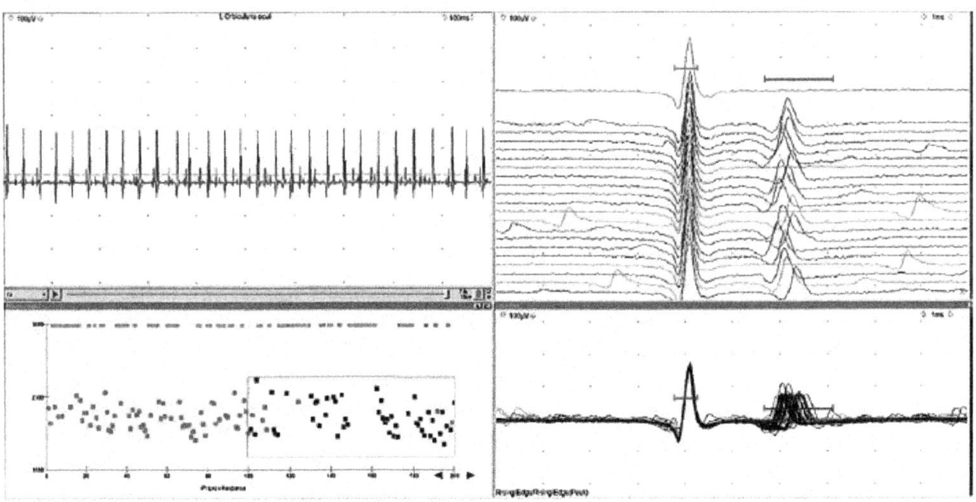

A. Normal jitter with blocking
B. Normal jitter with no blocking
C. Increased jitter with blocking
D. Increased jitter with no blocking
E. Decreased jitter with no blocking

231. A 70-year-old underwent a median sternotomy for coronary bypass surgery. Postsurgery he noticed numbness in his hands. He was referred for electrodiagnostic testing. On testing he was noted to have reduced ulnar sensory amplitude with preserved medial antebrachial cutaneous sensory amplitude. Which of the following tests would help diagnose ulnar neuropathy?
A. Needle electromyography (EMG) of the first dorsal interosseous (FDI) muscle
B. Needle EMG of abductor pollicis brevis (APB) muscle
C. Needle EMG of biceps muscle
D. Needle EMG of deltoid muscle
E. Needle EMG of extensor digitorum brevis muscle

232. In true neurogenic thoracic outlet syndromes, which of the following electrodiagnostic changes are noted?
A. Absent medial antebrachial sensory response and predominant denervation changes in thenar muscles
B. Absent medial antebrachial sensory response and predominant denervation changes in hypothenar
C. Absent medial antebrachial sensory response and no denervation changes in thenar muscles
D. Normal medial antebrachial sensory response and predominant denervation changes in thenar muscles
E. Normal medial antebrachial sensory response and no changes in thenar or hypothenar muscles

233. A 28-year-old man reports chronic fatigue and muscle weakness without any ocular symptoms. Neurological examination was essentially normal. Repetitive stimulation was normal. Further assessment with single fiber EMG was performed to evaluate for myasthenia gravis.

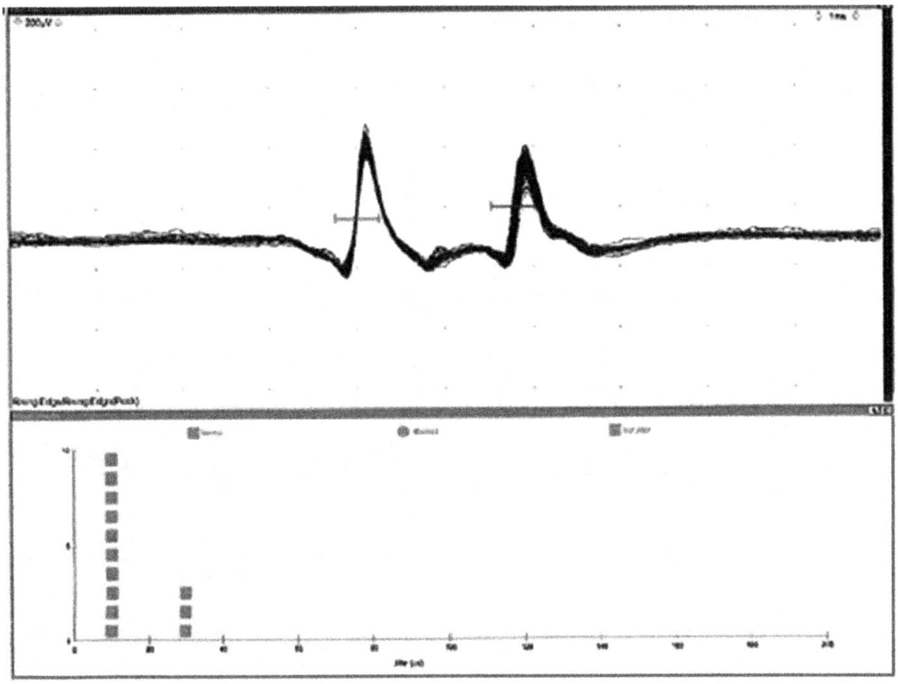

A. Increased jitter
B. Normal jitter but with blocking
C. Normal jitter and no blocking
D. Reduced jitter
E. This study is technically limited and therefore should not be interpreted.

234. Which of the following motor unit and recruitment patterns best supports the diagnosis of myopathy?
A. Baseline compound muscle action potential (CMAP) amplitudes
B. Changes in postexercise CMAP amplitudes
C. Slow repetitive stimulation
D. Fast repetitive stimulation
E. Deep tendon reflexes

235. A 25-year-old was evaluated for recent weakness and is suspected to have had a myopathy. Which of the following motor unit and recruitment patterns best supports the diagnosis of myopathy?
A. Long-duration, large-amplitude motor unit potentials with decreased recruitment
B. Long-duration, large-amplitude motor unit potentials with early recruitment
C. Long-duration, large-amplitude motor unit potentials with normal recruitment
D. Short -duration, small-amplitude motor unit potentials with early recruitment
E. Short-duration, small-amplitude motor unit potentials with decreased recruitment

236. A nerve conduction study is performed in a 20-year-old with severe distal weakness and sensory loss for many years. She is suspected to have hereditary polyneuropathy. Which of the following nerve conduction findings would best support the diagnosis of Charcot– Marie–Tooth (CMT) type 2a?

A. Severely prolonged distal latencies
B. Predominant changes in nerve amplitudes only in upper limbs
C. Normal sural responses
D. Severely reduced conduction velocities
E. Severe reduced sensory and motor amplitudes

237. A 55 year old presented with slowly progressive numbness in his feet for over 1 year. He does not report any weakness. On examination, he has sensory ataxia with absent reflexes. He also has a mild tremor in his hands. Routine lab testing was not revealing except abnormal paraproteinemia. Nerve conduction studies were performed, and below tibial motor response was found. What is the best next step?

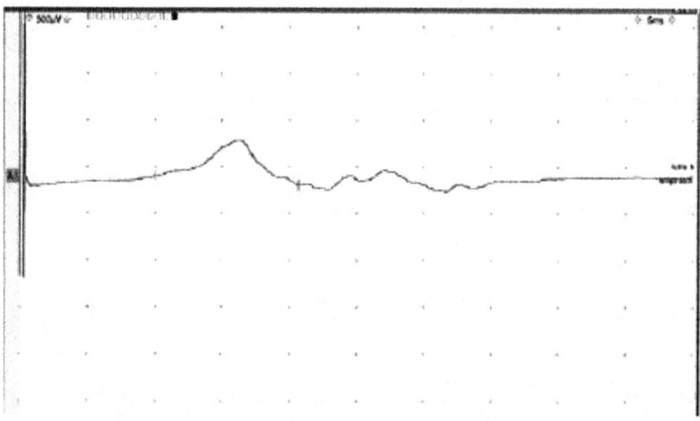

Site	Recording site	Latency	Amplitude	Duration	Area	Distance (mm)	Temp C
Ankle	AH	10.1	0.4	10.6	1.3	80	29

A. Spinal fluid analysis
B. Magnetic resonance (MR) lumbar spine
C. Test for myelin-associated glycoprotein (MAG) antibodies
D. Nerve biopsy
E. No need for further testing since this is likely an idiopathic neuropathy

238. What does the below median motor study reveal in a 50-year-old man with polyneuropathy?

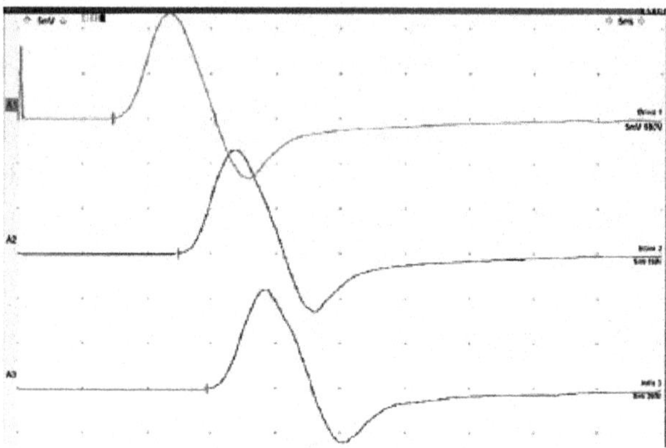

	Sites	Rec Site	Lat (ms)	Amp (mv)	Dur (ms)	Area (mvms)
A1	Wrist	APB	7.3	11.7	8.1	49.2
A2	Elbow	APB	12.4	11.5	8.2	48.8
A3	Axilla	APB	14.7	11.1	8.2	45.3

Segments	Dist (mm)	CV (ms)	Temp C
Wrist-APB	80		30.4
Elbow-Wrist	230	45	30.4
Axilla-Elbow	100	43	30.4

A. Normal latency, amplitude, and conduction velocity
B. Prolonged distal latency, normal amplitude, and conduction velocity
C. Prolonged distal latency, normal amplitude, and mildly reduced conduction velocity
D. Prolonged distal latency, reduced amplitude, and mildly reduced conduction velocity
E. Prolonged distal latency, normal amplitude, and mildly reduced conduction velocity in the setting of suboptimal limb temperature

239. A 33-year-old was referred to the neurodiagnostic lab for evaluation of a suspected myopathy. As the technician was starting the routine screening nerve conduction study, the patient questioned the utility of the nerve conduction study given the clinical suspicion of muscle disease. Which of the following statement best supports the rationale for doing nerve conduction study even if the clinical suspicion is a muscle disease?
A. Painful nerve stimulation should always be performed
B. Nerve conduction can help potential mimics such as Lambert–Eaton myasthenic syndrome (LEMS) or demyelinating neuropathies
C. If nerve conduction studies are normal, then needle electromyography (EMG) is not needed
D. Nerve conduction studies before needle EMG improves patient tolerance
E. Performing nerve conduction studies is justified, as referral was for both nerve conduction and needle EMG

240. A 44-year-old man noticed recent onset numbness in his feet and legs in addition to having difficulty with walking. Routine lab testing by his primary care physician for causes of neuropathy was not revealing. An examination by a neurologist revealed normal strength, distal sensory loss, absent reflexes, and a sensory ataxia. A routine nerve conduction study revealed normal motor and sensory responses. Needle electromyography (EMG) was also normal. He was diagnosed with an uncommon neuromuscular disease. Which of the following statements is most consistent with this diagnosis?
A. Sensory ataxia is likely because of proximal nerve root involvement
B. Magnetic resonance (MR) lumbar roots might reveal nerve root enlargement and enhancement with contrast
C. Somatosensory evoked potentials are absent
D. This condition might respond to intravenous immunoglobulin (IVIG)
E. All of the above

241. A 65-year-old man with poorly-controlled chronic diabetes and renal failure has progressive sensory loss and weakness. Which of the following statements best describes likely nerve conduction study findings in this patient?
A. Reduced or absent sural response
B. Motor conduction velocity slowing
C. Significant slowing across common compression sites
D. Denervation in weak distal muscles
E. All of the above

242. Which of the following statements is correct regarding selection of a nerve when considering nerve biopsy?

A. Usually a sensory nerve with absent sensory nerve action potentials (SNAP) should be biopsied
B. Usually a distal motor nerve is biopsied
C. Nerve biopsy is useful for most types of neuropathies
D. Usually a sensory nerve with normal SNAP should be biopsied
E. Nerve biopsy is not useful in vasculitis or amyloidosis

243. Which of the following features helps to differentiate chronic inflammatory demyelinating polyneuropathy (CIDP) from Lewis–Sumner syndrome?

A. Elevated cerebrospinal fluid (CSF) protein
B. Conduction block on motor nerve conduction studies
C. Nerve root enhancement on magnetic resonance (MR) imaging
D. Asymmetric changes on motor nerve conduction studies
E. Symmetrical changes on motor nerve conduction studies

ANSWERS

1. **C.** Monopolar needles give rise to increased variability of motor unit potentials. Monopolar needles record from large areas of muscle and produce larger motor unit action potentials. For these reasons, most centers prefer to use concentric needles. However, monopolar needles may cause less pain. There is no difference between monopolar and concentric needles regarding the time it takes to complete needle EMG study.

2. **B.** The clinical picture is consistent with radial nerve injury at the spiral groove. Intact distal amplitude and complete conduction block in the arm suggest a conduction block at the spiral groove consistent with a neuropraxic injury. If the patient had nerve transection or neurotmesis at the spiral groove, wallerian degeneration is expected to occur, leading to decreased CMAP amplitude on distal stimulation 12 days after an injury. Because distal CMAP is normal, a neuropraxic injury in the forearm is not likely. A submaximal proximal stimulation can always lead to erroneous conclusion of conduction block, but this clinical scenario this is not likely as patient has wrist drop suggesting a clear nerve injury.

3. **C.** Among the options presented in the question, increment on fast repetitive stimulation is only seen with botulism and LEMS. However, LEMS is not likely in this age group and increment in LEMS tends to exceed 100%. Decrement on slow repetitive stimulation is seen with congenital myasthenic syndromes and botulism. When reviewing repetitive stimulation data, it is important to pay close attention to the rate of stimulation.

4. **C.** The EMG depicts a decreased interference pattern as seen in a neurogenic process. In a normal patient, with maximal contraction, multiple motor units fire and it is not possible to distinguish individual motor units at this sweep speed (100 ms). In this case, with maximum activation, because of decreased number of motor unit action potentials seen in a neurogenic process, one is able to distinguish individual motor units. This type of interference pattern is also called a "picket fence" interference pattern and is suggestive of a neurogenic process. There is a clear motor unit activity however recruitment pattern is suggestive of neurogenic process. In myopathic and neuromuscular junction (NMJ) disorders, small motor units fire rapidly and it is not possible to distinguish individual motor units.

5. **B.** CMT type 1 is hereditary demyelinating polyneuropathy. In this study, there is profound slowing of the conduction velocity that is consistent with a primary demyelinating polyneuropathy such as CMT type 1. CMT type 2A typically leads to an axonal polyneuropathy and this nerve conduction study is not consistent with a primary axonal neuropathic process. Spinal muscular atrophy and distal myopathies may lead to decreased amplitude but do not cause severely decreased conduction velocity. Nerve conduction velocities in teenagers are same as adults.

6. **A.** Acute onset of weakness, severe pain, and swelling in the thigh in a man with poorly controlled diabetes is likely diabetic muscle infarction, and MRI of the thigh will reveal signal changes in the infarcted muscle. Obvious swelling in the thigh makes a diabetic lumbosacral plexopathy less likely, so MRI of the lumbar spine or lumbosacral plexus is not as useful. NCS/EMG will reveal distal symmetrical neuropathy and irritative myopathic changes in the affected muscles, but needle EMG can be quite painful in diabetic muscle infarction; therefore, an MRI of the thigh is a better choice. Muscle biopsy of the affected muscle will reveal edema, hemorrhage, and infarcts in muscle, but this is invasive. Diagnosis could potentially be determined with MRI of the thigh alone. Spinal fluid analysis would not be helpful for a diagnosis of diabetic muscle infarction.

7. **D.** Either excessive stimulation at the fibular head or submaximal stimulation at the ankle can lead to higher peroneal motor amplitude at the fibular neck compared to stimulation at the ankle. However, these findings are secondary to inappropriate study techniques. The accessory peroneal nerve can also lead to this picture on peroneal motor study, but this is a normal anatomical variant and can be confirmed by stimulating posterior to lateral malleolus while recording from the extensor digitorum brevis muscle. Intrinsic foot muscle atrophy would lead to low compound muscle action potential (CMAP) amplitudes at all sites of stimulation.

8. **E.** Acute quadriplegic myopathy is characterized by irritative changes and myopathic units on electromyography (EMG). There is characteristic myosin chain loss on electron microscopic evaluation of muscle biopsy. Prolonged steroid use (IV and oral), solid organ transplantation, and renal failure can be associated with a higher likelihood of myopathy. Opiate or benzodiazepine use for sedation is not considered a risk factor for acute severe myopathic weakness with quadriparesis.

9. **D.** In posterior cord brachial plexopathy, triceps and brachioradialis reflexes will be abnormal but biceps reflex will be normal.

10. **C.** EMG of the first dorsal interosseous muscle is not likely to cause any significant ulnar nerve injury as only the terminal branch of this ulnar nerve supplies first dorsal interosseous (FDI). Needle EMG of the other muscles can potentially injure the associated nerves.

11. **E.** Because MG causes facial and bulbar muscle weakness more than distal limb muscle weakness, SFEMG of frontalis is the most sensitive test. SFEMG is more sensitive than repetitive stimulation in MG. AChR antibody testing is also useful but SFEMG can be abnormal even in antibody negative MG. Icepack test is neither specific or sensitive for MG.

12. **A.** This nerve conduction study reveals conduction block across the fibular head with severely diminished conduction velocity. These features favor a compressive peroneal neuropathy at the fibular head, which can be seen after significant weight loss, but not with weight gain. Ankle or tibial fracture is not expected to cause compressive neuropathy at the fibular head. Conduction block at the fibular head is not suggestive of lumbosacral radiculopathy.

13. **C.** In both hereditary and acquired demyelinating neuropathies, prolonged distal latency and severely reduced conduction velocity are seen. However, abnormal temporal dispersion and conduction block are usually features of acquired demyelinating neuropathy. Severely reduced motor or sensory amplitudes or reduced recruitment patterns on needle EMG can be seen with both primary axonal and demyelinating neuropathies.

14. **D.** If neither ammonia nor lactate level increased as expected, then an insufficient effort from the patient is the most likely cause. In myoadenylate deaminase deficiency, ammonia levels do not increase but lactate level does. In all other diseases of glycolysis, ammonia levels increase but not the lactate level.

15. **A.** F-wave responses will not help with localization in this case. Because both median and ulnar motor fibers pass through medial cord, lower trunk, and C8–T1 roots, this additional information regarding motor fibers does not improve the localization any further. However, median and ulnar sensory responses will be helpful because the median sensory nerve action potentials will be normal in medial cord/lower trunk lesions. History of trauma does not preclude from performing F-wave studies.

16. **A.** Initial positive deflection in a motor nerve conduction study could indicate that the G1 is not on top of the belly of the muscle, so moving the G1 electrode toward the belly of the muscle would resolve the problem. Moving the G2 electrode does not change the initial positivity. Moving the stimulating electrode would not change the initial positivity as long as the same nerve is stimulated. It is not common to have an initial positive deflection in motor studies, and one should attempt to correct this and positive deflection with proximal stimulation still indicates inappropriate G1 position.

17. **C.** In patients with neurogenic thoracic outlet syndrome, generally the medial cord or lower trunk is primarily affected. Among the options provided in the question, first dorsal interosseous weakness and loss of sensation over the 5th digit best localize to the medial cord or lower trunk. Deltoid weakness with loss of sensation over the shoulder is consistent with axillary neuropathy. Finger extensor weakness and loss of sensation over the dorsum of the hand is seen with radial neuropathy. While abductor pollicis brevis muscle weakness may be seen with medial cord or lower trunk brachial plexopathy, loss of sensation over the lateral forearm is inconsistent with the above localization because the lateral forearm is supplied by the lateral antebrachial cutaneous nerve that originates from the lateral cord. Biceps weakness and sensory loss over the lateral aspect of forearm is suggestive of musculocutaneous nerve injury, not a feature of neurogenic thoracic outlet syndrome.

18. **B.** Motor unit potentials with large duration and amplitude indicate chronic reinnervation. Reduced recruitment can be seen with both acute and chronic denervation. Positive sharp waves and fibrillation potentials are indicative of active denervation changes. Fasciculation potentials are seen with acute or chronic denervation changes.

19. **E.** In severe critical illness weakness, it is sometimes not possible to differentiate neuropathy from myopathy. Compound muscle action potential (CMAP) amplitude may be decreased in both conditions. If sensory responses are normal, this favors critical illness myopathy. Occasionally, sensory studies are technically difficult to obtain in the ICU. In such cases, motor unit morphology and recruitment patterns on needle EMG may help. If this is not possible due to lack of activation from the patient, direct muscle stimulation and comparison of this response with nerve stimulation may help in differentiating these two conditions.

20. **D.** Myotonia congenita is a channelopathy presenting with myotonia, stiffness, and weakness in cold temperature. Patients with periodic paralysis usually have episodes of weakness. Patients with myotonic dystrophy have moderate to severe limb and facial weakness. Patients with Pompe disease have limb weakness and also develop neuromuscular respiratory insufficiency.

21. **D.** The most sensitive study and the earliest electrodiagnostic change in a patient with length-dependent axonal polyneuropathy is decreased or absent sural sensory response. Peroneal motor response changes are generally seen after sural sensory changes, and tibial motor changes occur later in the disease course. F-wave responses may be abnormal in both peripheral nerve and nerve root disorders.

22. **A.** Amyloid myopathy is frequently caused by hereditary amyloidosis (transthyretin or gelsolin) or primary amyloidosis (light-chain amyloidosis). It is not common in secondary amyloidosis. Even though patients have weakness, muscles may look hypertrophic. Peripheral neuropathy is not uncommon because of associated amyloid deposition. Creatinine kinase is elevated in amyloid myopathy. Electrodiagnostic studies usually reveal a combination of neuropathy and irritative myopathic changes. Muscle biopsy may reveal amyloid deposition.

23. **C.** Calculation of area and duration of the CMAP helps with identification of abnormal temporal dispersion on proximal stimulation. Conduction velocity and latency are measured from the initial negative deflection of CMAP, and therefore, are not affected by duration or area of CMAP. Stimulus intensity or duration should not affect these measures as long as they are supramaximal.

24. **A.** The patient has asymmetric finger flexion weakness and bilateral lower extremity weakness, predominantly affecting the quadriceps muscles. These features are most consistent with inclusion body myositis (IBM). EMG in IBM is typically myopathic in nature, and therefore, short-duration, small-amplitude motor units with early recruitment are likely to be seen. Rarely, large-duration motor units may be seen but overall the recruitment patterns will be early. Irritative features (fibrillation potentials and positive sharp waves) may be seen but since the weakness has been ongoing for more than 1 year, motor unit morphology is not expected to be normal.

25. **C.** Among the options given, only sympathetic skin response has a long-duration potential and is predominantly a low-frequency waveform; therefore, the low-frequency filter should be set at 0.5 Hz to visualize the waveform. Other options have higher frequency components and do not require the low-frequency filter to be set at 0.5 Hz.

26. **C.** The firing frequency of the waveform is about 80 Hz and the waveform pattern does not change during the recording. These features favor that this signal is probably an electrical artifact and likely related to the spinal stimulator. Morphology and amplitude of the waveform are not consistent with either positive sharp waves or fibrillation potentials or myokymia. Motor unit potentials do not usually fire at this frequency.

27. **D.** The baseline CMAP amplitude in this ulnar study is normal because amplitude above 5 mV is generally considered normal. In addition, the increment in amplitude is less than 30% after 15 seconds of exercise; such mild increase in amplitude can be seen in normal individuals, and therefore is not considered significant.

28. **B.** The study reveals a clear conduction block in the forearm with severely slowed conduction velocity. These features are suggestive of an acquired demyelinating disease, likely multifocal motor neuropathy. Other listed conditions only lead to axonal changes.

29. **D.** Severely decreased conduction velocity, severely prolonged distal latency, absent or prolonged F-wave responses may suggest a demyelinating polyneuropathy; however, they can be seen in both hereditary and acquired demyelinating polyneuropathies. Abnormal temporal dispersion pattern is a feature of acquired demyelinating polyneuropathy. Decreased compound muscle action potential amplitude can be seen in both axonal and demyelinating polyneuropathies.

30. **B.** There is severe decrease in compound muscle action potential (CMAP) amplitude and conduction velocity on stimulation in the axilla. This is suggestive of conduction block in the arm. Because both amplitude and area are equally decreased without much change in duration of the CMAP, abnormal temporal dispersion is not the correct answer. Demyelinating process is likely underlying physiology, but it is focal, not diffuse.

31. **E.** As only the median nerve passes through the carpal tunnel, comparison studies with ulnar or radial nerves can help find focal slowing within the carpal tunnel. Inching across the wrist while looking for abrupt change in latency will also help with localization of compression at the wrist in CTS.

32. **C.** These types of clinical scenarios are localized by reviewing the brachial plexus anatomy. Motor fiber innervating deltoid muscle arise from C5–C6 roots and pass through upper trunk followed posterior cord and axillary nerve. Motor fibers for triceps muscle originate in C6–C8 roots and pass through the posterior cord and radial nerve. Because biceps and pronator teres muscles were normal, it is unlikely that the lesion is in the C5, C6, or C7 roots or upper trunk. Fibers to pronator teres pass through the lateral cord.

33. **C.** Extensor indices proprius (EIP) is a radial nerve innervated muscle. Even though the fibers innervating EIP pass through C8 and the lower trunk, they are then directed to the posterior cord and then the radial nerve. Therefore, denervation in this muscle would indicate a lesion in the lower trunk, not the medial cord. All other muscles in this example are supplied by both the medial cord and lower trunk so they do not differentiate between these two conditions.

34. B. F-wave responses can be absent due to heavy sedation (e.g., propofol) and do not always indicate proximal demyelination. It is important to document the degree of sedation and agents used while performing electrodiagnostic studies in ICU patients. There is no clear evidence that this patient has GBS or a neuromuscular junction (NMJ) disease. SSEP will not help with the diagnosis of a peripheral process. Excessive electrical noise in ICU settings can affect nerve conduction studies technically but with appropriate attention, normal F-wave responses can be obtained.

35. B. The waveforms show repair of the decrement after exercise but without significant facilitation. Repair refers to improvement in the neuromuscular junction (NMJ) transmission after brief exercise, and consequently, improvement in decrement. Facilitation refers to significant increase in the compound muscle action potential (CMAP) amplitude after exercise. In this case, there is no significant increase in amplitude after exercise but there is clear improvement in the decrement after exercise. This was slow repetitive stimulation performed at 3 Hz as denoted in the figure.

36. B. The next step would be to warm the limb and repeat the test if the limb is significantly colder than 32°C. Higher rate of stimulation is not ideal to detect postsynaptic neuromuscular junction (NMJ) dysfunction. Giving pyridostigmine or edrophonium could mask an abnormal study and will not affect an already normal study. Higher amplifier gain would not affect the study results or conclusions. Other alternatives, not mentioned in the choices, would be to perform repetitive stimulation of the spinal accessory or facial nerve.

37. A. Only the stimulus artifact is considered to be a far-field potential. All types of motor and sensory nerve responses are near-field potentials.

38. A. In this peroneal motor study, there are two clear features suggesting that the patient has a demyelinating polyneuropathy: the distal latency is prolonged by 100% of normal; and distal compound muscle action potential (CMAP) duration is more than 9 ms. Decreased CMAP amplitude is not specific and can be seen in either demyelinating or axonal neuropathy. This study is not normal for any age. In this patient with severe sensory ataxia, distal demyelinating changes as seen here suggest an underlying demyelinating polyneuropathy. Needle EMG is not needed to interpret a single motor nerve conduction study. Needle EMG will help assessment of degree of secondary axonal changes.

39. D. Fasciculation potentials are secondary to random firing of the motor units. Positive sharp waves and fibrillation potentials are regular, arising from the muscle fibers. Complex repetitive discharges are also regular, arising from firing of adjacent muscle fibers. Myokymic discharges can be regular or semi-irregular and represent nonvoluntary firing of group of motor unit potentials.

40. D. Short-duration motor units, the so-called myopathic motor units, may be seen in polymyositis, or any severe muscle diseases such as critical illness myopathy, neuromuscular junction disorders such as LEMS, and during early reinnervation after severe denervation. ALS is a neuropathic condition, and therefore, long-duration motor units are likely to be seen.

41. **B.** History and examination are suggestive of a slowly progressive painless process with weakness in the lower cervical myotomes. In a South Asian man, this is likely to be monomelic amyotrophy. In this condition, motor amplitudes are decreased with evidence of active/chronic denervation and reinnervation changes in the affected muscles, along with long-duration motor unit potentials with reduced recruitment patterns. Sensory responses are normal in monomelic amyotrophy. Lack of sensory symptoms or pain makes brachial plexopathy unlikely, and so sensory responses are expected to be preserved. This case is not suggestive of a presynaptic neuromuscular junction disorder or a polyneuropathy, so options C and D are incorrect. Presentation is not typical of a myopathy and so short-duration motor unit potentials with early recruitment patterns is not likely.

42. **C.** Because CTS is a relatively common electrodiagnostic finding, it is important to recognize the unique features seen in patients with both MGA and CTS. Delayed distal latency is secondary to compression of the median fibers at the wrist. The spuriously increased conduction velocity and positive dip on proximal stimulation both are secondary to stimulation of the ulnar innervated muscles conducted through the ulnar nerve because of MGA. Because these fibers cross from the median to ulnar nerve in the forearm, they stimulate the thenar muscles earlier than the median-innervated thenar muscle fibers, leading to the unique electrophysiological findings. Median sensory responses are affected earlier than motor responses in patients with CTS.

43. **A.** Low-CMAP amplitudes are seen in many nonneurogenic conditions. Both LEMS and botulism, even though they are neuromuscular junction (NMJ) disorders, generally have low-CMAP amplitudes on motor studies. Severe myopathies or myopathies with significant distal weakness may have low-CMAP amplitudes. Low-CMAP amplitudes are also seen in periodic paralysis during the attack. However, low-CMAP amplitudes are not seen in predominantly proximal muscle disease such as adult-onset acid maltase deficiency.

44. **B.** Rise time refers to the duration of the rapid positive to negative inflection and is a measure of the distance between the muscle fibers and recording needle. The farther the muscle fibers are from the recording needle electrode, the greater the rise time. A rise time of less than 0.5 ms is considered optimal, and motor unit potentials with >0.5 ms rise time should not be analyzed because this would lead to falsely decreased duration and amplitude of the motor unit potentials. Duration, amplitude, phases, and firing frequency are all analyzed after evaluating rise time.

45. **D.** In root avulsion, sensory nerve responses are normal even though the patient will have loss of sensation in the dermatome. Other mentioned tests are all affected in both root avulsion and plexus lesions and do not differentiate between these two conditions.

46. **C.** Glucose 6-phosphate deficiency leads to Von Gierke's disease (type 1 GSD). This condition does not have any neuromuscular symptoms or weakness. In all the other options, various types of neuromuscular manifestations, especially exercise intolerance and weakness, can be seen. Acid alpha-glucosidase deficiency causes Pompe disease, which can present in infancy, juvenile period, or in adulthood with different types of neuromuscular, respiratory, and cardiac manifestations. Beta enolase deficiency causes type XIV GSD, and mainly leads to exercise intolerance. Aldolase deficiency causes type XII GSD and leads to exercise intolerance and weakness.

47. **B.** A close observation of the CMAP amplitude reveals that there is a small increase in amplitude with successive stimulations, which is depicted as a negative percentage decrement in the accompanying table. This mild increment is considered normal. There is no clear decrement in CMAP amplitude. Repair refers to a phenomenon where the decrement improves, and these waveforms do not show evidence of repair. Baseline is stable and the quality of the study is acceptable.

48. **D.** Note that the sweep speed is set at 20 ms for the top waveform and 100 ms for the bottom waveform. The bottom waveforms fire as a group of motor unit potentials at regular intervals with each burst firing at approximately 1.5 Hz. The frequency of motor unit firing within each burst is 25 to 50 Hz. These features suggest that the pattern and rate of firing are consistent with myokymia, and not tremor. Fasciculation potentials are single irregularly firing motor unit potentials. Fibrillation potentials are regularly firing potentials that originate at the muscle fiber level. Complex repetitive discharges seen with regular firing of adjacent motor fibers with ephatic transmission.

49. **A.** This patient likely has Miller Fisher syndrome with the classic triad of ophthalmoplegia, ataxia, and areflexia. Motor nerve conduction amplitudes and velocities is typically normal in these patients.

50. **B.** Based on the history of myalgias, tiredness, and proximal limb weakness, this patient likely has a myopathy. In certain muscle diseases, CPK is elevated along with ALT and AST. In this case, the ALT/AST elevation is likely related to muscle disease, and the appropriate testing would be CPK level followed by needle EMG to confirm a myopathic process if needed. Because transaminases are known to be elevated in muscle disease, a liver biopsy should not be done. Muscle biopsy should not be done before checking CPK level. Generally, genetic testing (e.g., for limb girdle muscular dystrophy) is performed after confirming that the patient has a muscle disease. Routine nerve conduction studies will not help in evaluating a likely muscle disease.

51. **C.** The figure shows a recording of H-reflex. During H-wave reflex studies, a submaximal stimulus is used and the stimulus intensity is gradually increased. With the increase in stimulus intensity the M-wave amplitude gradually increases, whereas the H-wave amplitude decreases.

52. **A.** The baseline repetitive stimulation revealed decrement that is more than 10% and is suggestive of neuromuscular junction (NMJ) dysfunction. Note that the maximum decrement was 13% on the baseline repetitive stimulation test and 2% after exercise, suggesting repair in decrement postexercise. The maximum amplitudes are the same both pre- and postexercise, so there is no significant facilitation.

53. **A.** Because each small division is 10 ms and the epoch has 20 divisions, the whole epoch accounts for 200 ms. As the same motor unit is seen at least four times during the 200 ms, it is therefore expected to fire 20 times per second and the firing frequency is 20 Hz.

54. **B.** The nerve conduction study supports ulnar neuropathy at the elbow. There is a severely slowed conduction velocity across the elbow and an obvious conduction block across the elbow. These are common findings in compressive ulnar neuropathy at the elbow. There is no slowing or conduction block in the forearm and ulnar latency is normal at the wrist; therefore, the other options are incorrect.

55. B. This blink reflex study shows that with right-sided V1 stimulation (top traces), there is no ipsilateral R1 or R2 response but there is a normal contralateral R2 response; therefore, it excludes a right trigeminal neuropathy. With left-sided V1 stimulation (bottom traces), ipsilateral R1 and R2 are normal but the contralateral R2 response is absent; therefore, it excludes a left trigeminal or facial neuropathy. These findings in combination suggest a right facial neuropathy. Technically this study is adequate.

56. C. This is a normal median sensory study. Unlike motor conduction studies, with antidromic sensory studies, it is not uncommon to have a significant drop in amplitude with proximal stimulation. This does not mean that there is conduction block or abnormal temporal dispersion. After sensory responses there are motor responses in the waveforms, but these are not used for assessment of latencies and amplitudes.

57. B. Even though the site of the compression is at the level of the sciatic nerve, the peroneal nerve fibers are more likely to be compressed than tibial nerve fibers, resulting in significantly decreased peroneal amplitude compared to tibial amplitude. Consequently, patients may only have a foot drop because of predominant peroneal nerve involvement. Sural response would be affected only with a significant degree of tibial nerve involvement. Tibial H-reflex would be absent or prolonged compared to the opposite normal side. Peroneal F-wave responses are more likely to be abnormal or absent before peroneal motor amplitudes are reduced.

58. D. The number of surrounding axons does not affect the conduction velocity of the action potential. Thickly myelinated nerve fibers and nerve fibers with a larger diameter conduct faster than nerve fibers with thinly myelinated axons. A longer distance between the nodes of Ranvier leads to faster conduction velocity because of saltatory conduction. Lower temperature leads to slowing of the conduction velocity.

59. B. Close attention to the sweep speed and gain makes this calculation relatively easy. Distal latency is less than 5 ms but is not less than half of the first division. It is marked just before the first division, so it is likely to be 4 ms. Distal amplitude is a little bit more than two divisions, and with the gain set at 5 mV per division, this is likely to be 12 mV. The difference in latencies is approximately 8 ms and therefore the conduction velocity is 400 mm / 8 ms = 50 m / sec.

60. A. Recruitment frequency is the frequency of firing of a motor unit when the next motor unit appears during activation. Recruitment frequency varies with the type of muscle and is usually around 16 Hz in a cranial muscle and 7 to 10 Hz in a limb muscle. Significantly, higher frequencies suggest a decreased number of available motor units and denervation.

61. B. This median motor study shows evidence of focal demyelination in the forearm. There is clear evidence of a conduction block in the forearm (greater than a 50% drop in amplitude on proximal stimulation) with severe slowing of conduction velocity. In the clinical context of multifocal painless weakness without sensory loss, this is most likely multifocal motor neuropathy. CTS does not cause conduction block or severe slowing of velocity in the forearm. Lower trunk brachial plexopathy may reveal evidence of an axonal process in the median motor study but not focal demyelination. Monomelic amyotrophy may lead to decreased median compound muscle action potential amplitude because of loss of motor nerves in C8–T1 myotomes but does not lead to focal conduction block. CMT is not likely because of recent onset asymmetric motor weakness with no sensory deficits.

62. A. In a 5-year-old boy with high CPK, enlarged calf muscles, and Gower's sign, an electrodiagnostic study is not needed to confirm that this is likely a myopathic process; in this case, genetic testing for Duchenne muscular dystrophy is appropriate. In a patient with fatigue, weakness, and ptosis, electrodiagnostic studies will help localize the pathology to the neuromuscular junction (NMJ). In a 15-year-old with possible hereditary sensorimotor neuropathy, nerve conduction studies are very helpful to differentiate axonal from demyelinating processes and to guide further genetic testing. Similarly, in a 22-year-old with suspected Guillain–Barré syndrome, electrodiagnostic testing would be appropriate to confirm the diagnosis. A 65-year-old with painless progressive weakness is concerning for motor neuron process and electrodiagnostic studies are indicated.

63. C. In myoadenylate deaminase deficiency, the lactate level increases during exercise but the ammonia level does not. In all the other options noted, ammonia level increases but the lactate does not, suggesting a glycogen storage disease or a disorder of glycolysis. In cases of suboptimal effort from the patient, neither ammonia nor lactate level increases.

64. C. This clinical picture represents chronic progressive external ophthalmoplegia with cardiac involvement, most likely Kearns–Sayre syndrome, in which case the needle EMG will reveal short-duration myopathic motor unit potentials. Decrement on slow repetitive stimulation or significant increment on fast repetitive stimulation are features of neuromuscular junction (NMJ) disorders. Although predominant manifestations are ocular and cardiac, since she has significant proximal limb muscle weakness, EMG is expected to reveal myopathic process with short-duration motor unit potentials.

65. C. Short-duration, small-amplitude polyphasic units in this patient likely represent "nascent motor unit potentials," seen mostly in the very early reinnervation process, as opposed to a new myopathic condition. The best way to differentiate these from short-duration motor unit potentials seen in a myopathy is to rely on the recruitment pattern. In neurogenic processes, the recruitment will be reduced, whereas in myopathic processes it will be either early or normal. Abnormal spontaneous activity may be seen in both neurogenic and myopathic diseases. Degree of activation does not differentiate neurogenic from myopathic diseases. Activation is generally reduced in central diseases. CPK level can be mildly elevated even in neurogenic disorders. Muscle biopsy is not indicated in this clinical scenario.

66. C. The figure in the question shows a polyphasic motor unit potential with a firing frequency of 10 Hz. The motor unit appears twice during the whole sweep of 200 ms (1/5th of a second), and would be expected to fire 10 times in a second; therefore, the firing frequency is 10 Hz.

67. B. The latency difference between the ankle and fibular head stimulations is 7.1 ms; therefore, the conduction velocity is 350 mm/7.1 ms, or approximately 49 m/sec. The latency difference between the knee and fibular head stimulations is 1.6 ms and conduction velocity in this segment is 90 mm/1.6 ms ~56 m/sec.

68. C. The figure reveals large-amplitude (~2 mV), long-duration (~20 ms) motor unit potentials with severely reduced recruitment. These findings suggest a chronic neurogenic process with reinnervation such as chronic polyradiculopathy. Myopathic conditions usually lead to short-duration, small-amplitude motor unit potentials. Motor unit potentials are either normal or have myopathic features in patients with LEMS. Motor unit potential morphology and firing pattern tends to be normal in myasthenia gravis except for motor unit variability.

69. **D.** While decremental response on slow repetitive stimulation is typically seen in neuromuscular junction (NMJ) disorders such as myasthenia gravis (MG), LEMS, or botulism, this has been reported in other conditions such as paramyotonia congenita and neomycin toxicity. This type of decremental response is not seen in Becker or Duchenne muscular dystrophies.

70. **B.** When the elbow is extended, the ulnar nerve is not taut, leading to underestimation of the ulnar nerve length across the elbow and consequently an artifactual decrease in conduction velocity across the elbow. Elbow position does not affect the CMAP amplitude or distal latency.

71. **C.** In H-reflex studies, the duration of the stimulus is increased but the stimulation intensity is submaximal so that Ia muscle spindle sensory afferents are stimulated. As the stimulation intensity is increased, H-reflex waveform disappears. All other motor and sensory studies are performed with supramaximal stimulations.

72. **C.** Each motor nerve has a spectrum of axons with various conduction velocities. CMAP is the summation of the responses from all axons with varying conduction velocities within the motor nerve. Therefore, the duration of CMAP reflects the temporal dispersion. In demyelinating diseases, there is either excessive or abnormal temporal dispersion because of selective or nonuniform demyelination. Due to these features, it is always important to measure the CMAP duration along with latency and amplitude. CMAP features are not related to patients ability to tolerate the study.

73. **A.** The figure shows many positive sharp waves and occasional fibrillation potentials. The gain is set at 50 μV, which is appropriate to record spontaneous activity. There are no complex repetitive discharges (repeated complex waveforms secondary to ephaptic transmission) or myokymia (spontaneous firing of grouped motor unit potentials). There are no motor potentials recorded in this epoch.

74. **B.** Motor unit morphology depends on multiple factors. Motor unit duration increases with age. Morphology of motor unit also depends on type of the muscle, with facial muscles generally having shorter duration compared to large limb muscles. Temperature also affects motor unit morphology, with lower muscle temperature decreasing the amplitude and increasing the duration. Another important feature to consider before analyzing motor unit features is the rise time, which is a reflection of proximity of the recording surface of the needle to the motor unit, but this is not related to the core or center of the muscle. There are mild changes in motor unit morphology in monopolar needle compared to concentric needle.

75. **B.** The EMG reveals a single motor unit firing very rapidly without the second or third motor unit being recruited. This is consistent with severely reduced recruitment and is seen in neurogenic processes. Early recruitment is seen with myopathic diseases. Synkinesis refers to aberrant reinnervation of the axons after facial nerve injury and does not correlate with reduced recruitment patterns on needle EMG. Firing pattern is not suggestive of fasciculation potentials.

76. **C.** The clinical description in this case likely suggests an acquired inflammatory myopathy with skin rash, most likely dermatomyositis. In myopathic disorders, short-duration and small-amplitude motor unit potentials are seen with an early recruitment pattern. Long-duration, large-amplitude motor unit potentials with decreased recruitment are seen in neurogenic conditions.

77. **B.** The waveforms seen between M-waves and F-waves are called A-waves or A-reflex. These additional waveforms are related to reinnervation fibers, leading to an additional firing of a small collection of motor fibers. A-waves are usually identified by the fact that they occur after M-waves and usually before F-waves, and unlike F-waves, they do not change in amplitude or minimal latency. A-waves are not artifacts, are not related to excess patient movement with stimulation or filter setting and have no relation to H-reflex.

78. **D.** In patients with NMJ disorders, jitter is increased and blocking may be seen in weak muscles. Even in normal healthy individuals, a jitter value can be measured but this is not prolonged. Abnormal jitter may be seen in various neurogenic conditions, and therefore, is not confirmatory of a NMJ disorder. Normal upper limit of jitter varies by muscle being tested.

79. **B.** Myotonic discharges are seen in acid maltase deficiency or Pompe disease. Duchenne muscular dystrophy, Miyoshi myopathy, steroid myopathy, and hypokalemic periodic paralysis do not cause myotonic discharges on needle electromyography (EMG). Hyperkalemic, not hypokalemic, periodic paralysis may be associated with myotonic discharges.

80. **B.** This waveform represents the classic finding of more than 100% increase in compound muscle action potential (CMAP) amplitude on fast repetitive stimulation. The frequency of stimulation is 50 Hz and is consistent with fast repetitive stimulation. These findings are suggestive of presynaptic neuromuscular junction (NMJ) dysfunction, likely Lambert–Eaton myasthenic syndrome.

81. **B.** Both F-wave and H-reflex have shorter latencies with proximal stimulation and longer latencies with distal stimulation. F-wave latency and amplitude vary with each stimulation. F-wave requires supramaximal stimulation but H-reflex requires submaximal stimulation. For F-waves, the afferent impulse travels through alpha motor neurons; for H-reflex, the afferent impulse travels through sensory fibers.

82. **C.** Because the injury is a few weeks old, positive sharp waves and fibrillation potentials are likely on needle EMG. Decreased recruitment patterns are also likely as the patient has weakness, and the cause of the weakness is neurogenic. Motor unit amplitude and duration are likely to be normal because adequate time has not passed for reinnervation to occur. Therefore, option C best explains the combination of acute neurogenic denervation changes with decreased recruitment.

83. **B.** The peroneal motor nerve study reveals two features suggestive of an underlying demyelinating neuropathy: distal latency is severely prolonged (increased by approximately 300%); and distal compound muscle action potential (CMAP) duration is quite prolonged (distal CMAP duration more than 9 ms is suggestive of a demyelinating process). Along with the clinical history of recent onset ataxia, sensory loss, mild weakness, and tremor, the patient most likely has neuropathy associated with anti-MAG

antibodies. With normal conduction velocity, PMP gene-related cause is less likely. This history and nerve conduction study is not suggestive of vasculitic neuropathy (choice C) or paraneoplastic neuropathy (choice D). Such severe distal slowing with normal conduction velocity is not typical of hereditary neuropathies and so exome sequencing is not going to be useful.

84. A. Fasciculation potentials are spontaneously firing motor unit potentials and have an irregular rhythm. Positive sharp waves, complex repetitive discharges, and fibrillation potentials have a regular rhythm. Myokymic discharges also regular pattern.

85. B. When calculating firing frequency, it is important to first review the sweep speed and measure the duration. In the figure, the sweep speed is 200 ms per division and the duration of the whole figure is 4 seconds (200 ms multiplied by 20 divisions). There are 17 grouped motor unit potentials firing before the recording stops, making the approximate firing frequency 4 to 5 Hz (17 divided by 4 seconds). This firing frequency is most likely a tremor. Failure to pay attention to sweep speed leads to incorrect conclusions.

86. D. Based on the data, it is not possible to come to a clear conclusion about polyneuropathy or radiculopathy in the patient. It is not uncommon for the sural sensory response to be absent in the elderly but not peroneal motor changes. Mild changes in peroneal motor response can also be age related or could represent either polyneuropathy or lumbosacral radiculopathy. In these instances, further studies in the upper limbs or needle electromyography (EMG) study should be used to differentiate axonal polyneuropathy from lumbosacral radiculopathy.

87. D. Cold temperature increases latency, increases amplitude, and decreases conduction velocity. Consequently, after rewarming one would expect the latency to decrease, amplitude to decrease, and the conduction velocity to increase. Among the options noted, only option D is likely.

88. A. The figure reveals positive sharp waves and fibrillation potentials. While these potentials are commonly seen in denervation, they can also be seen in various types of irritative myopathies including toxic myopathy, inflammatory or necrotizing myopathies, and certain glycogen storage disorders. These irritative changes are not seen in steroid-induced myopathy.

89. B. Both neuropathy and myopathy may be seen in patients on colchicine but this becomes significantly more likely if patients have concomitant renal failure. The possibility of toxic neuropathy or myopathy from colchicine does not change irrespective of the condition being treated, and is related to chronic usage and renal failure.

90. B. In subacute nerve injury, compound muscle action potential (CMAP) amplitude might be decreased. Spontaneous activity is likely to reveal positive sharp waves and fibrillation potentials. Motor unit morphology will be normal because reinnervation would not have occurred. However, the recruitment will be decreased. Choice C represents the pattern most likely to be seen with chronic nerve injury while choice D represents the pattern most likely to be seen in hyperacute nerve injury.

91. C. Fibrillations are due to regular depolarization of single muscle fiber. Irregular depolarization of single muscle fibers on needle EMG causes end-plate spikes. Regular firing of multiple adjacent muscle fibers is usually identified as complex repetitive discharge. Irregular firing of a single motor unit is likely to be a fasciculation potential.

92. **D.** The patient has the classical pattern of weakness for a femoral mononeuropathy, which is likely from a hematoma formation around the femoral nerve after arterial puncture for cardiac catheterization. In cases of severe femoral neuropathy, an electrodiagnostic study after 2 weeks will reveal decreased or absent femoral motor response, absent saphenous sensory response, and active denervation in the quadriceps muscles. Peroneal and tibial motor responses are expected to be normal if there is no evidence of lower lumbosacral plexopathy. Sural response is also expected to be normal if there is no sciatic neuropathy or lower lumbosacral plexopathy. Sensory only findings such as absent saphenous sensory response is not likely as there is severe knee extension weakness and femoral motor response is expected to be abnormal.

93. **C.** Neurotonic discharges are rapid irregular discharges and suggest nerve injury or excess irritation. This type of irregular firing pattern may be seen with nerve irritation or handling, but does not necessarily suggest a nerve injury. Positive sharp waves, fibrillation potentials, fasciculations, complex repetitive discharges, and myokymia are not features of hyperacute nerve injury from surgery.

94. **C.** Routine nerve conduction studies are normal in small-fiber neuropathy as the small-fiber nerves cannot be tested by routine nerve conduction studies. Needle EMG would be normal in a pure small-fiber neuropathy, as this condition does not cause muscle denervation. Radiculopathy may cause decreased motor amplitudes even though the sensory responses are normal. In patients with large-fiber neuropathy, nerve conduction studies are usually abnormal. Patients with LEMS usually have small-amplitude motor responses with normal sensory responses. Severe distal myopathy may also lead to small motor amplitudes.

95. **C.** F-wave latencies are shorter because limb length has a pronounced effect on the F-wave latencies. Conduction velocity reaches adult values by 3 years so this does not affect F-wave latency significantly. F-wave responses, similar to other motor nerve conduction responses, are present in children but technically difficult to perform because of the need for repeated supramaximal nerve stimulation but are not contraindicated.

96. **D.** The scenario best fits a situation in which a motor response is being done with the recording electrode far from the stimulated muscle. In general, motor responses do not have an initial positivity due to the waveform being produced directly underneath the recording electrode from the depolarizing muscle fibers. An initial positivity can be observed in sensory studies due to an approaching wavefront. But when a bipolar digital sensory study is done, the initial positivity is cancelled. A retreating wavefront would lead to positivity at the end and not at the beginning of the waveform. Initial positivity from a motor response is not feature of submaximal stimulus.

97. **B.** As all the median-innervated muscles including pronator teres are involved, the lesion is localized proximal to the innervation of pronator teres. Because ulnar- and radial-innervated distal muscles are normal, a lower trunk or medial cord brachial plexopathy is not likely.

98. **D.** Early in the course of acute demyelinating processes such as GBS, conduction block decreases the effective number of active motor nerve fibers, resulting in decreased motor

unit recruitment. Positive sharp waves and fibrillation potentials are seen approximately 2 weeks after the onset. Fasciculation potentials are not commonly seen in acute neuropathies. Needle EMG of a weak muscle is unlikely to be normal in patients with peripheral neurogenic diseases. Motor unit potentials with increased amplitude and duration are seen with chronic reinnervation changes.

99. C. The clinical picture is consistent with an acute superimposed on chronic neurogenic process. Long-duration and large-amplitude motor unit potentials are suggestive of a chronic neurogenic process. Positive sharp waves and fibrillation potentials are suggestive of active denervation. Decreased recruitment is seen in both acute and chronic neurogenic conditions as there is an overall reduction in number of motor unit potentials. Early recruitment is seen with myopathic diseases and not likely to be cause of weakness in this case. Other options do not include both active and chronic neurogenic process, hence are not likely choices.

100. B. Among the various electrodiagnostic findings in patients with AIDP, decreased CMAP amplitude is the most reliable indicator of poor prognosis. Severely prolonged distal latency or reduced conduction velocity suggest a demyelinating process, and these patients are more likely to have good recovery. Active denervation is less reliable as a predictor of poor prognosis compared to severely reduced CMAP amplitude.

101. D. Long thoracic nerve that innervates serratus anterior arises from C5, C6, and C7 roots directly; denervation in this muscle localizes to either the long thoracic nerve or cervical roots but not the brachial plexus. Nerves innervating other muscles, such as the deltoid (axillary nerve), biceps brachii (musculocutaneous nerve), and infraspinatus (suprascapular nerve), originate from the brachial plexus.

102. D. Decreased activation refers to a situation on needle EMG where only a few motor unit potentials are noted even though the recruitment pattern and frequency are normal. This could be a normal finding when testing very strong muscles. Pain from the needle EMG may also lead to poor activation. Pure upper motor neuron diseases such as primary lateral sclerosis or weakness in limb muscle after stroke may cause poor activation on needle EMG.

103. C. Chronic amiodarone usage may lead to myopathy; however, these patients have autophagic vacuoles but not necrotizing changes on muscle biopsy. EMG usually reveals irritative myopathic findings. Patients may also develop thyroid dysfunction from amiodarone use. Cyclosporine, HMG-CoA reductase inhibitors, propofol, and alcohol can lead to necrotizing myopathy.

104. C. The figure shows a late spike, distinct from the main potential that is time-locked to the main potential, and is called a satellite potential. The satellite potential is generated by a muscle fiber in a motor unit that has a longer nerve terminal or narrow diameter, leading to longer latency. Satellite potentials generally indicate a reinnervation process.

105. D. Variability of motor units (i.e., variation of a single motor unit potential amplitude or morphology during repeated firing) tends to be excessive in neuromuscular junction (NMJ) dysfunction. ALS and CIDP would lead to neurogenic changes such as long-duration and large-amplitude motor unit potentials, but these tend to be stable. Polymyositis may lead to short-duration units that are stable in appearance.

106. **B.** Ulnar nerve is prone to compression at the elbow (cubital tunnel) or the wrist (Guyon's canal). With compression at the wrist, the first dorsal interosseous muscle may be affected, but not the flexor carpi ulnaris muscle, because the innervation for this muscle arises proximal to the wrist. Median nerve may be compressed in the carpal tunnel, but not in the Guyon's canal. The common site of radial nerve compression leading to weakness is in the arm.

107. **B.** This median motor study reveals severely prolonged latency, severely reduced amplitude, and severely decreased conduction velocity. These features in combination suggest a demyelinating neuropathy. In severe carpal tunnel syndrome (CTS), latency may be severely prolonged along with severely reduced amplitude, but the conduction velocity is either normal or only mildly reduced. A conduction velocity of less than 20 m/sec is not seen with primary axonal neuropathy. This is an abnormal study, not a normal variant such as Martin–Gruber anastomosis. Limb temperature in this study is optimal.

108. **C.** F-wave amplitude is approximately 3% to 5% of the M-wave amplitude. Only about 3% to 5% of the available motor neurons are activated by their antidromic electrical impulse; hence, the F-wave amplitude is significantly smaller.

109. **B.** The afferent impulse travels from the knee proximally (orthodromic sensory) and the efferent impulse travels from spinal cord to gastrocnemius muscle (orthodromic motor).

110. **D.** This waveform reveals numerous positive sharp wave potentials. Positive sharp waves are spontaneous potentials originating from the muscle fibers and may be seen with neurogenic conditions such as motor neuron disease, axonal neuropathies, and some myopathic conditions such as inflammatory or toxic myopathies. GBS, also known as acute inflammatory demyelinating polyradiculoneuropathy, is predominantly demyelinating, not commonly associated with severe neuropathic changes; however, axonal variant of GBS may have severe neuropathic changes including positive sharp waves and fibrillations.

111. **D.** Even though denervation is seen predominantly in the peroneal-innervated muscles, medial gastrocnemius, a tibial nerve innervated muscle, is also affected. It is not uncommon to have predominant peroneal nerve changes even in clinical scenarios with a primary sciatic nerve lesion. Peroneal nerve lesion alone would not explain the changes seen in the medial gastrocnemius muscle. L5 radiculopathy is expected to cause denervation changes in the gluteus medius muscle and medial gastrocnemius muscle (an S1-innervated muscle) is expected to be normal in L5 radiculopathy. A S1 radiculopathy would not lead to predominant peroneal muscle denervation pattern.

112. **B.** Rise time of the motor unit potential is a direct reflection of the distance between the recording electrode and the nearest muscle fiber. Shorter rise time indicates that the needle is close to the motor unit. To perform quantitative analysis of the motor unit potential, it is important that the recording electrode is very close to the motor unit and have a short rise time.

113. **D.** The description of sensory loss after wearing a tight-fitting bracelet is suggestive of a superficial radial sensory neuropathy, and therefore it is ideal to test this nerve and compare it to the unaffected side. Antebrachial cutaneous nerves or median nerves do not

supply sensation to the dorsum of the hand. Because the symptoms are purely sensory, a radial motor study is not going to be helpful.

114. C. Delayed or absent F-wave response tends to be the first abnormal finding in patients with acute demyelinating polyneuropathy on nerve conduction study. Other demyelinating features, including decreased conduction velocity and conduction block or abnormal temporal dispersion, are seen later in the disease course. In the typical demyelinating form of the illness, axonal features such as reduced motor amplitudes appear later in the disease course.

115. B. This study reveals evidence of a severe demyelinating process (conduction velocity of less than 20 m/sec, a partial conduction block, and severely prolonged distal latency). While conduction block is a feature of acquired inflammatory demyelinating neuropathy, in this case, the partial conduction block is at a common entrapment site (i.e., elbow) and so is not diagnostic of an acquired process. Axonal neuropathies or motor neuron processes do not lead to the noted distal latency or conduction velocity changes. Electrophysiology in MMN usually reveals partial conduction block at a noncompressive site.

116. B. Motor unit potentials in infants are significantly smaller than in adults because of the small muscle fiber size. This is an important finding to remember, as otherwise normal motor unit potentials may be incorrectly called myopathic motor units in infants.

117. A. Among the options presented in the question, only a sensory response can differentiate brachial plexopathy from cervical radiculopathy because it can be abnormal in brachial plexopathy but not in root lesions. Median H-reflex and ulnar motor amplitudes as well as median somatosensory evoked potential can be abnormal in both conditions.

118. C. Myokymic discharges reflect spontaneously firing motor unit action potentials. Other discharges such as complex repetitive discharges, positive sharp waves, and fibrillation potentials are all generated from muscle fibers.

119. D. Active denervation changes may be seen in paraspinal muscles for a prolonged period after extensive lumbosacral spine surgery. Therefore, these changes are not indicative of recent radiculopathy, nonmusculoskeletal pain, or the need for surgery. Because these active denervation changes can result from the surgery itself, they do not necessarily add further information in the workup of radiculopathy after spine surgery. Denervation in lumbar paraspinal musculature is normal.

120. D. The patient presents with chronic symptoms of weakness, atrophy, and sensory loss in the hand muscles. A normal median sensory response with decreased median motor amplitude would be an unusual finding in CTS. MGA, a normal anatomical variant, does not lead to pathological changes such as atrophy. C7–C8 radiculopathy does not explain the findings as the ulnar sensory response was diminished because sensory responses are expected to be preserved in radiculopathy. In lower trunk or medial cord lesion, such as thoracic outlet syndrome, the median and ulnar motor responses will be affected along with the ulnar sensory response; the median sensory response is likely to be preserved as the median sensory fibers travel through the lateral cord and upper trunk. Ulnar neuropathy at the elbow should not cause reduced median motor amplitude.

121. **A.** The study reveals slow repetitive stimulation with significant decrement (35% in this case). Any decrement greater than 10% is considered significant. Stimulus frequency is 3 Hz (as noted in the table in the question). Faster repetitive stimulation is usually at a rate of 20 to 50 Hz. Significant decrement on slow repetitive stimulation can be seen in both presynaptic and postsynaptic neuromuscular junction (NMJ) dysfunction.

122. **C.** The axillary nerve supplies both deltoid and teres minor muscles. The triceps is supplied by the radial nerve. Teres major is supplied by the lower subscapular nerve.

123. **E.** Significant decrement on slow (2–3 Hz) repetitive stimulation can be seen in any of the noted neuromuscular junction (NMJ) disorders. In presynaptic NMJ disorders such as LEMS or botulism, a significant increment in motor amplitude is seen on fast (50 Hz) repetitive stimulation.

124. **B.** Fiber-type grouping is suggestive of the chronic reinnervation process which is characterized by large-amplitude, long-duration motor unit potentials on EMG. Fiber-type grouping is not seen with active denervation, which would be characterized by positive sharp waves and fibrillation potentials. Myopathic disease usually reveal small-amplitude, short-duration motor unit potentials with positive sharp waves and fibrillation potentials in irritative myopathies.

125. **C.** The overall clinical picture and electrodiagnostic findings are suggestive of a slowly progressive motor neurogenic process such as an adult-onset spinal muscular atrophy. Fiber-type grouping on muscle biopsy correlates with chronic reinnervation on needle EMG (large-amplitude and long-duration motor unit potentials). Other options suggest a primary myopathic process but there is no evidence of myopathic motor units on needle EMG. Rimmed vacuoles may be seen in inclusion body myositis, perifascicular atrophy is seen in dermatomyositis, and glycogen positive vacuoles are seen in Pompe disease. Necrotic fibers may be seen necrotizing myopathy, which usually presents with rapid onset weakness and high creatine phosphokinase (CPK).

126. **A.** The study is an example of common electrodiagnostic findings in patients with median mononeuropathy at the wrist and MGA. The distal latency is quite prolonged at 5.5 ms in this example, suggesting a median mononeuropathy at the wrist. In MGA, the anomalous fibers that innervate some of the thenar and hypothenar muscles pass through the ulnar nerve. These muscle fibers are activated before the median-innervated muscle fibers fire, leading to an initial positivity with elbow stimulation. Conduction velocity also tends to be spuriously fast for the same reason.

127. **D.** Only the biceps and brachioradialis reflexes (served by C5–C6) are expected to be absent in a pure upper trunk brachial plexus lesion. Triceps reflex tends to be normal.

128. **B.** The median distal latency is prolonged and median distal compound muscle action potential (CMAP) amplitude is mildly reduced. However, there is no clear evidence of conduction block or slowing of conduction velocity in the forearm. These features suggest that there is median neuropathy distal to stimulation at the wrist and not in the forearm. Additional information including sensory responses are useful but the motor study findings are suggestive of slowing across the wrist.

129. C. Adult conduction velocities are reached in children by the age of 3 to 5 years as myelination of the peripheral nerves is complete by this time. Before 2 years, the normal conduction velocity in a child is still lower than the adult range.

130. C. The largest motor unit only appears once in 200 ms (10 ms per division and there are 20 divisions in the figure in the question). So the firing frequency is 5 Hz ($1/200 \times 1{,}000 = 5$).

131. D. The figure reveals motor unit activity with multiple different motor units firing in groups, consistent with tremor. The frequency of tremor is 6 Hz as approximately six groups of motor unit firing is seen in 1 second (50 ms per division multiplied by 20 divisions). Complex repetitive discharges involve repetitive muscle fiber activity not motor unit activity, and the individual potentials tend to be uniform. In myokymia, a small group of the same motor unit potentials fire together at regular intervals (not different motor unit potentials as shown in this figure). This pattern of grouped motor unit potentials is not typical of diffuse fasciculation potentials and this motor unit firing pattern is not normal.

132. D. Scapular winging can be secondary to either neurogenic or myopathic causes. Common myopathic causes include fascioscapulohumeral muscular dystrophy and various types of limb girdle muscular dystrophies. Injury to the long thoracic nerve (weakness of serratus anterior), injury to the spinal accessory nerve (weakness of trapezius) and injury to dorsal scapular nerve (weakness of rhomboids) may also lead to scapular winging.

133. A. After a focal nerve injury, fibrillations and positive sharp waves indicate wallerian degeneration distal to the site of injury. The time it takes for these changes to appear is a reflection of the distance between the site of nerve injury and muscle being tested.

134. C. This nerve conduction response is most likely seen in hereditary demyelinating polyneuropathy. Other mentioned conditions are acquired causes of demyelinating polyneuropathy, which are unlikely to cause such profound impairment in latency or conduction velocity. In addition, there is no clear evidence of a conduction block or temporal dispersion on this study to support the diagnosis of an acquired demyelinating neuropathy.

135. D. Musculocutaneous nerve innervates the elbow flexors (biceps brachii, brachialis, and coracobrachialis muscles) and terminates as the lateral antebrachial cutaneous nerve. Because other C5–C6-innervated muscles are strong, cervical radiculopathy or upper trunk brachial plexopathy is not likely. With lateral cord brachial plexopathy, the patient will be expected to have weakness in the pronator teres and flexor carpi radialis muscles along with weakness of elbow flexion. Medial cord brachial plexopathy will result in hand weakness and sensory loss. Therefore, this patient's presentation is most consistent with musculocutaneous neuropathy.

136. A. Recording from digit 3 in reference to digit 5 is a referential recording, and it would result in an initial positive deflection due to the approaching wavefront. Moving the reference to digit 3 would be a bipolar recording that would result in an initial negative deflection because the approaching wavefront is sensed by both electrodes and gets cancelled out (similar to having recording and reference electrode over digit 2. Switching the recording electrode to digit 5 and referencing digit 3 results in a waveform that is initially negative and morphologically opposite to the correct answer. If the anode and cathode were reversed, then the stimulation would move proximally up the arm and the distal stimulation could be blocked.

137. **A.** Disulfiram, typically used to treat alcoholism, can cause polyneuropathy. Chloroquine, amiodarone, clofibrates, and colchicine can cause a combination of neuropathy and myopathy associated with vacuolar changes on biopsy.

138. **C.** The most likely localization based on the limited data is the femoral nerve. Because the patient has significant weakness along with sensory loss, a pure sensory neuropathy is not likely. This, along with the absent right saphenous sensory response (saphenous nerve is the terminal branch of the femoral nerve), suggests femoral neuropathy. Sciatic nerve or lower lumbosacral plexus lesion is unlikely as the peroneal, tibial, and sural responses are normal and similar to the opposite side. The lateral femoral cutaneous nerve is a purely sensory nerve and is not expected to cause weakness. L2 to L4 radiculopathy is not likely as saphenous sensory response is absent and sensory responses are usually preserved in primary radiculopathy.

139. **D.** Flexion contracture of the elbow is not a common feature of Pompe disease. Pompe disease is caused by lysosomal acid alpha-glucosidase deficiency. Adult-onset Pompe disease presents with progressive limb and respiratory muscle weakness along with cardiac abnormalities. In addition, some patients have dilated arteriopathy, which can lead to intracranial aneurysms and subarachnoid hemorrhage.

140. **D.** Isolated neck extensor myopathy (INEM) typically presents with severe neck extension weakness without significant involvement of other muscle groups. Creatine phosphokinase (CPK) can be normal or mildly elevated, and EMG reveals myopathic features in cervical paraspinals and proximal limb muscles. While head drop can be one of the features of motor neuron disease, usually there is evidence of weakness in different muscle groups. Myasthenia gravis (MG) can also cause head drop but patients also complain of fatigue, ptosis, or bulbar weakness. Pompe disease can cause significant proximal weakness, but isolated neck extensor weakness makes this diagnosis less likely. Inclusion body myositis causes a unique pattern of weakness with predominant involvement of quadriceps and finger flexor muscle.

141. **C.** Progressive proximal limb weakness with worsening respiratory function should raise the possibility of Pompe disease (acid maltase deficiency), especially in a patient with limb girdle pattern of weakness. EMG of the thoracic paraspinal muscles might reveal myotonia in Pompe disease; therefore, this should be performed. A dried blood spot might help confirm the diagnosis of Pompe disease without having to perform a muscle biopsy. Diaphragmatic EMG is not needed in this patient. Long exercise testing is usually preformed to assess for channelopathies or nondystrophic myotonias, but this clinical presentation is not suggestive of those disorders.

142. **A.** Decreased distal CMAP amplitude indicates wallerian degeneration, and therefore is not consistent with isolated neuropraxic injury. Decreased proximal CMAP amplitude and conduction block are suggestive of focal demyelination as seen in neuropraxic injury. With a pure neuropraxic injury, motor units firing may not be seen on needle EMG; however, evidence of active denervation is less likely. Severe neuropraxic injuries

leads to absent F-wave responses as there is lack of transmission across the neuropraxic injury site.

143. C. The firing frequency is calculated based on sweep speed and the number of times the waveform is seen in the epoch. In the waveform displayed in the question, the largest single motor unit fires two times in 200 ms. So, the firing frequency is 10 Hz (expected to fire 10 times in 1 second). Motor unit amplitude is the maximum peak-to-peak amplitude of the main spike of motor unit potential. Since each small vertical box is 1 mV and the largest motor unit amplitude is approximately 7.5 mV.

144. C. The motor terminal branch of the radial nerve, the posterior interosseous nerve, may be prone to compression at the Arcade of Frohse and can cause weakness in the distal muscles, such as exor carpi radialis. Other nerves do not go through the Arcade of Frohse, and so are not sites of compression at the location.

145. D. Medial aspect of the leg is supplied by the saphenous nerve, which is a branch of the femoral nerve rather than the sciatic nerve and is, therefore, expected to be normal after sciatic nerve injury. Other parts of the leg and foot given as options are supplied by branches of the sciatic nerve: dorsum of the foot and lateral part of the calf is supplied by the superficial peroneal nerve; the sole of the foot is supplied by the distal tibial nerve; the first web space between the great toe and second toe is supplied by the deep peroneal nerve; and lateral aspect of the foot is supplied by sural nerve.

146. C. The clinical description and examination findings in the question are classical for Guillain–Barré syndrome (GBS). In patients with GBS, F-waves and H-reflexes are the first responses to become abnormal. After this, motor and sensory changes are seen. Occasionally, sural response remains normal even though median or ulnar sensory amplitudes are decreased ("sural sparing phenomenon"). Slow repetitive stimulation is expected to be normal since GBS is not a neuromuscular junction disorder.

147. D. HIV infection can lead to multiple types of neuropathy, the most common being the distal symmetrical polyneuropathy, presenting with numbness in toes and feet as well as pain in feet. AIDP can be seen with HIV infection, mostly during the seroconversion phase. Clinically, AIDP with HIV infection might not be distinguishable from the idiopathic form but cerebrospinal fluid (CSF) is expected to have a high white blood cell (WBC) count (with lymphocytic pleocytosis), along with high protein, raising a possibility of a viral infection. Chronic inflammatory demyelinating polyneuropathy (CIDP) may develop anytime with HIV infection. Other less common forms of neuropathy seen with HIV infection include sensory neuronopathy or ganglionopathy and autonomic neuropathy. Multifocal motor neuropathy is not typically associated with HIV infection. It should be noted that some of the retroviral medication used to treat HIV can also cause sensory neuropathy. Autonomic neuropathy is seen with HIV-positive status with sympathetic and parasympathetic involvement.

148. B. This figure reveals abundant positive sharp waves and occasional fibrillation potentials. Both of them originate at the muscle fiber. Spontaneous potentials such as fasciculation potentials originate from the anterior horn cells or motor nerve. Complex repetitive discharges originate from the muscle fibers due to ephaptic transmission.

149. B. The clinical history is suggestive of a progressive disorder with spasticity and neuropathy. The patient's brother also has similar manifestations (suggesting a potential X-linked dominant pattern of inheritance). This raises the possibility of adrenomyeloneuropathy (AMN), which is associated with peripheral neuropathy. On nerve conduction studies, these patients have predominant axonal changes with sensory and motor nerve involvement and mild slowing. Primary demyelinating neuropathy is not a common feature of AMN.

150. B. The nerve conduction study reveals severely prolonged duration and profoundly diminished conduction velocity along with severely reduced amplitude, suggestive of a hereditary demyelinating neuropathy. Among the options presented in the question, PMP mutation analysis, which tests for Charcot–Marie–Tooth (CMT) type 1A or hereditary neuropathy with liability to pressure palsy (HNPP), will be the most appropriate. MFN mutations usually present with axonal features on nerve conduction studies. Abnormal very long-chain fatty acids are useful in adrenomyeloneuropathy; however, this usually does not lead to this degree of demyelination on nerve conduction studies. Spinal fluid analysis is more likely to be helpful in chronic inflammatory demyelinating polyneuropathy (CIDP), a type of acquired demyelinating neuropathy, not hereditary demyelinating neuropathy as shown in the question's figure. Diabetes can cause neuropathy, but this degree of slowing is not seen with diabetic neuropathy.

151. B. The clue to arriving at the correct answer lies in noticing the sweep speed and gain setting. Although 100 uV of gain may be occasionally (normally 50 uV) used to assess spontaneous activity, sweep speed is set for 500 ms and the whole epoch is 10 seconds long (500 ms multiplied by 20). Once these values are considered, it becomes obvious that the firing pattern is suggestive of normal active breathing. Motor unit morphology or abnormal spontaneous activity cannot be identified at this sweep speed; therefore, it is not possible to differentiate between a neurogenic or myopathic process. Paying attention to sweep speed again avoids confusion with myotonia.

152. C. A nerve conduction velocity in the range of 25 to 26 m/sec is considered normal in a 25-day-old infant. The velocity is lower than that of adults because the myelination is not complete; however, this does not mean that the infant has demyelinating neuropathy. It is not possible to infer if the infant has myopathy based on the conduction velocity. Neuromuscular junction diseases cannot be diagnosed solely based on normal nerve conduction velocity.

153. C. Rapid or early recruitment on needle EMG indicates a disease of muscle fiber such as muscular dystrophies and is not a neurogenic feature. ALS and CMT diseases are neurogenic conditions that cause denervation and lead to decreased recruitment patterns on needle EMG. Needle EMG in a patient with periodic paralysis in between episodes of weakness is normal and during an episode of weakness may cause mild irritative change. Hereditary spastic paraparesis is likely to reveal normal needle EMG patterns or reduced activation, but no changes on recruitment.

154. B. Bulbar and facial weakness with significant decrement on repetitive study is suggestive of myasthenia gravis (MG). Lack of response or worsening of symptoms with pyridostigmine along with normal AChR antibody testing should prompt additional testing for muscle-specific kinase (MuSK) antibody testing. This case is not suggestive of Lambert–Eaton myasthenic syndrome (LEMS), so voltage-gated calcium channel antibody is not going to be useful. The patient already has significant decrement on repetitive stimulation, so single-fiber EMG is not needed. Muscle biopsy is not useful in neuromuscular junction (NMJ) disorders. Although clinical history is suggestive of neuromuscular junction disorder, this is not likely congenital myasthenic syndrome since onset and progression are suggestive of acquired NMJ disorder.

155. C. This peroneal motor study reveals the presence of an accessory peroneal nerve, a normal anatomical variant. In the presence of an accessory peroneal nerve, the compound muscle action potential (CMAP) amplitude will be higher with stimulation at the fibular head than at the ankle because the accessory peroneal nerve supplies the lateral half of the extensor digitorum brevis muscle. Stimulation posterior to the lateral malleolus will confirm the presence of accessory peroneal nerve. There is no evidence of peroneal neuropathy at any site on this study. Accessory peroneal nerve does not indicate an underlying tibial neuropathy.

156. D. Because this is an acute neurogenic process, even though there is weakness, spontaneous activity may remain normal for 7 to 10 days. Motor unit morphology changes will take a few weeks to become obvious. However, recruitment pattern tends to be decreased even during the acute phase and is an early EMG abnormality in patients with GBS.

157. B. Diffuse myokymia is seen in Isaac's syndrome and voltage-gated potassium channel antibody titer may be elevated in this condition. Voltage-gated calcium channel antibody is associated with Lambert–Eaton myasthenic syndrome (LEMS); AChR antibody is seen with myasthenia gravis (MG); GM1 antibody is elevated in with multifocal motor neuropathy; NT5C1A antibody is associated with inclusion body myositis; and none of these four conditions is known to cause diffuse myokymia.

158. C. There is evidence of conduction block across the elbow without any evidence of a distal axonal process (note that the distal latency and amplitude are normal). Therefore, this nerve conduction study is suggestive of a focal demyelinating process at the elbow. In focal demyelinating lesions, EMG may reveal reduced recruitment patterns but not early recruitment process, as this is associated with myopathic process. Positive sharp waves and fibrillation potentials indicate active denervation, while large-amplitude and long-duration motor unit potentials indicate chronic reinnervation; these are seen with axonal processes, not with focal demyelinating causes.

159. C. This is a normal study. There is no significant decrement, defined as more than a 10% decrease in amplitude. There is no evidence of facilitation. Because there was no significant decrement, repair is not expected.

160. B. In peroneal nerve studies, the reference electrode does not contribute significantly to the resulting waveform. Recall that the resulting waveform after nerve stimulation is the difference between what the recording and reference electrodes sense. In an ideal scenario, the recording electrode would be contributing the entire waveform and the reference electrode would sense no response. For the most part, this is what occurs in motor studies of the median and peroneal nerves. Only a subset of the muscles in the region is stimulated, allowing the reference electrode to be relatively uninvolved in the field. Volume conduction is negligible. However, motor studies of the tibial, ulnar, and radial nerves tend to stimulate a large subset of the muscles in the region, resulting in an actively involved reference electrode contributing significantly to the resulting waveform.

161. C. End-plate spikes are seen because of nerve twig irritation by the needle electrode. End-plate spikes can be morphologically similar to fibrillation potentials but they subside when the needle is moved away from the end-plate region. Positive sharp waves have predominant positive (downward) spikes and are not usually confused with fibrillation potentials. Fasciculation potentials are large, irregular firing motor unit potentials. Tremor is because of a group of motor units firing in a regular pattern and is not generally confused with fibrillation potentials. Motor unit potential amplitude is much larger than fibrillation potentials and is seen with active muscle contraction only unlike fibrillation potential which is usually assessed at rest.

162. B. Recruitment frequency of 30 Hz is very high and is seen with neurogenic conditions. After poliomyelitis, the surviving motor nerves reinnervate, and this leads to long-duration and large-amplitude motor units with significantly increased recruitment frequency. In a complete traumatic nerve injury with no reinnervation, no motor unit activity is seen. In neuromuscular junction (NMJ) disorders such as LEMS or MG, variability in the motor unit amplitude may be seen but not increased recruitment frequency. In polymyositis, irritative myopathic changes and an early recruitment pattern are seen.

163. A. The clinical description of this case is suggestive of myotonic dystrophy. Chronic facial weakness, ptosis, and limb weakness with postanesthesia worsening of symptoms is typical of myotonic dystrophy. While myasthenia gravis (MG)-related symptoms can be worse after anesthesia, a 10-year history and distal weakness makes this less likely. Abnormal increment on fast repetitive stimulation suggests a presynaptic disease such as Lambert–Eaton myasthenic syndrome (LEMS), but the phenotype described is not consistent with it. Other myopathic disorders, such as mitochondrial diseases, can also cause ptosis and myopathic motor unit potentials on EMG; however, the clinical description is not typical of mitochondrial disease. Chronic neurogenic changes with reduced recruitment patterns are seen with neurogenic syndromes, but this clinical history is not typical of any neurogenic diseases.

164. A. F estimate is calculated on the basis on the distal latency, the conduction velocity, and the distance between the stimulator electrode and the spinal cord. Height or limb length essentially reflects the distance between stimulator and spinal cord. F estimate does not depend on the CMAP amplitude. F estimate is helpful in determining whether the delayed F-wave latency is primarily due to a decrease in conduction velocity and prolongation of distal latency or due to an underlying demyelination in the proximal segment of the nerve.

165. A. After remyelination, the length of the internode decreases. Longer internodes correspond to faster conduction velocity, which would not be expected in cases of incomplete recovery from GBS. Shorter internodes, onion bulb formation, and decrease in the nerve fiber density on skin biopsy are typical pathological findings after incomplete recovery from GBS. Muscle biopsy will reveal a neurogenic process including loss of checkerboard pattern.

166. B. Type 2b, not type 1 or type 2a, muscle fiber atrophy is seen in steroid myopathy. Creatinine kinase tends to be normal. Irritative changes are not common with steroid myopathy, unlike inflammatory or toxic myopathy. Flourinated corticosteroids are more likely to cause myopathy than nonfluorinated corticosteroids.

167. B. The patient most likely has an upper trunk brachial plexopathy. Denervation is only seen in the muscles supplied by the upper trunk. Normal median motor and ulnar motor and sensory studies as well as normal EMG of FDI and APB muscles make a lower trunk or medial cord lesion unlikely. His lateral antebrachial sensory response is absent, which makes radiculopathy less likely. EMG of the serratus anterior is normal and this argues against C5–C6–C7 root lesion. Posterior cord lesion is not expected to cause weakness in the biceps muscle.

168. B. Tabulated nerve conduction study reveals absent motor responses with normal sensory responses. This is suggestive of a motor nerve, root, or anterior horn cell disease. The preceding viral illness before the onset of limb weakness makes West Nile-associated poliomyelitis type syndrome the likely diagnosis. Monomelic amyotrophy (Hirayama's disease) leads to very slowly progressive weakness and takes a few years to manifest. Focal weakness after a viral illness makes spinobulbar muscular atrophy or ALS unlikely. Although multifocal motor neuropathy does cause focal motor neuropathy and reduced or absent chronic inflammatory demyelinating polyneuropathy (CMAP) and normal sensory responses, the disease course is not typical of MMN.

169. B. Hydroxychloroquine can lead to a neuropathy and myopathy. Electrodiagnostic studies will reveal axonal neuropathy and myopathic motor units on needle electromyography (EMG). Muscle biopsy may reveal vacuolar myopathy with curvilinear bodies seen on electron microscopy. Metronidazole, isoniazid, cisplatin, and phenytoin typically cause axonal polyneuropathy.

170. B. Very early in compressive or traumatic neuropathies, distal motor and sensory responses are generally normal. Within 24 hours of a nerve injury, responses on distal stimulation are likely to be normal as well. Therefore, it is not possible to exclude a focal neuropathy by distal stimulation alone early in the course of a nerve injury. Comparing distal response with the opposite limb is not going to help since distal response might be normal.

171. B. When selecting a muscle for biopsy in patients with suspected myopathy, it is ideal to select a muscle that is mildly weak. Severely weak muscle (MRC 3 or less) might have significant end-stage muscle changes on biopsy and the results might not be diagnostic. Biopsy of completely atrophic muscle is not going to be diagnostic either as muscle fibers are likely replaced by fibrous tissue. Similarly, a muscle with normal strength will also have decreased diagnostic yield. There is no consensus that an MRI of the muscle is needed before biopsy but few physicians use MRI scans to help identify the muscle with maximal changes, especially in cases of inflammatory myopathy.

172. C. The most likely neuromuscular manifestations of amiodarone include both neuropathy and myopathy. Neuropathy characteristically tends to be axonal in nature. Muscle biopsy may reveal autophagic vacuoles and phospholipid inclusions. Amiodarone is not associated with neuromuscular junction dysfunction or motor neuron pathology.

173. C. Active and chronic denervation changes are seen in deltoid and triceps muscles. No clear denervation changes are seen in the biceps, first dorsal interosseous, and abductor pollicis brevis muscles. Even though the deltoid is supplied by the axillary nerve and the triceps is supplied by the radial nerve, both these nerves arise from the posterior cord. Because biceps are normal, lateral cord or upper trunk involvement is less likely. As first dorsal interosseous and abductor pollicis brevis muscles are normal, medial cord or lower trunk involvement is less likely.

174. C. The patient most likely has spinobulbar muscular atrophy. Slowly progressive predominant flaccid bulbar weakness followed by limb weakness, decreased reflexes, and fasciculation potentials are suggestive of spinobulbar muscular atrophy (Kennedy's disease). Unlike ALS, SMA, or PLS, sural sensory amplitude is either severely diminished or absent in spinobulbar muscular atrophy. Upper motor predominant ALS does not cause flaccid limb weakness or fasciculations.

175. A. The latency for the wrist stimulation is almost 5 ms and the onset latency for the elbow stimulation is approximately 17 ms. Therefore, the difference in the latencies is approximately 12 ms, and the conduction velocity is clearly less than 20 m/sec (225 mm/17 ms). In addition, there is a clear drop in amplitude on proximal stimulation without significant increase in duration, suggestive of partial conduction block and not abnormal temporal dispersion. In combination, this study is consistent with an acquired demyelinating neuropathy.

176. C. Among the choices given in the question, C5 or C6 root injury is not likely because both median and radial sensory responses were abnormal. Spinal accessory nerve injury does not lead to sensory nerve changes in the median or radial nerve. Upper trunk brachial plexopathy is the most likely cause. Lower trunk brachial plexopathy does not cause reduced median and radial sensory nerve amplitudes.

177. C. Decrement on repetitive stimulation study would suggest a neuromuscular junction (NMJ) dysfunction. However, decrement is usually found in weak muscles. Because the patient does not have any distal limb weakness, it is not surprising that repetitive stimulation of the ulnar nerve is normal. In such cases, repetitive stimulation of the facial or spinal accessory nerves will likely reveal significant decrement. Giving pyridostigmine would mask findings and is not recommended. Using higher frequency of repetitive stimulation will not help with diagnosis of MG. Warming the limb, while useful in increasing the yield of repetitive stimulation, is helpful only when the limb is cold. Single-fiber EMG is certainly an option, but this is generally performed if repetitive stimulation is not diagnostic and repetitive stimulation is mostly diagnostic in the weak muscles only.

178. C. Decreased temperature leads to prolonged latency, decreased conduction velocity, and may lead to increased amplitude. While it is possible to correct for decreased temperature by various correction factors, the examiner should always make an attempt to warm the lower limb to an acceptable temperature before performing the study. The ideal temperature for the lower limb is at least 30°C; for an upper limb, it is 32°C. As an electrodiagnostic physician, one should always aim to perform a technically appropriate study and not leave it to referring physician to interpret a technically limited study.

179. A. Clinical history is suggestive of periodic paralysis. In between episodes, EMG in periodic paralysis will be normal. During an episode of weakness, an increased insertional activity may be seen. Recruitment patterns remain normal in periodic paralysis in between episodes.

180. A. The first repetitive stimulation performed at baseline reveals a significant decrement with 19% reduction in amplitude. Postexercise (only after 15 seconds), there is a repair of the decrement with the maximum decrement less than 10%. These features suggest both significant decrement and repair of the decrement after exercise, consistent with a neuromuscular junction defect. There are no obvious technical limiting factors on this study.

181. C. In neuromuscular junction (NMJ) disorders such as MG, there is intermittent failure of some muscle fibers within a motor unit to fire due to blocking. This leads to variation in motor unit amplitude. Large-amplitude polyphasic motor unit potentials and motor unit potentials with increased recruitment frequency are seen in neurogenic conditions. Positive sharp waves and fibrillation potentials are seen in neurogenic and in irritative myopathic processes but not in MG.

182. B. Needle EMG reveals very large motor units (approximately 5 mV in amplitude) and increased duration. These features favor a chronic neurogenic process with reinnervation changes. Among the options presented in the question, only chronic polyradiculopathy could lead to this type of motor unit potential morphology. Acute neuropathies such as AIDP can lead to active denervation changes but not chronic reinnervation changes. Myopathies, toxic or steroid induced, lead to small, short-duration motor unit potentials but not motor unit potentials. Neuromuscular junction disorders do not cause significant changes in motor unit morphology.

183. D. Biceps, triceps, and brachioradialis reflexes are served by C5–C6–C7 roots, so these are not affected in a pure lower trunk lesion. This is important to remember, as normal deep tendon reflexes in the affected upper limb will not rule out a lower trunk brachial plexopathy.

184. C. Among the options given in the question, suprascapular neuropathy is most likely in volleyball players because of the tethering of the nerve near the suprascapular notch. Suprascapular neuropathy can lead to pain and weakness (abduction and external rotation) in the shoulder. Therefore, needle EMG of the supraspinatus and infraspinatus is going to be most helpful.

185. B. The correct answer is the trapezius, which is supplied by the spinal accessory nerve. Spinal accessory is one of the superficial nerves in the neck and is likely to be damaged. Nerves supplying other muscles are deeper in the cervical triangle area and are less likely to be injured during lymph node biopsy.

186. B. Tibialis posterior is supplied by the L5 root and tibial nerve and not the peroneal nerve. The short head of the biceps femoris and peroneus brevis are supplied by the L5 root and peroneal nerve. Medial gastrocnemius muscle is supplied by the S1 root and tibial nerve. Tibilias anterior is innervated by peroneal nerve and predominantly has L4/L5 fibers. Therefore, among these options, only tibialis posterior can differentiate L5 radiculopathy from peroneal mononeuropathy.

187. B. Perifascicular atrophy is a characteristic feature on dermatomyositis. Rimmed vacuoles are seen in inclusion body myositis. Myofiber necrosis and endomysial inflammatory infiltrates may be seen in polymyositis. Cox negative fibers is a feature of mitochondrial disorders and while it can be seen in inflammatory myopathies, it is not a characteristic finding of dermatomyositis.

188. D. Typical findings in botulism include low-CMAP amplitude, increment on fast repetitive stimulation (or more than 100% facilitation after brief exercise), decrement on slow repetitive stimulation, and active denervation potentials in weak muscles. Such active denervation changes are not usually seen in other neuromuscular junction (NMJ) disorders such as myasthenia gravis (MG) or Lambert–Eaton myasthenic syndrome (LEMS).

189. D. Decreased recruitment of motor unit potentials is the earliest feature. Positive sharp waves and fibrillation potentials are seen later in the course, usually about 10 to 14 days after disease onset. Complex repetitive discharge and polyphasic motor unit potentials are usually features of chronic denervation. Short-duration motor unit potentials is a feature of myopathic disorders.

190. C. Less than 10% drop in amplitude on proximal stimulation is normal because of normal temporal dispersion. In MGA, there is generally an increase in amplitude on proximal stimulation in median motor study and an abnormal decrease in amplitude with proximal ulnar stimulation.

191. C. During needle EMG study, if the insertional activity lasts less than 300 ms after moving the concentric EMG needle, it is considered normal. It is due to transient membrane instability caused by the probing needle electrode. Insertional activity lasting more than 300 ms is considered abnormal.

192. B. The EMG shows both positive sharp waves and fibrillation potentials, suggesting active denervation and is never a normal finding even in older individuals. In addition, there were motor unit potentials with increased duration and amplitude which suggests chronic reinnervation. These features in combination suggest that the patient has both active denervation and chronic reinnervation changes in the right tibialis anterior muscle.

193. B. GBS cannot be ruled out because normal sural response is not uncommon in GBS. This is the so-called sural sparing phenomenon seen in GBS. It is not possible to rule out GBS just because sural response is normal, and not all types of neuropathies lead to abnormal sural sensory response. Only length-dependent axonal sensorimotor neuropathies initially affect the sural response. If the rest of the clinical picture and other diagnostic studies such as spinal fluid analysis are suggestive of GBS, a nerve conduction study is not always needed to start treatment in patients with GBS. Routine sedation under anesthesia is not recommended in GBS as this may precipitate ventilator failure.

194. C. Excess vitamin B6 or pyridoxine toxicity typically causes numbness and ataxia without weakness. Nerve conduction studies typically reveal a sensory neuropathy with absent sensory nerve responses. Motor neuropathy or myopathies are not seen with vitamin B6 toxicity. B6 toxicity does not lead to myopathy.

195. B. The clinical picture is suggestive of a myopathy, and because of recent onset and fast progression, an acquired inflammatory myopathy is possible. Short-duration and small-amplitude motor units are suggestive of a myopathic process. Early recruitment pattern is seen in myopathic processes. Positive sharp waves and fibrillation potentials are suggestive of irritative myopathy. Long-duration motor units are commonly seen in neurogenic process.

196. B. Bifid sensory nerve action potentials in children can be a normal variant as not all fibers are myelinated to the same degree. As myelination becomes complete, the bifid morphology disappears. This is not related to poor technique and is not suggestive of neuropathy. Bifid sensory nerve action potentials is not a feature of axonal or demyelinating neuropathy.

197. B. The median and ulnar motor responses and ulnar sensory responses are affected. These nerve fibers pass through the lower trunk and medial cord. Median sensory fibers are preserved because they originate in the C5–C6 roots and pass through the upper trunk and lateral cord. C8–T1 roots are not likely to be involved because the sensory responses will be normal in isolated root lesions (note that the ulnar sensory response was absent in this patient).

198. C. Positive sharp waves/fibrillation potentials and short-duration motor unit potentials are usually seen in inflammatory myopathies such as polymyositis, dermatomyositis, and toxic myopathies. Long-duration motor unit potentials are typically seen in chronic neurogenic processes. Rarely, in some myopathies, long-duration motor unit potentials may be seen after reinnervation but with early recruitment pattern. Early recruitment pattern is a major feature in myopathic conditions in weak muscles.

199. D. The clinical presentation in the question is most consistent with injury to the distal deep palmar motor branch of the ulnar nerve in the palm. This nerve supplies the interossei and third and fourth lumbricals in the hand. This nerve does not have any sensory fibers, and therefore patients do not experience any sensory loss. As abductor digiti minimi is not affected, the nerve supply to the hypothenar muscles is likely normal. His median-innervated muscles are not affected so anterior interosseous neuropathy or medial cord brachial plexopathy is not likely. An ulnar neuropathy in the forearm or at the elbow is not likely as the ulnar sensory response and ulnar motor response to hypothenar muscles are normal.

200. C. Presentation with asymmetrical ptosis, facial weakness, weakness of neck flexion, and proximal limb weakness is suggestive of a NMJ dysfunction. Peripheral nerve disease generally causes distal weakness but proximal weakness can occur in conditions such as Guillain–Barré syndrome, which would be expected to have absent reflexes as well. Muscle diseases can cause facial and proximal limb weakness, but asymmetrical ptosis is unusual. Acute anterior horn disease is unusual, will be associated with weakness, and usually does not cause ptosis. It would be unusual to have acute multiple cranial neuropathies causing ptosis and facial weakness but not cause any extra ocular movement deficits.

201. C. CPK levels are more useful in patients with inflammatory muscle disease and not neuromuscular junction (NMJ) dysfunction. Routine nerve conduction study will help with neuropathy but not NMJ dysfunction, the exception being Lambert–Eaton myasthenic syndrome (LEMS) where small compound muscle action potential (CMAP) amplitudes are seen. While acetylcholine receptor (AChR) antibody tests are confirmatory when positive, they usually will take a few days to return. Needle EMG testing might reveal motor unit variability in NMJ disorder, but this finding is not used to diagnose NMJ disease. Spinal fluid analysis is used in nerve root or cranial nerve disorders. In this context, repetitive nerve stimulation can confirm the diagnosis quickly.

202. B. The study shows a normal slow (3 Hz), not fast repetitive stimulation. The peak amplitude and area of each motor response does not decrease by more than 10%. This is not surprising as the patient does not have any distal weakness. Significant decrement (>10% decrease in amplitude) in MG is usually seen in the weak muscles. There is no decrement or increment seen in this study. Abnormal increment is seen in LEMS with fast repetitive stimulation.

203. A. The study is abnormal showing decrement (more than 10% decrease in amplitude) on slow (3 Hz) repetitive stimulation of the spinal accessory nerve. Significant decrement on slow repetitive stimulation is consistent with a neuromuscular junction (NMJ) dysfunction. In this case, because of recent onset ocular, facial, and proximal limb weakness, this is most likely secondary to MG. Repetitive stimulation below 5 to 10 Hz is considered slow repetitive stimulation.

204. B. When the repetitive nerve stimulation study is suggestive of myasthenia gravis (MG), the next most appropriate step is to check AChR antibodies to confirm the diagnosis and CT scan of the chest to rule out thymoma. MuSK antibody should be considered if the AChR antibody is negative. The case is not consistent with Lambert–Eaton myasthenic syndrome (LEMS), so voltage-gated calcium channel antibody is not going to be helpful. MRI brain is normal in patients with myasthenia gravis (MG). Paraneoplastic panel and PET scan are not routinely performed in patients with MG. MR spine and spinal fluid analysis again will be normal in patients with MG.

205. C. This patient has all the manifestations of peripheral nerve disease, including distal more than proximal weakness, distal atrophy, sensory loss, and areflexia. There is no evidence of any central dysmyelination syndrome such as spasticity or cognitive impairment. Predominant distal pattern of weakness makes a root localization unlikely.

206. A. While the clinical scenario described suggests neuropathy as the most likely diagnosis, nerve conduction studies are helpful in differentiating between the types of neuropathy (e.g., demyelinating vs. axonal) and guide genetic testing. Repetitive stimulation will not be useful in this case. Performing needle electromyography (EMG) may not be useful as this is a primary neurogenic process, although it can be performed after nerve conduction studies to ascertain the extent of denervation. MRI of the brain and spine or spinal analysis will not be useful as the patient likely has a pure peripheral nerve disease.

207. A. The nerve conduction study shows demyelinating neuropathy with profoundly diminished conduction velocity and a partial conduction block. However, the partial conduction block is across the elbow, a common compressive site. The conduction velocity is clearly in the demyelinating range in this case, and therefore a primary axonal neuropathy is unlikely. The drop in amplitude across the elbow meets the criteria for conduction block (greater than 50% drop in both amplitude and area across the elbow).

208. B. This patient most likely has hereditary demyelinating polyneuropathy. Long history suggests a hereditary process. Examination is consistent with severe neuropathy, and nerve conduction study is suggestive of a hereditary demyelinating process. Even though there is conduction block, it is across a common entrapment site such as the elbow. While a distal myopathy causes distal weakness, the presence of sensory loss on examination and absent sural response do not favor a distal myopathy. Severe slowing in conduction velocity is not consistent with axonal neuropathy.

209. A. This patient has clear evidence of severe demyelinating neuropathy suggestive of an underlying hereditary process. Additional conduction block across the elbow could suggest hereditary neuropathy with liability to pressure palsy (HNPP), which is characterized by evidence of diffuse polyneuropathy with conduction block across common entrapment sites. Alternatively, this case could represent the most common form of hereditary demyelinating neuropathy, Charcot–Marie–Tooth (CMT) type 1A, in which the underlying genetic abnormality is PMP deletion in 70% of cases. MFN mutation is seen in axonal neuropathy. Spinal fluid analysis and sural nerve biopsy will not be useful. Muscle biopsy would not help in differentiating the causes of neuropathy. Repetitive nerve stimulation might be useful in congenital myasthenic syndrome but not in CMT.

210. B. Slowly progressive proximal limb and facial weakness along with myalgia is suggestive of muscle disease. The patient's examination only reveals proximal weakness, which is typical of most acquired muscle diseases. Lack of distal weakness, normal reflexes, and sensory examination makes primary peripheral nerve localization unlikely. Neuromuscular junction (NMJ) disorders such as myasthenia gravis (MG) cause proximal and facial weakness but generally do not cause any pain. Clinical picture is not consistent with spinal cord or anterior horn cell localization.

211. C. This is a normal nerve conduction study of the left tibial nerve. The amplitude and conduction velocity are in the normal range. Demyelinating neuropathy is not likely as the latency and conduction velocity are normal. Proximal motor latency depends on limb length and conduction velocity is an appropriate measure of proximal nerve conduction.

212. C. At rest, the spontaneous activity revealed positive sharp waves and fibrillations (trace A). On activation, short-duration motor units were seen (trace B). The duration, if measured, would be less than 5 ms. Long-duration motor unit potentials are more than 15 to 20 ms. All of these features favor an irritative myopathy.

213. C. The motor unit potentials look "myopathic" with short duration and small amplitude. Because the whole epoch is filled with different motor units with minimal effort, it is consistent with early recruitment that is indicative of myopathic disorders. Decreased recruitment pattern is usually seen in neurogenic processes.

214. B. Ptosis and proximal weakness may be seen with either NMJ or muscle disorders. Furthermore, proximal weakness with absent deep tendon reflexes suggest Lambert–Eaton myasthenic syndrome (LEMS), an NMJ disorder, as the likely cause. By the same token, absent tendon reflexes and dry mouth are not common features in most muscle diseases. While some inflammatory neuropathies may cause proximal weakness with absent reflexes, normal sensory examination makes this less likely. Anterior horn cell disease or multiple root involvement typically does not cause ptosis and tends to cause both proximal and distal weakness.

215. C. Presynaptic disorders such as Lambert–Eaton myasthenic syndrome (LEMS) commonly cause reduced motor amplitude. Absent sensory responses are typically seen with neuropathies. Decreased conduction velocity or absent F-wave responses are a feature of nerve diseases. Positive sharp waves and fibrillation potentials are typically seen in denervation in neurogenic processes and in inflammatory myopathies.

216. C. This nerve conduction study reveals a 10-second postexercise test. The second stimulation reveals a greater than 100% increment in motor amplitude compared to baseline stimulation. Such a high degree of increment is characteristic of a presynaptic disorder such as Lambert–Eaton myasthenic syndrome (LEMS). In a normal post-10-second exercise test, there is no or very minimal increase in motor amplitude (<10%). Motor amplitude on repeat test is clearly higher than the baseline test and a 10-second exercise test is as sensitive as 50 Hz stimulation. This study is not technically limited and proximal stimulation is not needed to show a postexercise increment in CMAP amplitude.

217. A. This patient has a presynaptic neuromuscular junction (NMJ) disorder with Lambert–Eaton myasthenic syndrome (LEMS) being the most likely cause. Diagnostic workup for LEMS should involve checking for voltage-gated calcium channel antibodies, followed by others including CT scan of the chest and PET scan. AChR antibodies and MuSK antibodies are tested in patients with myasthenia gravis (MG) and are not expected to be useful in this case. A complete paraneoplastic panel and PET scan will be less useful because the syndrome is most consistent with LEMS in this case and focused testing is more efficient and economical. Spinal fluid analysis and MR brain are not helpful with diagnosis of LEMS.

218. B. This patient most likely has Lambert–Eaton myasthenic syndrome (LEMS), which can be either paraneoplastic or autoimmune. Some patients with LEMS do not have an underlying neoplastic cause and are expected to have relatively normal life expectancy if their disease is well controlled. In patients with an underlying malignancy, treatment of the malignancy would be the most appropriate option. If no malignancy is found after extensive workup, immunotherapy is helpful. 3,4-diaminopyridine (3,4 DAP) can provide symptomatic treatment, but response to therapy might be incomplete and patients may require extensive immunotherapy.

219. C. This study reveals low-CMAP amplitude with >100% increase in CMAP amplitude after brief exercise. This degree of facilitation after exercise is suggestive of presynaptic NMJ disorders such as Lambert–Eaton myasthenic syndrome (LEMS). Baseline CMAP amplitude is low in LEMS and it is always appropriate to repeat stimulation after brief exercise to look for facilitation if CMAP amplitudes are low during nerve conduction studies. Conduction velocity and distal latencies are normal in this study.

220. B. This motor nerve conduction study revealed clear prolongation of distal latency, and severely reduced conduction velocities. Additionally, there is a clear abnormal temporal dispersion on proximal stimulation. These features are suggestive of a demyelinating neuropathy. Axonal neuropathies and motor neuron diseases usually only lead to reduced amplitude and mild slowing. Distal myopathies may cause low compound muscle action potential (CMAP) amplitudes.

221. B. History of ocular and limb weakness which improved with prednisone and recurrence is concerning for neuromuscular junction (NMJ) disorder. Slow repetitive stimulation at 2 Hz of spinal accessory nerve reveals >10% decrement at baseline after exercise and is suggestive of neuromuscular junction dysfunction. This is not a fast repetitive stimulation study.

222. B. This is a slow repetitive stimulation with significant decrement. Additionally, there is evidence of significant facilitation after exercise (shown twice in this series). While decrement is obvious on repetitive stimulation, there is a clear evidence of facilitation after exercise, so option A is incorrect. This is not a normal study.

223. B. This is likely Parsonage Turner syndrome, inflammatory brachial plexopathy, frequently seen after recent viral infections or after surgeries with pain and predominant motor nerve involvement. Neuropraxic injury is not likely, as single nerve injury does not explain elbow flexion weakness and scapular winging. There is no history to suspect traumatic brachial plexopathy or cervical radiculopathy. Postsurgical inflammatory neuropathy is typically an inflammatory neuropathy within the vicinity of the surgery, but not directly related to any surgical intervention.

224. C. The adductor longus muscle is innervated by the obturator nerve which originates from the lumbo- sacral plexus. The iliopsoas and vastus lateralis muscles are innervated by the femoral nerve and the lumbo-sacral plexus. Lumbosacral paraspinals or gluteal muscles are not supplied by the femoral nerve or the lumbosacral plexus.

225. E. Neuromuscular ultrasound is increasingly used for diagnosis of peripheral nerve and muscle diseases. In focal neuropathies, multiple changes might be seen including increase in nerve cross sectional area, hypoechogenicity, reduced mobility of the nerve, and, on doppler, increased vascularity of the nerve.

226. C. Single-fiber EMG, fast and slow repetitive stimulations are performed for neuromuscular junction (NMJ) disorders. Short exercise testing can help with nondystrophic myotonias. Long exercise testing helps with diagnosis of periodic paralysis. The clinical history is suggestive of periodic paralysis.

227. E. Radiation induced brachial plexopathy can have a delayed onset and tends to present with painless progressive weakness predominantly in upper trunk. Characteristically patients have myokymic discharges. In contrast, malignancy recurrence leading to brachial plexopathy typically causes severe pain and generally tends to involve lower trunk. Imaging studies are also utilized to help differentiate these two subtypes.

228. A. MAG neuropathy is a slowly progressive distal sensory, ataxic neuropathy with distal demyelination changes. Patients tend to have severe ataxia and mild weakness. AIDP and CIDP can have significant proximal weakness. AMSAN, a variant of Guillain–Barré syndrome (GBS), can have severe proximal weakness and has diffuse axonal loss. MMN can asymmetric and might only involve upper limbs at the onset.

229. E. Abnormal temporal dispersion and conduction block are features of acquired demyelinating polyneuropathy and AIDP fits this description. CMT1A causes hereditary demyelinating polyneuropathy with severe slowing. CMT2 cause axonal polyneuropathy. Diabetes and renal failure cause axonal polyneuropathy, albeit with more prominent slowing in patients with who have both diabetes and renal failure.

230. C. This is single-fiber EMG study. Close observation reveals clearly increased jitter (right lower box). Additionally, there is intermittent blocking as the second waveform does not appear occasionally (right upper box). Absolute jitter values are not needed to appreciate these changes.

231. B. This patient likely postmedian sternotomy plexopathy. However, nerve conduction studies are unusual because of only ulnar sensory is abnormal with normal medial antebrachial cutaneous response. This may occur in poststernotomy plexopathy because of predominant C8 anterior ramus damage during this surgical procedure and C8 anterior ramus predominantly has ulnar sensory fibers. This condition can be frequently misdiagnosed as ulnar neuropathy if the electrodiagnostician is not careful. Needle EMG of other C8 muscles as APB will help differential C8 root involvement. Needle EMG of the FDI does not help differentiate ulnar neuropathy from C8 root involvement. Needle EMG of other non-C8 muscles does not help with diagnosis.

232. A. In true neurogenic thoracic outlet syndromes, the medial antebrachial sensory response is almost always abnormal. Thenar group of muscles are more likely to be affected rather than hypothenar muscles.

233. C. This is normal single-fiber EMG. Visual analysis reveals normal jitter with no clear blocking. Further attention to the lower box data reveals absence of blocking or increased jitter. Most of time, blocking is associated with increased jitter.

234. C. Slow repetitive stimulation reveals abnormal decrement in both LEMS and MG and does not always differentiate these two conditions. Baseline CMAP are low in LEMS with postexercise facilitation. Fast repetitive stimulation in LEMS reveals significant increment and no significant changes in MG. Deep tendon reflexes tend to be absent in LEMS.

235. D. Short-duration and small-amplitude motor unit potentials are typically seen with myopathic process. In myopathies, typically early recruitment patterns are noted. Large duration and large-amplitude motor unit potentials with reduced recruitment is seen with neurogenic process. Occasionally in chronic myopathies, long-duration motor unit potentials are seen in myopathic diseases.

236. E. CMT2a causes severe axonal polyneuropathies with predominant changes in lower limbs followed by upper limbs. Sural responses tend to be absent. Severely reduced conduction velocities and prolonged distal latencies are mostly seen in demyelinating neuropathies.

237. C. This tibial motor study reveals severely prolonged distal latency, prolonged distal duration. These features are seen with distal predominant demyelinating neuropathies. In a patient with progressive sensory loss, ataxia, absent reflexes, tremor, and paraproteinemia, MAG neuropathy should be suspected. MR lumbar spine does not help with diagnosis in MAG neuropathy. Cerebrospinal fluid (CSF) studies and nerve biopsy might reveal abnormalities, but these will not be diagnostic of MAG neuropathy.

238. E. With nerve conduction studies, it is important to look at all the information. There is clear prolongation of distal latency (7.3 ms) and, in addition, conduction velocity is mildly reduced (44 and 45). Additionally, upper limb temperature is only 30.4C. This is less than optimal for upper limb studies. Recommended minimum skin temperature for lower limb studies is 30C and for upper limbs is 32C.

239. B. The correct explanation in these situations is to rule out potential mimics, such as LEMS or demyelinating neuropathies with predominant motor manifestations. It is not mandatory to perform painful procedures and testing should always be designed to the clinical question while making sure it is tolerable. Performing nerve conduction studies does not improve tolerance. Normal nerve conduction study does not rule out the need for EMG, as nerve conduction studies are normal in most myopathies.

240. E. This patient likely has chronic immune sensory polyradiculopathy (CISP), which is a rare immunotherapy responsive neuropathy with involvement of sensory nerve roots in cauda equina. Patients with CISP present with sensory symptoms and sensory ataxia but have normal strength. CSF reveals elevated protein. Unlikely classical CIDP, NCS, and EMG might be normal and abnormalities on MR lumbar spine or SSEP might reveal evidence of this condition. Since this is immunotherapy responsive, it is imperative that clinician consider this condition.

241. E. Patients with chronic poorly controlled diabetes and renal failure tend to have severe axonal polyneuropathy with higher incidence of further slowing across the compressive sites. In addition, slowing at noncompressive sites can be more severe than other axonal polyneuropathy and therefore can be confused with chronic inflammatory demyelinating polyneuropathy (CIDP).

242. A. A sensory nerve with absent SNAP or very low SNAP amplitude should be considered for biopsy. Distal motor nerve is not a common site for nerve biopsy. Nerve biopsy is mostly useful in patients with vasculitis and amyloidosis and not in routine polyneuropathies.

243. D. Lewis–Sumner syndrome (LSS) is an immune-mediated polyneuropathy with many features overlapping with CIDP, including demyelinating changes, elevated CSF protein, and nerve root enhancement on MR imaging. However, LSS tends to present with asymmetrical upper limb involvement, unlike CIDP which tends to present with fairly symmetrical findings.

4

Electroencephalography

QUESTIONS

1. All of the following statements regarding the evolution of photic driving response are true *except:*
   A. The initial photic driving appears at 1 year of age
   B. Best driving response in preschool children occurs at lower (less than 8 Hz) flash frequencies
   C. Best driving response in older children and adolescents occurs at medium (6–16 Hz) flash frequencies
   D. Paroxysmal response to flicker can be seen in normal school-age children
   E. Photoconvulsive response may be seen in healthy adolescents

2. Which of the following is most likely to occur as part of syncope?
   A. Multifocal myoclonus
   B. Prominent tonic activity
   C. Postictal confusion lasting more than a minute, especially with prolonged syncope
   D. EEG flattening at the onset of unconsciousness
   E. All of the above

ANSWERS TO THIS SECTION CAN BE FOUND ON PAGE 236

The figures in this chapter can be viewed in a larger size by accessing the digital version of this chapter found on Springer Publishing Company Connect™. Refer to the front of this book for access instructions.

3. An EEG from a 15-year-old male with focal cortical dysplasia in the right posterior quadrant, admitted for video-EEG monitoring, is shown below (filter 1–70 Hz). The waveforms highlighted in the box are most consistent with:

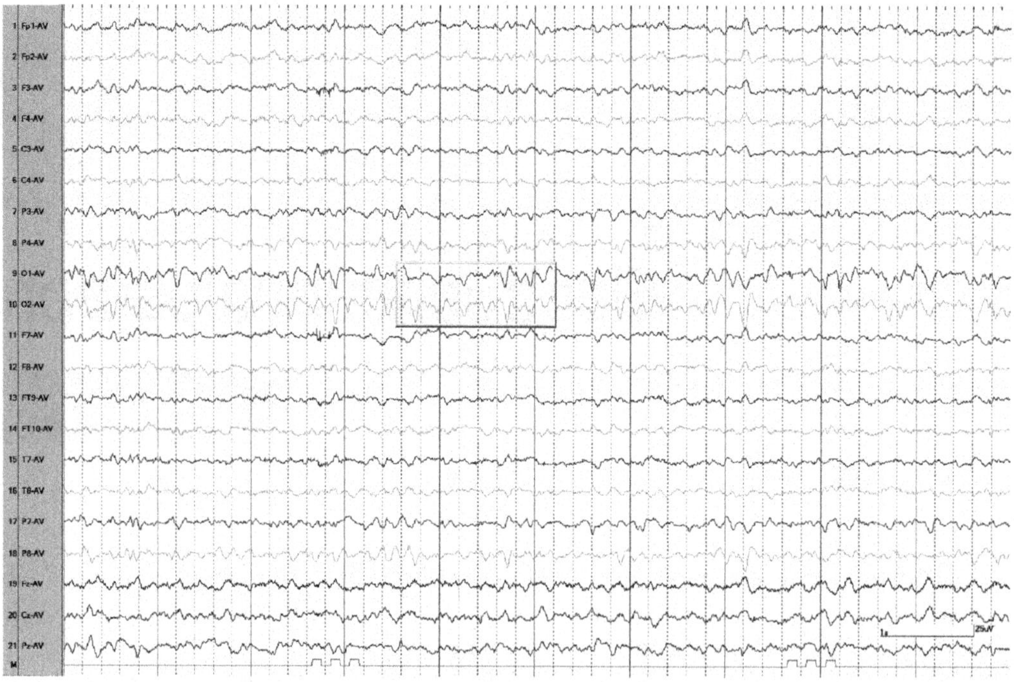

A. Posterior slow waves of youth
B. Positive occipital sharp transients of sleep (POSTS)
C. Lambda waves
D. Periodic lateralized epileptiform discharges (PLEDs)
E. Interictal epileptiform discharges (IEDs)

4. Which of the following statements best describes the evolution of vertex waves and K-complexes?
A. Both appear simultaneously by age 3 months
B. Vertex waves appear at a much earlier age than K-complexes
C. Vertex waves appear at a much later age than K-complexes
D. Vertex waves may have frontal predominance during infancy
E. Both have smaller amplitudes in children than adults

5. Which of the following statements is true about shut-eye waves?
A. They are predominantly seen in the fronto-polar leads
B. They are triggered by eye blinking
C. They are typically seen in adolescents over the age of 12 years
D. They tend to be low-amplitude and spike-like in morphology
E. They are surface-positive

6. Which of the following features is least likely to be seen following normal arousal from sleep?
   A. Diffuse 4 to 6 Hz activity with intermixed slower frequencies in children
   B. Frontal rhythmic sharp and spiky activity in adolescents
   C. Shorter duration, diffuse theta activity in older children
   D. Rapid transition to posteriorly-predominant alpha activity in adolescents
   E. Occipital rhythmic sharply contoured, surface-positive waveforms

7. What is the main difference between active sleep (AS) and quiet sleep (QS) around 37 to 40 weeks of conceptional age?
   A. AS consists of low-voltage irregular (LVI) pattern, while QS consists of a tracé alternant pattern
   B. AS consists of irregular theta and delta frequencies, while QS consists of a tracé discontinu pattern
   C. AS consists of an LVI pattern, while QS consists of a tracé discontinu pattern
   D. AS consists of a high-voltage slow (HVS) pattern, while QS consists of a tracé alternant pattern
   E. AS consists of LVI pattern with superimposed slow waves, while QS consists of a tracé discontinu pattern

8. What is the best interpretation of the posterior activity seen on the following EEG (filter 1–70 Hz; sensitivity 15 μV/mm; solid vertical lines are 1 second apart) of a 4-year-old boy?

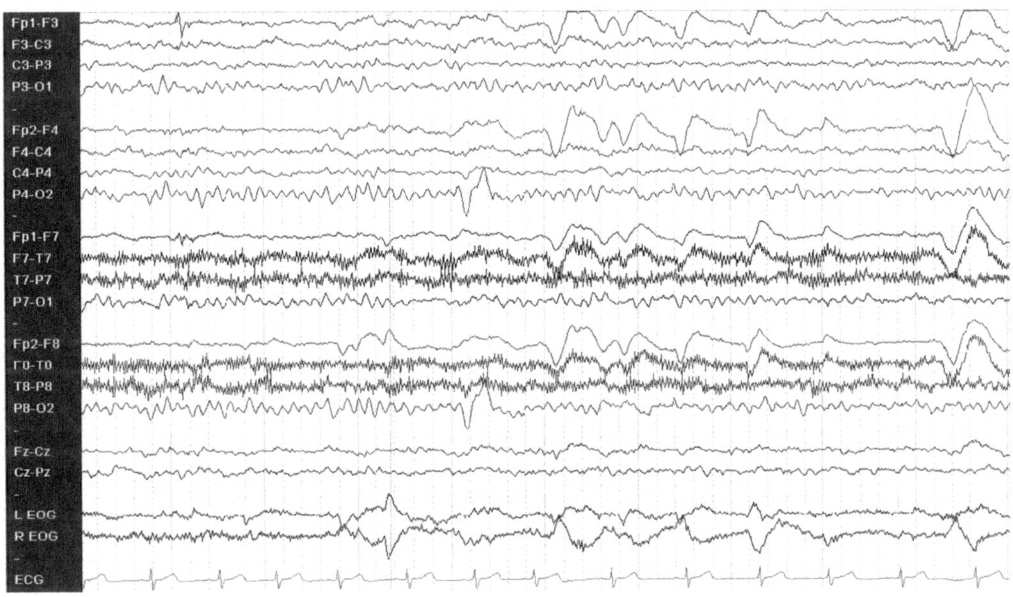

   A. Frontal spike-wave discharges
   B. Lambda waves
   C. Occipital spike-wave discharges
   D. Normal posterior dominant rhythm (PDR)
   E. Positive occipital sharp transients of sleep

9. Which of the following changes seen during hyperventilation (HV) is considered abnormal?
   A. Diffuse polymorphic delta activity in children
   B. Diffuse rhythmic delta activity in children
   C. Bifrontal delta activity in adults
   D. Bitemporal delta activity in adults
   E. Unilateral focal slowing in adults

10. Which of the following features is seen in primary generalized epileptic myoclonus?
   A. It is triggered by voluntary movement
   B. Myoclonus is usually asynchronous
   C. It is usually associated with giant somatosensory evoked potentials
   D. It is preceded by generalized fronto-central activity on the EEG time-locked to the myoclonus
   E. It is believed to arise from subcortical structures

11. Which of the following features is least likely to be associated with subclinical rhythmic electrographic discharge in adults (SREDA)?
   A. It is typically in the theta frequency range
   B. It could present as rhythmic sharply contoured activity with evolution
   C. It can last 1 to 2 minutes
   D. It has been correlated with seizures
   E. It is commonly seen in the temporal or parietal regions

12. A 6-year-old girl has multiple seizures that involve facial contraction. Her EEG showed centrotemporal spikes. Which part of the EEG is likely to demonstrate accentuation of these abnormalities?
   A. Wakefulness
   B. Photic stimulation
   C. Hyperventilation
   D. NREM sleep
   E. REM sleep

13. Which of the following EEG findings is seen in Angelman syndrome?
   A. Low-voltage fast activity
   B. Background resembling hypsarrhythmia
   C. Normal posterior dominant rhythm
   D. Tremor associated with 10-Hz rhythmic EEG activity
   E. Spells of laughter associated with ictal discharge

14. A 58-year-old woman has a history of staring spells since age 14 years. Her first generalized convulsion was at age 26 years, and she continues to have them intermittently. What is the most likely diagnosis based on the EEG (filter 1–70 Hz) shown below?

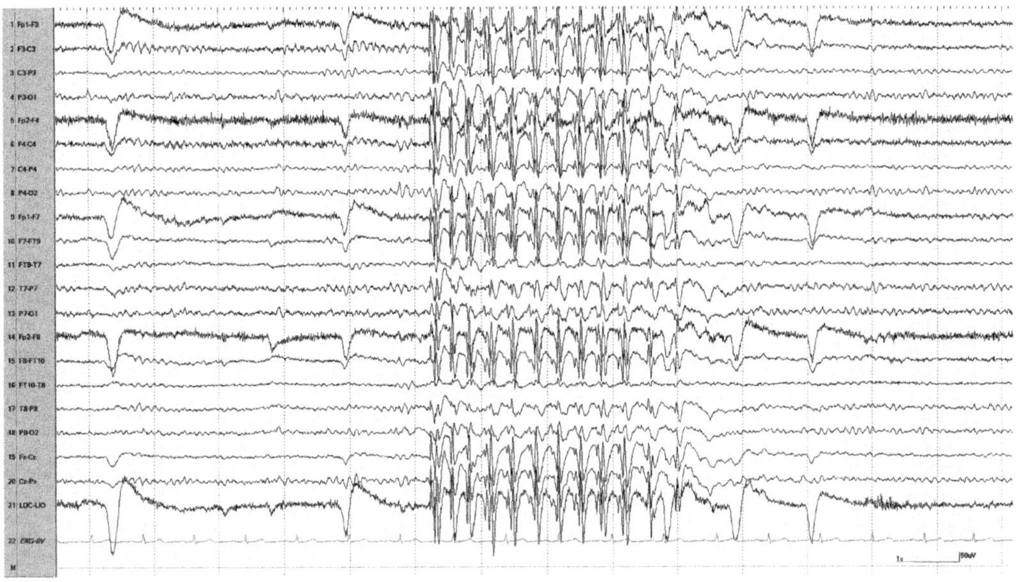

A. Childhood absence epilepsy (CAE)
B. Juvenile myoclonic epilepsy (JME)
C. Symptomatic generalized epilepsy
D. Focal epilepsy with secondary bilateral synchrony
E. Frontal lobe epilepsy

15. EEG in a patient with progressively deepening coma can show:
A. Reactive high-voltage delta activity
B. Reactive background attenuation with stimulation
C. Nonreactive high-voltage delta activity
D. Nonreactive background attenuation
E. All of the above

16. Which of the following features is least likely to be seen in an absence seizure?
A. Rhythmic eye blinking
B. Repetitive oral automatisms
C. Retropulsion of the head
D. Loss of postural control
E. Impairment of working memory

17. The EEG frequency bands described by Hans Berger include:
A. Alpha
B. Alpha and beta
C. Alpha, beta, and gamma
D. Alpha, beta, and theta
E. Alpha, beta, theta, and delta

18. A 10-year-old boy was undergoing hyperventilation (HV) during EEG recording as shown below (filter 1–70 Hz; sensitivity 15 μV/mm; solid vertical lines are 1 second apart). What does it show?

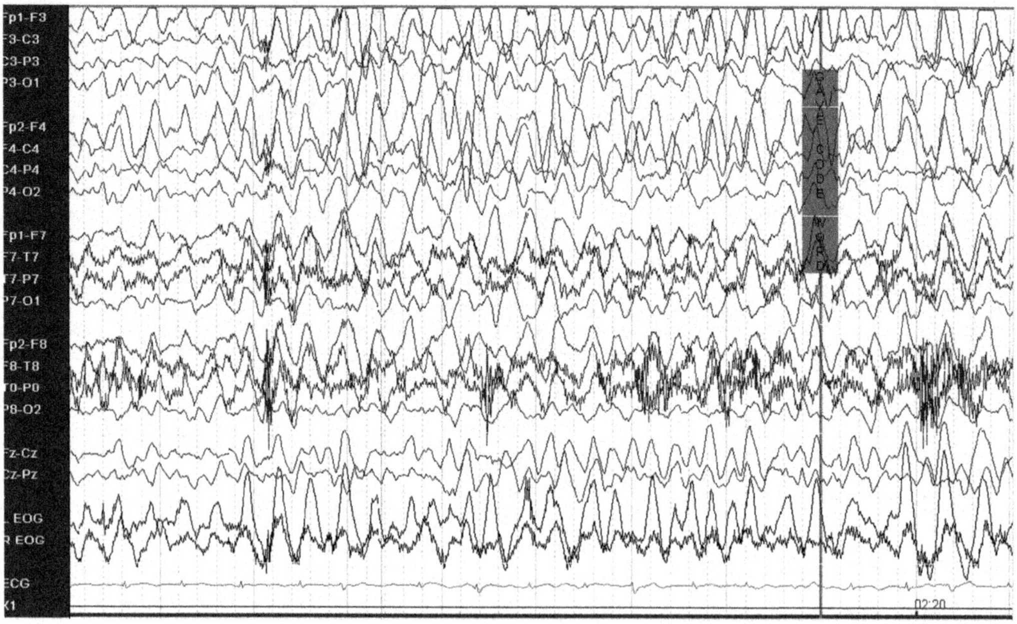

A. Seizure
B. Frontal intermittent rhythmic delta activity (FIRDA)
C. Normal response
D. Irregular generalized spike-wave discharges
E. Artifact from head movement

19. Which of the following statements best characterizes the psychomotor variant?
A. It is abnormal in adults, being associated with temporal lobe seizures
B. It is typically seen in slow-wave sleep
C. It tends to evolve into alpha or beta frequencies
D. It is comprised of 5 to 7 Hz sharply contoured rhythmic bursts
E. It consists of polymorphic waveforms

20. Which of the following statements best describes the normal evolution of the frequency of the posterior dominant rhythm (PDR)?
A. It is 3 Hz by age 3 months
B. It is 4 Hz by age 12 months
C. It is 6 Hz by 3 years
D. It is 8 Hz by 5 years
E. It is 10 Hz by 8 years

21. A 12-year-old boy with Lennox–Gastaut syndrome (LGS) presents with tonic and atonic seizures. An ambulatory EEG was done to assess the frequency of the seizures. When the electroencephalographer reviewed the study, the video did not appear to record properly. Which of the following features helps to distinguish a tonic seizure from an atonic seizure?
A. Electrodecremental response
B. Muscle activity obscuring the EEG activity
C. 2 Hz spike-wave ictal discharge
D. 3 Hz spike-wave discharge
E. Hypsarrhythmia

22. Age-related EEG slowing in the elderly is characterized by:
A. 4 to 5 Hz activity
B. Diffuse 2 to 3 Hz activity
C. Greater predominance over the right temporal region
D. Occurrence in trains of 7 to 10 theta waves lasting 1 to 2 seconds
E. Disappearance with light sleep

23. An 11-year-old boy with learning disability had a single nocturnal seizure associated with subtle facial twitching and hypersalivation. What abnormality would you expect to see?
A. Centrotemporal spikes
B. Frontal spikes
C. Parietal spikes
D. Occipital spikes
E. Generalized spikes

24. Which of the following features is characteristic of physiologic hyperventilation (HV)-induced EEG slowing?
A. Abrupt buildup of diffuse delta activity
B. Gradual buildup of focal delta activity
C. Resolution within 3 minutes of stopping the HV effort
D. Bifrontal predominance in children
E. Rhythmic delta activity in the temporal region in the elderly

25. What EEG pattern is expected to be present in neonates starting at 29 weeks of conceptional age?
A. Tracé discontinu
B. Tracé alternant
C. Burst suppression
D. Isoelectric
E. Continuous delta activity with superimposed beta frequencies

26. Which of the following features is seen around 35 to 37 weeks of conceptional age?
A. Absence of EEG reactivity during wakefulness and active sleep (AS)
B. Absence of EEG reactivity during quiet sleep (QS)
C. Absence of delta brushes in quiet sleep
D. Presence of tracé alternant instead of tracé discontinu pattern during AS
E. Replacement of multifocal sharp transients by frontal sharp transients

27. A 45-year-old male with a history of heart disease status postcoronary artery bypass graft (CABG) surgery, and a left parietal meningioma status postresection, was brought to the emergency department (ED) unresponsive after collapsing and prolonged CPR. What is the most likely cause for the EEG findings shown below (filter 1–70 Hz, vertical lines are 1 second apart)?

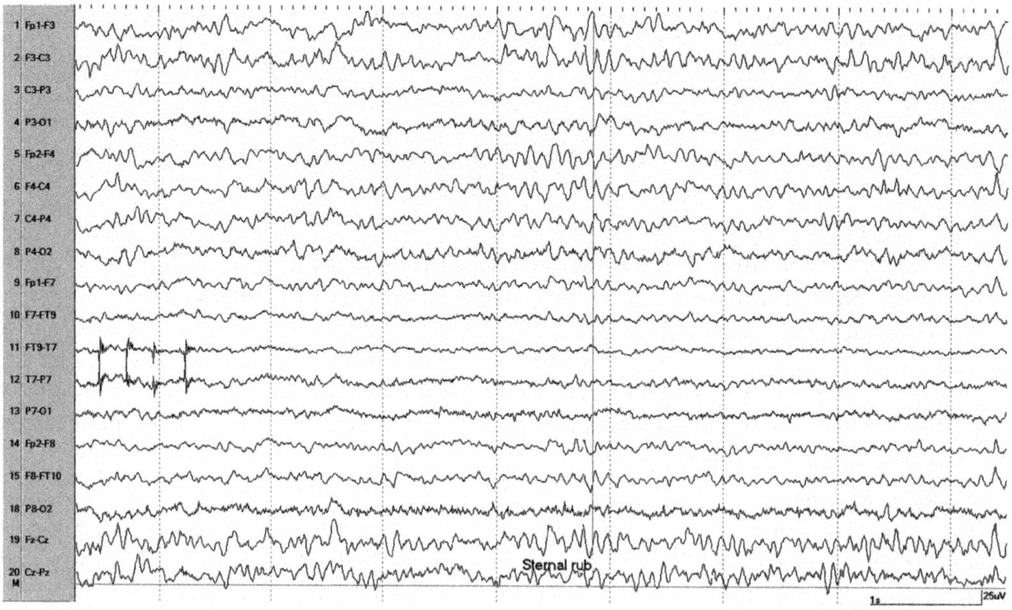

A. Anoxic injury
B. Anesthetic effect
C. Benzodiazepine effect
D. Skull defect
E. 60 Hz electrical noise artifact

28. A 13-year-old boy had a seizure in the setting of playing a video game. When the neurophysiologist was reading his EEG, she saw that there were EEG changes during photic stimulation. All of the following statements correctly describe the possible changes that can be seen during photic stimulation *except:*

A. Photoparoxysmal response (PPR) refers to any EEG change without clinical correlation
B. Photoconvulsive response refers to spike-wave discharges correlated to clinical manifestations
C. Photomyoclonic response refers to widespread muscle twitching timed to the stimulus
D. Photoelectric response refers to changes in a channel that disappear with shielding the electrode from the light
E. Photic driving response refers to activity in the posterior head regions time-locked to the photic stimulus

29. A 58-year-old male presents with new-onset acute weakness in the setting of chronic left-sided weakness and has the following EEG findings (filter 1–70 Hz). Which of the following scenarios is most likely?

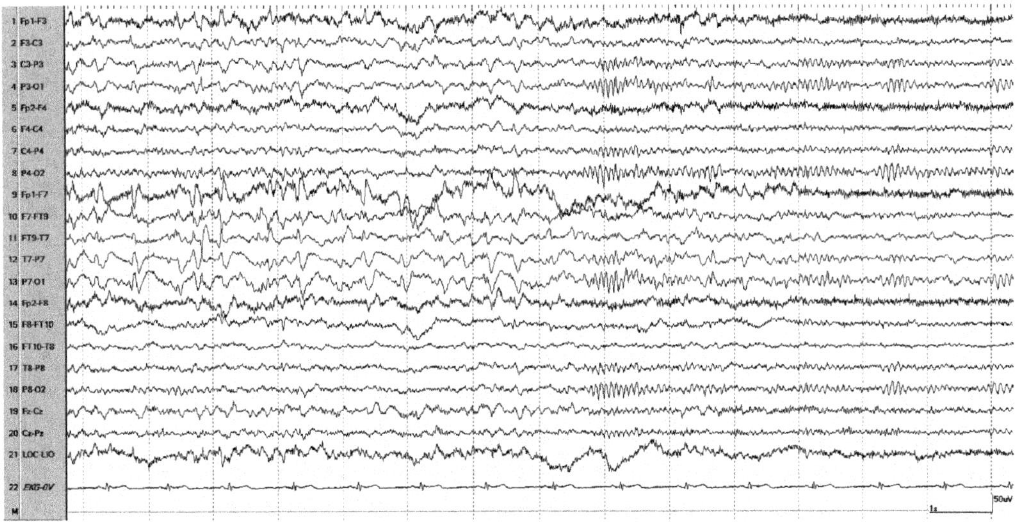

A. Mesial temporal sclerosis in the setting of childhood febrile seizures
B. Acute middle cerebral artery (MCA) infarction in the setting of prior infarction
C. Todd's paralysis after a focal motor seizure
D. Herpes simplex virus (HSV) infection, causing cerebral and spinal cord dysfunction
E. Acute relapse of multiple sclerosis (MS)

30. Which of the following statements is true regarding interictal epileptiform discharges (IEDs)?
A. They occur only in individuals with seizures
B. Spikes are generated by synchronous depolarization of neurons within 2 cm^2 of the cortex
C. Sharp waves result from synchronous depolarization of neurons further away from the recording electrode
D. In a spike-and-wave discharge, the slow wave represents prolonged depolarization of cortical neurons
E. Only spikes and spike-wave discharges, but not sharp waves, are associated with seizures

31. Which of the following syndromes is considered to have a more favorable prognosis?
A. Epilepsy with generalized tonic-clonic seizures (GTCs) on awakening
B. Neonatal myoclonic encephalopathy
C. West syndrome
D. Lennox–Gastaut syndrome (LGS)
E. Atypical benign partial epilepsy of childhood

32. How far along in a patient's course with Creutzfeldt–Jakob disease (CJD) would the following EEG pattern be expected to be seen?

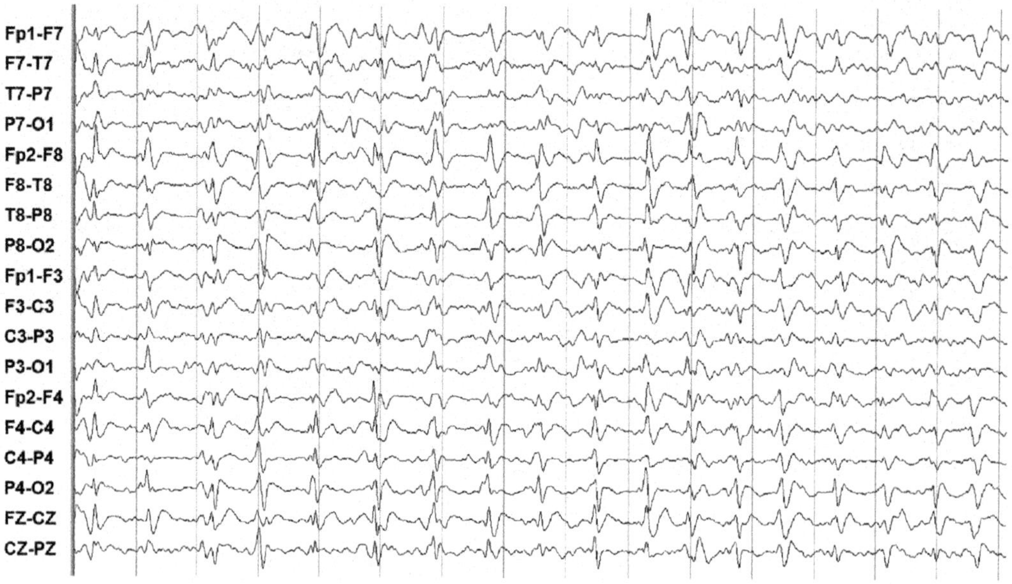

A. Prior to symptom onset
B. In the early stage of the disease
C. In the middle of the disease course
D. Only in the very late stages
E. Throughout the entire disease course

33. A 53-year-old male with a history of drug and alcohol abuse presented to the emergency department (ED) with fluctuating mental status with hallucinations, bizarre behavior, and urinary incontinence. A routine EEG (filter 1–70 Hz) without video was obtained as shown below. What does his EEG show?

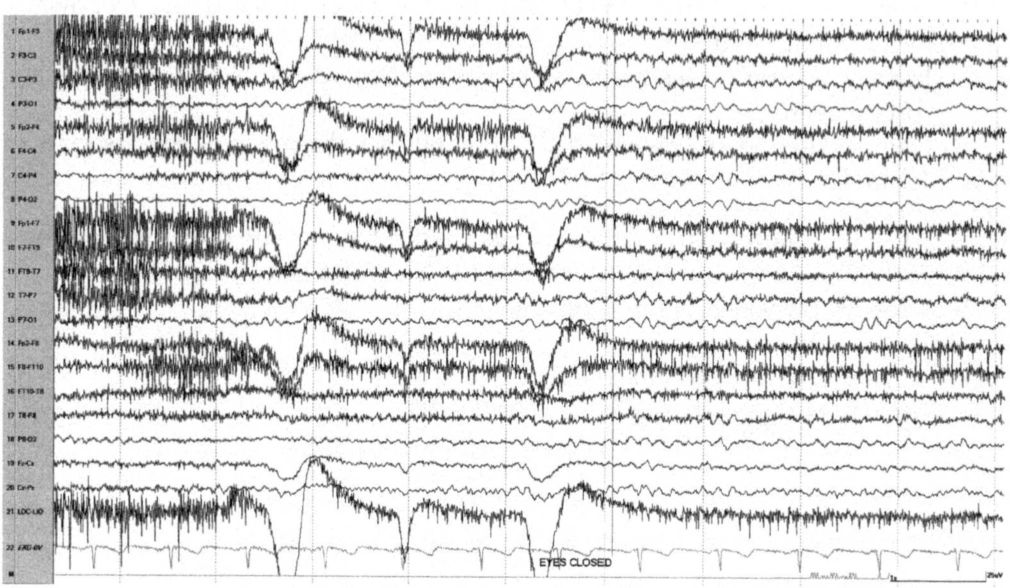

A. Normal findings
B. Mild cerebral dysfunction
C. Nonconvulsive status epilepticus
D. Temporal lobe epilepsy
E. Psychogenic nonepileptic spell

34. What is the chance that the first routine EEG will be nondiagnostic for epilepsy?
A. 10%
B. 20%
C. 50%
D. 80%
E. 90%

35. Generalized, 4 to 6 Hz polyspike-and-wave discharges during photic stimulation are diagnostic of which of the following conditions?
A. Childhood absence epilepsy
B. Juvenile absence epilepsy
C. Juvenile myoclonic epilepsy
D. Frontal lobe epilepsy with secondary bilateral synchrony
E. Neuronal ceroid lipofuscinosis type 2

36. A 43-year-old male with intractable epilepsy underwent right temporal lobectomy with electrocorticography (ECoG; sampling rate 1,000 Hz, filters 1–300 Hz) using a 6-contact subdural strip placed subtemporally with electrode 1 medial and electrode 6 lateral. What is the prominent finding on the ECoG shown below?

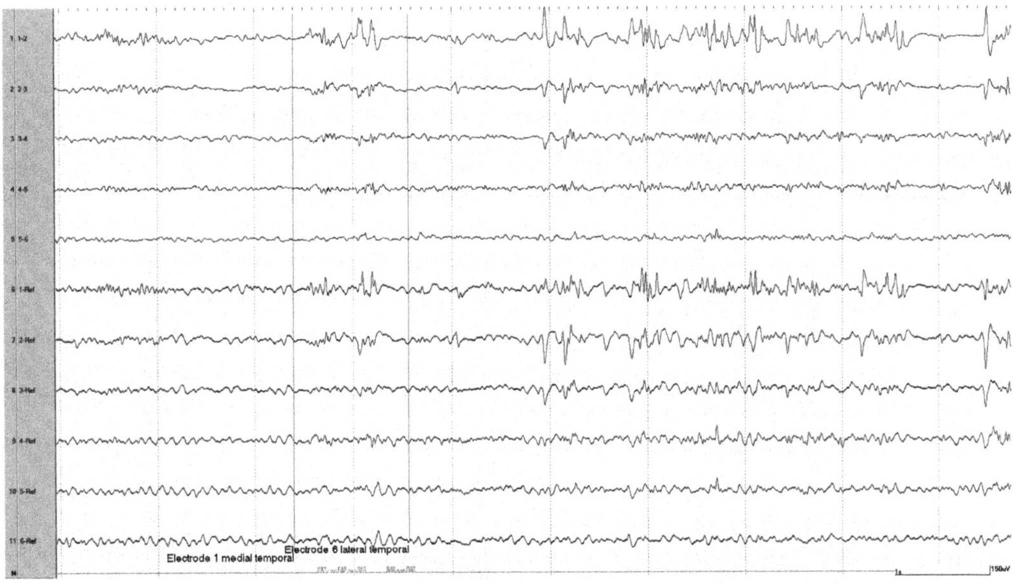

A. Sharply contoured slowing
B. Pulse artifact
C. Mesial temporal spikes
D. Burst suppression from anesthesia
E. Fast ripples

37. Which of the following statements is true regarding frontal intermittent rhythmic delta activity (FIRDA)?
   A. It is thought to reflect diffuse white matter dysfunction
   B. It is more common in chronic neurologic conditions
   C. It is more common in encephalopathy related to structural causes
   D. It is more common in children than adults
   E. It is often mistaken for eye movement artifacts

38. Which of the following statements is NOT characteristic of the EEG abnormalities seen in patients with brain tumors?
   A. Focal slowing can be seen with hyperventilation (HV)
   B. Focal slowing suggests white matter involvement
   C. Intermittent rhythmic delta activity (IRDA) suggests thalamic involvement
   D. Background attenuation suggests low-grade glioma
   E. Background attenuation suggests extensive peritumoral edema

39. Which of the following EEG findings is characteristic of Landau–Kleffner syndrome (LKS)?
   A. Epileptiform and slow abnormalities in non-REM sleep
   B. Epileptiform abnormalities in REM sleep
   C. Slow spike-wave discharges in wakefulness
   D. Burst suppression
   E. Normal background

40. Which of the following statements is true about the alpha rhythm?
   A. It reaches its mean adult frequency of 10 Hz around age 10 years
   B. Its frequency remains unchanged in the elderly
   C. Its frequency can decrease transiently with eye closure
   D. It has higher amplitude over the left hemisphere
   E. It has higher amplitude in right-handed subjects

41. The following is an EEG from an 11-year-old girl, on no medications, with progressive alteration of mental status. What is the most likely diagnosis?

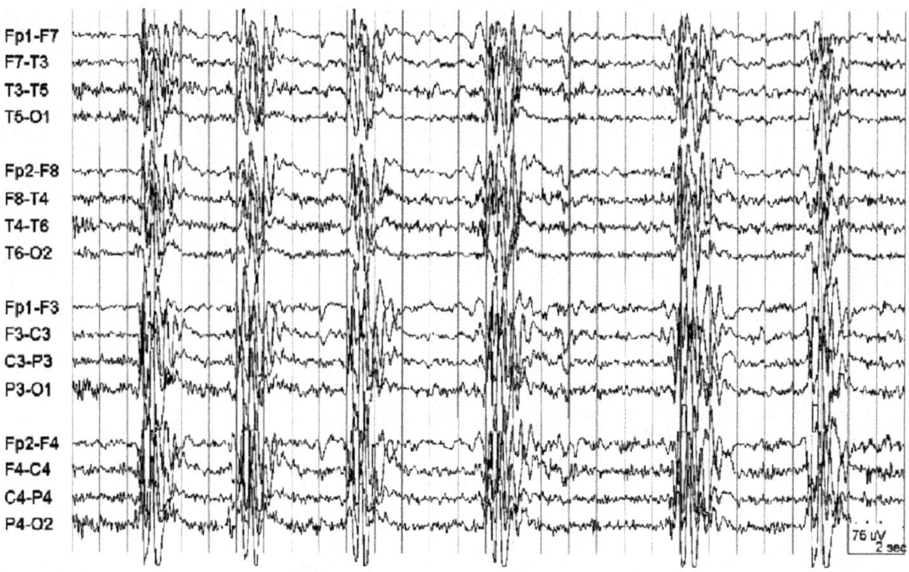

A. Subacute sclerosing panencephalitis (SSPE)
B. Creutzfeldt–Jakob disease (CJD)
C. Anesthetic effect
D. Anoxic injury
E. Chewing artifact

42. What would be the clinical significance of the following EEG pattern (filter 1–70 Hz) if seen in different distributions as outlined below?

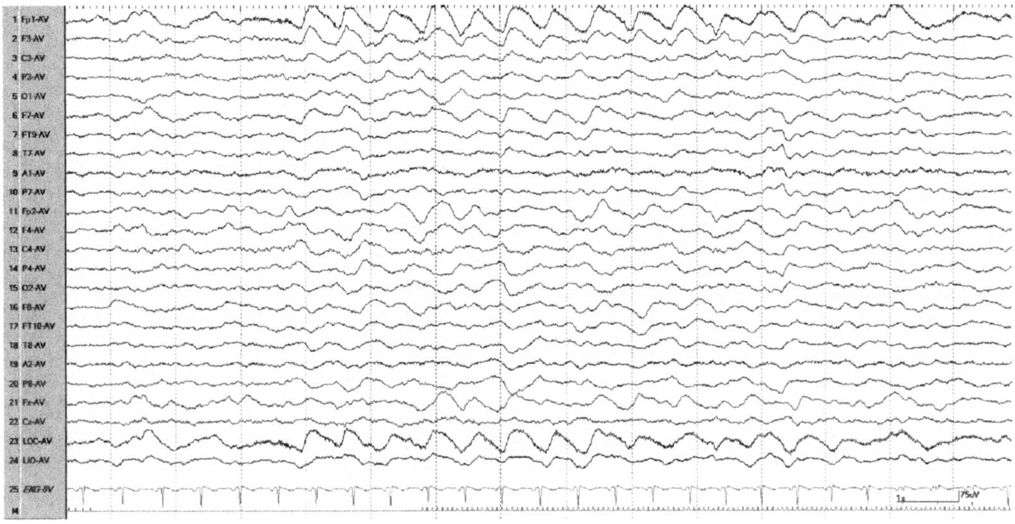

A. If occipital, is highly associated with absence epilepsy
B. If frontal, is associated with a structural lesion
C. If temporal, is highly associated with nonspecific dysfunction
D. If central, is considered a normal sleep variant
E. If generalized, is associated with poor prognosis

43. Which of the following conditions is not associated with EEG described findings?
A. West syndrome: High-amplitude, disorganized slow activity with multifocal spikes and generalized electrodecrements that can be associated with spasms
B. Infantile ceroid lipofuscinosis: Occipital spikes in the setting of photic stimulation
C. Eyelid myoclonia with absences: Eyelid myoclonia immediately after eye opening in the dark and brief bilateral spike-wave discharges
D. Lennox–Gastaut syndrome (LGS): Slow spike wave with fast activity in sleep
E. Dravet syndrome: Generalized polyspike-wave complexes with unilateral predominance

44. What is the earliest conceptional age at which active sleep (AS) and quiet sleep (QS) can be distinguished from one another?
A. 28 weeks
B. 30 weeks
C. 32 weeks
D. 35 weeks
E. 40 weeks

45. Which of the following statements is true about the 14- and 6-Hz positive bursts?
A. They are most common in school-age children and adolescents.
B. They can be positive or negative in polarity
C. The bursts typically last 3 to 4 seconds
D. They tend to be maximal in the parietal regions
E. They are usually symmetric

46. A 26-year-old female presented with new-onset seizures characterized by "dizziness, light-headedness, spacing out prior to falling to the floor." What is the most likely finding in the occipital region on her EEG (filter 1–70 Hz) shown below?

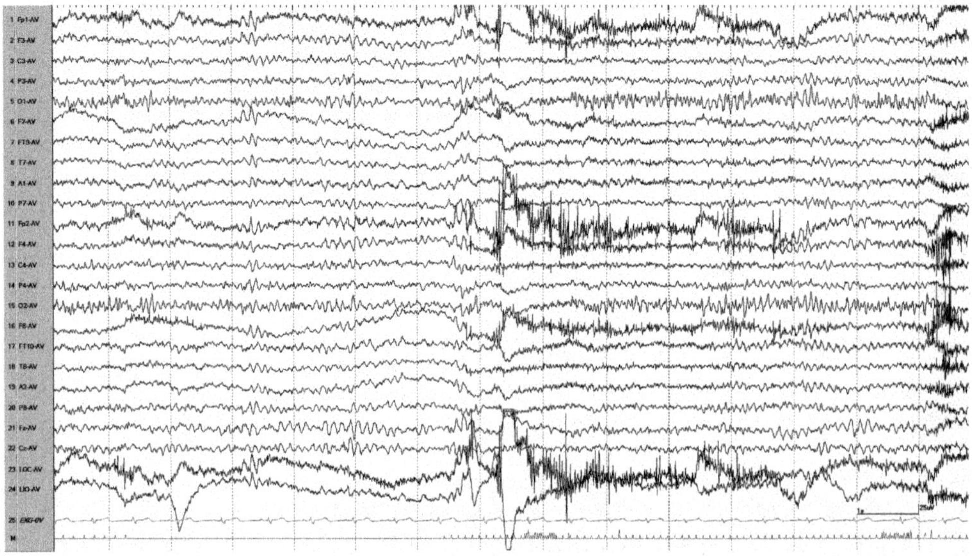

A. Positive occipital sharp transients of sleep (POSTS)
B. Occipital seizure
C. Normal activation response
D. Slow alpha variant
E. Fast alpha variant

47. Around 32 to 34 weeks of conceptional age, the background during active sleep (AS) and quiet sleep (QS) tends to be
A. Tracé discontinu in both states
B. A more continuous pattern in AS and tracé discontinu in QS
C. Tracé discontinu in AS and a more continuous pattern in QS
D. More continuous patterns in both states
E. Tracé alternant in both states

48. During a routine EEG, the technologist asks the patient to spell the word "gladiolus" (the first National Spelling Bee-winning word in 1925). Which of the following EEG activities can be expected to appear or enhance?
A. Alpha rhythm
B. Mu rhythm
C. Theta rhythm
D. Beta rhythm
E. Lambda waves

49. Which of the following statements is true regarding stereotactic depth electrodes?
A. They have low impedance
B. They are most useful for recording seizures arising from the frontotemporal convexity
C. They are immune to muscle artifacts
D. They are routinely used to map eloquent cortex
E. They need to be removed within a week of implant

50. A 12-year-old boy presents with Reye's syndrome. Which of the following EEG findings has been associated with the syndrome?
A. 14- and 6-Hz positive spikes
B. Rhythmic mid-temporal theta bursts
C. Triphasic waves
D. Phantom spike waves
E. Lambda waves

51. A 36-week-old infant was noted to have right temporal sharply contoured activity. What normal finding could this represent?
A. Delta brushes
B. Positive sharp waves
C. Small sharp spikes (SSS)
D. Benign epileptiform transients of sleep (BETS)
E. Rhythmic temporal theta bursts

52. Which of the following statements is true regarding the development of REM sleep during the first year of life?
A. Low-voltage irregular (LVI) pattern changes into the REM sleep pattern
B. Quiet sleep is the precursor of REM sleep
C. The percentage of time spent in REM increases during the first year of life
D. REM sleep tends to be more prominent in the second half of the night in infants
E. Transition from wakefulness into REM sleep is common in infants up to 12 months of age

53. Which of the following statements best describes the 10 to 20 system of EEG electrode placement as shown below?

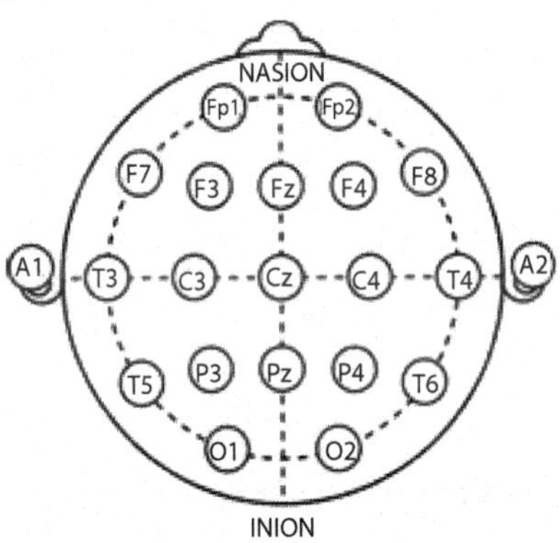

A. It is only applicable to the North American EEG laboratories
B. It mandates that either 10 or 20 electrodes be used for the recording
C. It only refers to the location but not the name of the electrodes
D. Electrodes are placed at a distance from each other equal to 10% or 20% of the total front-to-back or side-to-side distance
E. It fails to account for the individual differences in the size of the skull

54. In a patient with myoclonic seizures, which of the following features is least likely to be helpful in differentiating juvenile myoclonic epilepsy (JME) from Lennox–Gastaut syndrome (LGS)?
A. EEG background
B. Frequency of the spike-wave discharge
C. Presence of polyspikes
D. Age of onset
E. Response to antiseizure medications

55. A 7-year-old boy, who had normal development, started to have difficulty with language. Which of the following statements is true regarding the EEG findings in this child?
A. Epileptiform discharges over the posterior temporal regions
B. Worsening of the EEG abnormalities in slow wave sleep
C. Background attenuation over the left frontotemporal region
D. A and B are correct
E. A, B and C are correct

56. Which of the following statements is true regarding positive occipital sharp transients of sleep (POSTS)?
A. They are periodic, surface negative waveforms in the occipital region
B. They can be seen during deeper stages of slow-wave sleep
C. They can persist into REM sleep
D. They become less prominent in adults after age 20 years
E. They can be seen in blind, otherwise healthy individuals

57. The slow activity on the EEG in brain tumors can be described by all of the following statements *except:*
A. Focal delta activity can be associated with well-circumscribed tumors in the white matter
B. Focal slowing can be seen in cortical tumors
C. Generalized delta activity can be seen with a small thalamic tumor
D. Hemispheric slowing can be seen with a large thalamic tumor
E. Generalized slowing can be seen with a tumor in the midbrain tegmentum

58. Which of the following is a characteristic feature of subclinical rhythmic electrographic discharge of adults (SREDA)?
A. It is consistent with subclinical seizures
B. It is most common in adolescents
C. It is characterized by a sudden buildup of alpha range activity
D. It is typically maximal in the temporoparietal regions
E. It typically lasts less than 5 seconds

59. Which of the following statements is true regarding epileptic spikes?
A. Their duration is 70 to 100 ms
B. They are felt to be related to desynchronization of neuronal firing.
C. They are usually surface negative
D. They increase in frequency before and after seizure
E. Their rate increases with decrease in antiseizure medication levels

60. Which of the following statements best describes EEG evaluation of suspected brain death?

A. The recommended term for "flat line EEG" is electrocerebral silence
B. In all patients over 1 year of age, a minimum of two EEGs 24 hours apart should be obtained for confirmation
C. Integrity of the recording system should be checked by touching each electrode with a cotton swab to produce an artifact potential
D. EEG reactivity to noxious somatosensory stimuli need not be checked as long as there is no discernible electrical activity at 2 μV/mm sensitivity
E. The minimum recording time is 60 minutes

61. Which of the following is the characteristic finding in the following EEG (filter 1–70 Hz; sensitivity 10 μV/mm) from a 10-month-old infant during sleep?

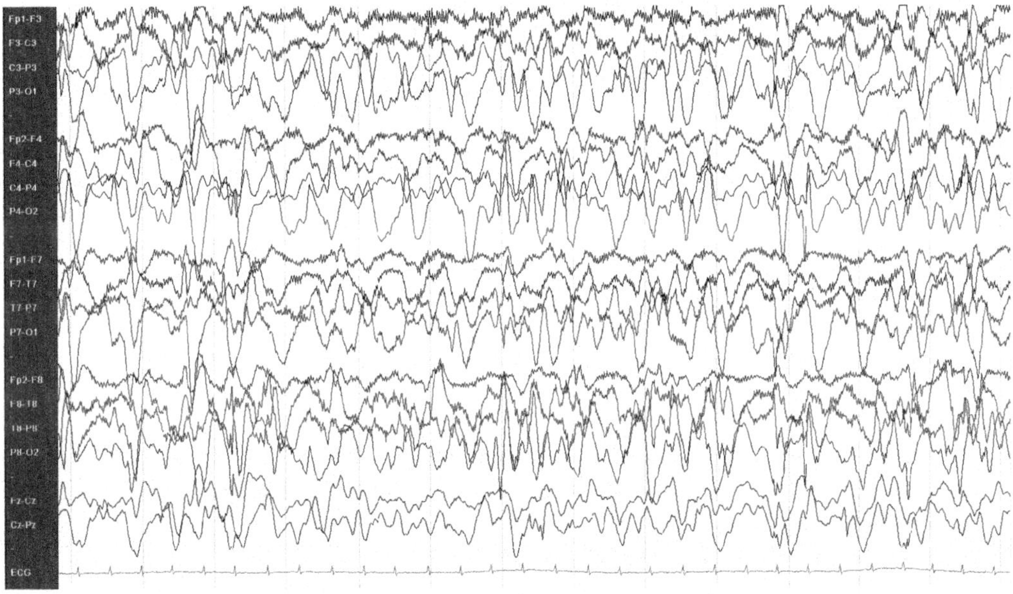

A. Organized background
B. Normal slow-wave sleep
C. Bilaterally synchronous spikes and sharp waves
D. Disorganized background in slow-wave sleep
E. Disorganized background in REM sleep

62. A 70-year-old nursing home resident developed acute altered mental status. An MRI of the brain showed no acute changes. Based on the following EEG (filter 1–70 Hz), what is the most likely etiology?

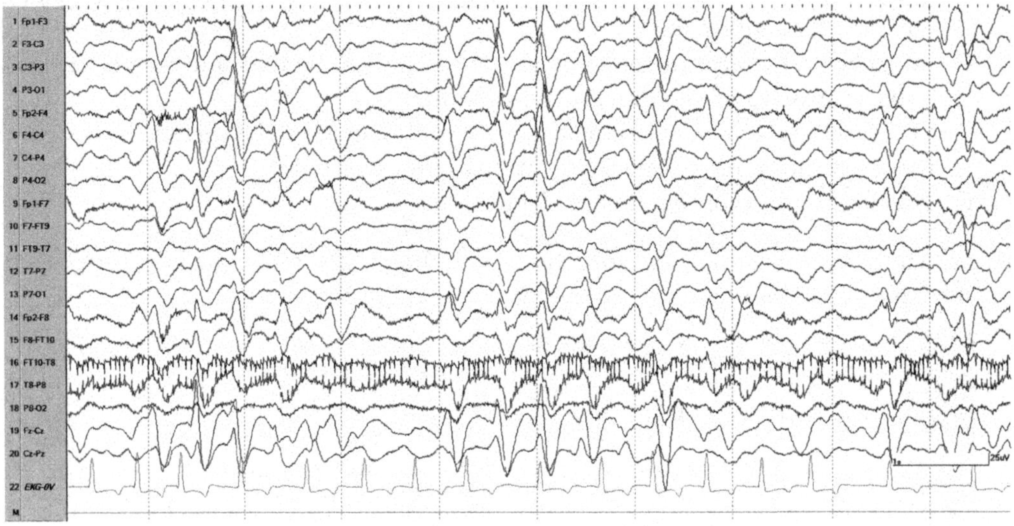

A. Stroke
B. Herpes simplex encephalitis (HSE)
C. Focal status epilepticus
D. Toxic-metabolic encephalopathy
E. Cruetzfeldt–Jakob disease (CJD)

63. A 27-year-old male has moderate cognitive impairment with lifelong history of intractable epilepsy including tonic seizures. Which of the following features is most likely to be seen on his EEG?
A. Normal posterior dominant rhythm (PDR)
B. Generalized fast spike-and-wave discharges
C. Generalized slow spike-and-wave discharges
D. Focal polyspikes
E. Hypsarrhythmia

64. The 6-Hz phantom spike and waves are characterized by all of the following *except:*
A. They are seen predominantly in young children
B. They occur in up to 2.5% of EEG records
C. They can be seen in wakefulness
D. They disappear in deep sleep
E. They occur in bursts lasting 1 to 2 seconds

65. A 20-year-old female presents with spells of daytime sleepiness leading to a car accident. At night, she is noted to move her legs in sleep. What is the likely interpretation of the EEG (filter 1–70 Hz)?

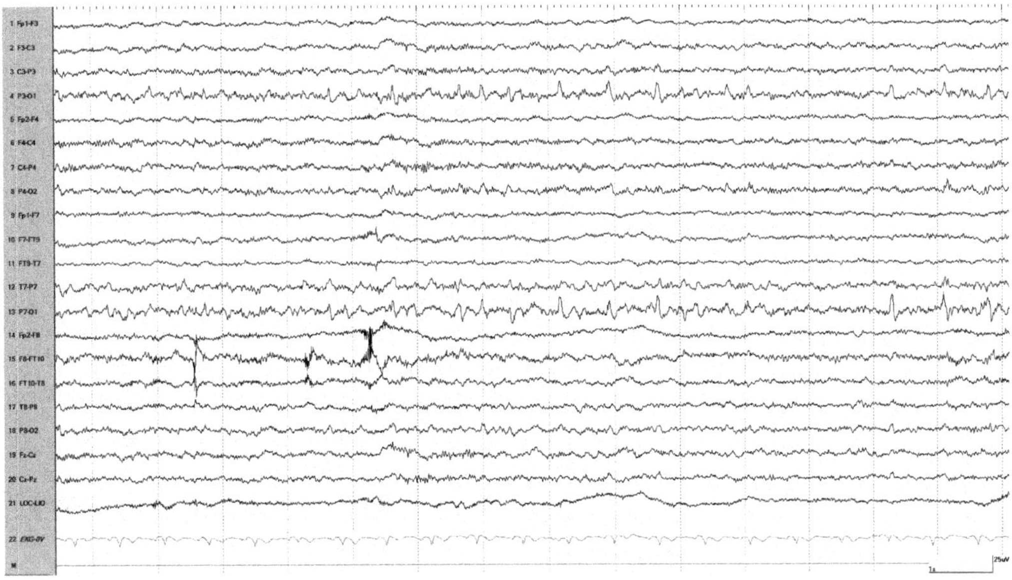

A. Restless leg syndrome
B. Normal sleep
C. Potential epileptogenicity predisposing to seizures
D. Focal seizure
E. Localized cerebral dysfunction

66. Which of the following statements is true regarding the classic 3 Hz spike-wave complexes?
A. They have high correlation with clinical absences
B. They are a marker for both typical and atypical absences
C. The wave component is inhibitory
D. Burst durations of 10 seconds or more are associated with clinical absences
E. They are generalized and bisynchronous, with equal antero-posterior field distribution

67. Which of the following statements is true regarding the EEG features during 32 to 34 weeks of conceptional age?
A. Quiet sleep (QS) consists of tracé alternant pattern
B. The interburst intervals during QS typically last 20 to 30 seconds
C. Delta brushes are confined to QS
D. Temporal theta evolves into alpha frequencies
E. Background reactivity is absent

68. Which of the following findings is least likely to be associated with increased risk for seizures?

A. Unilateral temporal intermittent rhythmic delta activity (TIRDA)
B. Bilateral TIRDA
C. Bilateral frontal intermittent rhythmic delta activity (FIRDA)
D. Bilateral occipital intermittent rhythmic delta activity (OIRDA)
E. Generalized intermittent rhythmic delta activity (GIRDA)

69. Which of the following features are characteristic of low-voltage EEG records?

A. They are rare in children
B. They are seen in 5% of adolescents
C. They are seen in 12% of adults
D. They are dominated by beta range activity
E. All of the above

70. In a term infant, how does the predominant sleep pattern change during the first 6 weeks of life?

A. At term, the total amount of time spent in sleep is 70% to 80%
B. At term, active sleep (AS) predominates, while at 46 weeks, quiet sleep (QS) predominates
C. At term, QS predominates, while at 46 weeks, AS predominates
D. AS predominates at term and during the first 6 weeks
E. QS predominates at term and during the first 6 weeks

71. The following EEG (filter 1–70 Hz; sensitivity 5 μV/mm; vertical lines are 1 second apart) is of a 17-year-old boy who was noted to be daydreaming at school. What is the sharply contoured activity seen?

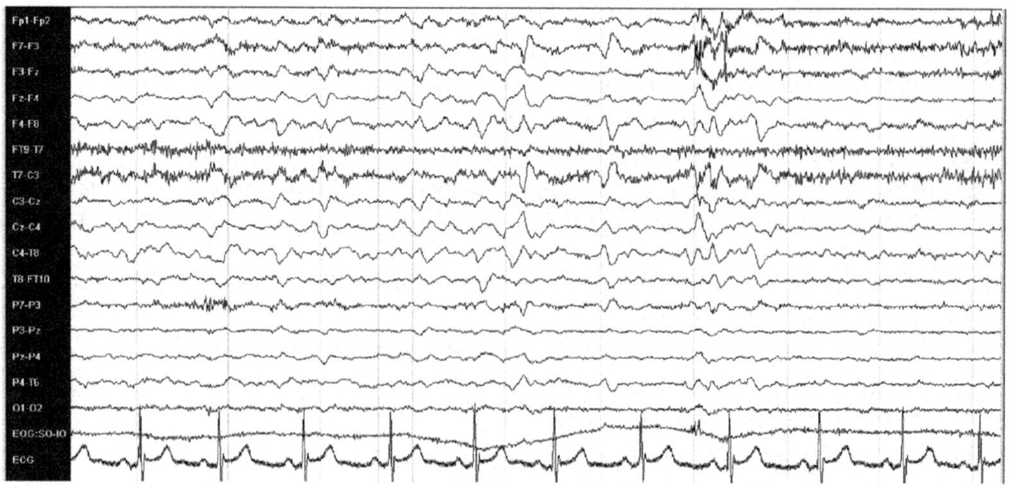

A. Spike-wave discharges
B. Pathological slowing
C. Normal sleep architecture
D. Mu rhythm
E. Positive occipital sharp transients of sleep (POSTS)

72. Alexander disease is likely to be associated with which of the following EEG findings?
A. Bifrontal slowing
B. Generalized periodic discharges (GPDs)
C. Temporal spikes
D. Burst suppression
E. Photosensitivity

73. Which of the following activation techniques is least helpful in increasing the yield of epileptiform abnormalities on EEG?
A. Photic stimulation
B. Hyperventilation
C. Loud noise
D. Intravenous saline administration
E. Sleep

74. An adult clinical neurophysiology fellow begins his first block of rotation with the pediatric epilepsy group. Which of the following EEG features in a 6-year-old child should he be concerned about as being possibly abnormal?
A. Posterior dominant rhythm (PDR) of 8 Hz
B. Hypnagogic hypersynchrony
C. Sleep spindles with duration of 1 second
D. Low-voltage record
E. Posterior slow waves of youth

75. Which of the following conditions is least likely to be associated with the presence of subclinical rhythmic electrographic discharge in adults (SREDA)?
A. Resting state
B. Drowsiness
C. Photic stimulation
D. Hyperventilation (HV)
E. Elderly subjects

76. Which of the following statements best describes the mu rhythm?
A. Its frequency tends to be in the alpha and theta range
B. It is best seen over the centro-parietal head regions
C. It is associated with the prefrontal cortex
D. It is asymmetrical and asynchronous in distribution
E. Bilateral rhythm can be attenuated by eye opening

77. An 8-year-old boy was admitted to the intensive care unit (ICU) for an asthma exacerbation and was noted to have an episode of unresponsiveness. A routine EEG (filter 1–70 Hz; sensitivity 7 μV/mm; vertical lines are 1 second apart) was done while the patient was drowsy, as noted by the technologist. What is the most likely interpretation of the rhythmic activity over the right temporal region?

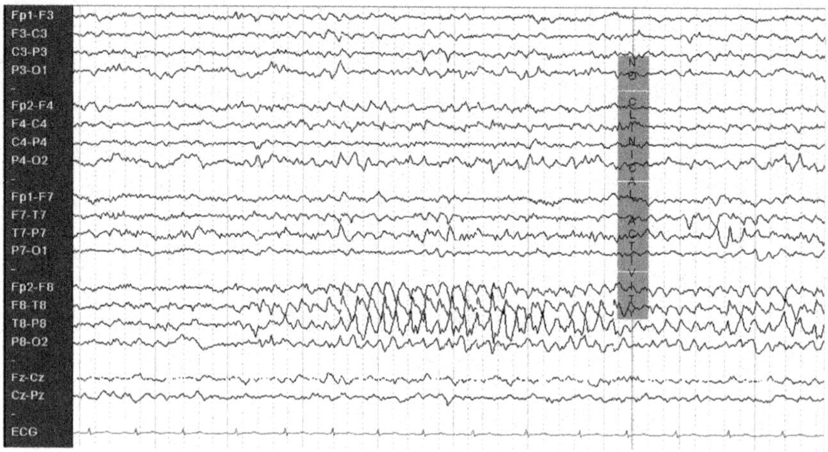

A. Temporal intermittent rhythmic delta activity (TIRDA)
B. Normal variant
C. Ciganek rhythm
D. Seizure discharge
E. Artifact

78. An epileptiform spike is characterized by which of the following features?
A. Steep upslope and steep downslope
B. Duration of 70–120 ms
C. Wider field in REM sleep compared with Stage 2 sleep
D. Horizontal dipole
E. All of the above

79. A 2-month-old term infant who had a normal doctor's visit a week ago was noted by her parents to have an episode of arm stiffening lasting 2 to 5 seconds. What does her EEG (filter 1–70 Hz; sensitivity 10 μV/mm; solid vertical lines are 1 second apart) show?

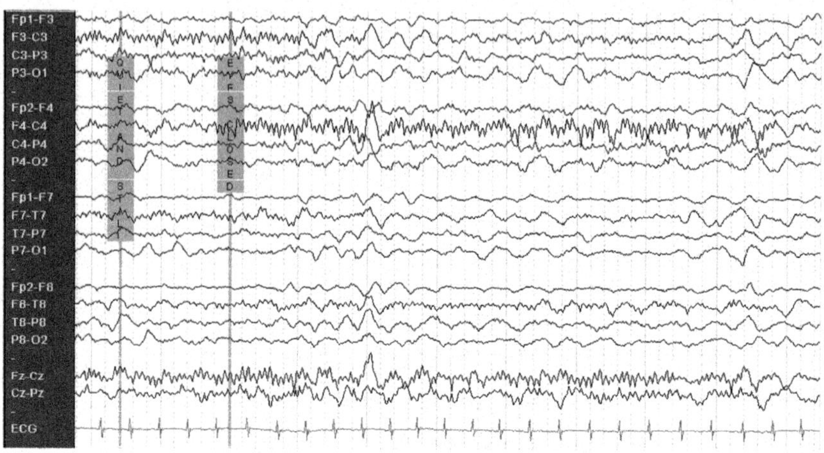

A. Seizure discharge
B. Normal sleep
C. Patting artifact
D. Electrode artifact
E. Drug effect

80. A 37-year-old woman has had multiple visits to the emergency department (ED) with generalized convulsions, incontinence, and tongue biting. She had a typical event during photic stimulation lasting 7 minutes, characterized by motionless staring, as noted by the EEG technologist. The video file was corrupted and could not be reviewed. What is the interpretation of the captured episode based on the EEG (filter 1–70 Hz) below, which depicts the activity 4 minutes into the spell?

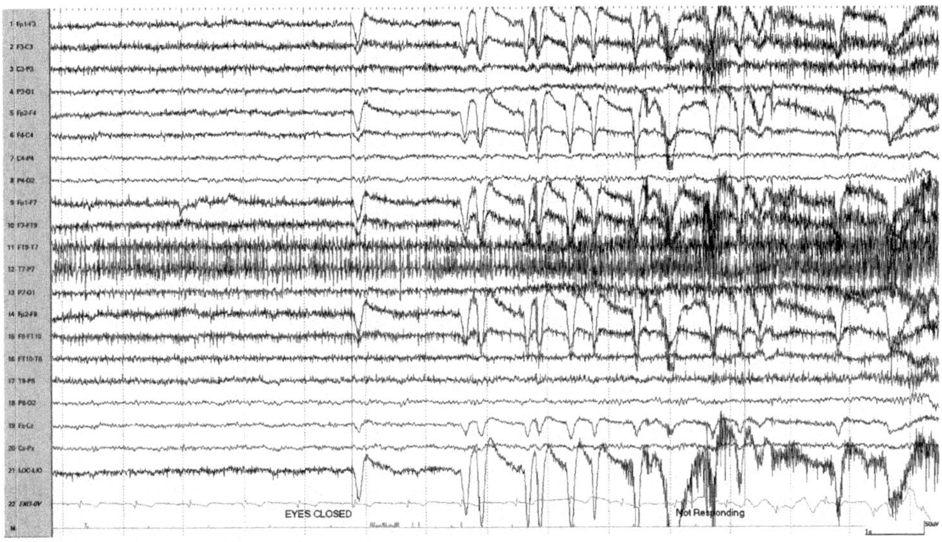

A. Absence seizure
B. Psychogenic nonepileptic event
C. Scalp EEG negative epileptic seizure
D. Frontal lobe seizure
E. None of the above

81. Which of the following EEG features is considered abnormal in a neonate of 37 to 40 weeks conceptional age?
A. Delta brushes during active sleep (AS)
B. Encoches frontales during transition between AS and quiet sleep (QS)
C. Monorhythmic frontal delta activity during transition between AS and QS
D. Rare, sporadic multifocal sharps
E. High-voltage slow (HVS) waves during QS

82. Which of the following EEG findings is least likely to be associated with in mitochondrial disorders?
A. Sharp waves with bifrontal predominance
B. Sharp waves with bioccipital predominance

C. Enhancement of sharp waves with photic stimulation
D. Epilepsia partialis continua
E. Periodic or pseudoperiodic sharp waves

83. Which of the following features is considered to be outside the normal developmental evolution of the EEG in a 1-year-old child?
A. 6 Hz posterior dominant rhythm (PDR)
B. Hypnagogic hypersynchrony
C. Sleep spindles with vertex predominance
D. Discernible photic driving response
E. All of the above

84. Which of the following features are characteristic of the triphasic waves?
A. Triphasic morphology with a prominent negative phase in the middle
B. Generalized bilaterally symmetric and synchronous distribution
C. Monotonous waveforms with 1.5 to 2.5 Hz frequency
D. B and C
E. A, B, and C

85. Which of the following statements best describes the occipital intermittent rhythmic delta activity (OIRDA)?
A. It is most commonly seen in children younger than 5 years of age
B. It is suppressed by hyperventilation
C. It is attenuated by eye closure
D. It is activated by photic stimulation
E. It is invariably associated with an underlying seizure disorder

86. An 8-year-old child with history of right eye blindness since birth had an EEG after he fainted while playing outside in the summer. Which of the following findings should prompt additional workup?
A. Left occipital spikes
B. Right occipital spikes
C. Asymmetric slowing of the right posterior dominant rhythm (PDR)
D. Loss of photic driving
E. Loss of lambda waves

87. How are spikes and sharp waves typically interpreted in a 34-week-old neonate?
A. As epileptiform if they are rare and multifocal
B. As normal if they are focal
C. As nonspecific cerebral dysfunction if they are frequent and multifocal
D. As of unknown significance if they are multifocal
E. As of unknown significance in all cases

88. Which of the following clinical conditions is least likely to be associated with the EEG pattern (filter 1–70 Hz) shown below?

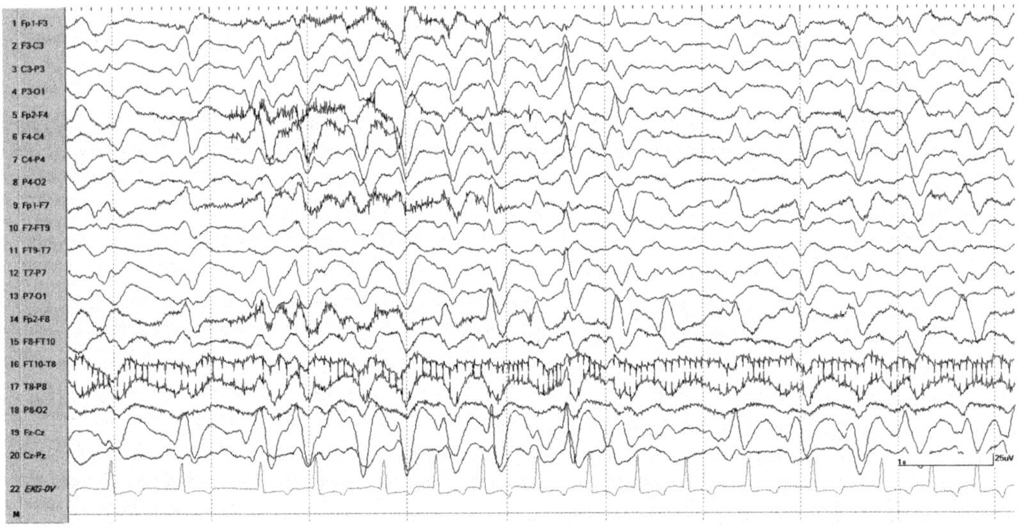

A. Baclofen toxicity
B. Lithium toxicity
C. Bismuth subsalicylate toxicity
D. Creutzfeldt–Jakob disease (CJD)
E. Uremia

89. At 29 weeks of conceptional age, the majority of delta brushes are:
A. Predominant during wakefulness
B. Predominant during active sleep (AS)
C. Predominant during quiet sleep (QS)
D. Fairly equally distributed between the 3 states
E. Equally predominant in AS and QS

90. Which of the following typically presents with periodic complexes with the longest period?
A. Creutzfeldt–Jakob disease (CJD)
B. Subacute sclerosing panencephalitis
C. Baclofen toxicity
D. Liver failure
E. Landau–Kleffner syndrome (LKS)

91. Which of the following statements regarding Landau–Kleffner syndrome (LKS) and continuous spike waves of sleep (CSWS) is true?
A. The EEG discharges in LKS are more bitemporal and/or biparietal versus more diffuse in CSWS
B. There is global behavioral regression in LKS versus language regression in CSWS
C. Epileptiform activity in LKS is activated in both NREM and REM sleep versus only in NREM sleep in CSWS
D. Carbamazepine may improve the EEG pattern in CSWS but not in LKS
E. Steroids may improve the EEG pattern in LKS but not in CSWS

92. A 36-year-old male was admitted to the surgical intensive care unit (ICU) after cardiac arrest in the emergency department (ED). The EEG below was done a month after initial insult (filter 1–70 Hz). At that time, the patient had minimal brainstem reflexes and no withdrawal to painful stimuli in any of the extremities. What is the likely diagnosis based on the clinical and EEG findings?

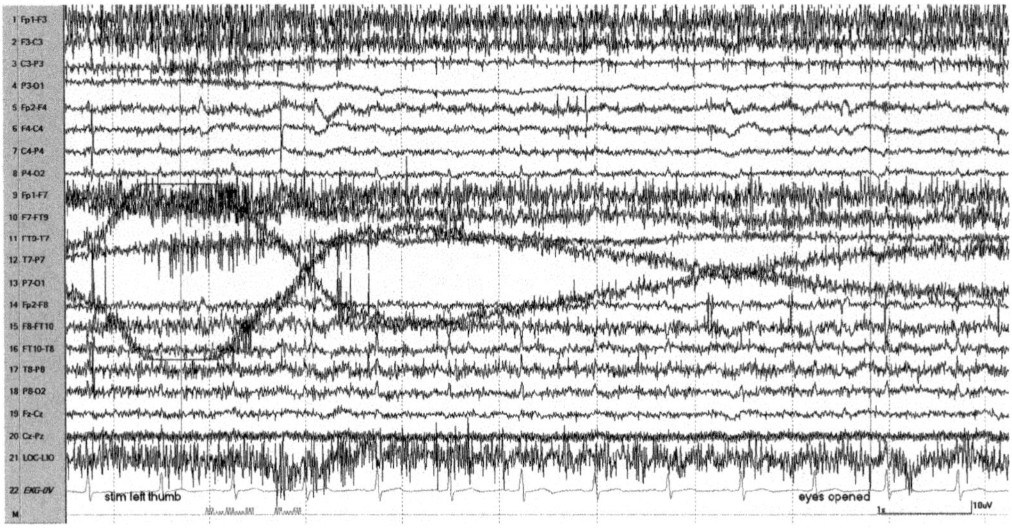

A. Vegetative state
B. Locked-in syndrome
C. Minimally responsive state
D. Brain death
E. Akinetic mutism

93. Which of the following statements is true regarding the modified combinatorial nomenclature (MCN) of EEG electrode placement?
A. Extra electrodes are added using the 10% or 20% division
B. Extra letter codes are introduced to designate more specific regions of the underlying cortex
C. Extra letter codes eliminate the need for designating the midline electrode positions
D. T3 and T4 are renamed as T7 and T8, respectively
E. P3 and P4 are renamed as P7 and P8, respectively

94. Which of the following statements is true of photoparoxysmal response (PPR)?
A. It is equally common in generalized and focal seizures
B. It can be seen in subjects without an underlying seizure disorder
C. It is most likely to be elicited by a flash frequency of 9 to 12 Hz in photosensitive epilepsy
D. It is more likely to occur upon eye opening
E. Its presence is pathognomonic of occipital lobe epilepsy

95. Which of the following statements best describes the sleep architecture in active sleep (AS) vs quiet sleep (QS) at 30 weeks of conceptional age?

A. Background is discontinuous throughout with shorter interburst intervals in AS versus QS
B. Background is discontinuous throughout with shorter interburst intervals in QS versus AS
C. Background is discontinuous throughout with similar duration of interburst intervals in AS versus QS
D. Background is continuous in AS but discontinuous in QS
E. Background is discontinuous with prominent delta brushes in both AS and QS

96. Which of the following ictal patterns is least likely to be seen at the onset of a generalized tonic–clonic seizure?

A. Voltage attenuation
B. Paroxysmal beta activity
C. Rhythmic alpha activity
D. Generalized polyspike-wave discharges
E. Rhythmic 3 Hz sinusoidal activity

97. A 16-year-old girl with intractable epilepsy was admitted for intracranial EEG evaluation. Her semiology is characterized by an epigastric aura, salivation, and swallowing along with concomitant clonic facial movements. Which area is likely to be in the ictal onset zone?

A. Supplementary motor area
B. Frontal operculum
C. Cingulate gyrus
D. Hippocampus
E. Amygdala

98. The EEG shown below was obtained in a neonate of 38 weeks conceptional age. Which of the following is the best interpretation?

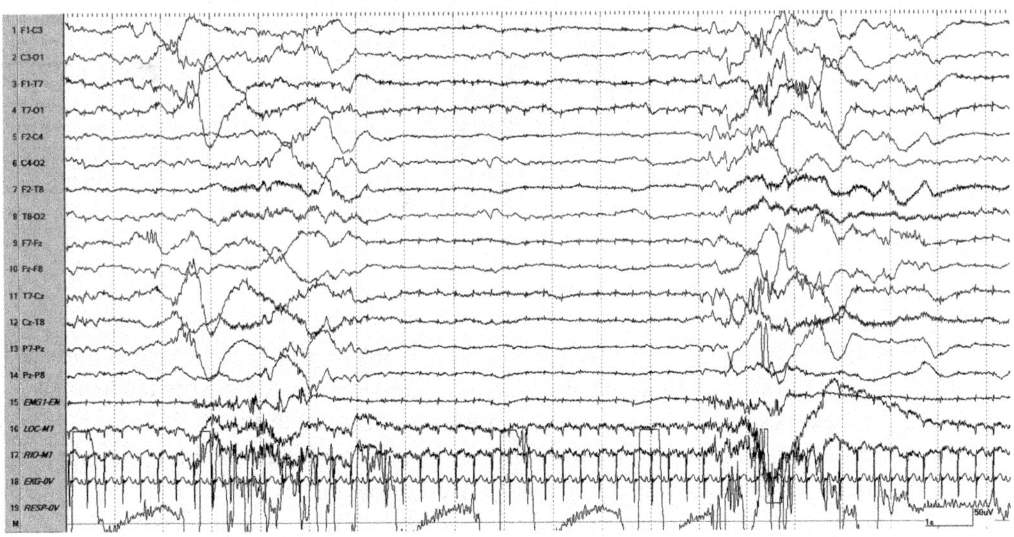

A. Dysmature EEG
B. Normal for gestational age
C. Severe encephalopathy
D. Increased risk for epileptic seizures
E. Electrodecremental seizure

99. Which of the following statements best describes the process of transition of quiet sleep (QS) into NREM sleep?
A. High-voltage slow (HVS) pattern completely disappears at term
B. Rhythmic, monophasic occipital slow waves appear at term
C. Cone waves are characteristically seen in NREM sleep during infancy
D. Vertex waves are well developed at term
E. K complexes are well developed at 3 months of age

100. Which of the following statements is true about occipital sharp transients?
A. They can be seen in blind individuals without seizures
B. They can disappear with eye closure
C. They can disappear with eye opening
D. They may be associated with epilepsy in young children
E. All of the above

101. A 10-year-old, developmentally normal boy with a 4-year history of seizures has an EEG (filter 1–70 Hz) shown below. Which of the following is the best interpretation of the EEG finding?

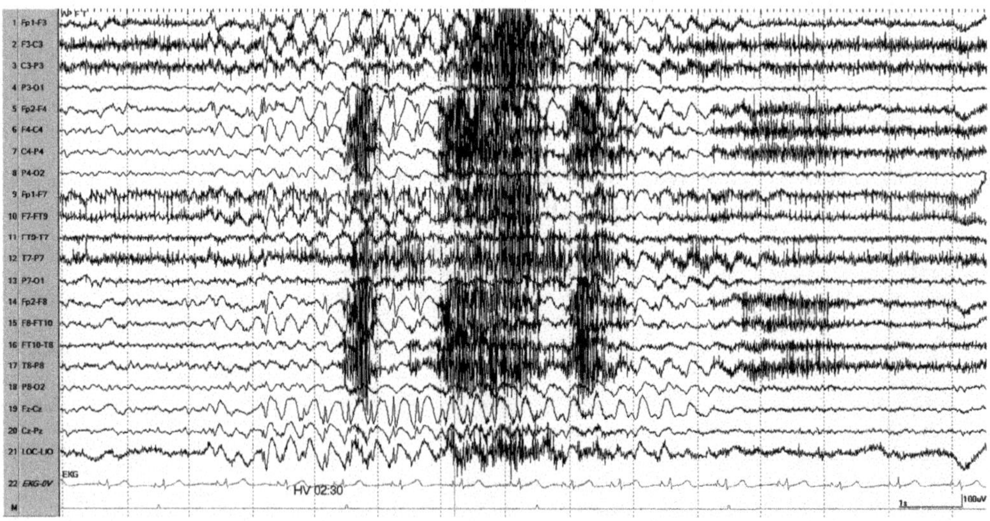

A. It suggests an epilepsy syndrome that is typically associated with myoclonic jerks
B. It is associated with an epilepsy syndrome that is likely to become refractory
C. It can be associated with seizures characterized by eye flutter
D. It is a normal hyperventilation (HV) response not associated with epilepsy
E. It represents movement artifact due to head nodding

102. Which of the following EEG patterns is considered abnormal in a term infant 1 month after birth?
A. Centrally predominant, nonreactive, rhythmical theta activity in wakefulness
B. Relatively symmetrical and synchronous background
C. Continuous slow waves during quiet sleep (QS)
D. Tracé alternant with asynchronous bursts during QS
E. Tracé alternant with synchronous bursts during QS

103. In a bipolar montage, if G1 is negative and G2 is positive, the waveform deflection in channel G1–G2 will be
A. Upward
B. Downward
C. Flat
D. Equipotential
E. C and D

104. The eye movements immediately following markers 1 and 2 are

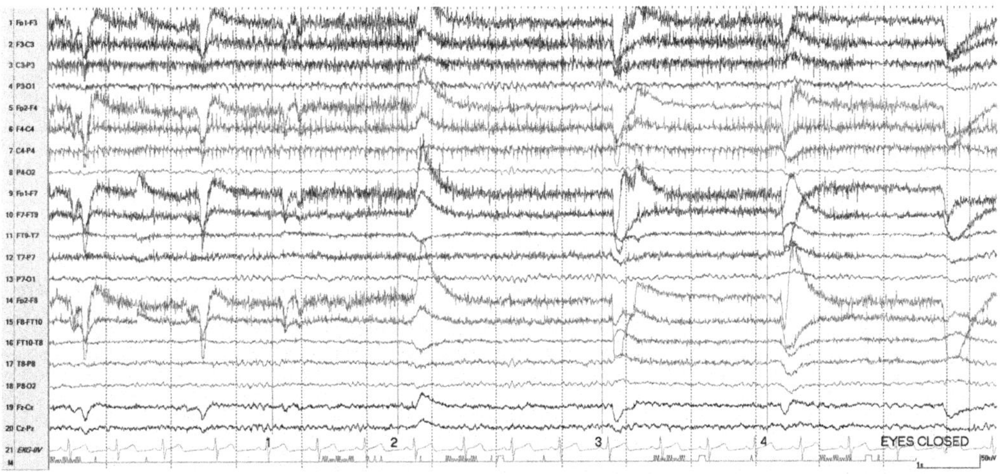

A. Up, down
B. Down, up
C. Left, right
D. Right, left
E. Up, left

105. Which of the following is NOT characteristic of delta brushes?
A. They appear at about 26 weeks of conceptional age
B. They are analogous to K-complexes seen in adults
C. They tend to be seen mainly over the central head region
D. They occur asynchronously
E. They appear in quiet sleep (QS) at an earlier stage than active sleep (AS)

106. Which of the following statements is true regarding the finding shown in the following EEG (filter 1–70 Hz)?

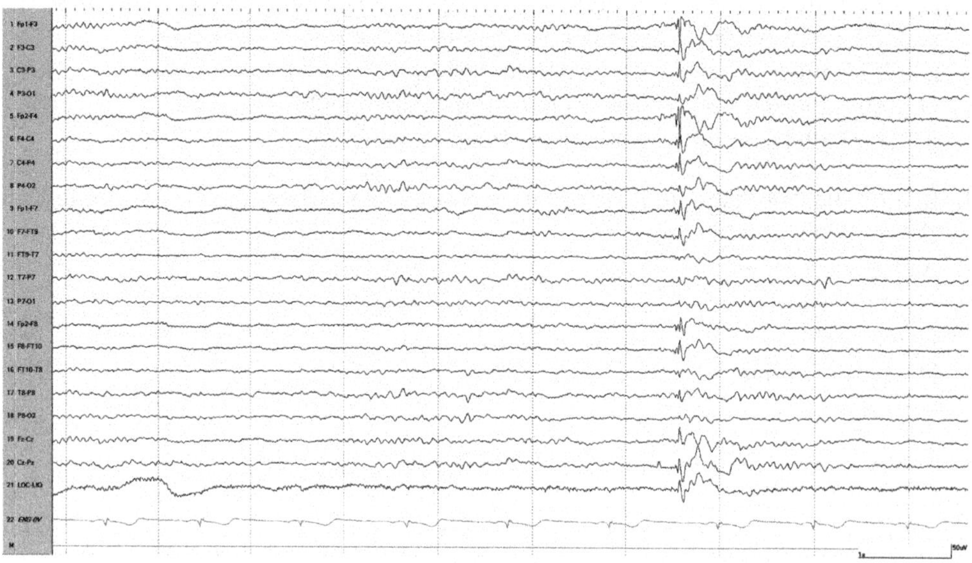

A. It is associated with a higher seizure threshold
B. It can be seen in patients without epilepsy
C. It is common in patients with simple febrile seizures
D. A and B
E. A, B, and C

107. The following EEG (filter 1–70 Hz; sensitivity 20 μV/mm; solid vertical lines are 1 second apart) was obtained from a 19-month-old girl during sleep. Which of the following scenarios is likely to be associated with this EEG finding?

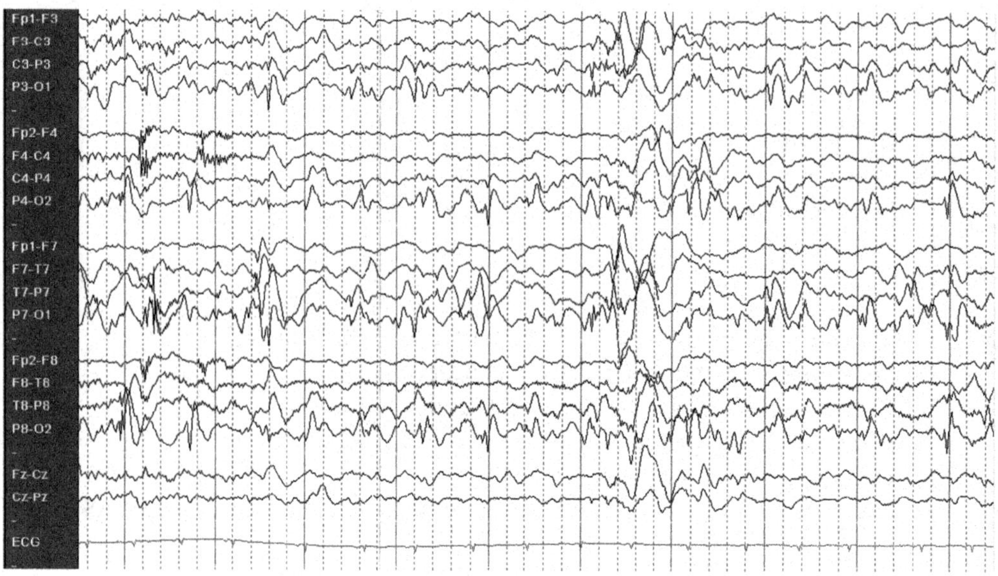

A. Auditory verbal agnosia
B. Electrographic seizures in sleep
C. Clinical seizures during daytime
D. A and B
E. A, B, and C

108. Which of the following statements is true regarding the amplitude of the EEG activity?
A. It does not exceed 50 μV on the scalp
B. It does not exceed 500 μV on electrocorticograms
C. It is typically measured from peak to trough
D. It depends on the interelectrode distance
E. It does not depend on the montage

109. While doing an EEG on a 2-year-old boy, the technologist accurately documents the "time since the last meal." Which of the following statements provides the rationale for such documentation?
A. Low blood glucose may enhance hyperventilation (HV)-induced slowing
B. Low blood glucose may provoke photoparoxysmal response (PPR)
C. Low blood glucose can trigger generalized EEG abnormalities.
D. A and B
E. A and C

110. In the following EEG showing a left temporal discharge, the relative polarities of the electrodes Fp1 relative to F7 and electrode P7 relative to T7 are:

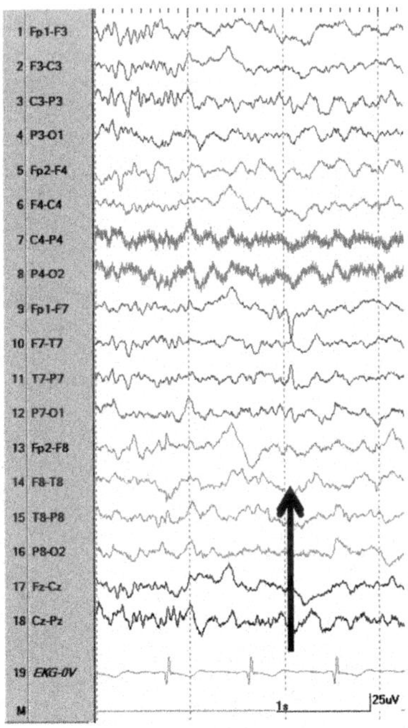

A. Negative; Negative
B. Negative; Positive
C. Positive; Negative
D. Positive; Positive
E. Cannot be determined in the given montage

111. Which sleep state is least likely to show epileptiform abnormalities?
A. N1
B. N2
C. N3
D. REM
E. NREM

112. Around 37 to 40 weeks of conceptional age, wakefulness is characterized by:
A. Features of sleep-onset REM
B. Presence of rhythmic theta waves
C. Features of active sleep (AS)
D. Presence of low-voltage irregular (LVI) activity
E. All of the above

113. Which of the following features of small sharp spikes (SSS) is helpful in distinguishing it from epileptiform discharges?
A. Disappearance during deeper stages of sleep
B. Steep ascending limb
C. Presence of aftergoing slow waves
D. Disruption of background
E. Broad field with temporal predominance

114. The following EEG (filter 1–70 Hz; sensitivity 10 μV/mm; solid vertical lines are 1 second apart) is most consistent with which of the following epilepsy syndromes?

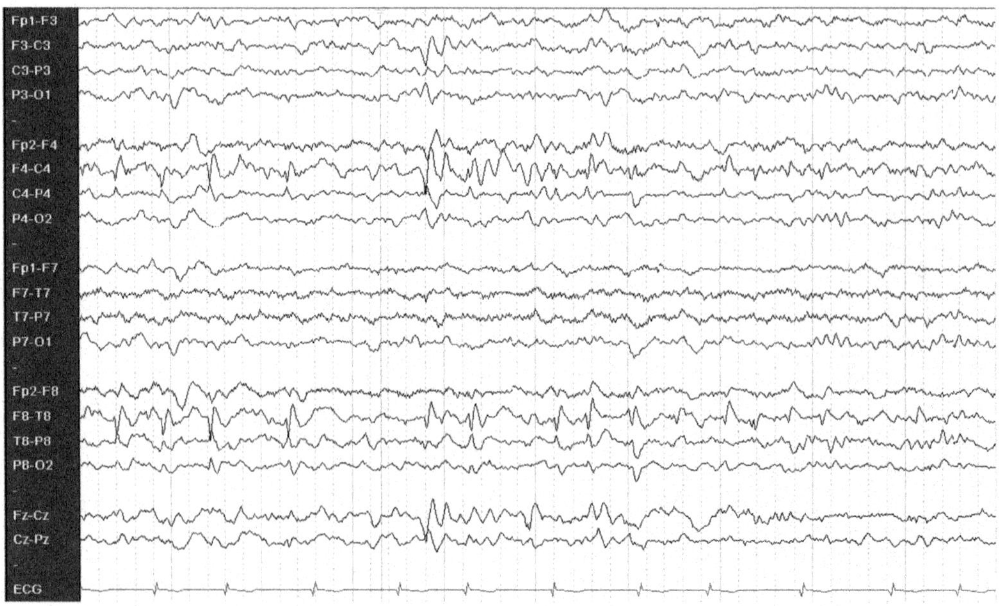

A. Autosomal dominant nocturnal frontal lobe epilepsy
B. Mesial temporal lobe epilepsy
C. Benign rolandic epilepsy (BRE)
D. Cingulate epilepsy
E. Lennox–Gastaut syndrome

115. A 43-year-old male, otherwise healthy, was running a 10K marathon when he had a witnessed generalized tonic–clonic seizure. He was able to stand and walk to the car with minimal support but was noted to be "not himself." When he arrived to the closest emergency department (ED), 30 miles away, he was able to follow simple commands but remained confused. A stat EEG (filter 1–70 Hz), as shown below, was done. Considering the clinical scenario and EEG findings, which of the following is the most likely etiology for his presentation?

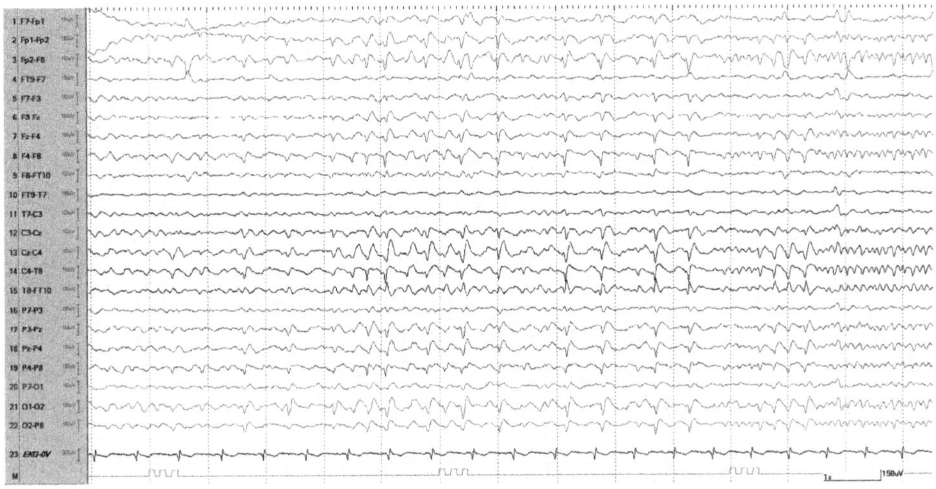

A. Herpes simplex virus (HSV) type I
B. HSV type II
C. Autoimmune disorder
D. Stroke
E. Anoxic brain injury

116. Obtaining serial EEGs can increase the sensitivity of detecting epileptiform abnormalities. What would be the sensitivity after three EEGs?
A. 10%
B. 20%
C. 30%
D. 50%
E. 90%

117. Which of the following statements is true regarding hypsarrhythmia?
A. It is associated with an organized high-amplitude background
B. It consists of irregular, low-amplitude, fast activity
C. It disappears during an infantile spasm
D. It is the most characteristic EEG finding in Lennox–Gastaut syndrome (LGS)
E. All of the above

118. Absence seizures are least likely to be potentiated by which of the following?
A. Hyperglycemia
B. Hypoglycemia
C. Hyperventilation (HV)
D. Intermittent photic stimulation (IPS)
E. NREM sleep

119. Which of the following statements is true regarding the Rolandic spikes?
   A. They can be seen in healthy siblings of children with benign rolandic epilepsy (BRE)
   B. They typically resolve by age 8 years
   C. They exhibit horizontal dipoles with central negativity and temporal positivity
   D. They are suppressed during sleep
   E. All of the above

120. Which of the following statements regarding malignant epilepsy syndromes is incorrect?
   A. Neonatal myoclonic encephalopathy may present with complex bursts of spikes and sharp waves with periods of discontinuity with evolution to hypsarrhythmia
   B. Early infantile epileptic encephalopathy may present with tonic spasms with a burst-suppression EEG pattern
   C. Severe myoclonic seizures of infancy may present as myoclonic seizures initially and progress to nonfebrile clonic seizures with generalized spike-wave and polyspike-wave discharges
   D. Myoclonic astatic epilepsy may present with febrile seizures in patients with normal development progressing to multiple seizure types with generalized spike-wave discharges in the setting of diffuse theta activity
   E. Ohtahara syndrome may present with tonic seizures and burst-suppression EEG pattern with subsequent progression to hypsarrhythmia

121. Which of the following findings is least likely to be seen in a patient with progressively worsening encephalopathy when serial EEGs are performed?
   A. A 6 Hz, medium voltage, reactive posterior dominant rhythm (PDR)
   B. A 9 Hz, low-voltage, reactive PDR
   C. A 7 Hz, medium voltage, nonreactive PDR
   D. Frontal intermittent rhythmic delta activity (FIRDA)
   E. Continuous generalized asynchronous delta activity

122. What does "paradoxical alpha rhythm" refer to?
   A. Presence of posterior alpha frequencies when the eyes are closed
   B. Appearance of posterior alpha frequencies when the eyes are open during drowsiness
   C. Presence of alpha frequencies anteriorly rather than posteriorly
   D. Appearance of alpha activity during slow-wave sleep
   E. Appearance of alpha activity during REM sleep

123. Which of the following statements regarding infant sleep is true?
   A. Infants typically sleep 8 to 10 hours during a 24-hour period
   B. Proportion of REM sleep increases at the expense of N2 sleep during infancy
   C. Transition from wakefulness into REM sleep is common until 1 year of age
   D. Sleep time decreases during the first few months of life
   E. All of the above

124. A 9-year-old girl with staring spells had an EEG that showed high-amplitude, 3 to 4 Hz sharply contoured delta activity. In which of the following scenarios would this finding be always considered pathological?
A. Hyperventilation (HV)
B. Drowsiness
C. Photic stimulation
D. Slow-wave sleep
E. A and C

125. A 32-year-old woman with a long history of intractable epilepsy undergoes an EEG (filter 1–70 Hz) as shown below. Which of the following statements is true regarding the finding shown in the figure?

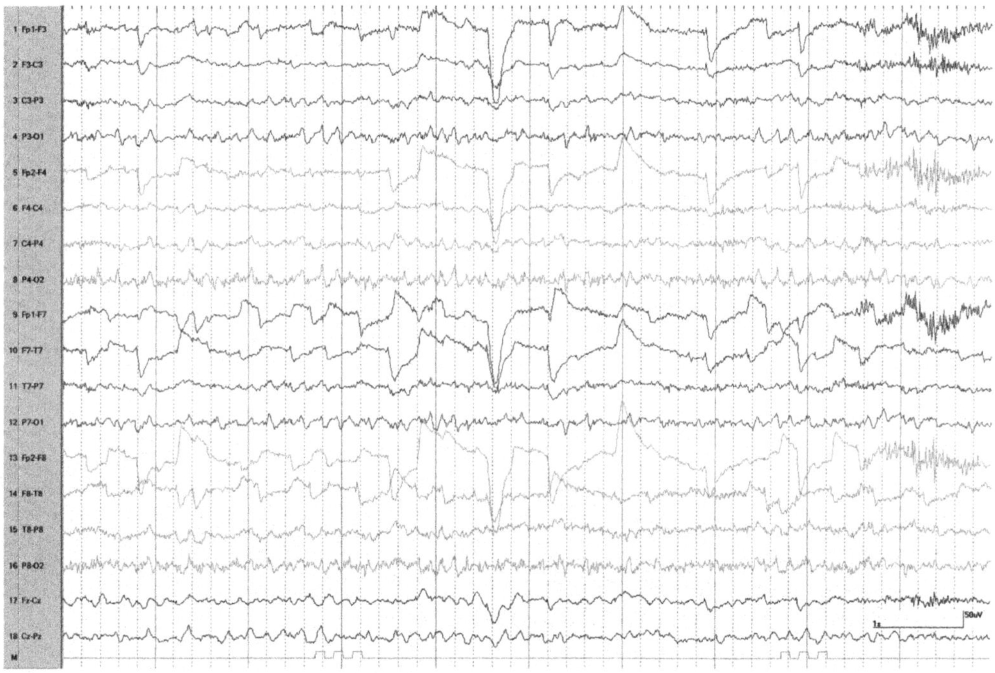

A. The patient has nystagmus
B. The patient has eye flutter
C. The patient is in REM sleep
D. The patient is reading a book
E. The patient is having a focal seizure involving the bioccipital region

126. Small sharp spikes (SSS) are
A. Seen in wakefulness
B. Most prominent in childhood
C. Controversial with respect to risk of epileptic seizures
D. Predominant in the temporo-occipital region
E. Typically between 60 and 100 microvolts

127. The generalized periodic discharges (GPDs) in Creutzfeldt–Jakob disease (CJD) are characterized by all of the following *except:*
A. They tend to disappear during sleep
B. They can be confined to the occipital region
C. They can be unilateral
D. They have a sensitivity of over 95%
E. They occur typically between 0.5 and 2 Hz

128. A 47-year-old male with HIV presents with fever and new-onset seizure. What does his EEG (filter 1–70 Hz) below show?

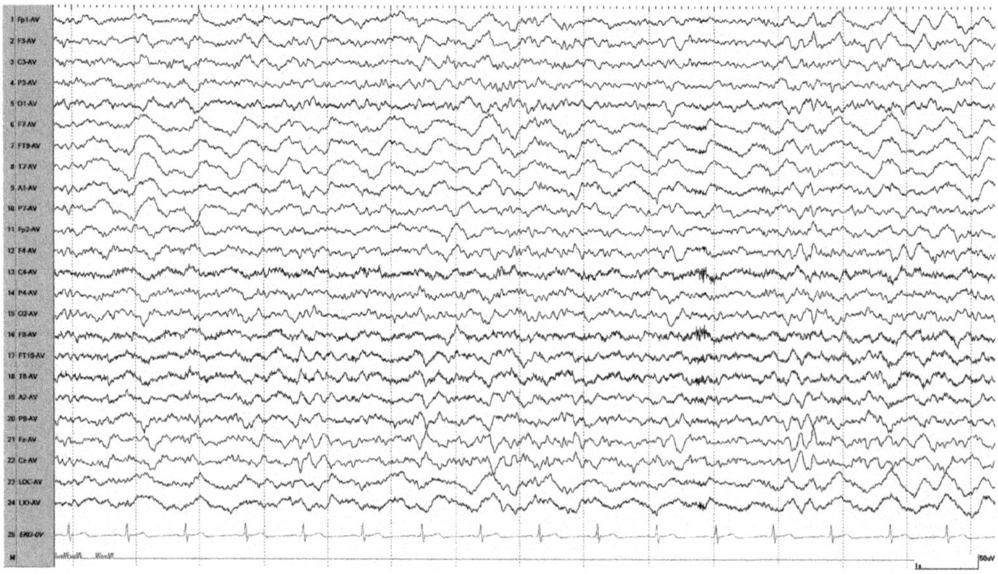

A. Lateralized periodic discharges (LPDs)
B. Intermittent rhythmic delta activity (IRDA)
C. Breach rhythm
D. Seizure
E. Pulse artifact

129. Which of the following EEG findings is most consistent with a diagnosis of encephalopathy?
A. An 8.5 Hz posterior dominant rhythm (PDR)
B. Temporal intermittent rhythmic delta activity (TIRDA)
C. Lateralized periodic discharges (LPDs)
D. Subclinical rhythmic electrographic discharge of adults (SREDA)
E. Frontal intermittent rhythmic delta activity (FIRDA)

130. What is the posterior activity seen in the following EEG (filter 1–70 Hz; sensitivity 7 μV/mm; vertical lines are 1 second apart) in a 48-year-old woman with a history of seizures since childhood?

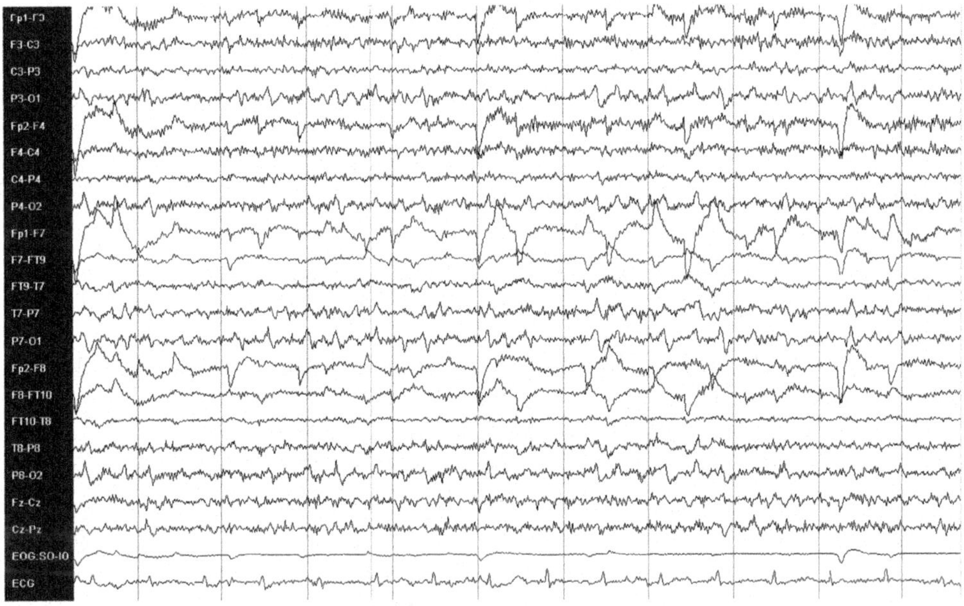

A. Lambda waves
B. Positive occipital sharp transients of sleep (POSTS)
C. Spike-wave discharges
D. Posterior slow waves of youth
E. Photic driving

131. A 25-year-old male with intractable epilepsy had seizure onset at age 15 years with grand mal seizures. He also has a history of bipolar disorder and prior suicide attempt. Which of the following findings is not seen in his EEG (filter: 1–70 Hz)?

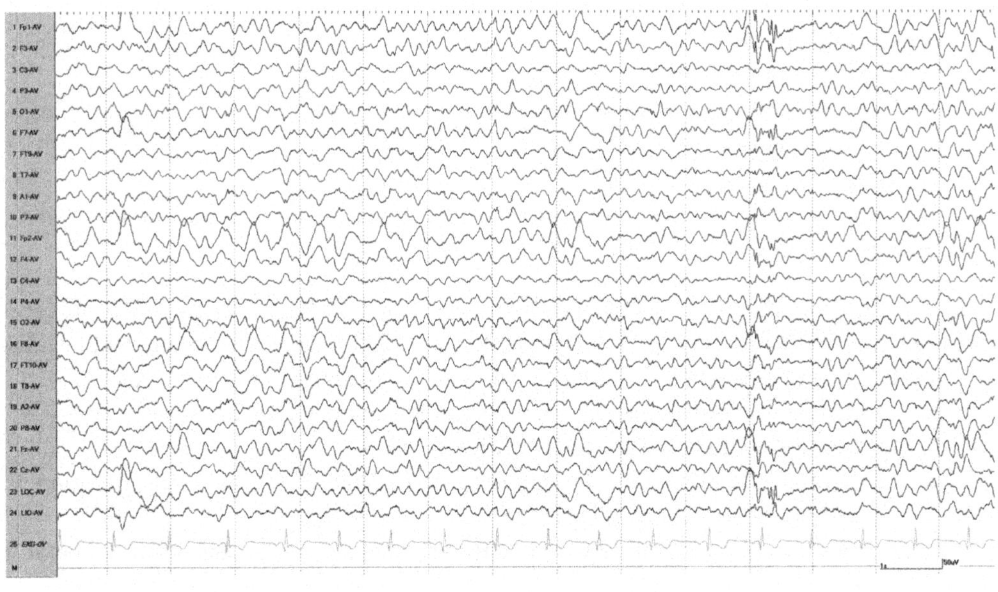

A. Generalized spike-wave discharges
B. Generalized theta slowing
C. Generalized polymorphic delta slowing
D. Lateralized intermittent rhythmic delta activity
E. Slow posterior dominant rhythm (PDR)

132. Which of the following statements is true regarding the use of chloral hydrate in recording EEG?
A. It can be routinely administered in most EEG laboratories
B. It accentuates epileptiform activity in wakefulness
C. It is slowly metabolized
D. It can frequently cause paradoxical excitation and irrational behavior
E. It can be used when natural sleep cannot be achieved

133. In which of the following clinical scenarios is hyperventilation (HV) considered unsafe and contraindicated?
A. An 8-year-old boy who frequently daydreams in school
B. A 58-year-old male with a remote history of right-sided hemiplegia
C. A 27-year-old female with a history of significant psychosocial stressors and nonstereotyped intractable seizures
D. A 30-year-old female with seizures characterized by déjà vu and lip smacking
E. A 15-year-old female with history of chronic strokes due to known moyamoya disease

134. Which of the following statements best describes generalized spike-and-wave discharges?
A. They are symmetric in morphology between anterior and posterior head regions
B. They can be rarely seen in patients with focal seizures
C. Frequency of less than 4 Hz in children is invariably associated with good prognosis
D. They may be activated by hyperventilation (HV), but not photic stimulation
E. They can be more readily classified as interictal or ictal activity compared to focal discharges

135. Which of the following statements best describes the evolution of sleep spindles in infants and children?
A. They first appear by age 6 months
B. They exhibit centro-parietal predominance rather than midline predominance throughout infancy
C. They reach a frequency of 14 Hz by 12 months
D. Faster spindle activity with paroxysmal traits is considered normal in infants
E. Spindle activity is symmetric by 12 months

136. Which of the following is NOT a criterion according to the American Clinical Neurophysiology Society (ACNS) guidelines for recording EEG in suspected brain death evaluation?
A. Recording at a sensitivity of 2 μV/mm for a minimum of 30 minutes
B. Electrode impedance greater than 10 and less than 10,000 ohms
C. Interelectrode distance should be at least 10 cm
D. Low-frequency filter should not be greater than 1 Hz and high-frequency filter should not be less than 30 Hz
E. There should be a lack of EEG reactivity to auditory, somatosensory, and visual stimuli

137. A technologist was performing an EEG on a 9-year-old girl and noted that hyperventilation (HV) led to altered awareness. Which of the following clinical observations by the technologist is NOT consistent with HV-induced high-amplitude rhythmic slowing (HIHARS)?
A. Fidgeting
B. Yawning
C. Staring
D. Eyelid flutter
E. Smiling

138. A 64-year-old female with rapidly progressive dementia and myoclonus is being evaluated with an EEG. Which of the following EEG abnormalities is most consistent with a specific diagnosis based on the clinical scenario?
A. Triphasic waves
B. Bitemporal independent lateralized periodic discharges (LPDs)
C. Bisynchronous generalized periodic discharges (GPDs)
D. Frontal intermittent rhythmic delta activity (FIRDA)
E. Generalized intermittent rhythmic delta activity (GIRDA)

139. Which of the following statements regarding the development of REM sleep is true?
A. REM sleep constitutes 30% of sleep at birth
B. REM sleep is characterized by the presence of occipital sharp transients during infancy
C. Apneic periods during REM sleep in normal infants are pathological
D. REM sleep shows increasing desynchronization by 3 years of age
E. REM latency is longest in the early morning hours during infancy

140. Which of the following is most consistent with an ictal EEG pattern?
A. Semirhythmic delta activity for 2 seconds followed by increase in frequency and decrease in amplitude
B. Sharply contoured theta activity followed by increase in frequency and increase in amplitude
C. Repetitive spikes at 3 Hz frequency for 3 seconds followed by rhythmic theta activity
D. Single 1 Hz slow spike-wave followed by a generalized electrodecremental pattern with superimposed fast activity
E. All of the above

141. Which of the following is NOT an expected feature in the EEG of a normal 3-month-old infant?
A. 3 Hz posterior dominant rhythm (PDR)
B. Hypnagogic hypersynchrony
C. Sleep spindles
D. Photic driving
E. None of the above

142. A neonate of 36 weeks conceptional age (CA) was found to have respiratory arrest shortly after birth. Upon extubation, the child clinically stable. An EEG was done for suspected seizures as shown below (filter 1–70 Hz; sensitivity 15 μV/mm; the solid vertical lines are 1 second apart). The patient was noted to be resting quietly at time of recording. What is the best interpretation of the findings seen?

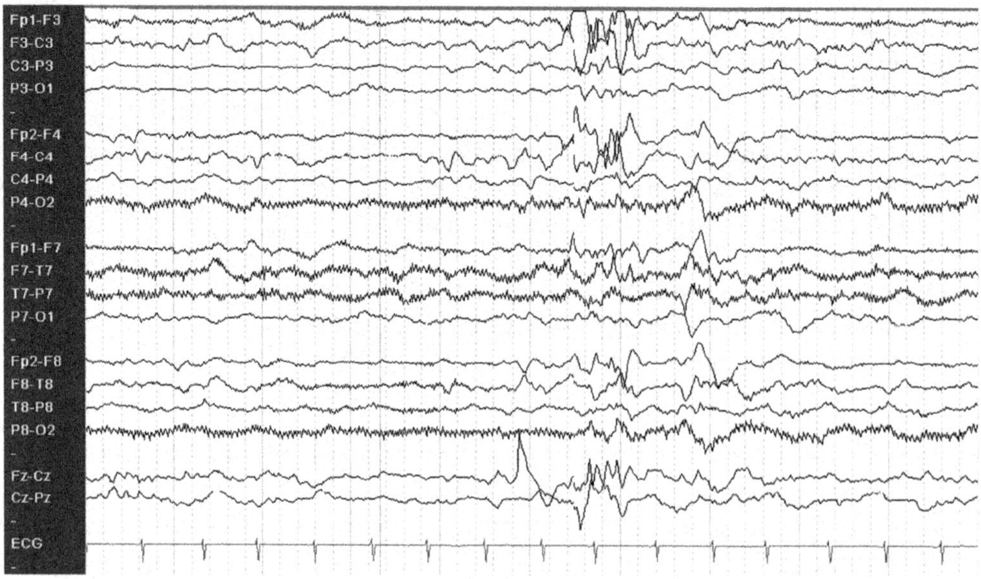

A. Epileptiform activity
B. Artifact
C. Encephalopathy
D. Normal awake finding
E. Normal sleep finding

143. Which of the following is NOT usually considered to have a bipolar montage configuration?
A. Longitudinal
B. Transverse
C. Hatband
D. Laplacian
E. Double banana

144. Which electrode placement system is shown in the figure below?

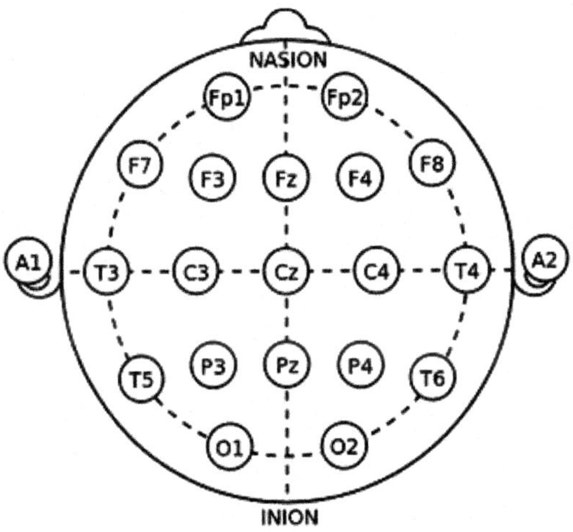

A. International 10 to 5 system
B. International 10 to 10 system
C. International 10 to 20 system
D. Modified combinatorial nomenclature (MCN)
E. American Clinical Neurophysiology Society (ACNS) system

145. Twitching of which of the following muscles is most associated with the photomyogenic effect seen on EEG?
A. Orbicularis oris muscle
B. Temporalis muscle
C. Frontalis muscle
D. Mentalis muscle
E. Buccinator muscle

146. A normal variant is shown in the following EEG (filter 1–70 Hz). What are its typical state, distribution, and synchrony?

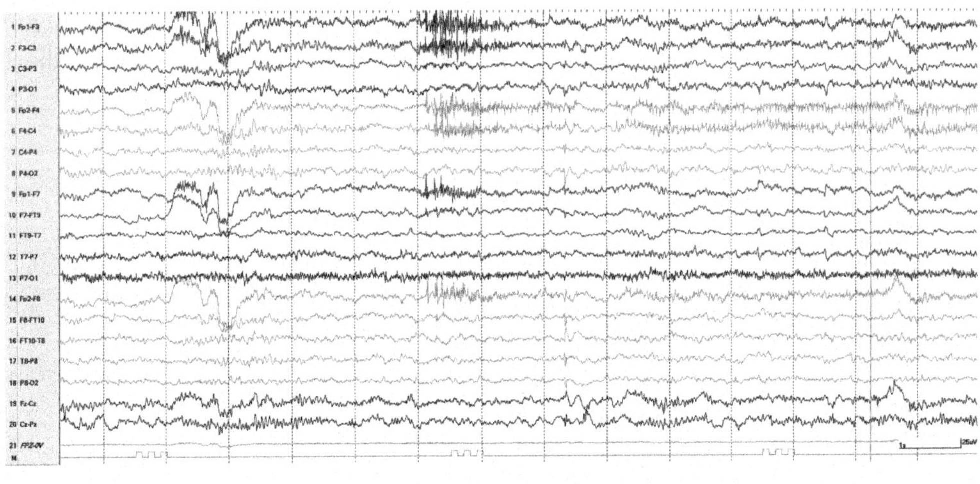

A. Drowsy; temporal; asynchronous
B. Stage N2 sleep; diffuse; asynchronous
C. Drowsy; midline; asynchronous
D. REM; temporal; synchronous
E. Awake; multifocal; synchronous

147. Which of the following best describes the distribution of the periodic discharges in the following EEG (filter: 1–70 Hz)?

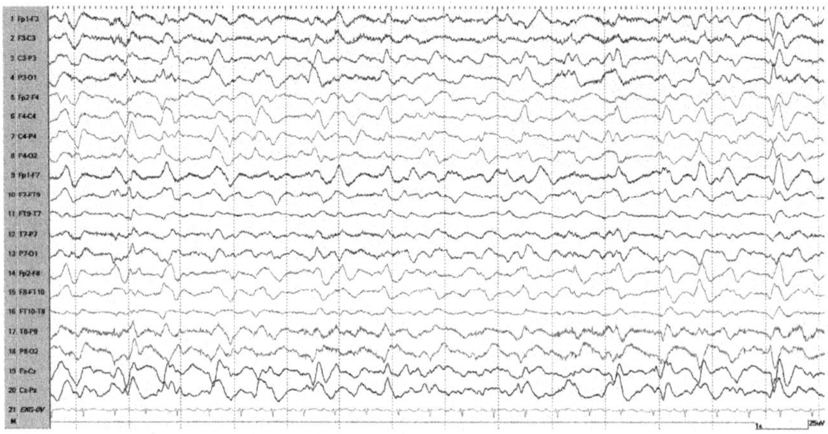

A. Generalized
B. Lateralized
C. Lateralized and bilaterally independent
D. Nonlateralized
E. Midline

148. On postoperative day 2 after a renal transplant, a 12-year-old boy with a history of a ventriculoperitoneal (VP) shunt became febrile and developed altered mental status. The patient had normal intracranial pressure (ICP) and cerebrospinal fluid (CSF) was sent for analysis. He was placed on antibiotics and continuous video-EEG monitoring was obtained as shown below (filter 1–70 Hz; sensitivity 10 μV/mm; solid vertical bars are 1 second apart). Six hours into the monitoring session, a relatively abrupt decrease in EEG amplitude was seen as shown below. His vital signs and ICP were stable. What is the most likely cause of the change?

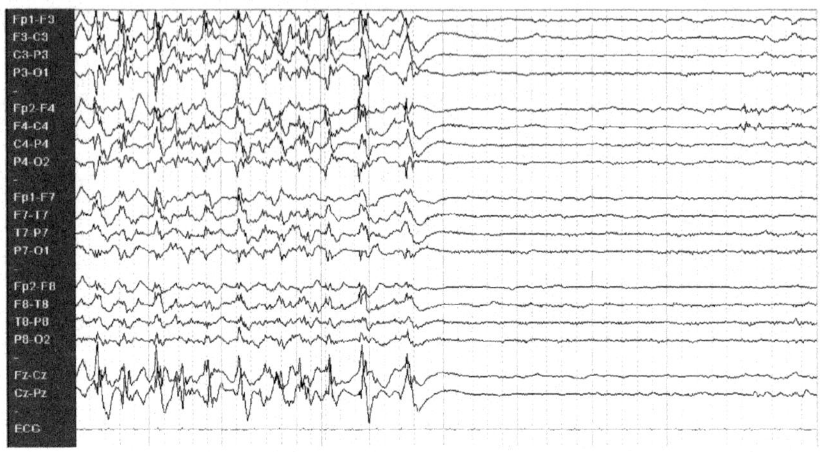

A. Cessation of a generalized seizure discharge
B. Suctioning the patient
C. Cerebral hypoperfusion
D. Turning off propofol
E. The reference electrode fell off

149. EEG findings in coma can include all of the following *except:*
A. Generalized burst suppression is invariably associated with poor prognosis regardless of etiology
B. Diffuse monomorphic nonreactive alpha activity can be associated with brainstem lesions or hypoxic-ischemic injury
C. Normal sleep features such as spindles may be seen with cyclic variability
D. A pattern of low-voltage irregular (LVI) activity alternating with high-voltage slowing may be seen in patients with Cheyne–Stokes breathing
E. EEG may show signs of reactivity without associated clinical response to the same external stimulus

150. Which of the following statements is true regarding lambda waves?
A. They are not seen outside the occipital region
B. They are most common in children and adolescents
C. They can be triggered by eye closure immediately after scanning a complex picture
D. They are usually asynchronous and asymmetric
E. Their polarity is typically negative

151. A 25-year-old male had an EEG (filter 1–70 Hz; sensitivity 5 μV/mm; the solid vertical lines are 1 second apart) as part of the workup for syncope. During the recording as shown below, the technologist noted focal rhythmic activity in the left central region, which went away when the patient wiped his nose with his right hand. Which of the following statements is true regarding this activity?

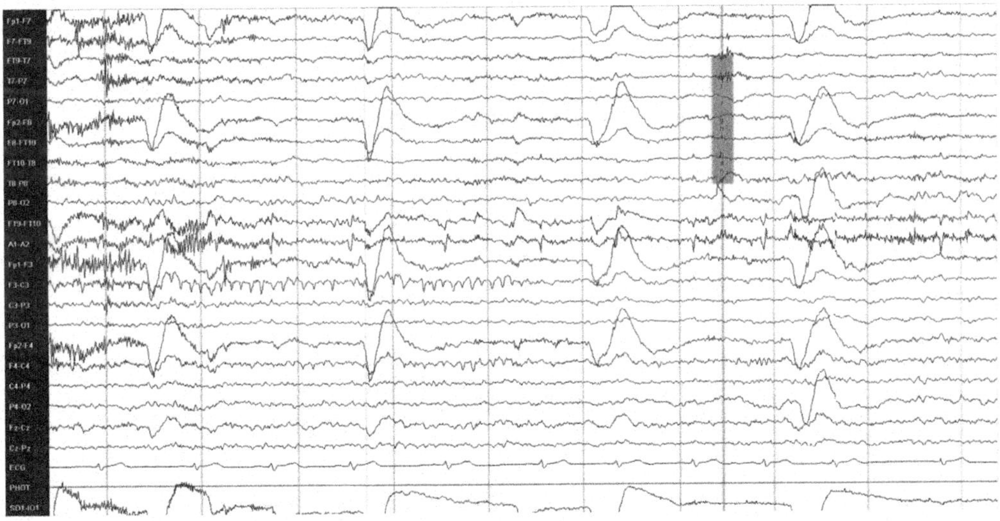

A. Its frequency is in the theta range
B. Nose wiping with the right hand has no relation to the activity
C. It represents the resting rhythm of the Rolandic cortex
D. It represents a brief ictal discharge that may have originated in the temporal region
E. It is most prominent in deep sleep

152. The characteristics and evolution of a drowsy pattern on EEG consists of:
A. Appearance of hypnagogic hypersynchrony by age 3 months
B. Disappearance of hypnagogic hypersynchrony by age 6 years
C. Dropout of the posterior dominant rhythm (PDR) by age 3 years
D. Mature pattern with alpha dropout and diffuse low-voltage with intermixed slow and fast activity by adolescence
E. All of the above

153. Which of the following features is NOT a characteristic of NREM sleep in infants?
A. NREM sleep features emerge and are well developed by age 2 months
B. Vertex waves (V-waves) tend to be high amplitude, sharply contoured, and may occur in trains
C. K-complexes tend to have a longer duration than V-waves
D. K-complexes can be elicited with auditory stimulation
E. V-waves are synchronous from birth but may be asymmetric during early stages of sleep

154. Characteristics of sleep spindles in infants include all of the following *except:*
A. They are clearly seen by age 3 months
B. They become synchronous by age 1 year
C. Early on they typically occur in runs lasting seconds
D. They are comb-shaped rather than sinusoidal
E. They can appear as early as 46 to 48 weeks gestational age (GA)

155. A 33-year-old female with meningoencephalitis had a stroke with left facial droop. She presents with new episodes of dizziness and right facial twitching. She had two witnessed seizures described as "shaking all over." She is back to baseline with proper mentation and no appreciable twitching. An EEG was then done. What is the most prominent finding seen on the EEG (filter 1–70 Hz)?

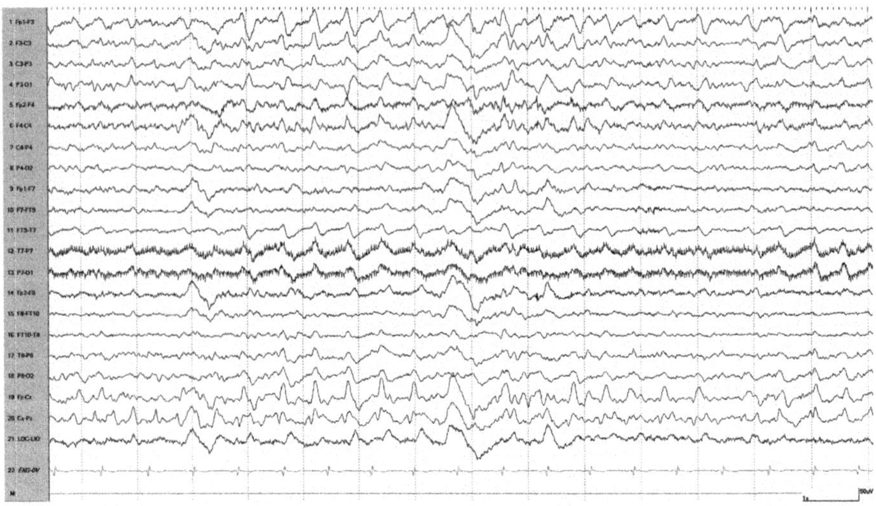

A. Lateralized periodic discharges (LPDs)
B. Intermittent rhythmic delta activity (IRDA)
C. Sharply contoured polymorphic delta slowing
D. Seizure discharge
E. EKG artifact

156. Intermittent rhythmic delta activity (IRDA) is:
A. Typically predominant in the frontal region in children
B. Can be associated with predisposition to seizures
C. Activated by sleep
D. Activated by eye opening
E. Attenuated by hyperventilation (HV)

157. Compared with the scalp electrodes, the subdermal needle electrodes are characterized by which of the following statements?
A. They have a smaller contact area
B. They have higher input impedances
C. They are more susceptible to noise
D. They are less likely to cause skin breakdown
E. All of the above

158. Which of the following statements best describes the clinical significance of interictal epileptiform discharges (IEDs)?
A. About 66% of patients with epilepsy show IEDs on the first routine EEG
B. IEDs may not be seen in certain forms of temporal lobe epilepsy on scalp recordings
C. Frequency of IEDs correlates roughly with seizure frequency
D. Hyperventilation (HV) activates generalized IEDs but not focal IEDs
E. Landau–Kleffner syndrome (LKS) has a dramatic increase in abundance of IEDs in wakefulness

159. Which of the following is true regarding the nomenclature of EEG activity?
A. Sigma rhythm refers to 15 to 20 Hz activity
B. Rho waves refer to positive occipital sharp transients of sleep (POSTS)
C. Phi rhythm refers to temporal rhythmic delta activity in children
D. Ripples refers to 50 to 80 Hz activity
E. High-frequency oscillations refers to 250 to 500 Hz activity

160. Which of the following is NOT a feature of Ciganek rhythm?
A. Presence in the bitemporal region
B. Presence during both wakefulness and drowsiness
C. Activation by mental task
D. Notched morphology
E. Theta frequency range

161. A 48-year-old male with a history of seizures has an EEG as shown below. During the recording, the patient is noted to be drowsy by the technologist. What is the best interpretation of his EEG (filter 1–70 Hz)?

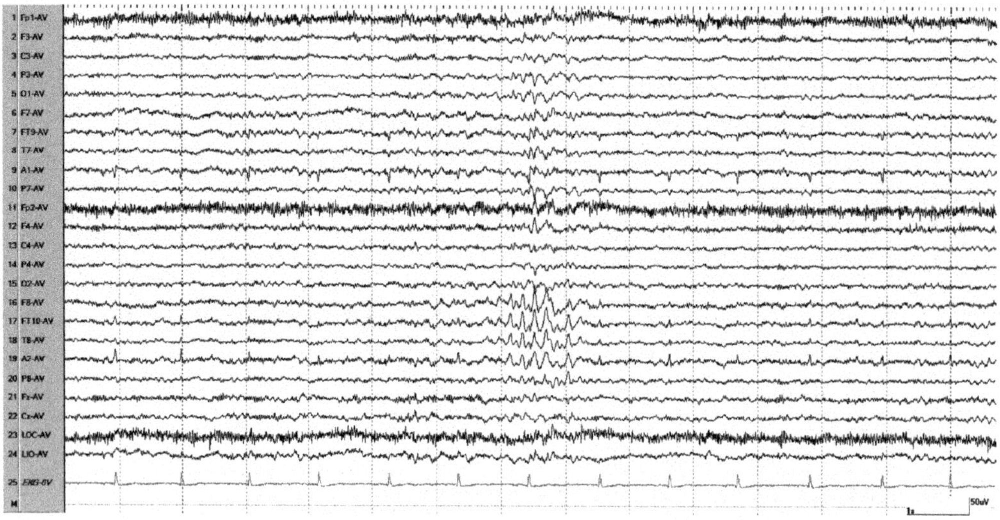

A. Psychomotor seizures
B. Mild encephalopathy
C. Temporal lobe seizures
D. Breach rhythm
E. None of the above

162. All of the following statements regarding the EEG abnormalities after acute stroke are true *except:*
A. Absence of delta activity within the infarcted region predicts a benign course
B. Frontal intermittent rhythmic delta activity (FIRDA) suggests a large infarct causing midline shift
C. Lateralized periodic discharges (LPDs) are more likely after acute thrombotic strokes
D. Vertebrobasilar stroke can be associated with an alpha coma pattern
E. Diffuse slowing in the ischemic region suggests predisposition to develop cerebral edema

163. Which of the following is true regarding wicket spikes?
A. They usually occur in adults over 30 years of age
B. They have a strong association with seizures when seen in adolescents
C. They are common patterns seen in up to 25% of EEG records
D. They are seen in wakefulness and REM sleep but absent during drowsiness
E. They frequently have an after-going slow wave

164. Lambdoid waves are:
A. Surface-positive waveforms
B. Seen during both wakefulness and light sleep
C. Triggered by scanning complex visual patterns
D. Relatively rare, being encountered in less than 10% of the healthy population
E. Believed to represent a "playback" of information to the temporal cortex

165. Which of the following is NOT considered as EEG reactivity to auditory or tactile stimulation in a term infant?

A. Diffuse flattening
B. Burst of generalized theta activity
C. Burst of generalized delta activity
D. Occipital rhythmic activity occurring at the same frequency as the respiratory rate
E. Discernible change in amplitude, frequency, or continuity

166. All of the following statements regarding focal slow activity are true *except:*

A. Continuous focal arrhythmic polymorphic delta activity can be seen in a brain tumor
B. Continuous focal arrhythmic polymorphic delta activity can be seen during a migraine attack
C. Continuous focal rhythmic monomorphic theta activity suggests an underlying white matter lesion
D. Intermittent focal rhythmic monomorphic delta activity can be seen in epilepsy
E. Gray matter lesions can result in different slowing patterns than white matter lesions

167. Which of the following findings would most likely be seen in Rasmussen syndrome?

A. Burst suppression
B. Generalized periodic discharges (GPDs)
C. Electrographic status epilepticus
D. Diffuse low voltage
E. Regional rather than hemispheric abnormalities

168. The following EEG (filter 1–70 Hz; sensitivity 10 μV/mm; solid vertical lines are 1 second apart) is from a 9-year-old boy with intractable epilepsy with psychiatric comorbidities. What medication is likely causing the diffuse changes?

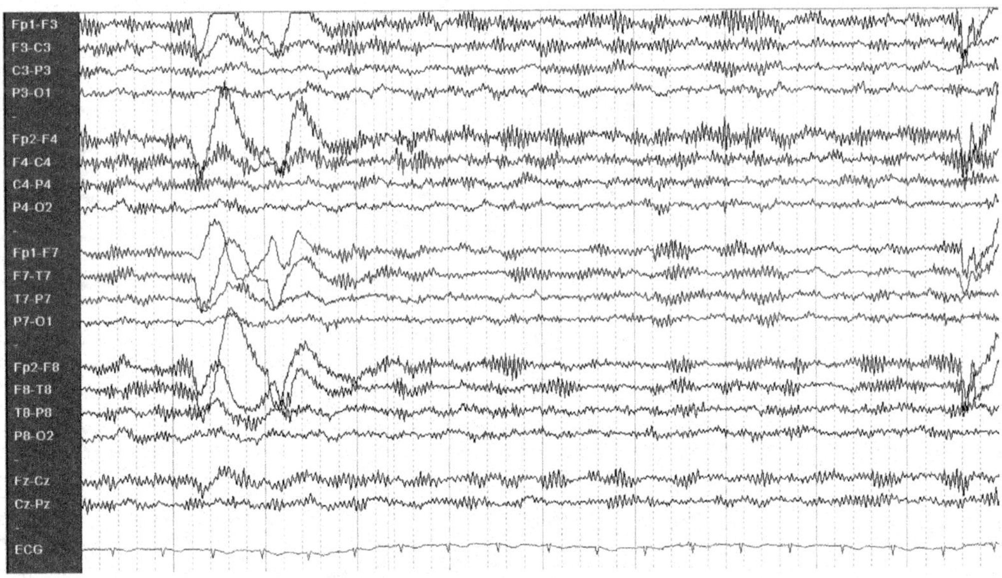

A. Antidepressant
B. Anxiolytic
C. Antipsychotic
D. Analgesic
E. None of the above

169. As infants grow, the posterior dominant rhythm (PDR) changes. All of the following regarding evolution of the PDR are true *except:*
A. 1 month: No clear PDR
B. 2 months: A PDR is first appreciable
C. 3 months: 3 Hz
D. 5 months: 5 Hz
E. 12 months: 12 Hz

170. Which of the following statements is true regarding sphenoidal electrodes?
A. They are positioned medial to the foramen ovale
B. They may pick up posterior–temporal potentials better than surface electrodes
C. They are felt to pick up similar potentials as FT9 and FT10
D. They require placement under fluoroscopic guidance
E. Clean but not sterile technique is required for placement

171. Which of the following ictal patterns is least likely to be associated with generalized seizures?
A. A 10 Hz spike-and-wave discharge at the onset of a generalized tonic–clonic seizure
B. An electrodecremental pattern during a tonic seizure
C. A 2 Hz spike-and-wave discharge during a staring spell
D. An electrodecremental pattern followed by a high-voltage slow wave during an infantile spasm
E. Generalized polyspike pattern often obscured by muscle and movement artifact during a tonic seizure

172. What is the anterior slow activity seen in the following EEG (filter 0.1–70 Hz)?

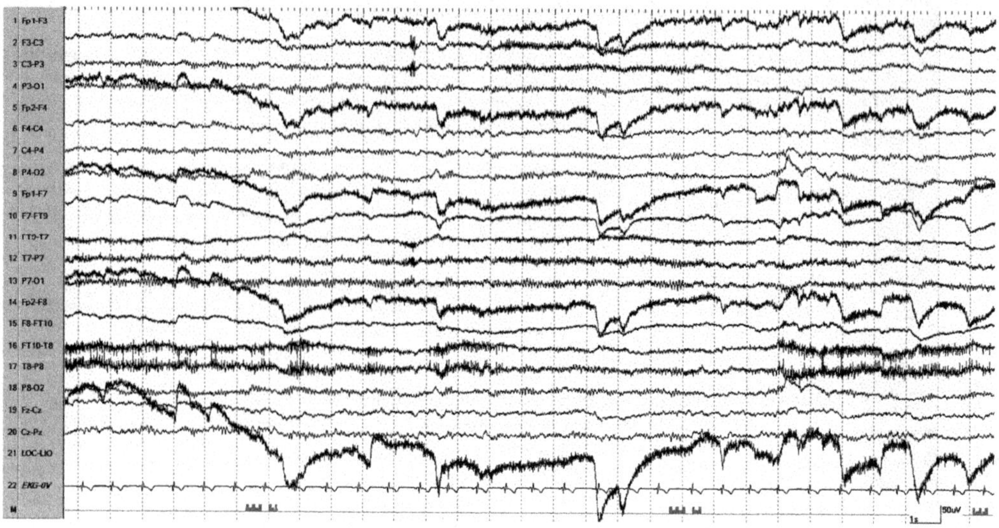

A. Lateral eye movements
B. Sweat artifact
C. 60 Hz artifact
D. Frontal intermittent rhythmic delta activity (FIRDA)
E. Glossokinetic artifact

173. Which of the following EEG patterns is highly specific for an underlying seizure disorder?
A. Triphasic waves
B. Temporal intermittent rhythmic delta activity (TIRDA)
C. Frontal intermittent rhythmic delta activity (FIRDA)
D. Generalized intermittent rhythmic delta activity (GRDA)
E. Generalized periodic discharges (GPDs)

174. From term to 3 months of age, drowsiness typically consists of:
A. Eyes open state
B. Increase in amplitude
C. Temporal slowing
D. A and B
E. A, B and C

175. Which of the following statements is true regarding periodic discharges on the EEG?
A. They occur at a frequency of 0.5 to 2 Hz in subacute sclerosing panencephalitis (SSPE)
B. They occur in a generalized distribution in herpes simplex encephalitis (HSE)
C. They occur every 4 to 16 seconds in Creutzfeldt–Jakob disease (CJD)
D. They may be associated with contralateral motor phenomena
E. All of the above

176. The standard paper speed for EEG recording in the United States is:
A. 10 mm/sec
B. 15 mm/sec
C. 30 mm/sec
D. 45 mm/sec
E. 60 mm/sec

177. A 22-year-old male with a 4-month history of seizures has an EEG shown below (filter 1–70 Hz). What is the most likely diagnosis?

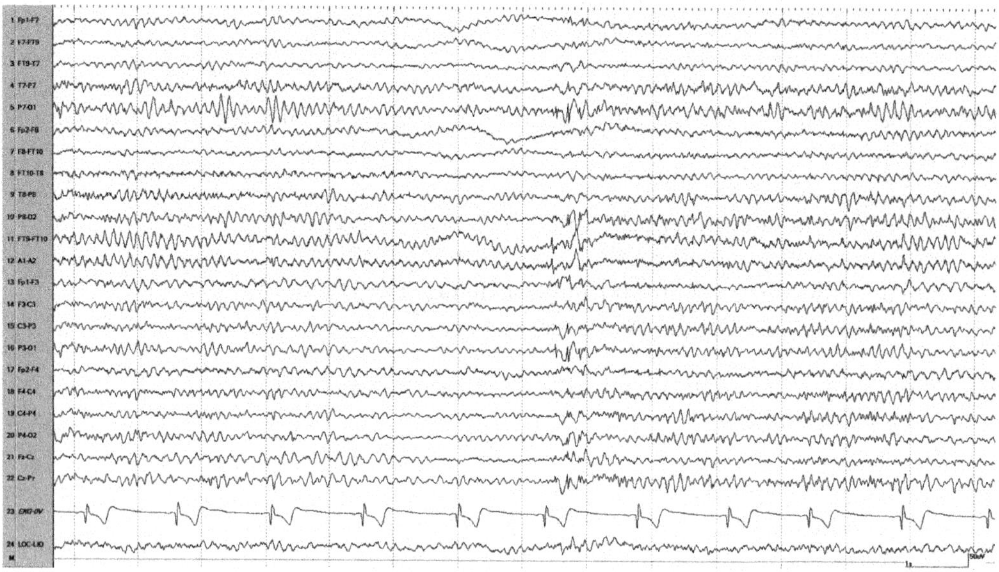

A. Panayiotopoulos syndrome
B. Normal awake recording
C. Partial (focal) epilepsy
D. Idiopathic generalized epilepsy with bioccipital predominance
E. Lennox–Gastaut syndrome

178. A 49-year-old male with a history of a childhood traumatic brain injury presents with seizures and migraines. What is the most likely reason for the asymmetrical frontal activity noted on his EEG (filter 1–70 Hz) below?

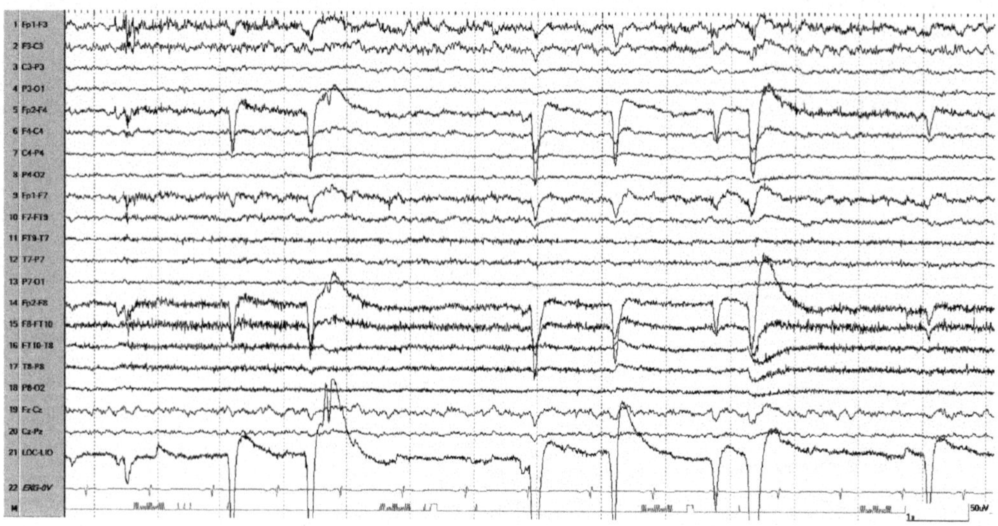

A. REM sleep
B. Enucleation
C. Misplaced Fp1 electrode
D. Bell's palsy
E. Sweat artifact

179. Which of the following statements regarding hypnagogic hypersynchrony is true?
A. It is most commonly seen in children age 6 to 12 years
B. It is characterized by high amplitude, synchronous, rhythmic activity
C. It occurs at the transition from sleep to wakefulness
D. The activity is brief, typically less than 1 second
E. The activity has a typical frequency of 8 to 12 Hz

180. Which of the following statements regarding lateralized periodic discharges (LPDs) is true?
A. They occur at a frequency of 0.05 to 2 Hz
B. They are strictly distributed unilaterally
C. The background between the discharges is typically normal
D. The morphology of the discharges is monophasic
E. They are difficult to suppress with antiseizure medications

181. Hypnagogic hypersynchrony refers to:
A. Intermittent diffuse slowing during arousal
B. Intermittent bifrontally predominant slow activity upon falling asleep in children
C. Serial runs of K-complexes and spindles
D. High-amplitude slowing intermixed with multifocal sharp waves
E. High-amplitude, hypersynchronous background slowing during hyperventilation

182. The posterior dominant rhythm (PDR) in adults is characterized by all of the following *except:*
A. It is predominant in the occipital region but may extend into parietal, central, and temporal regions
B. It is attenuated by visual, auditory, tactile, and other somatosensory stimuli
C. It is enhanced by mental activity such as solving arithmetic problems
D. It is affected by menstrual cycle
E. It may present as a frequency harmonic of itself

183. By 3 months of age, what is the frequency of the posterior dominant rhythm (PDR)?
A. 2 Hz
B. 3 Hz
C. 5 Hz
D. 6 Hz
E. 8 Hz

184. Ctenoids are:
A. Rhythmic sinusoidal waveforms
B. Surface positive waveforms
C. Frontal in distribution with shifting predominance
D. More common in adults than children
E. Seen typically in wakefulness

185. Which of the following statements is true regarding epilepsy associated with brain tumors?
A. Solid tumors are highly epileptogenic by themselves
B. The seizure focus always localizes to the vicinity of the tumor
C. Low-grade glial tumors are more epileptogenic than high-grade tumors
D. EEG abnormalities in solid tumors are directly related to the tumors themselves
E. Lateralized periodic discharges (LPDs) are not likely in tumor-related epilepsy

186. Which of the following statements is true regarding posterior slow waves of youth?
A. They are predominant in the parietal region
B. They consist of waveforms with a frequency of 5 to 7 Hz
C. They are best seen during relaxed wakefulness
D. They disappear with eye closure
E. They are typically seen in children less than 2 years of age

187. Which of the following statements is true regarding hyperventilation (HV) performed during an EEG?
A. It may induce cerebral hypoxia
B. Persistence of HV-induced slowing beyond 30 seconds after stopping HV is almost always abnormal
C. HV-induced slowing is enhanced by recumbent position
D. HV-induced slowing is enhanced by high blood glucose
E. HV is more likely to trigger focal seizures than generalized seizures

188. The accepted nomenclature of EEG electrodes includes all of the following *except:*
A. Even numbers over the right hemisphere
B. Odd numbers over the left hemisphere
C. The letter "z" refers to midline electrode
D. M1 and M2 refer to the earlobe electrodes
E. TP refers to intermediate electrode placement between T and P electrodes

189. What would the sensitivity be if there is 2 mm deflection in the FP1–F3 channel where FP1 is −60 μV and F3 is −50 μV?
A. 5 μV/mm
B. −5 μV/mm
C. 55 μV/mm
D. 75 μV/mm
E. 7.5 μV/mm

190. A 39-year-old male presents with a 2-week history of intermittent right index finger twitching. What is the most likely interpretation of his EEG (filter 1–70 Hz), shown below?

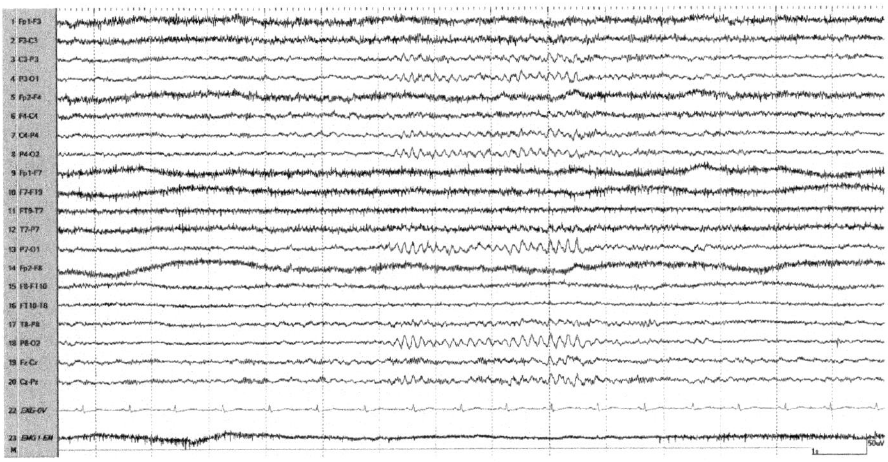

A. Psychogenic nonepileptic event
B. Scalp-negative epileptic seizure discharge
C. Slow alpha variant
D. Occipital intermittent rhythmic delta activity (OIRDA)
E. Positive occipital sharp transients of sleep (POSTS)

191. An electrodecremental ictal EEG pattern can be seen in:
A. Myoclonic seizure
B. Tonic seizure
C. Atonic seizure
D. B and C
E. A, B and C

192. A 43-year-old woman with lupus and hypertension presents for an EEG (filter 1–70 Hz), shown below after a witnessed seizure. Which of the following can be part of the patient's ictal clinical semiology?

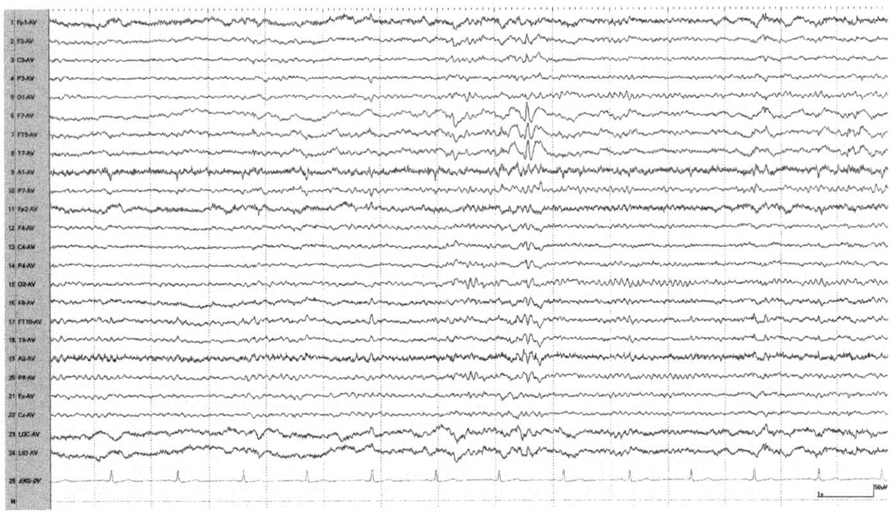

A. Grunting
B. Left hand dystonic posturing
C. Bilateral asymmetric posturing
D. Left hand rhythmic ictal nonclonic hand (RINCH) movements
E. Postictal nose wiping with the left hand

193. A 62-year-old female, status postresection of a left hemispheric glioblastoma, was noted to have altered mental status on postoperative day 1. What is the most prominent finding on her EEG shown below (filter 1–70 Hz, sensitivity 10 μV/mm)?

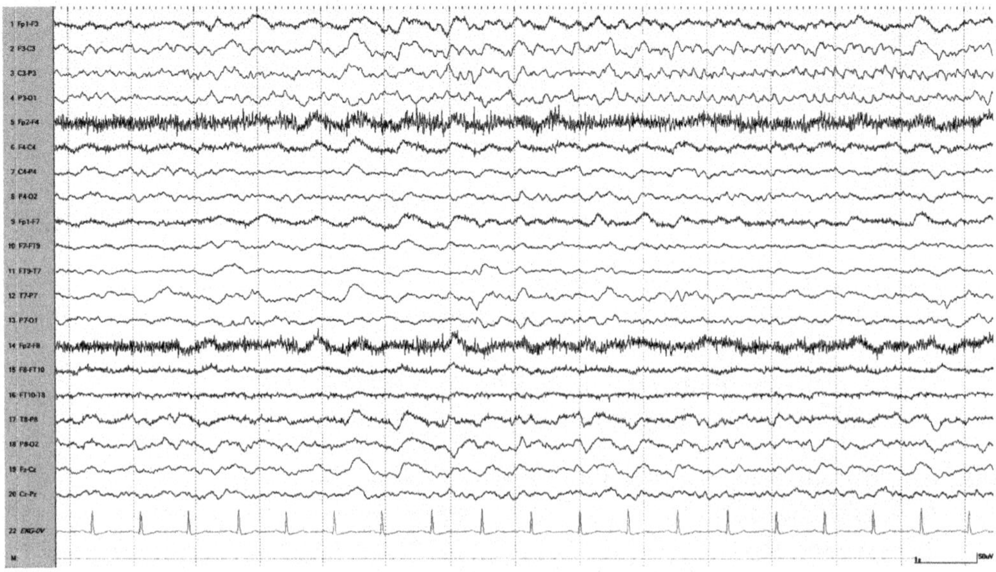

A. Lateralized periodic discharges (LPDs)
B. Continuous rhythmic delta activity
C. Breach rhythm
D. Seizure discharge
E. Asymmetric posterior dominant rhythm (PDR)

194. What is the interpeak duration of a normal posterior dominant rhythm (PDR) in a 15-year-old child?
A. 25 ms
B. 70 ms
C. 100 ms
D. 150 ms
E. 200 ms

195. What clinical scenario could lead to the following EEG pattern (filter 1–70 Hz)?

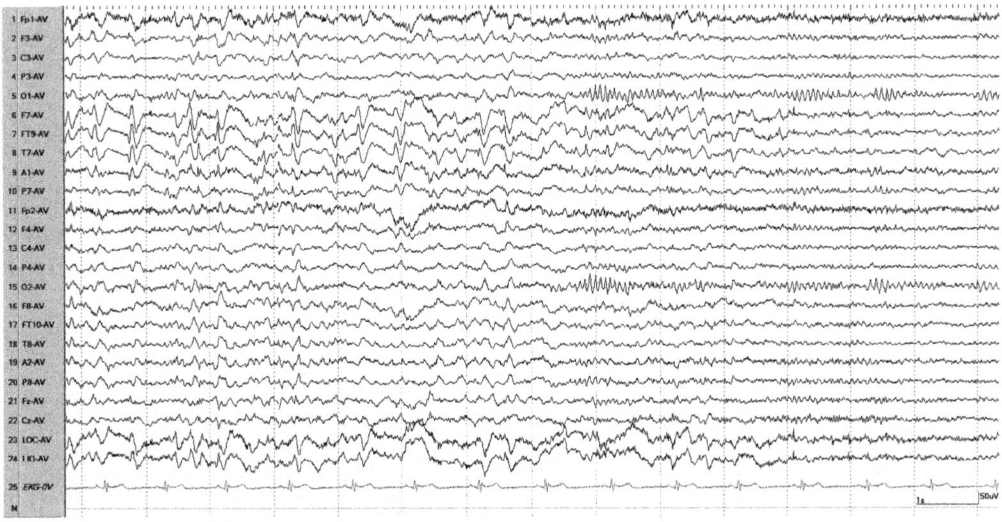

A. A 29-year-old male with acute left middle cerebral artery (MCA) stroke
B. An 18-year-old male with lithium overdose
C. A 61-year-old female with early-onset Alzheimer's disease
D. A 2-year-old boy with brainstem glioma
E. A 1-year old girl with left temporal ganglioglioma

196. Which of the following is true regarding benign occipital epilepsy of childhood?
A. The late-onset type presents with extra-occipital spikes more frequently than the early-onset type
B. The early-onset type presents with rhythmic alpha seizure discharge
C. Occipital paroxysms are activated by elimination of visual fixation rather than darkness
D. The epileptiform discharges are always bilateral and synchronous
E. The interictal discharges attenuate with eye closure and reoccur with eye opening

197. Reliable predictors of death or persistent vegetative state after cardiac arrest include all of the following *except:*
A. Absent N20 responses
B. Electrographic status epilepticus
C. Burst-suppression pattern
D. Low-voltage pattern
E. Spindle coma pattern

198. What should be the duration of an EEG in order to qualify for an electrocerebral inactivity (ECI) recording according to the American Clinical Neurophysiology Society (ACNS) guidelines?
A. At least 20 minutes
B. At least 30 minutes
C. At least 45 minutes
D. At least 60 minutes
E. None of the above

199. Which of the following is NOT a characteristic of frontal arousal rhythm (FAR)?

A. It may be associated with cerebral dysfunction
B. It consists of trains of delta waves
C. It appears during sleep-to-wake transitions
D. It is mainly seen in children
E. It can last as long as 20 seconds

200. A 29-year-old female, status-postmeningeal repair for cerebrospinal fluid (CSF) leak, presented with new-onset seizure and ataxia. Her EEG and CT scan images are shown below. What is the most prominent finding on her EEG (filter 1–70 Hz) shown below?

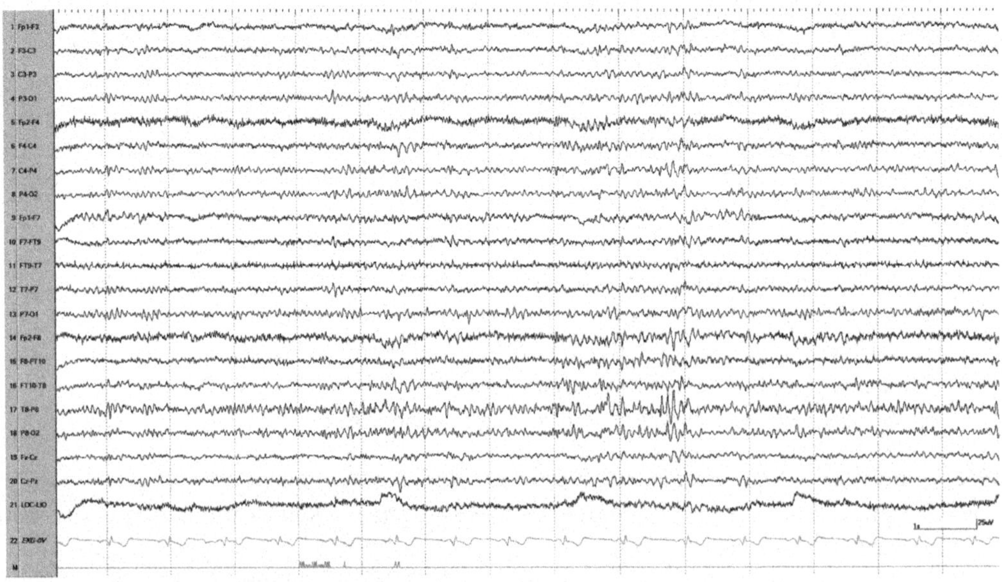

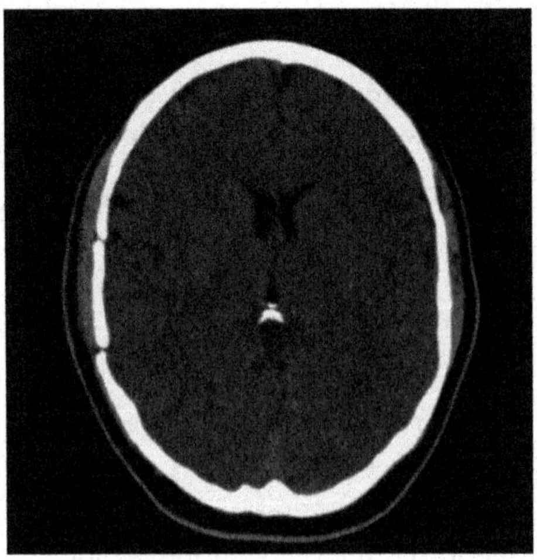

A. Lateralized periodic discharges (LPDs)
B. Paroxysmal fast activity
C. Breach rhythm
D. Seizure
E. Interictal epileptiform discharges (IEDs)

201. Which of the following is true regarding neonatal seizures?
A. They can be seen as early as 28-week conceptual age
B. Ictal discharges most commonly arise from the occipital region
C. They are never generalized
D. The background is frequently normal
E. They are never multifocal

202. The phantom spike-and-waves are generally considered to be a normal EEG variant. Which of the following statements best describes them?
A. They are typically asymmetric and asynchronous in distribution
B. They tend to be of lower amplitude in the frontal region
C. They are felt to be associated with seizures only when found in the occipital region
D. They may show gender differences in their distribution
E. They have a frequency of 8 to 12 Hz

203. Which of the following referential montages is least likely to be helpful to evaluate changes in the temporal region?
A. Cz
B. Ipsilateral ear
C. Contralateral ear
D. Average
E. Laplacian

204. A 64-year-old man with a history of hypertension, seizures, dementia, and resection of a brain tumor 35 years ago was admitted for bizarre behavior noted at the nursing home. His wife stated that his last seizure, described as a staring spell, was 7 years ago. His MRI brain showed a left posterior–temporal lobe meningioma along with evidence of a prior right temporal lobe resection. Twelve hours into the monitoring session (filter 1–70 Hz), a dramatic decrease in EEG amplitude was seen as shown below in 5 consecutive epochs. What is the most likely cause of the change?

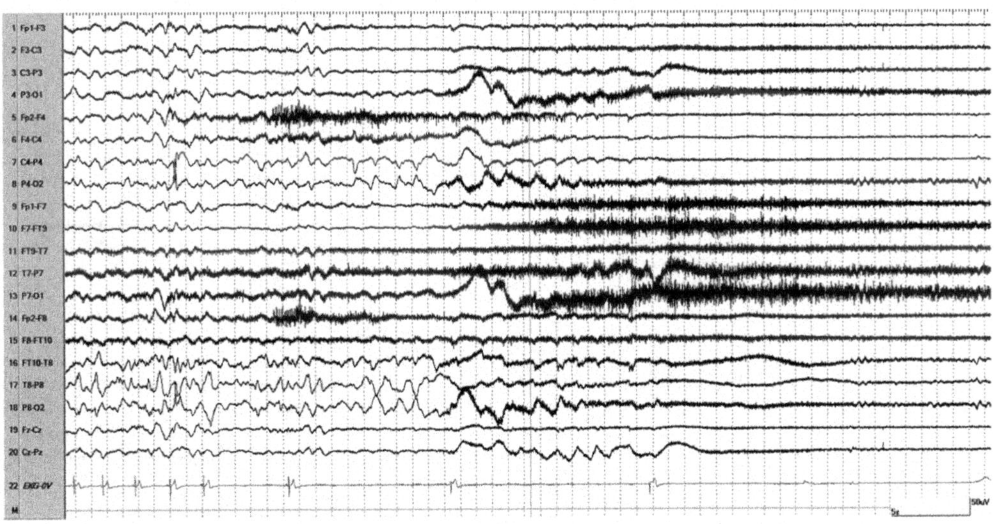

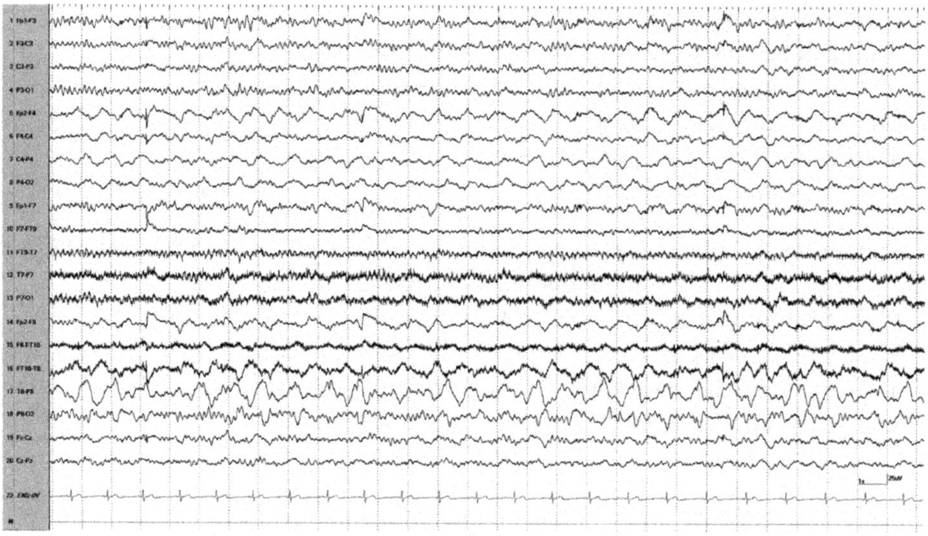

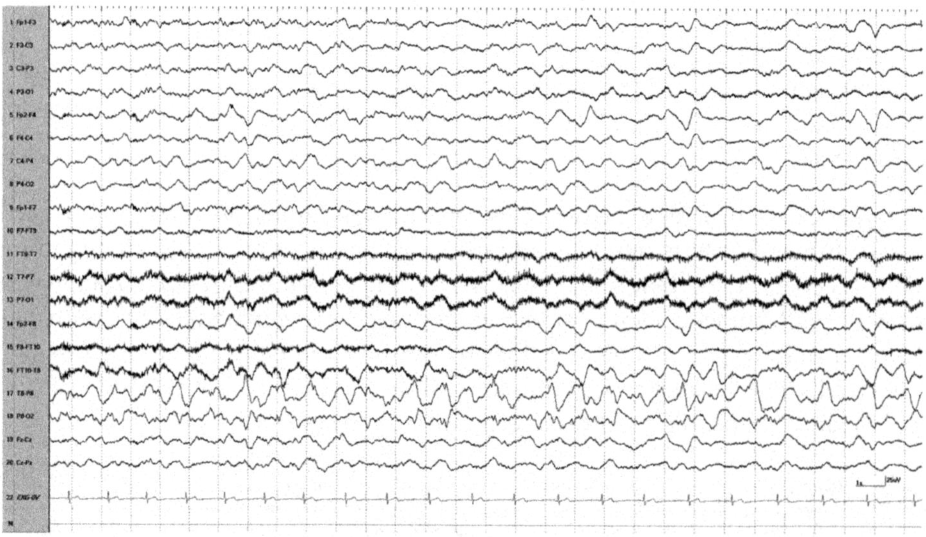

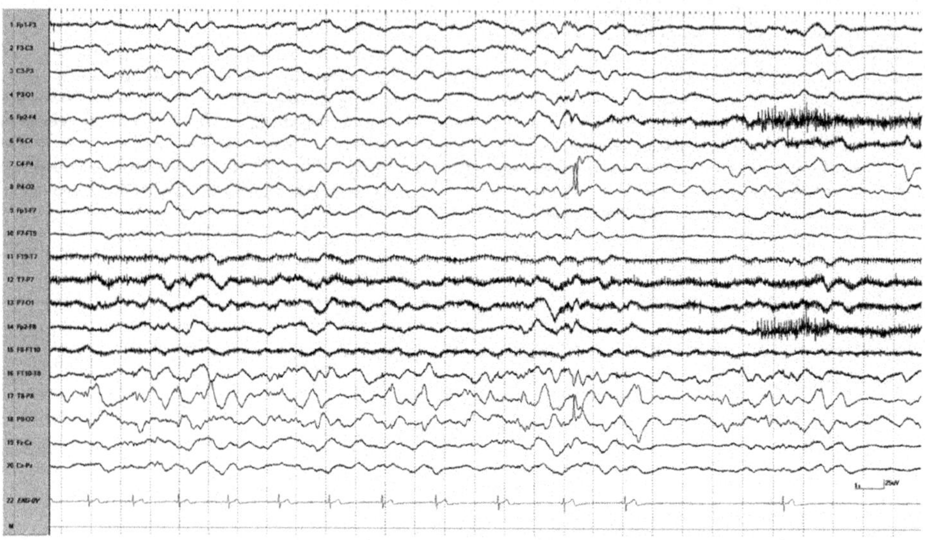

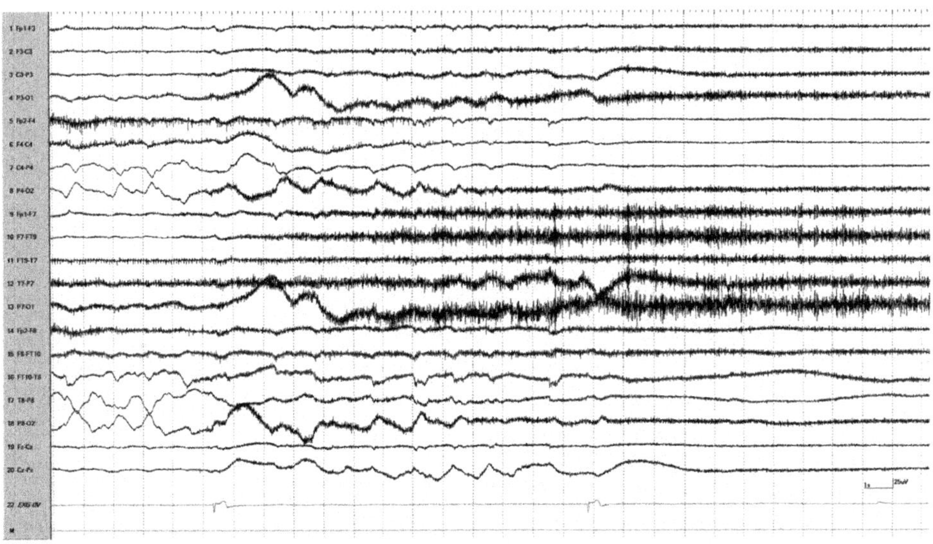

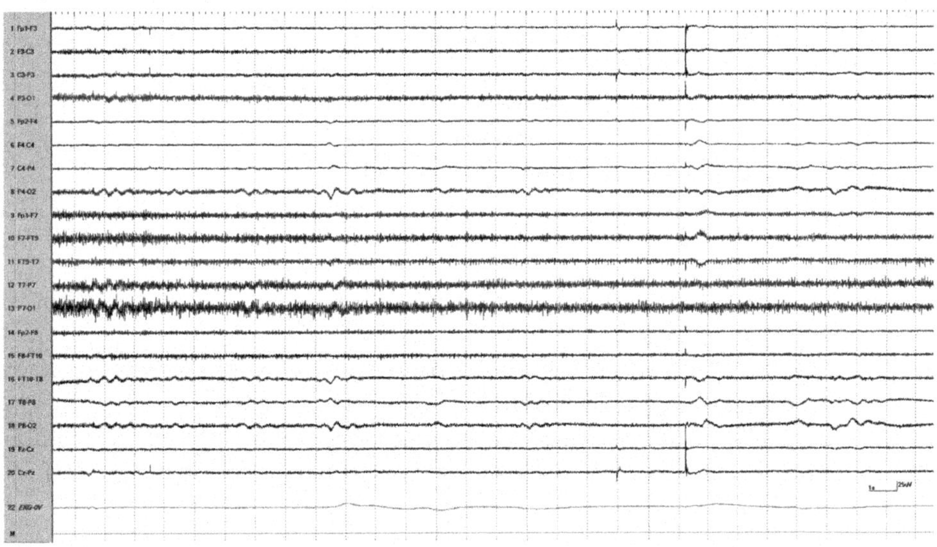

A. Cessation of a generalized seizure discharge
B. Suctioning the patient
C. Cerebral hypoperfusion
D. Starting propofol infusion without a bolus
E. The reference electrode creating a salt bridge with an adjacent electrode

205. Which of the following statements is true about the alpha variant?
   A. It is best seen with eye opening
   B. It is associated with increased risk of seizures
   C. It can occur at subharmonic or supraharmonic frequency of the posterior dominant rhythm (PDR)
   D. It is typically seen in the anterior head regions
   E. It is also known as alpha squeak

206. Neuronal ceroid lipofuscinosis (NCL) is characterized by
   A. High amplitude EEG
   B. Occipital spike-wave discharges in response to 1 to 2 Hz photic stimulation
   C. Generalized spike-wave discharges in response to 13 Hz photic stimulation
   D. Normal visual evoked potentials
   E. Normal somatosensory evoked potentials

207. Which of the following features of wicket spikes differentiates them from epileptiform spikes?
   A. Their occurrence in deeper stages of sleep
   B. Their occurrence in trains
   C. Their sharp monophasic morphology
   D. Their high amplitude of up to 200 μV
   E. Their disruption of the underlying background

208. Which of the following periodic patterns is least pathognomonic of an underlying neurological disorder?
   A. Periodic generalized sharp waves occurring at 1 Hz frequency and accompanied by occasional myoclonic jerks
   B. Periodic generalized sharp waves occurring every 10 to 15 seconds and accompanied by occasional myoclonic jerks
   C. Bitemporal independent periodic lateralized sharp waves at 1 to 1.5 Hz frequency
   D. Left parieto-central periodic lateralized epileptiform discharges (PLEDs) at 1 Hz frequency
   E. Periodic generalized sharp waves occurring at 0.5 to 1 Hz frequency with triphasic morphology and anterior-posterior lag

209. Which of the following statements regarding subdural electrodes is true?
   A. They can be used to map eloquent cortex
   B. They are susceptible to the filtering effects of the dura
   C. They can remain implanted for weeks without any morbidity
   D. They cannot be used in conjunction with stereotactically implanted depth electrodes
   E. They are highly susceptible to motion and muscle artifact

210. Which of the following EEG abnormalities is associated with a risk for seizures?
   A. Frontal phantom spike-wave discharges
   B. Occipital phantom spike-wave discharges
   C. Rudimentary spike-wave discharges (pseudo petit mal discharges)
   D. Needlelike occipital spikes
   E. All of the above

211. Which of the following features best describes cone waves?

A. They are surface-positive waves
B. They are seen when sleep transitions from the quiet sleep (QS) pattern to the active sleep (AS) pattern
C. They are seen in term infants less than 4 weeks of age
D. They are typically seen in the fronto-central region
E. They increase the risk for epileptic seizures in childhood

212. Where is the maximal negativity in the following EEG (filter 1–70 Hz)? Note that the 2 frames display the same 3-second EEG in 2 separate montages.

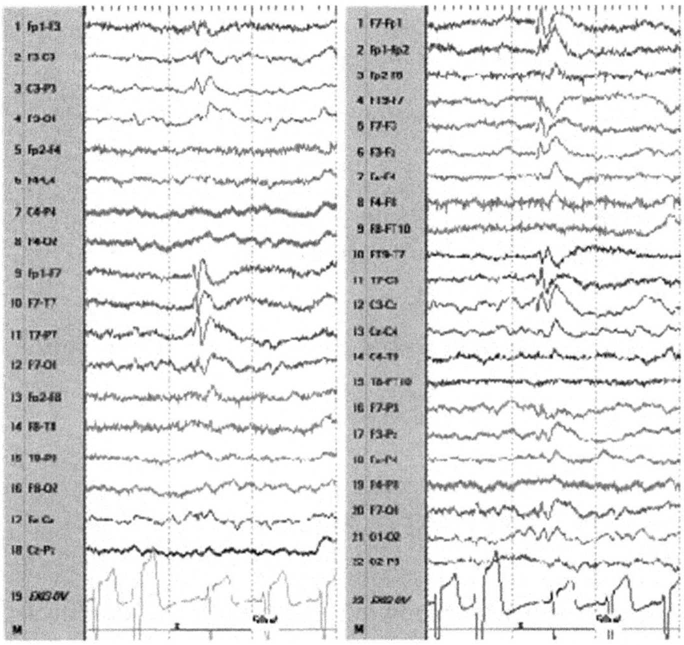

A. F3
B. C3
C. F7
D. T7
E. P7

213. Which of the following is NOT considered a normal feature in the EEG of a 15-year-old child?

A. 10 Hz posterior dominant rhythm (PDR)
B. Gradual dropout of posterior alpha at the onset of drowsiness
C. Rhythmic midline frontal sharply contoured activity upon arousal
D. Occasional photoconvulsive response
E. Photic driving response between 6 and 16 Hz

214. Which of the following physiological changes are seen during hyperventilation (HV)?
A. Both $PaCO_2$ and PaO_2 decrease
B. Both $PaCO_2$ and PaO_2 increase
C. $PaCO_2$ decreases, but PaO_2 increases
D. $PaCO_2$ decreases, but PaO_2 increases only after cessation of HV
E. $PaCO_2$ increases, but PaO_2 decreases

215. All of the following are true regarding neonatal seizures *except:*
A. They can be seen as early as 30 weeks' conceptional age (CA)
B. They are focal in onset
C. They can start in one hemisphere and terminate in the opposite hemisphere
D. They can manifest as brief periods of apnea
E. They typically start in the central or temporal regions

216. Which of the following statements is true regarding small sharp spikes (SSS)?
A. They are common in all age groups
B. They tend to occur in trains
C. They have an amplitude of 50 to 100 microvolts
D. They can be seen in up to 25% of normal individuals
E. They increase the risk of epileptic seizures

217. Which of the following statements best describes frontal intermittent rhythmic delta activity (FIRDA)?
A. It is considered abnormal after hyperventilation (HV)
B. It is considered abnormal in the elderly
C. It tends to have an interval between consecutive waveforms
D. It tends to have a polymorphic morphology in young adults
E. It can be seen in sepsis

218. Which of the following responses is least likely to be seen during intermittent photic stimulation (IPS)?
A. Photic driving
B. Photomyogenic response (PMR)
C. Photoparoxysmal response (PPR)
D. Photoelectric response
E. Photosensitive response

219. Which of the following statements best describes the EEG waveforms that occur after scanning a complex pattern in a brightly lit room?
A. They occur predominantly in the fronto-central regions
B. They are monophasic positive waveforms
C. They are not time-locked to the saccadic eye movements
D. They cannot be triggered by mental imagination of a complex picture
E. They are felt to represent the planning process of the impending eye movements

220. A 42-year-old female with a 3-month history of seizures presents with symptoms of alcohol withdrawal. The patient describes her events as "loss of consciousness with a terrible, helpless feeling that lasts 30 to 40 seconds." She has a history of alcohol abuse. What is the best interpretation of her EEG shown below (filter 1–70 Hz; sensitivity 7 μV/mm; vertical lines are 1 second apart)?

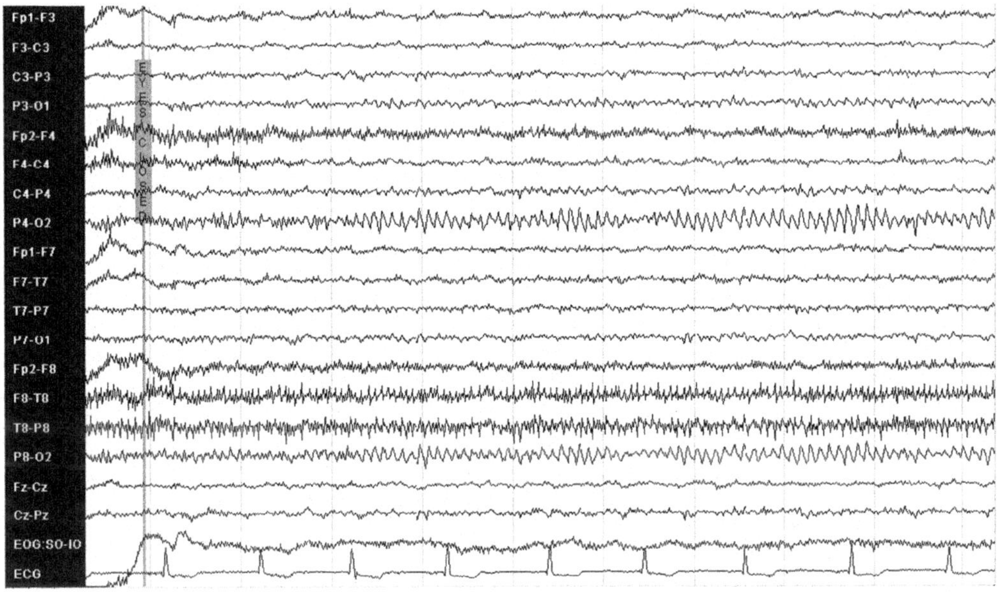

A. Seizure discharge
B. Breach rhythm over the right occipital region
C. Left hemispheric dysfunction
D. Rhythmic temporal theta bursts of drowsiness
E. Interictal epileptiform abnormality

221. A 22 year-old male underwent EEG after an episode of syncope at a basketball game. He told the technologist that he got bored and counted the holes in the ceiling tiles during the recording. Which of the following findings is likely to be seen on his EEG?
A. Bioccipital, surface-positive, sharp waves
B. Bitemporal, asynchronous, intermittent rhythmic theta activity
C. Bursts of midline theta activity
D. Bursts of bitemporal positive spikes at 6 Hz or 14 Hz
E. None of the above

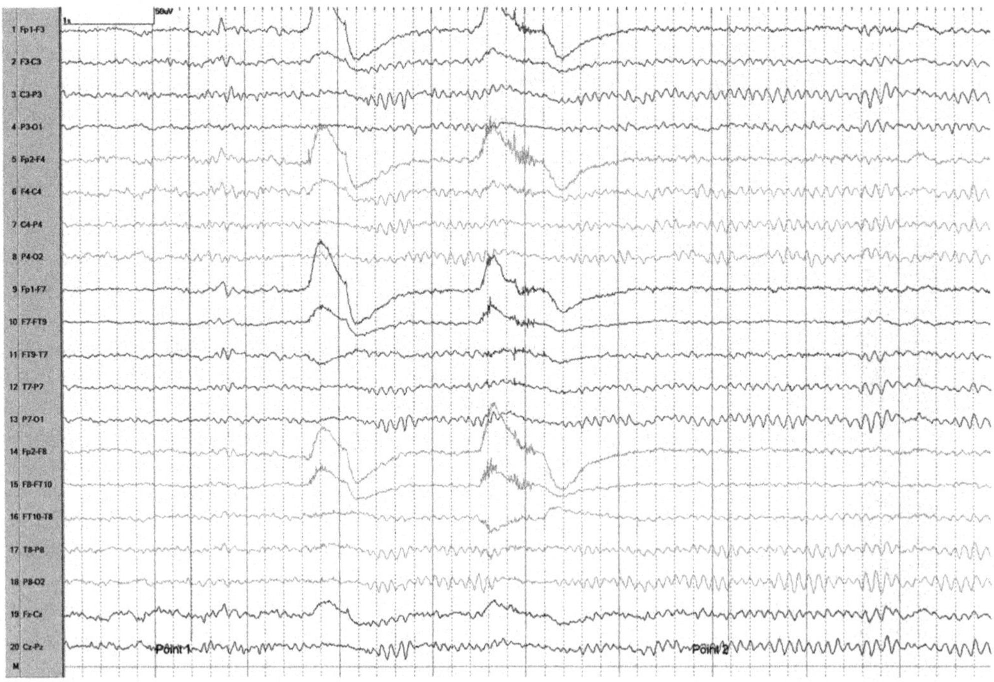

222. A 29-year-old female has a 1-year history of seizures and undergoes the routine EEG shown above (filter 1–70 Hz; sensitivity 7 microvolts/mm; vertical lines are 1 second apart). What are most likely depicted at Points 1 and 2, respectively?
A. Eyes open, eyes closed
B. Eyes open, eyes open
C. Eyes closed, eyes closed
D. Awake, REM sleep
E. Awake, drowsy

223. Which of the following is least likely to alter the activity seen at Point 2 in the above EEG?
A. Opening eyes
B. Increasing age
C. Follicular phase of the menstrual cycle
D. Ambient light
E. Varying cerebral blood flow (CBF)

224. In a normal subject, the activity seen at Point 2 in the above EEG can be appreciated in which of the following channels?
A. Temporal
B. Parietal
C. Occipital
D. Central
E. All of the above

225. The activity seen at Point 2 in the above EEG was noted to have an amplitude asymmetry with the amplitude being 80 to 110 μV on the left side and 100 to 130 μV on the right. Which of the following statements is true about the amplitude of the depicted activity?
A. It is always asymmetric, being higher on the left side

B. Amplitude asymmetry of more than 25% between the two sides is considered abnormal
C. It tends to diminish with age
D. It can be increased by doing simple math
E. It can be decreased with eye closure

226. Which of the following statements best describes the EEG findings in encephalopathy?
A. Agitated delirium may present with no EEG reactivity
B. EEG patterns in encephalopathy have high specificity for an underlying etiology
C. An increase in delta activity during stimulation is suggestive of poor prognosis
D. Continuous EEG provides little added benefit if the routine EEG already shows encephalopathic patterns
E. A slow posterior dominant rhythm (PDR) may be the only finding in mild encephalopathy

227. In assessing the severity of encephalopathy, which of the following conditions is discordant with the EEG findings described?
A. Mild encephalopathy may have preservation of some sleep architecture
B. Moderate encephalopathy has loss of state changes
C. Severe encephalopathy can have periods of background attenuation
D. Severe encephalopathy can have frequencies faster than delta range present
E. Electrocerebral inactivity (ECI) has EEG activity no greater than two microvolts

228. A 41 year old female has the following EEG (filter 1–70 Hz; sensitivity 7 microvolts/mm; vertical lines are 1 second apart). Which of the following etiologies best fits with the EEG findings?

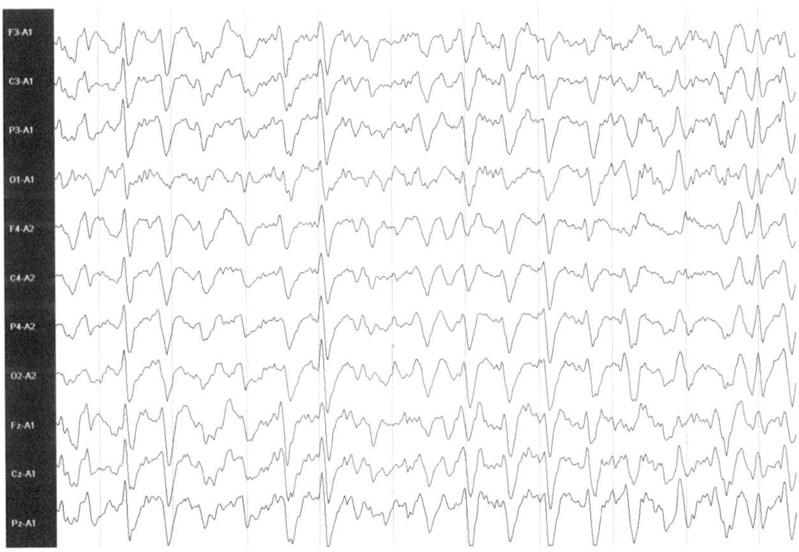

A. Postanoxia
B. Renal impairment
C. Nonconvulsive status epilepticus
D. Hyperkalemia
E. Baclofen toxicity

229. A 96 year old female has the following EEG (filter 1–70 Hz; sensitivity 7 microvolts/mm; vertical lines are 1 second apart). Which of the following interpretations best describes the EEG?

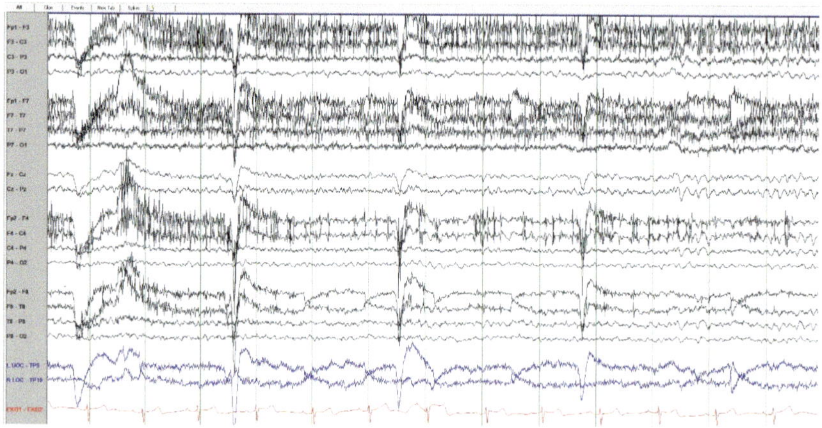

A. Normal awake pattern
B. Normal drowsiness pattern
C. Normal sleep pattern
D. Abnormal awake pattern
E. Abnormal sleep pattern

230. Which of the following neurophysiologic abnormalities is commonly seen in Huntington's disease?
A. Low-voltage background on EEG
B. Enhanced visual evoked potential (VEP) amplitudes
C. Delayed bilateral median somatosensory evoked potential (SSEP) latencies
D. Accentuation of the alpha rhythm with hyperventilation during EEG
E. Accentuated sleep architecture on EEG

231. Which of the following is most likely associated with the EEG below (filter 1–70 Hz; sensitivity 7 microvolts/mm; vertical lines are 1 second apart)?

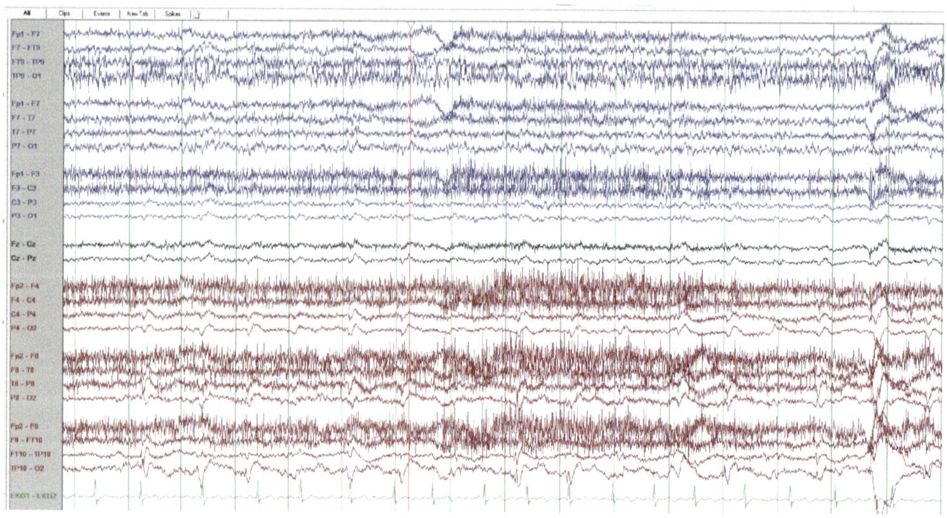

A. There is significant EKG artifact in the EEG channels
B. The patient has had a stroke
C. The patient has an increased risk for primary generalized seizures
D. The patient is having a tonic seizure
E. The patient is comatose

232. Continuous EEG monitoring least likely to be helpful in which of the following clinical scenarios?

A. Monitoring depth of coma: 18-year-old male admitted with polysubstance abuse, currently intubated and sedated for agitation
B. Detecting nonconvulsive seizures: 12-year-old girl admitted after a single prolonged generalized tonic-clonic seizure with continued altered mental status in the setting of medication noncompliance
C. Ischemia monitoring: 72-year-old female admitted with headache and found to have aneurysmal subarachnoid hemorrhage (SAH) in the intensive care unit (ICU)
D. Diagnosing conversion disorder: 31-year-old male admitted with 4 months of daily convulsive seizures lasting 10 to 15 minutes per episode with no postictal amnesia
E. Diagnosing brain death: 56-year-old female admitted with altered mental status, found to have diffuse traumatic SAH (Hunt and Hess Grade V) with diffuse cerebral edema and no brainstem reflexes

233. A 68-year-old male presents after a cardiac arrest and is undergoing hypothermia protocol. The patient is on sedation and the paralytic is about to be given. No movement has been noted thus far. Which of the following statements is true regarding the EEG below?

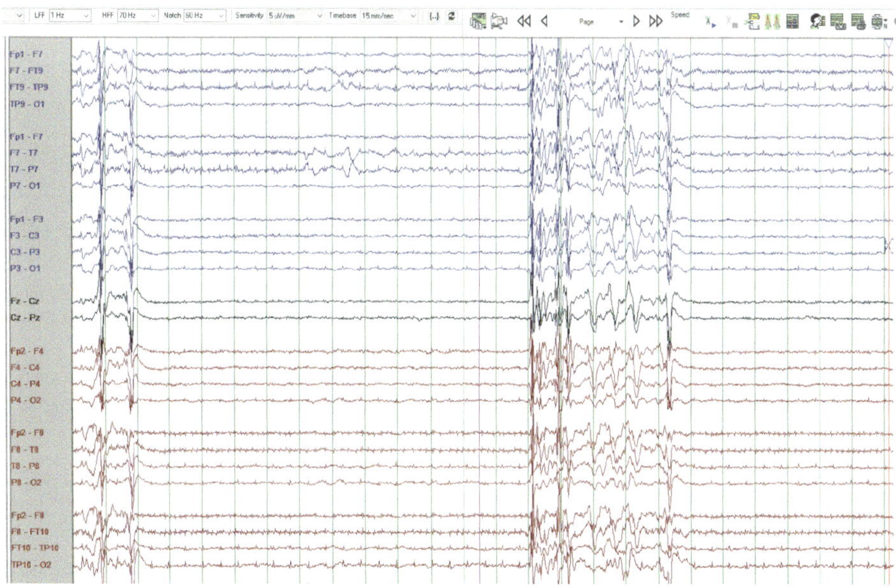

A. The interburst interval is 5 seconds
B. The suppression ratio is greater than 50%
C. The electrodecremental pattern is due to hypothermia and sedation
D. The large amplitude bursts represent artifact caused by agitation
E. The patient is in myoclonic status epilepticus

234. A 19-year-old female presents with refractory status epilepticus. She required intubation and anesthesia to stop the myoclonic jerks. Currently the patient is off propofol but is on pentobarbital. Which of the following best classifies the following EEG?

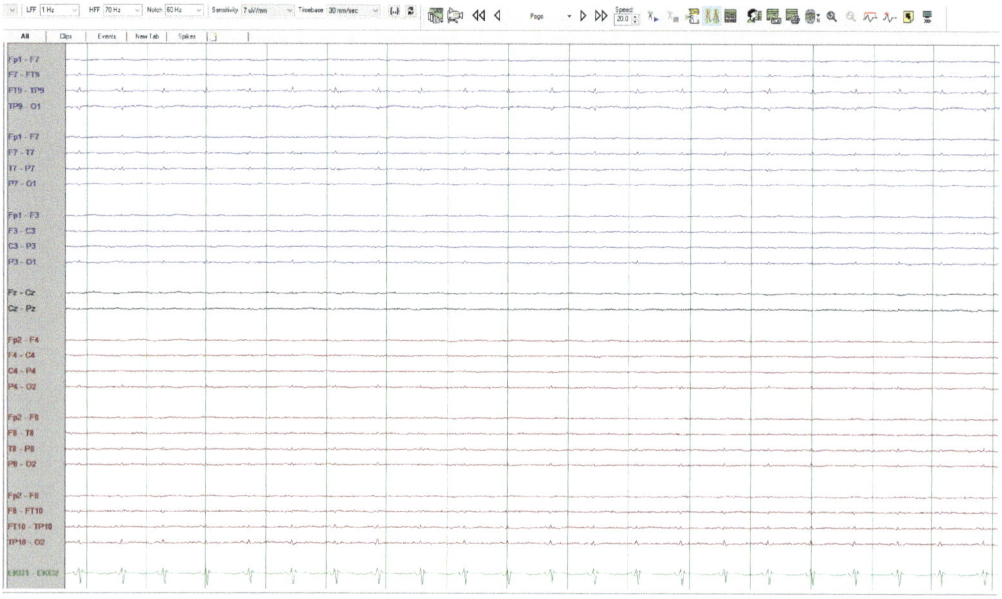

A. Lack of cerebral perfusion
B. Severe cerebral dysfunction
C. Brain death
D. Malignant status epilepticus
E. Artificial suppression due to sensitivity set too high

235. A patient is being placed under anesthesia for burst suppression for treatment of refractory status epilepticus. The anesthesia was being titrated when the EEG appeared flat for an entire epoch. What should the monitoring EEG technologist do to be able to visualize at least one burst per epoch?
A. Reduce the timebase
B. Increase the timebase
C. Increase the paper speed
D. Increase the sensitivity
E. Change to a Laplacian montage

236. A 7-year-old girl, who has a history of measles, was noted to have intellectual decline and presented to a neurologist. Her EEG showed periodic bursts concerning for subacute sclerosing panencephalitis (SSPE). Which of the following is the typical interburst interval seen in this condition?
A. 0.33 seconds
B. 0.5 seconds
C. 1 seconds
D. 10 seconds
E. 20 seconds

237. Which of the following clinical scenarios can present with unresponsiveness but still have a preserved and reactive posterior dominant rhythm?

A. Locked-in syndrome
B. Catatonia
C. Bithalamic strokes
D. Psychogenic coma
E. All of the above

238. Which of the following statements best describes the EEG features in regarding Creutzfeldt–Jakob disease (CJD)?

A. Periodic sharp wave complexes (PSWC) are seen in variant CJD (vCJD) and not sporadic CJD (sCJD)
B. Nonspecific findings such as diffuse reactive slowing and frontal rhythmic delta activity (FIRDA) are characteristic of late stages of sCJD
C. PSWC are seen in the early stages of sCJD
D. Alpha coma is never seen in sCJD
E. The World Health Organization has included EEG into its diagnostic classification criteria of CJD

239. All of the following statements regarding the periodic sharp wave complexes (PSWC) in Creutzfeldt–Jakob disease (CJD) are correct *except:*

A. They can be lateralized or generalized
B. They occur in two-thirds of patients with variant CJD (vCJD)
C. They are rare in patients with valine homozygosity at codon 129 of the prion protein gene
D. They disappear in sleep
E. They can be confined to the site of inoculation in iatrogenic CJD

240. An obese 65-year-old male presented in malignant status epilepticus, requiring complete EEG suppression with pentobarbital. After being off anesthetic sedation for 3 days, the EEG remained diffusely suppressed. The intensive care unit (ICU) team told the family that the EEG shows brain death. Which of the following statements best describes the clinical correlation of the EEG findings?

A. The EEG is consistent with brain death
B. The EEG is consistent with severe cerebral dysfunction
C. The level of cerebral dysfunction cannot be determined by the EEG
D. The EEG is consistent with anesthesia
E. No clinical correlation should be made regarding the EEG patterns in the EEG report

241. Which of the following statements is NOT supported by the American Academy of Neurology (AAN) Guidelines for determining brain death?

A. EEG is considered an ancillary test
B. EEG can be used with there is uncertainty about the reliability of the neurological examination
C. EEG can be used to shorten the duration of the observation period
D. EEG can replace the neurological examination in adults
E. Electrocerebral inactivity (ECI) protocol must be followed for a proper assessment of brain death

ANSWERS

1. **A.** The photic driving response can be seen as early as 3 to 4 months. Driving is best seen below 8 Hz flash frequency in children 3 to 5 years of age and at 6 to 16 Hz in children 6 to 12 years of age. Paroxysmal responses to flicker are more likely to occur in school-age children, including normal children. Healthy adolescents may occasionally exhibit photomyoclonic as well as photoconvulsive responses.

2. **A.** The frequency of myoclonic or tonic activity during syncope is high (approximately 70%–90%). Myoclonus associated with syncope tends to be asynchronous, multifocal rather than generalized, and brief (less than 30 seconds). Tonic movements are less frequent and less pronounced in syncope, and more common after profound cerebral hypoxia (e.g., prolonged asystole, breath-holding spells). Even after a prolonged syncope lasting 1 to 2 minutes, the postictal confusion rarely lasts more than 30 seconds. Thus, longer-lasting disorientation suggests an epileptic seizure, although an exception would be frontal lobe seizures, which can be associated with very brief postictal periods. EEG during syncope shows a sequence of changes: diffuse high-amplitude slowing at the onset of unconsciousness; suppression; reappearance of slow activity; and return of normal background activity. This sequence represents the final common path for global cerebral hypoxia, and is independent of the mechanism of syncope and of the clinical presentation as convulsive or nonconvulsive syncope.

3. **B.** The waveforms highlighted in the box are positive and confined to the bioccipital region. The background is slow and there is no posterior dominant alpha rhythm, consistent with drowsiness or light sleep. These features suggest that the waveforms are most likely POSTS. Posterior slow waves of youth occur in wakefulness as delta waves interrupting the posterior dominant rhythm (PDR). Lambda waves are positive and occipital in location but they occur when the patient is actively reading or scanning, which typically occurs during wakefulness. The highlighted waveforms are discrete, surface-positive, and do not have the epileptiform features (sharp-and-slow wave morphology) to suggest PLEDs or IEDs.

4. **D.** Vertex waves and K-complexes first appear around the age of 5 months. Initially, the K-complexes have high amplitude but the initiating sharp component is poorly developed and somewhat "blunted." The vertex waves may be frontally predominant or extend into the lateral frontal regions (they are often referred to as F-waves). In school-age children, vertex waves may show amplitude asymmetry with asymmetric spread into the vicinity. The amplitude of vertex waves and K-complexes tend to be higher in children and adolescents than adults.

5. **B.** Shut-eye waves are seen in the occipital region following the onset of eye blinks. They are seen in children younger than 10 years of age. They occur singly as surface negative, high-amplitude (100–200 μV), broad (200–400 ms), monophasic or diphasic, sharply contoured waves.

6. **B.** In children, arousal from sleep can be characterized by prolonged, diffuse, high-voltage 4 to 6 Hz with intermixed slower frequencies, called hypnopompic hypersynchrony. In addition, prolonged rhythmic sharp or spiky activity over the midline frontal region, called frontal arousal rhythm (FAR), can be seen. FAR is seen in children between ages 2 to 4 years, not adolescents. Although FAR is rare (occurring in 0.22% of children) and considered to be a normal variant, one study showed that FAR was associated with epileptic seizures in 70% of cases while another study reported the occurrence of a clinical seizure consisting of eyelid flutter and chewing with FAR. By 6 to 12 years, arousal is characterized by shorter duration of high-voltage theta activity. Mature pattern of arousal with rapid transition from sleep to waking rhythm, in the form of posteriorly-predominant alpha activity, is seen in adolescents. Occipital rhythmic sharply contoured, surface-positive waveforms, also known as POSTS (positive occipital sharp transients of sleep) are seen in light sleep.

7. **A.** AS consists of either LVI or a mixed pattern of irregular theta and delta frequencies. In QS, tracé alternant is the dominant pattern. However, if QS persists longer, an HVS pattern can be seen with delta waves mixed in. The bursts in tracé alternant are 100% synchronous at this age.

8. **D.** The posterior rhythm has a frequency of 9 Hz, which in a 4-year-old is consistent with a normal PDR. There are no lambda waves, positive occipital sharp transients of sleep or spike-wave discharges seen.

9. **E.** Normal HV responses in children include high amplitude diffuse polymorphic or rhythmic delta waves that can occur in bursts or runs. In adults, normal HV responses include mild diffuse, bifrontal, or bitemporal slowing. Unilateral focal slowing or epileptiform activity is considered abnormal during HV.

10. **D.** Primary generalized epileptic myoclonus is seen in primary generalized epilepsy, and is believed to arise in the frontal lobe, especially the supplementary motor area. It involves small myoclonus of fingers or large whole-body jerks. They are not triggered by voluntary movement, unlike cortical reflex or reticular reflex myoclonus. However, they can be precipitated by photic stimulation. The myoclonus is bilaterally synchronous. Somatosensory evoked potentials are unremarkable in epileptic myoclonus but have large amplitude in cortical reflex myoclonus. It is preceded by generalized surface negative fronto-central activity on the EEG time-locked to the myoclonic movement.

11. **D.** SREDA is best seen in older adults in the temporoparietal region. The rhythm has theta range frequencies with a sharply contoured morphology. It usually occurs during rest, drowsiness, or hyperventilation (HV). The pattern can evolve into rhythmic activity lasting over 1 minute (average 40–80 seconds). Although the pattern can be misinterpreted as ictal, it is considered nonspecific. Abrupt onset and termination may help distinguish SREDA from an ictal discharge. SREDA pattern is never associated with symptoms or postictal slowing, unlike a seizure pattern.

12. **D.** This patient likely has benign rolandic epilepsy (BRE), which is characterized by the presence of centrotemporal spikes with a horizontal dipole, activated particularly in NREM sleep. Although the spikes may be present in wakefulness and activation phases (photic stimulation and hyperventilation), they are not known to activate the spikes. Spikes are rarely, if ever, seen in REM sleep.

13. **B.** In Angelman syndrome, EEG background resembles hypsarrhythmia, but unlike true hypsarrhythmia, it does not show fragmentation during sleep. Runs of rhythmic, high-amplitude (greater than 300 μV), delta or theta activity can be seen over the frontal regions. Multifocal epileptiform discharges can be intermixed. Tremor is common, and it correlates with 4 to 10 Hz electromyography (EMG) bursts, not EEG activity. Similarly, the spells of laughter have no ictal EEG correlate, and are not felt to represent gelastic seizures.

14. **B.** This patient most likely has JME given the EEG shows generalized spike-wave and polyspike-wave discharges in the setting of a normal background of 9 Hz. Her seizure onset is beyond the typical age for CAE, which is 4 to 10 years of age. It is unlikely that she has symptomatic generalized epilepsy given the normal EEG background. Although there is a possibility that the patient has focal epilepsy (i.e., frontal lobe epilepsy) with secondary bilateral synchrony, the history of staring spells, suggestive of absence seizures, makes this less likely.

15. **E.** The patterns in the question can be seen in different stages of coma. In general, the EEG becomes less reactive as the coma deepens.

16. **D.** Absence seizures can be associated with some motor manifestations including rhythmic eye blinking, retropulsion of the head, and repetitive oral automatisms (swallowing, chewing, lip smacking, and lip licking). Postural control is usually maintained, but swaying may be seen in the standing patient. It is felt that the loss of consciousness during the classic absence is due to transient impairment of the working memory attributed to the accentuation of spike-wave discharges in the frontal cortex. This phenomenon is believed to underlie the immediate restoration of the working memory along with consciousness at the end of the absence episode.

17. **B.** The alpha and beta bands were described originally by Berger. The gamma rhythm was subsequently described by Jasper and Andrews to designate frequencies greater than 30 Hz. The term "delta" was initially introduced to designate all frequencies below the alpha range by Walter, who subsequently introduced the term "theta" to specifically designate the 4 to 7.5 Hz activity.

18. **C.** The EEG shows diffuse slowing, which is consistent with a normal HV response. There is no convincing evolution to support a seizure. FIRDA can be brought out during HV but the changes in the above EEG are too diffuse. No spikes are noted to support interictal epileptiform discharges. The activity is too rhythmic and uniform to be artifact from head movement.

19. **D.** Psychomotor variant is also known as rhythmic mid-temporal theta bursts of drowsiness or rhythmic temporal theta bursts of drowsiness. Although historically felt to be associated with seizures, recent data disputes this. It is rare, and seen in less than 2% of

records. This pattern consists of rhythmic theta range activity, which can be sharply contoured or notched. It is seen in drowsiness or light sleep, sometimes during wakefulness. It is best seen in the mid-temporal region but may be distributed in the parasagittal or occipito-temporal regions. Although the pattern can last longer than a minute, it is monomorphic and does not evolve in frequency.

20. A. The frequency of the PDR evolves from infancy to adolescence. It is 3 Hz by age 3 months, 6 Hz by age 12 months, 8 Hz by 3 years, and 10 Hz by 10 to 15 years.

21. B. The EEG during a tonic seizure may be obscured by muscle activity, which can help distinguish it from an atonic seizure. Tonic seizures typically present with a longer ictal discharge than atonic seizures. Both seizure types present with an electrodecremental pattern. A 2 Hz spike-wave discharge is characteristic of an atypical absence seizure, whereas a 3 Hz spike-wave discharge is seen in a typical absence seizure. Hypsarrhythmia is the high-voltage background seen in West syndrome, and is not ictal.

22. A. Low-voltage, intermittent temporal theta in the elderly is felt to be an age-related pattern, and has been estimated to occur with an incidence of approximately 35%. It is usually in the range of 4 to 5 Hz in the temporal region, but more prevalent over the left hemisphere. It is felt to represent a subharmonic of the 8 to 10 Hz background rhythm, which is often seen in the elderly. However, this rhythm is distinct from the alpha rhythm in that it persists with eye opening and even into drowsiness and light sleep. Hyperventilation (HV) augments its voltage and persistence. Temporal theta in the elderly usually occurs as a brief fragment lasting only 2 to 3 waves, rarely more than 7. The clinical significance of this pattern remains controversial. Some regard these waveforms as normal variants but others have suggested that they signify underlying subclinical vascular insufficiency.

23. A. The description in the question is most suggestive of benign Rolandic epilepsy (BRE), which is one of the common partial epilepsy syndromes in childhood, typically affecting children between 5 and 12 years of age. Centrotemporal spikes are the hallmark of BRE. Although the prognosis for seizure remission is great, there is a high incidence of learning disability and attention deficit disorder. The seizures are typically focal and usually involve hemifacial sensorimotor symptoms, oropharyngolaryngeal manifestations, speech arrest, and hypersalivation. Frontal lobe seizures could also lead to facial twitching but hypersalivation is not common. Hypersalivation, on the other hand, has been considered an autonomic symptom, and has also been associated with insular and temporal lobe seizures. Parietal spikes are expected to be associated with sensory phenomena. Occipital spikes would typically present with visual auras. Generalized spikes are seen in generalized epilepsies, which are not associated with the described clinical features.

24. A. HV-induced slowing is associated with buildup of diffuse theta and delta activities for several minutes. This buildup may be abrupt or gradual, rhythmic and of high amplitude (up to 500 μV). It typically resolves within 1 minute after stopping HV effort. This slowing is more prominent posteriorly in children and anteriorly in young adults. This phenomenon is highly age-dependent, being common in children and adolescents, less common in young adults, and uncommon after the age 30. However, any focal slowing or epileptiform activity induced by HV is considered pathological. Rhythmic temporal delta activity (i.e., temporal intermittent rhythmic delta activity, TIRDA) at any age is felt to be pathological and suggests underlying temporal lobe epilepsy.

25. A. At 29 weeks of gestation, the EEG tends to be very discontinuous (tracé discontinu pattern) and consists of long periods (typically 10–20 seconds) of nearly flat background interrupted by synchronous diffuse high-amplitude bursts that may be posteriorly predominant. Occasional bursts of rhythmic occipital delta and temporal theta activity are noted during this discontinuity. Delta brushes are characteristic at this stage; they are infrequent, and central or posterior dominant. There are relatively no behavioral changes to distinguish awake and sleep except a few gross body movements. Eye movements are very rare, and respiration is irregular. As there is no differentiation between awake and sleep, it is difficult to accurately determine the age of the neonate.

26. E. Around 35 to 37 weeks, multifocal sharp transients are scarce and seem to be replaced by frontal sharp transients. Frontal sharp transients occur most often in sleep. Anterior slow dysrhythmia is present at this age as well. EEG reactivity is present in all states, appearing as diffuse flattening. The continuous pattern of AS and wakefulness develop into a low-voltage irregular (LVI) pattern. The increase in reactivity marks the distinction between wakefulness and AS. QS is still discontinuous, but is considered as tracé alternant as the amplitude during interburst intervals increases to more than 25 μV. The bursts are 85% synchronous between the hemispheres. Delta brushes become less frequent, and are seen only in QS. Temporal alpha bursts disappear as well.

27. A. This EEG shows diffuse alpha range frequencies that are nonreactive to stimulation (note that there is no change in the EEG pattern after sternal rub) consistent with alpha coma. The relative low voltage over the left temporal region could be related to prior resection in that area. Of note, alpha coma can present with other frequencies, such as theta, resulting in alpha–theta coma (as seen here), and it can evolve into other coma patterns, including delta or burst-suppression. Alpha coma was felt to be associated with poor outcome; however, the current thought is that prognostication is dependent on the underlying etiology. Alpha coma can be seen after anoxic brain injury (typically unfavorable outcome) although it can also be seen in head trauma, brainstem stroke, and toxic-metabolic dysfunction (typically more favorable outcome). Some reports claim alpha coma to be the most common rhythmic coma pattern in children. Other coma patterns include spindle coma and beta coma, both of which tend to have more favorable outcomes. The effect of anesthesia on EEG can vary widely, including increased amount of beta activity, diffuse slowing, voltage attenuation, and burst-suppression patterns; however, alpha coma is not a typical pattern seen with anesthesia. Benzodiazepines also result in diffuse low-voltage beta activity. Breach rhythms occur in the area of skull defects, tend to be more focal or regional in distribution, and typically present as faster, sharper, and high-amplitude EEG activity. Although 50 or 60 Hz electrical noise artifact can lead to diffuse activity, the frequency seen on the EEG is lower than that and does not equal a harmonic frequency of the electrical noise either.

28. A. PPR refers specifically to generalized spike-wave discharges without clinical correlation. If there is any clinical response with such changes, then the term "photoconvulsive response" should be used. Other paroxysmal, noncerebral EEG changes can be seen. Photomyoclonic (i.e., photomyogenic) response refers to widespread muscle twitching timed to the stimulus representing a heightened brainstem-mediated reflex. Photoelectric (i.e., photochemical) response occurs if there are changes in the anterior channels that resolve with shielding the electrode from the light, representing a reaction of the light with the electrode-paste complex. Photic driving response refers to activity in the posterior head regions time-locked to the photic stimulus and occurring at the same or harmonic frequency of the stimulus frequency.

29. **B.** Acute MCA infarction in the setting of prior infarction is the most likely scenario. The EEG shows widespread left hemispheric slowing. More focal ipsilateral temporal slowing can be seen in mesial temporal sclerosis but clinical weakness is unlikely in that condition. Typically, more focal frontal slowing can be seen contralateral to the clinical jerking. In this case, there is no mention of a focal motor seizure. HSV infections, depending on the type, can involve the brain as well as the spinal cord, and has a predilection for the temporal lobes, which would typically lead to unilateral or bilateral temporal slowing. Although acute relapse of MS is clinically compatible, the EEG in MS shows sporadic slowing rather than widespread left hemispheric slowing as seen here.

30. **C.** Although IEDs are one of the specific electrophysiologic markers for seizures, they can be seen in patients without seizures, for example, siblings of patients with benign Rolandic epilepsy (BRE). IEDs consist of different morphologic types, such as spikes, sharp waves, and spike-and-wave discharges, all of which are associated with predisposition to seizures. Spikes are generated by synchronous depolarization of neurons within 6 cm^2 of the cortex. Sharp waves result from synchronous depolarization of a small pool of neurons or neurons further away from the recording electrode. Spike-and-wave complexes are more specific for underlying epilepsy because the slow wave represents prolonged hyperpolarization (not depolarization) of cortical neurons.

31. **A.** Epilepsy with GTCs on awakening is considered to have a more favorable prognosis. It is characterized by some as similar to juvenile myoclonic epilepsy (JME) but without the myoclonus. The remaining answer choices are examples of malignant epilepsy syndromes. Neonatal myoclonic encephalopathy (also known as early myoclonic encephalopathy) is associated with high mortality during the first year of life. West syndrome is characterized by intractable seizures and may require unconventional antiseizure therapies. LGS is characterized by intractable epilepsy with multiple seizure types. Atypical partial benign epilepsy of childhood has features similar to benign Rolandic epilepsy (BRE) but then evolves into periodic atonic seizures, with brief absences and GTCs; it has EEG findings similar to LGS and has been referred to as "pseudo-LGS."

32. **C.** The EEG pattern shows periodic complexes that are typically seen in the middle of the disease course. EEG patterns evolve over time (typically 6 months) in CJD. Initially, there can be intermittent diffuse slowing, evolving to the appearance of periodic complexes, evolving to more continuous diffuse slowing with periodic complexes, and finally evolving to loss of the periodic complexes with persistent slowing in the late stages of the disease. Of note, the periodic complexes seen in CJD may subside with state changes (e.g., drowsiness) and recur with stimulation, which are not typical of periodic complexes due to hypoxic-ischemic injury or status epilepticus.

33. **B.** The EEG in the question shows posterior background slowing with a posterior dominant rhythm (PDR) of 7 to 8 Hz, consistent with mild cerebral dysfunction. Prolonged monitoring would be needed to confirm nonconvulsive status epilepticus as this epoch does not show evidence of any ictal activity. There are no focal abnormalities in the

temporal region to support temporal lobe epilepsy. Although psychogenic nonepileptic spell could be a consideration, video would be needed to correlate with typical semiology.

34. **C.** A few studies have looked into the sensitivity of a single routine EEG in capturing any ictal or interictal epileptiform activity. It is generally accepted that the first routine EEG may be nondiagnostic for epilepsy 30% to 55% of the time.

35. **C.** The fast spike-and-wave and polyspike-and-wave discharges triggered by photic stimulation raise suspicion and can be considered diagnostic of a primary generalized epilepsy syndrome, such as juvenile absence epilepsy. Due to the high specificity for the diagnosis, it is felt that the interictal activity is sufficient for the diagnosis in the context of appropriate clinical picture. Absence epilepsy is associated with 3 Hz spike-and-wave discharge. Although generalized epileptiform discharges can be due to secondary bilateral synchrony, those occurring during photic stimulation are not usually diagnostic of frontal lobe epilepsy. Neuronal ceroid lipofuscinosis type 2 is associated with photosensitivity, characterized by a photoparoxysmal response (PPR) at low flicker rates of 1 to 3 Hz.

36. **C.** The ECoG in the question demonstrates mesial temporal spikes and polyspikes in channel 1 (this is because contact 1 is medial). This activity is mixed with some slowing but does not represent sharply contoured slowing per se. Pulse artifact can be present in ECoG but it is typically rhythmic, occurring at a frequency equal to the heart rate. EEG is continuous, and therefore incompatible with burst suppression. Fast ripples are high frequency oscillations with a frequency of 250 to 500 Hz. To evaluate fast ripples, the sampling rate has to be around 2,000 Hz with the filters typically set at 50 to 600 Hz; neither of these was done with the ECoG in the question; so it is not possible to infer the presence of fast ripples.

37. **E.** FIRDA is seen in adults and is thought to reflect acute or subacute diffuse cortical or subcortical gray matter dysfunction. It is more common in metabolic encephalopathy as opposed to structural disorders. Because of its frontal predominance, it is often mistaken for eye movement artifacts although the distinction can be easily made by using separate eye leads in the EEG.

38. **D.** Slow-growing tumors, meningiomas, and midline tumors may not be associated with any EEG abnormalities although HV may bring out focal slowing. Focal delta and/or theta activity correlates with white matter involvement by the tumor. IRDA suggests involvement of the thalamus or frontal deep white matter. Background attenuation is usually seen in the setting of high-grade gliomas with thalamic involvement (not low-grade gliomas) or with extensive peritumoral edema.

39. **A.** In LKS (also known as acquired epileptic aphasia), abundant high-voltage epileptiform activity (e.g., temporal, bitemporal, generalized) with intermixed slow activity is seen exclusively in sleep initially. At later stages of the illness, these abnormalities are accentuated in slow-wave sleep. The EEG typically has an abnormal background but not burst suppression. The presence of epileptiform discharges in wakefulness is not characteristic of the syndrome.

40. **A.** The mean frequency of alpha rhythm in adults is 10 Hz, and it is attained at the age of 10 years. The frequency tends to decline in elderly individuals, likely reflecting some degree of vascular or degenerative pathology. Immediately after eye closure, the alpha frequency may increase transiently ("squeak effect"). Alpha rhythm shows amplitude asymmetry with higher voltage over the right hemisphere. This suggests that the alpha rhythm has greater amplitude over the nondominant hemisphere, but no convincing conclusion concerning handedness can be determined from this asymmetry.

41. A. The EEG is most consistent with SSPE. SSPE usually presents 5 to 15 years after a primary measles infection with progressive psychoneurological deterioration, including personality change and seizures. The EEG is very characteristic, consisting of periodic complexes made in part by high-amplitude bisynchronous and symmetrical delta waves occurring once every 5 to 7 seconds (note the time scale calibration). Besides periodic complexes, several atypical EEG findings can also be also noted including frontal rhythmic delta activity in intervals between the periodic complexes, electrodecremental periods following EEG complexes, paroxysms of bisynchronous spike-wave activity, random spikes over frontal regions, and focal abnormalities such as spikes and slow-wave foci. In CJD, the periodic discharges occur once every 1 to 2 seconds. Anesthetic effect and anoxic brain injury can produce a similar EEG changes, but the patient is not on any medication and there is no history suggestive of anoxia. The EEG changes are too diffuse to be consistent with chewing artifact.

42. A. The EEG pattern demonstrates intermittent rhythmic delta activity (IRDA). If frontal (i.e., frontal intermittent rhythmic delta activity [FIRDA]), as shown in the figure, it suggests metabolic encephalopathy as opposed to a structural lesion. If occipital (i.e., occipital intermittent rhythmic delta activity [OIRDA]), it is more commonly seen in children and associated with absence epilepsy. If temporal (i.e., temporal intermittent rhythmic delta activity [TIRDA]), it is highly associated with increased risk for partial onset temporal seizures; in this case, it is not usually considered nonspecific. Central (i.e., CIRDA) and generalized (i.e., GIRDA) have no specific associations and are likely related to nonspecific dysfunction; there is growing evidence, however, that GIRDA may be associated with an increased risk of seizures, especially when seen in critically ill patients.

43. C. Eyelid myoclonia with absences typically occurs immediately after eye closure, is more frequent in bright light and does not occur in the dark, and is associated with brief bilateral spike-wave discharges. Progressive myoclonic epilepsies, such as infantile ceroid lipofuscinosis, can have occipital spikes elicited by photic stimulation. West syndrome is associated with high-amplitude, disorganized slow activity with multifocal spikes (termed hypsarrhythmia) and generalized electrodecrements; when associated with a clinical spasm, there is typically an initial generalized spike or sharp wave followed by diffuse EEG attenuation. West syndrome can progress into LGS, which presents with slow spike-wave discharges but can have faster, beta range activity in sleep, some of which may be associated with clinical tonic seizures. Dravet syndrome is characterized by generalized polyspike-wave complexes, which may be prominent unilaterally and occur in clusters.

44. D. EEG becomes continuous during wakefulness and AS at a conceptional age of 35 to 37 weeks, whereas QS still shows discontinuous background, thus making the states distinguishable from one another.

45. A. 14- and 6-Hz positive bursts (also called ctenoids) appear around age 3 to 4 years, but are more commonly seen in children and adolescents, especially those aged 13 to 14 years. Of note, the 6-Hz positive spikes predominate in children younger than 1 year and in adults older than 40 years, whereas the 14-Hz positive spikes predominate or combine with 6-Hz spikes in the other age groups. The reported incidence is 58% in normal teenagers and 12% in healthy adults. The bursts are of medium amplitude (20–60 μV), and occur at 14 and 6 cycles/sec (Hz). They are best seen in the posterior–temporal regions, unilaterally or bilaterally, with shifting predominance. They are typically seen during drowsiness or light sleep. Their morphology is similar to sleep spindles with sharply contoured positive (i.e., downgoing) spikes, alternating with a rounded negative component. They occur in short trains of less than 2 seconds. The 14- and 6-Hz positive spikes may be distinguished from temporal spikes by their characteristic positive polarity (compared to the negative polarity of epileptiform discharges) as well as their typical frequency.

46. C. Among the choices, a normal activation response such as photic driving at a supraharmonic frequency is the most likely possibility (note that the last channel in the EEG named "M" contains photic stimulation information with up ticks corresponding to photic stimuli). The patient is awake as noted by the presence of eye blinks and the posterior dominant rhythm (PDR), so POSTS are not likely. Although the activity in the posterior head region appears rhythmic, there is no clear, robust evolution to suggest an ictal discharge. A slow alpha variant can be seen in patients and presents at a subharmonic frequency, typically half of the PDR. Similarly, there can be a fast alpha variant, which presents at supraharmonic frequency, typically double the PDR. These alpha variants are blocked with eye opening unlike what is seen here.

47. A. AS and QS can be distinguished from one another around 35 to 37 weeks of conceptional age. Prior to that, both AS and QS exhibit trace discontinu pattern.

48. C. Theta activity is defined as activity in the 4 to 7 Hz range, and can be interpreted as normal (e.g., drowsiness) or abnormal (e.g., encephalopathy). Although some intermittent low-voltage theta activity is seen over the frontal–central region in healthy people while resting and awake, this is usually not well developed or regular. Under circumstances in which the subject is performing some moderately difficult mental task, such as spelling or arithmetic, one can occasionally see a well-developed theta rhythm in the frontal midline region. A small amount of left temporal theta activity during wakefulness is also expected as a normal finding with aging, starting around the age of 50 years. Of note, the alpha rhythm tends to attenuate during mental tasks. Lambda waves can be seen in the setting of visual scanning but not mental tasks. Mu rhythm (which is in the beta frequency range) can attenuate with the thought of or actual motor movement of the contralateral limb.

49. A. Stereotactically implanted depth electrodes are used to detect activity from the deeper structures, such as the mesial temporal or mesial frontal regions. They tend to have low impedances. Rarely, artifact from jaw muscle contraction can be seen in the depth electrodes. Subdural, not depth, electrodes are routinely used to stimulate or map eloquent cortex. Depth electrodes can remain implanted for a couple of weeks or longer, if required, for diagnostic purposes.

50. A. 14- and 6- Hz bursts have a particular association with Reye's syndrome, which is a potentially fatal syndrome affecting many organs, including the brain and liver; it has been associated with aspirin use in children. Fourteen- and six-Hz bursts have also been described in patients in stupor or coma (e.g., hepatic encephalopathy), although these bursts are felt to be a benign epileptiform variant seen mainly in teenagers during drowsiness and light sleep. Rhythmic mid-temporal theta bursts, phantom spike-waves, and lambda waves are normal EEG variants. Triphasic waves are associated with diffuse encephalopathies, which are typically metabolic or infectious in nature.

51. B. These are likely positive temporal sharp waves, which can be a normal finding in neonates 32 to 36 weeks, and tend to disappear subsequently. However, in pathological groups (e.g., asphyxia, metabolic disorders, intracranial hemorrhages, cystic periventricular leukomalacia), the finding tends to be persistent and is abnormal. Delta brushes are seen more commonly in the central head region, and consist of delta waves with superimposed beta frequencies. Although BETS (also called SSS) are seen over the temporal regions and have sharply contoured morphology, they are not typically seen in individuals less than 10 years of age. Rhythmic temporal theta bursts, a normal variant, are seen in drowsiness and light sleep in adults.

52. A. During the first year of life, several changes occur with sleep activity. Active sleep (AS) develops into REM sleep, transforming the low-voltage irregular (LVI) pattern into the asynchronous low-amplitude mixed frequencies of the adult REM sleep. The time spent in REM decreases from 40% of the sleep cycle at 3 months to 30% by the end of the first year of life. Newborns transition from wakefulness to REM sleep; after 3 months of age, REM sleep onset occurs after 40 to 50 minutes are spent in NREM sleep.

53. D. The 10 to 20 system is an internationally recognized method to name and apply the location of scalp electrodes that ensures standardized reproducibility over time and between subjects. The "10" and "20" refer to the actual distances between adjacent electrodes, which are either 10% or 20% of the total front-to-back or right-to-left distance of the skull.

54. C. The EEG background in LGS tends to be abnormal, whereas in JME it tends to be normal, and therefore, it is helpful. LGS tends to have slow spike-wave and/or polyspike-wave discharges (usually 1.5–2.5 Hz), whereas JME presents with fast spike-wave and/or polyspike-wave discharges (usually 4–6 Hz); therefore, the frequency of the discharge, not just the mere presence of polyspikes, is a helpful differentiating feature. Age of onset is helpful as JME typically develops in late childhood and adolescence, whereas LGS tends to develop much earlier. Response to antiseizure medications is also helpful as LGS tends to be medically refractory.

55. D. Based on the description provided, this boy has Landau-Klefner syndrome (LKS), in which the EEG shows epileptiform discharges over the posterior temporal regions, markedly activated by slow wave sleep. EEG can assist not only in the diagnosis of LKS but also in monitoring treatment of the disorder. The extent of language and cognitive regression is related to the duration of the continuous spike waves that tend to activate in sleep. Of note, LKS is a separate syndrome than continuous spikes and waves during slow-wave sleep (CSWS).

56. B. POSTS, as the name implies, are surface-positive, triangular waves that occur in the bilateral occipital region during light and deeper stages sleep but not in REM sleep. They are similar if not identical to lambda waves in morphology and distribution, and are sometimes referred to as lambdoid waves. They are relatively common, being seen in 50% to 80% of healthy adults. They are usually symmetric and can occur in runs at a frequency of 4 to 5 Hz. They can be seen in children as young as 4 years old but are most commonly seen in those aged 15 to 35 years. It is believed that POSTS might represent a "playback" of information to the visual cortex in order to reexamine visual material collected during the day. They are absent in blind or severely amblyopic individuals.

57. **C.** Focal slowing can be seen in association with tumors in the white matter or cortex. A small thalamic tumor can be associated with focal slowing, whereas a large lesion can be associated with diffuse hemispheric slowing. Generalized slowing can be seen with tumors in the midbrain tegmentum.

58. **D.** SREDA is not a seizure discharge and does not increase the risk of epileptic seizures. It is usually seen in older adults, typically at rest (including drowsiness) or during activation (i.e., hyperventilation [HV]). The activity is maximal over the temporoparietal region, and is characterized by a relatively sudden buildup of rhythmic, monomorphic theta activity that evolves and wanes. They typically last more than 30 seconds.

59. **C.** A spike is a transient with a pointed peak, clearly distinguishable from the background activity. Its main component is generally negative, duration is 20 to 70 ms, and the amplitude is variable. Spikes are felt to be hypersynchronous events caused by excessive simultaneous neuronal discharge. It has been shown that the spikes increase in frequency after a seizure either during wakefulness or sleep, but there is no apparent increase prior to a seizure. Generally, drug levels have little influence on the rate of spikes.

60. **C.** The recommended term for "flat line EEG" is electrocerebral inactivity (ECI). In infants less than 2 months, two EEGs 48 hours apart need to be obtained. In infants 2 to 12 months old, 2 EEGs 24 hours apart need to be obtained. In adults, one EEG is enough as long it is properly acquired and interpretable. In brain death evaluations, it is important to check the integrity of the recording system by touching each electrode with a cotton swab to produce an artifact. Reactivity should always be checked and presence of any reactivity argues against brain death. The minimum recording time is 30 minutes.

61. **D.** The EEG pattern is consistent with hypsarrhythmia, a pattern seen during NREM sleep in children with infantile spasms. It is characterized by a high-amplitude, disorganized background with multifocal spikes and sharp waves. It can improve or disappear during REM sleep and wakefulness.

62. **D.** The EEG in the question shows generalized periodic pattern with triphasic morphology and an antero-posterior gradient. This pattern can be seen in toxic-metabolic encephalopathies such as renal and liver failure, lithium toxicity, treatment with certain third generation cephalosporins among others. Although a similar pattern could be seen in generalized status epilepticus, the bilateral nature of the waveforms makes focal status epilepticus unlikely. Stroke typically would present with slowing, voltage attenuation, or lateralized periodic discharges (LPDs). HSE usually presents with epileptiform and nonepileptiform changes unilaterally or bilaterally in the temporal region. CJD can present with a generalized periodic pattern but the history of acute onset is inconsistent with it.

63. **C.** The patient most likely has Lennox–Gastaut syndrome (LGS), which is associated with generalized slow spike-and-wave discharges and tonic seizures. Given the moderate cognitive impairment, the chance seeing of a normal PDR is low. Presence of generalized fast spike-and-wave discharges is suggestive of juvenile myoclonic epilepsy (JME), which is typically associated with normal cognitive development, and myoclonic, absence, and generalized tonic–clonic seizures (rather than tonic seizures). Focal polyspikes are less likely, but multifocal polyspikes may be seen. Hypsarrhythmia refers to the high-voltage disorganized background seen in West syndrome, which is unlikely at this age.

64. **A.** The 6-Hz phantom spike-wave pattern is usually seen in adolescents and adults with an incidence of 1% to 2.5%. They tend to occur during relaxed wakefulness and drowsiness but disappear during deeper stages of sleep, a feature differentiating it from interictal epileptiform discharges. They tend to occur in bursts lasting 1 to 2 seconds with a frequency of 5 to 7 Hz. The spike component tends to be of short duration (less than 30 ms) and low amplitude (less than 30 μV), and tends to be overshadowed by the aftergoing slow wave, which is usually of higher amplitude (50–100 μV); this quality of the spikes gives rise to the term "phantom spike and wave."

65. **B.** The EEG in the question shows activity over the posterior head region, most consistent with positive occipital sharp transients of sleep (POSTS). POSTS are normal sleep phenomena, and can appear rhythmic or periodic, and should not be confused with epileptiform activity or localized dysfunction. The diagnosis of restless legs syndrome is made clinically, not based on EEG.

66. **C.** The 3 Hz spike-wave discharges are most pronounced in children with typical absence seizures; atypical absence seizures (e.g., as seen in Lennox–Gastaut syndrome) are associated with <3 Hz spike-wave discharges. The correlation between interictal spike-wave discharges and the occurrence of absences is only modest (16% according to some investigators). The spike-wave complex is not simply an association of a spike and a slow wave. It is believed that the surface negative spike is the result of excitatory postsynaptic potentials (EPSPs) on the apical dendrites of vertically oriented pyramidal type neurons, whereas the surface negative slow wave is the result of inhibitory postsynaptic potentials (IPSPs) on or near the soma of similar pyramidal cells. Thus, the slow-wave component is felt to be inhibitory, and the spike-wave discharge likely represents alternating excitation and inhibition. Clinical absences usually occur when the burst duration is greater than 5 seconds. Almost all spike-wave bursts are generalized and bisynchronous, although the synchrony may not be perfect; however, they typically show bifrontal predominance with a smaller field distribution over temporal and occipital regions.

67. **D.** Around 32 to 34 weeks conceptional age, QS still presents as tracé discontinu, but the bursts are 80% synchronous and interburst intervals are less than 10 seconds long. Delta brushes are present in active sleep (AS) and wakefulness over the occipital and central regions; at this stage, they can also be seen in QS. Temporal theta continues but transitions into temporal alpha bursts. Infrequent multifocal sharp transients appear in all states. There is increase in eye movements and decrease in EMG during AS. Stimulation, mostly auditory and tactile, causes reactive attenuation of the EEG around 34 weeks.

68. **C.** Bilateral FIRDA has not been associated with epilepsy; it is mainly suggestive of encephalopathy. There is growing evidence that unilateral intermittent rhythmic delta activities (IRDAs) as well as GIRDA are associated with an increased risk for seizures, especially in critically ill patients. Unilateral TIRDA has been associated with temporal lobe seizures while OIRDA has been associated with absence epilepsy.

69. **E.** Low-voltage EEG records are rare in children. They are seen in 5% of healthy adolescents and 12% of healthy adults. Such records are typically dominated by beta frequencies.

70. **B.** At term, the total amount of time spent in sleep is 50%, most of which will be in AS. By 46 weeks of conceptional age, QS predominates. This shift in sleep parallels the adult transition from wakefulness to NREM sleep. Sleep spindles may be present (typically first seen at 6–8 weeks of life) but will be underdeveloped and asynchronous.

71. **C.** The EEG shows normal drowsiness. The sharply contoured activity in the central head region is consistent with a run of vertex sharp waves. The activity is periodic, not consistent with pathological slowing. The activity lacks the morphological features of spike-wave discharges. Although mu rhythm can occur in the same region, the frequency tends to be in the alpha range with a morphology described as flat-topped notching. POSTS are surface positive and seen in the occipital region.

72. **A.** Alexander disease is a leukodystrophy and thus affects the white matter, which would most likely lead to slowing. The anterior predominance of the illness would likely lead to bifrontal slowing.

73. **D.** Hyperventilation has been used to trigger generalized seizures, particularly absence seizures. Similarly, intermittent photic stimulation can trigger abnormalities associated with generalized seizures, particularly those associated with photosensitive epilepsies. Startling caused by loud noise can trigger reflex seizures, which may be generalized or focal. Sleep, especially after sleep deprivation, can increase the yield of epileptiform discharges. Intravenous saline administration has been shown to provoke psychogenic nonepileptic seizures but not epileptiform abnormalities, although the ethical basis of this method is questionable.

74. **D.** The typical frequency of the PDR is 8 Hz by 3 years and 10 Hz by 10 to 15 years. Hypnagogic hypersynchrony, consisting of theta activity, appears as a drowsy pattern around 6 months and tends to disappear by 3 years although it may rarely persist into late childhood. Sleep spindles usually appear around age 3 months and acquire vertex predominance around age 2 to 3 years. Initially the spindle duration tends to be longer, and it decreases to around 1 second by age 6 to 12 years. Posterior slow waves of youth are typically seen in adolescents 6 to 12 years old, and are rare before age 2 years or after 21 years. On the other hand, low-voltage EEG records are rare in children.

75. **C.** SREDA is best seen in older adults (average age: 61 years) in the temporoparietal region. It usually occurs during rest, drowsiness, or HV. It has not been reported during photic stimulation.

76. **D.** The mu rhythm is a normal variant seen over the central head regions (e.g., C3, Cz, C4), is associated with the sensorimotor cortex. It tends to be in the alpha range, although

beta range frequencies could be seen. Although bilateral, it can be asymmetrical and asynchronous. Of note, unlike the posterior dominant rhythm (PDR), mu rhythm is not attenuated by eye opening but it is attenuated by planned or actual movement of the contralateral arm.

77. B. The EEG finding is consistent with rhythmic mid-temporal theta burst of drowsiness (RMTD), a normal variant, which can present as a long train of activity in children. Ciganek rhythm, also a normal variant, consists of theta activity seen predominantly in the midline region (vertex or Cz) in wakefulness and drowsiness. TIRDA is unlikely because the frequency of the rhythmic activity is in the theta, not delta, range. There is no evolution of the activity to suggest a seizure discharge. This activity could be artifact, but it is less likely given the large field involved.

78. D. Morphologically, an epileptiform spike usually has a steep upslope but a gradual downslope. It is less than 70 ms in duration. Epileptiform abnormalities tend to have a wider field of distribution in non-REM sleep than REM sleep. Thus, the extent and laterality of interictal epileptiform discharges during REM sleep can be useful in localizing or confirming the epileptogenic focus. Occasionally, a horizontal dipole may be seen, as in the case of the centrotemporal spikes of benign rolandic epilepsy (BRE).

79. B. The EEG shows asynchronous beta activity maximal over the central head regions consistent with sleep spindles, which constitute normal sleep architecture. When sleep spindles appear at the age of 2 months, they can be of long duration and asynchronous. They can continue to be asynchronous until the age of 2 years. Although neonatal seizures can occur even in a single channel and migrate from one channel to the other (as seen in the epoch), the activity is unlikely to be a seizure because there is no evolution. Patting artifact has variable EEG manifestations but tends to be of slower frequency and more widespread distribution. This activity is less likely to be an electrode artifact as it has a well-established field distribution. Beta activity related to the administration of benzodiazepines or barbiturates tends to be generalized rather than regional.

80. E. There is no ictal discharge seen on the EEG, which would be expected in a person with motionless staring or absence seizure. Although the spell is suggestive of a nonepileptic event (e.g., psychogenic), video correlation is mandatory for making this diagnosis. Partial seizures with dyscognitive features (complex partial seizures) are usually associated with EEG findings on scalp recording. Frontal lobe seizures can present with a wide variety of semiologies. Although motionless staring is typically associated with temporal lobe involvement, orbitofrontal seizures can present with a similar semiology and may not have a scalp ictal EEG correlate but the duration is typically less than 2 to 3 minutes, far shorter than the episode witnessed by the EEG technologist. Therefore, the episode is best interpreted as a recorded event not consistent with any of the other answer choices.

81. A. Around 37 to 40 weeks, delta brushes are typically restricted to QS. Encoches frontales (frontal sharp transients) and monorhythmic frontal delta are predominant during transition between AS and QS. Sporadic multifocal sharps are considered normal but they tend to be rare. HVS pattern can be seen as the predominant background during QS.

82. A. Mitochondrial disorders, such as MELAS (mitochondrial myopathy, encephalopathy, lactic acidosis and stroke) and MERRF (myoclonus, epilepsy, ragged red fibers) are characterized by a variety of neurologic abnormalities. EEG findings include epileptiform abnormalities with occipital (not bifrontal) predominance or generalized epileptiform discharges, which can be enhanced by photic stimulation. Periodic or pseudoperiodic sharp waves or epilepsia partialis continua can be seen in MELAS. Myoclonus can occur in conjunction with epileptiform discharges in MERRF.

83. C. The frequency of the PDR reaches 6 Hz by age 12 months. Drowsiness is characterized by the appearance of hypnagogic hypersynchrony at age 6 to 8 months, consisting of rhythmic theta activity around 4 Hz with gradual increase to 6 Hz over the next few years. Sleep spindles usually appear around 2 to 3 months, being well formed in amplitude and duration by 3 months. They reach a frequency of 12 to 15 Hz by 2 to 3 years, with 14 Hz being most commonly encountered. Throughout infancy, spindles are maximal over the centro-parietal region with shifting asymmetry but they do not exhibit clear-cut vertex predominance until age 2 to 3 years. The photic driving response appears around age 3 to 4 months, with driving best seen at low flash rates.

84. D. Morphology of triphasic waves consists of initial and terminal negative phases with a prominent positive phase in the middle. They are generalized, bilaterally symmetric and synchronous, monotonous waveforms with 1.5 to 2.5 Hz frequency. On bipolar montage, an antero-posterior lag may be noted.

85. D. OIRDA (also known as the "phi rhythm") is best seen in children and adolescents aged 6 to 16 years. It consists of rhythmic, high-voltage 3 to 4 Hz activity over the occipital region and its immediate vicinity. The slow waves sometimes have a "notch" appearance. OIRDA is activated by hyperventilation, photic stimulation, eye closure, and drowsiness. It can be seen in those with or without a seizure disorder.

86. A. Ipsilateral, not contralateral, occipital spikes can be seen in someone with unilateral blindness since birth. Similarly, slowing of the PDR, loss of photic driving, and loss of lambda waves can also be seen. However, the presence of left occipital spikes (contralateral to the blind eye) should raise suspicion for an underlying seizure disorder and prompt further workup.

87. C. In a 34-week-old neonate, if spikes and sharp waves are frequent and multifocal, they are typically associated with and underlying nonspecific encephalopathy. Rare spikes are not usually interpreted as epileptiform unless they are focal. They can be considered as normal or of unknown significance only if they are rare and multifocal.

88. C. The EEG in the question shows generalized periodic complexes (some with triphasic morphology), which can be seen in baclofen and lithium toxicities, uremia, and CJD. Bismuth subsalicylate toxicity may lead to prolonged encephalopathy, but the EEG is typically characterized by diffuse slowing without any epileptiform or periodic activity.

89. B. The majority of delta brushes are observed in AS at 29 weeks of gestation.

90. B. Subacute sclerosing panencephalitis, a rare chronic, progressive illness caused by persistent measles infection, presents with periodic complexes with the longest period (defined as the duration of one cycle in a repeating event and the reciprocal of frequency); typically, the period is 4 to 20 seconds, which is longer earlier in the disease and shortens over time. Creutzfeldt–Jakob disease (except the new variant type) and baclofen toxicity also can present with periodic discharges but with a shorter period (i.e., higher frequency), on the order of 1 to 2 seconds. Periodic discharges with triphasic morphology can be seen with liver failure, but tend to be continuous or have very short periods. LKS does not present with periodic complexes.

91. A. Although both LKS and CSWS are epilepsy syndromes with clinical regression and sleep-activated epileptiform EEG patterns in NREM sleep, there are some distinguishing features. The discharges are more bitemporal and / or biparietal in LKS, whereas they are more diffuse in CSWS. The regression in CSWS is more global behavior, whereas in LKS it is typically limited to language. Both syndromes present with intractable epilepsy and may require multiple antiepileptic agents. Of note, steroids have been noted to help with both conditions but carbamazepine has been noted to worsen the EEG patterns in both.

92. A. This slow, low-voltage (5–10 μV), minimally (if any) reactive EEG in the setting of some brainstem reflexes with no clear purposeful movements is consistent with a vegetative state. Note that in the vegetative state, the patients can open their eyelids occasionally and demonstrate sleep–wake cycles but completely lack cognitive function. A technically adequate electrocerebral inactivity (ECI) recording with absence of both EEG activity and brainstem reflexes would be consistent with (not diagnostic of) brain death. ECI with intact brainstem reflexes is consistent with cortical death. Minimally responsive slow EEG with some purposeful behavior and intelligible verbalization is consistent with a minimally conscious state. Clearly reactive, normal or mildly slow EEG with limited preserved brainstem reflexes is consistent with locked-in syndrome. Brainstem reflexes will be intact in akinetic mutism.

93. D. When recording a more detailed EEG with more electrodes, extra electrodes are added using the 10% division, which fills in intermediate sites halfway between those of the existing 10 to 20 system. This new electrode-naming system is called the MCN. MCN system uses 1, 3, 5, 7, and 9 for the left hemisphere (and similar even numbers for the right hemisphere) which represent 10%, 20%, 30%, 40%, and 50% of the inion-to-nasion distance, respectively. The introduction of extra letter codes allows the naming of intermediate electrode sites, although these new letter codes do not necessarily refer to an area on the underlying cerebral cortex. The new letter codes for intermediate sites are: AF, intermediate between Fp and F; FC, between F and C; FT, between F and T; CP, between C and P; TP, between T and P; and PO, between P and O. Also, the MCN system renames 4 electrode positions of the 10 to 20 system: T3, T4, T5, and T6 are renamed as T7, T8, P7, and P8, respectively.

94. B. PPR is typically seen in patients with generalized seizures (53%) but can also be seen on rare occasions in patients with focal seizures (3%). Of note, PPR can be seen in the photosensitive form of occipital lobe epilepsy. Some studies have suggested that the presence of PPR may be inherited as a genetic trait; therefore, it can be seen in patients without epilepsy. Intermittent photic stimulation (IPS) at 15 to 18 Hz frequency is considered to be most epileptogenic in eliciting PPR in patients with photosensitive epilepsy. PPR is most likely to occur immediately after eye closure. Eye closure is felt to produce activation by suddenly eliminating the visual pattern and by causing the field of vision to become red-hued.

95. A. At 30 weeks of conceptional age, although the EEG is still discontinuous, there is an electrographic difference between wakefulness/AS vs QS. In QS, the tracé discontinu pattern is more prominent, and the occipital-dominant bursts become asynchronous. Monorhythmic occipital delta and temporal theta activities persist. During AS and wakefulness, the interburst intervals are shorter than in QS. The majority of delta brushes are observed in AS. Rapid eye movement, obvious body movements, and occasional regular respirations help to differentiate the stages, although much of the recording tends to be in transitional sleep. During transitional or intermediate periods, features of both sleep states are apparent, and precise classification is often not possible.

96. E. At the onset of a generalized tonic–clonic seizure, there may be voltage attenuation (desynchronization, electrodecremental pattern). Fast activity (20–40 Hz) may be seen in all leads. In primary generalized epilepsy, a generalized burst of polyspike-wave discharges may be seen. Following voltage attenuation, rhythmic 10 Hz sinusoidal activity may be seen (i.e., epileptic recruiting rhythm). About 10 seconds after onset, slower frequencies in the theta and delta range occur. The clonic activity corresponds to the polyspike bursts at each jerk. The end of clonic activity is followed by postictal suppression and irregular delta activity before the return of the baseline alpha rhythm.

97. B. Frontal operculum seizures fit this semiology. Other symptoms that can be seen include mastication, fear, gustatory hallucinations, and speech arrest. Supplementary motor area seizures typically present with a somatosensory aura followed by unilateral or asymmetrical bilateral tonic posturing. Vocalizations, facial grimacing, and automatisms (e.g., laughing or kicking) can be present. Cingulate gyrus seizures can present with complex behaviors (sometimes misdiagnosed as psychogenic) characterized by agitation, gestural automatisms, repetitive motor activity (e.g., pelvic thrusting, pedaling, or thrashing), strong emotional feelings, vocalizations, laughter, and crying. Mesial temporal seizures can present with the semiology presented above except that the clonic facial movements would occur later in the ictal period as the seizure spreads from the mesial temporal to the frontal opercular regions.

98. A. This EEG is dysmature for a 38-week conceptional age neonate due to the presence of tracé discontinu, which is expected to resolve by 36 weeks of conceptional age. EEGs are considered dysmature if they contain patterns that are at least 2 weeks immature for the conceptional age. With serial EEGs, clinical concern may only arise if the dysmature patterns persist. A tracé discontinu pattern would not be a marker of severe encephalopathy until beyond 38 weeks conceptional age when the term "dysmature" can no longer be used. Tracé discontinu is not an epileptiform pattern, and therefore does not denote a seizure or increased risk for seizures.

99. C. HVS pattern, seen in neonates, subsequently develops into a more generalized, posterior dominant delta activity. This pattern is accompanied by occasional, isolated (not rhythmic), monophasic, occipital slow waves called cone waves. Cone waves appear in infancy and persist through mid-childhood, and are prominent in N2 and N3 sleep. While vertex waves and K-complexes may be apparent in a neonatal EEG, they are not well developed until 5 to 6 months of age.

100. E. There are many types of occipital sharp transients. In young children, they are likely to be associated with benign epilepsy that may remit in later life; in other words, presence of occipital spikes does not necessarily indicate intractable epilepsy. Lambda waves are occipital sharp transients that occur as a result of scanning objects, and they disappear with eye closure. Spikes associated with benign occipital epilepsy of childhood attenuate with eye opening. In blind individuals, occipital spikes can be seen without history of seizures.

101. C. This EEG shows typical generalized 3 Hz spike-and-wave activity likely triggered by HV, and possibly associated with an absence seizure. Given the patient is a child and is normal, this EEG is likely to be consistent with childhood absence epilepsy (CAE; age of onset 4–10 years), which is not typically associated with myoclonic jerks, but can present with automatisms and eye flutter. There is a high chance of the CAE going into remission. Although there is a wide spectrum of normal HV response variants, including synchronous notched delta activity, the presence of spike-wave discharges makes this EEG abnormal. Similarly, the finding does not represent movement artifact either.

102. D. An infant born between 37 and 42 weeks of conceptional age is considered a term infant. During this age, neonatal patterns gradually disappear, and are replaced by elementary adult patterns. When the infant is awake, the low-voltage irregular (LVI) pattern develops into a background of centrally dominant, nonreactive, rhythmical, 4 to 6 Hz activity. These waves appear synchronous and symmetrical by 1 month of age. During QS, continuous slow-wave sleep replaces tracé alternant as the dominant pattern. If tracé alternant is present, the bursts are 100% synchronous and the interburst intervals are less than 4 seconds.

103. A. There is a polarity convention that is universally accepted in EEG. In a bipolar montage channel G1–G2, the resultant voltage equals the difference between G1 and G2. According to the convention, if the G1 input is more negative than the G2 input, the pen deflection will be upward. It follows that either a negative event at G1 or a positive event at G2 would lead to an upward deflection. A positive event at G1 or a negative event at G2 leads to a downward deflection. A flat (i.e., an equipotential) deflection occurs if both G1 and G2 have equal inputs.

104. A. The eye movements corresponding to the markers 1 through 4 are up, down, left, and right respectively. Eye movements are appreciated on scalp EEG due to the dipole effect of the eyeball (the cornea is relatively positive compared to the retina). Vertical eye movements lead to deflections of the same polarity on the homologous anterior channels (i.e., FP1/FP2), whereas the lateral eye movements lead to deflections of the opposite polarities on the homologous anterior channels (i.e., FP1/FP2, F7/F8). In the figure, the signals after marker 1 have positive (downward) deflections in FP1 and FP2, consistent with upward movement of the eyes; the signals after marker 2 have negative (upward) deflections in FP1 and FP2, consistent with downward movement of eyes.

105. E. Delta brushes are present in the premature infant beginning at 26 weeks of conceptional age. Delta brushes are analogous to K-complexes in the adult; however, they typically occur asynchronously in the neonate. Delta brushes consist of a mixture of medium- to high-voltage delta activity intermixed with low- to medium-voltage fast activity, commonly with 18- to 22-Hz maximum in the central region. Delta brushes are a prominent feature in AS by 29 to 33 weeks of conceptional age; by 33 to 38 weeks of conceptional age, they are expressed maximally in QS; they can occur in REM sleep until 40 weeks.

106. B. The EEG in the question shows epileptiform activity combined with vertex waves and sleep spindles, also known as dyshormia. Although it can be seen in patients with and without epilepsy, it may indicate a lower seizure threshold. Children with simple febrile seizures typically have a normal EEG but they can have hypnagogic paroxysmal spike-wave activity with epileptiform activity embedded into hyperventilation (HV) or hypnagogic hypersynchrony; dyshormia is not typically seen in simple febrile seizures.

107. E. The EEG shows near-continuous epileptiform abnormalities in sleep. This EEG abnormality in a child should raise the possibility of Landau–Kleffner syndrome (LKS). LKS is a childhood syndrome characterized by language regression, which typically starts with auditory verbal agnosia. Although they can be associated with clinical seizures, many only present with an electrographic seizure pattern which activates in sleep, referred to as electrographic status epilepticus of sleep (ESES).

108. D. The amplitude of the scalp EEG tends to be 10 to 100 μV (in adults, it is usually 10–50 μV). On electrocorticograms, the amplitude tends to be 500 to 1,500 μV or higher. The EEG amplitude is measured from peak to peak. Precise determination of the amplitude of each wave is unnecessary because it is affected by too many confounding variables (e.g., interelectrode distance, type of montage). Therefore, reporting the amplitude as a range (e.g., "PDR of 20–30 μV") or qualitatively (e.g., "medium-voltage activity") would be sufficient.

109. E. Low blood glucose may enhance HV-induced slowing and trigger generalized EEG abnormalities; however, there is no relation between blood glucose level and PPR. Certain diets (e.g., ketogenic diet) can be used to treat seizures, and therefore, can affect the yield of the EEG abnormalities.

110. D. Both relationships are relatively positive based on the concept that the voltage in a channel G1–G2 is given by the equation G1–G2. Given that channel Fp1–F7 is positive (downgoing defection), Fp1 has to be more positive (i.e., less negative) than F7. Similarly, given that channel T7–P7 is negative (upgoing deflection), P7 has to be more positive (i.e., less negative) than T7.

111. D. The effect of sleep on epilepsy was recognized in the 1800s. Since then, more studies have been done to evaluate this further. It has been shown that REM sleep is the least likely and that N3 (slow-wave sleep) is the most likely to show epileptiform discharges. The increased synchronization during slow-wave sleep and the relative desynchronization during REM sleep are felt to be the underlying mechanisms.

112. E. Around 37 to 40 weeks of conceptional age, there is a clear distinction between wakefulness and quiet sleep (QS). However, wakefulness may resemble AS because the LVI pattern can be seen in both. EEG activity during wakefulness may resemble sleep-onset REM but appears more organized with some rhythmic theta waves.

113. A. SSS are also known as benign epileptiform transients of sleep (BETS) or benign sporadic sleep spikes (BSSS). They typically occur in drowsiness or light sleep and tend to disappear in deeper stages of sleep. They tend to have a broad field of distribution with anterior or mid-temporal predominance. They are unilateral, bilaterally independent, or bilaterally synchronous in distribution. The morphology tends to be monophasic or diphasic with a steep descending limb, unlike epileptiform discharges, which tend to have a steep ascending limb and a gradual descending limb. Although they may be associated with an aftergoing slow wave, they do not disrupt the EEG background, unlike epileptiform discharges. On a transverse montage, they may exhibit a transverse oblique dipole with opposite polarities in the two hemispheres, which is not typical for epileptiform discharges.

114. C. The EEG in the question shows centrotemporal spikes which are seen in BRE. Autosomal dominant nocturnal frontal lobe epilepsy and cingulate epilepsy typically present with frontal spikes or a normal EEG. Mesial temporal sclerosis would typically present with temporal spikes. Lennox–Gastaut syndrome presents with slow spike-wave discharges or generalized paroxysmal fast activity, neither of which is seen.

115. C. The clinical picture suggests nonconvulsive seizures and possibly nonconvulsive status epilepticus. The EEG is supportive showing right temporal epileptiform discharges with an ictal discharge beginning at the end of the epoch. Although nonconvulsive status epilepticus can be the result of many of the listed answer choices, the most likely cause is an autoimmune disorder given that the patient was previously in good health. More cases of autoimmune epilepsy are being recognized, the most common subset being paraneoplastic phenomena. Numerous antibodies have been identified, including antibodies to Hu, CRMP-5, Ma2, VGKC, GAD65, N-methyl-D-aspartate (NMDA) receptor, gamma-aminobutyric acid (GABA) B receptor, and alpha-amino-3-hydroxy-5-methyl-4-isoxazolepropionic acid (AMPA) receptor. The EEG patterns vary patient to patient, and can include multifocal interictal discharges. Although HSV type I can present with temporal lobe seizures in an otherwise healthy person, there is usually a prodromal phase with fever and headache, with the seizures involving the mesial temporal or orbitofrontal structures. HSV type II tends to cause a transverse myelitis or affect the brainstem rather than limbic encephalitis. Although seizures and multifocal discharges can be seen in the setting of stroke and anoxic brain injury, the clinical scenario does not support these diagnoses.

116. E. The sensitivity of detecting epileptiform abnormalities after three routine EEGs approaches 90%.

117. C. Hypsarrhythmia is an interictal pattern consisting of irregular, high-amplitude generalized spikes and waves in the setting of a chaotic and disorganized background. It is frequently seen in infants with infantile spasms. Hypsarrhythmia typically disappears or improves during the ictal spasms and/or REM sleep. It rarely persists beyond age 24 months. There are five variants of the hypsarrhythmia pattern, and the type with increased interhemispheric synchronization (e.g., those with West syndrome) can evolve clinically to LGS.

118. A. HV, IPS, NREM sleep, and hypoglycemia (not hyperglycemia) can activate the 3 Hz spike-wave discharge with or without associated clinical absences.

119. A. Rolandic spikes are seen in children with BRE as well as in healthy siblings of such children. They are prominent during sleep and they typically resolve by age 16 years (typically around puberty). They exhibit horizontal dipole with centrotemporal negativity and frontal (not temporal) positivity.

120. C. Severe myoclonic seizures of infancy may present with generalized or unilateral febrile clonic seizures within the first year of life and then progress to myoclonic seizures. The febrile seizures may be long and recurrent. The EEG will show generalized spike-wave and polyspike-wave discharges, early photosensitivity, and focal abnormalities. The other options are correct.

121. B. A 9-Hz PDR is considered to be normal despite low voltage and does not suggest encephalopathy. A slow PDR (reactive or nonreactive), FIRDA, and continuous slowing can all be seen in a patient with progressively worsening encephalopathy.

122. B. Paradoxical alpha rhythm represents an alerting response characterized by the appearance of posterior alpha frequencies in the setting of opened eyes and drowsiness.

123. D. The total daily sleep time for infants over a 24-hour period is typically 14 to 16 hours. During the first several months of life, sleep time decreases and consolidates into an overnight period with at least 1 daytime nap. REM sleep in infants represents a larger percentage of total sleep at the expense of Stage N3 (not N2). Until age 3 to 4 months, transition from wakefulness into REM sleep is common; after that, wakefulness begins to transition into NREM sleep.

124. C. Delta range slowing is always abnormal when seen during photic stimulation. However, it is important that the activity, if seen during photic stimulation, is not misinterpreted as photic driving or eye blinking artifact. Intermittent slowing may not necessarily be pathological during HV, drowsiness or slow-wave sleep.

125. D. The figure in the question shows lambda waves, which are positive waves in the bilateral occipital region. Careful inspection shows relatively rapid lateral eye movements preceded by lateral rectus spikes, most prominently in the Fp1-F7/F7-T7 and Fp2-F8/F8-T8 channels. These two findings suggest that the patient is mostly reading or scanning rather than having nystagmus. The patient is clearly awake. The lambda waves in the occipital region are discrete, not sustained or evolving like in a focal seizure.

126. C. SSS, also known as benign epileptiform transients of sleep (BETS), are rather inconspicuous discharges with a spiky character. They are typically less than 50 microvolts and 50 milliseconds. They are seen in a widespread distribution with frontotemporal predominance occurring synchronously or asynchronously. They are seen in drowsiness or light sleep in adults. It has a prevalence of about 1%. In one study, two-thirds of the patients had a history of epileptic seizures; among people without epilepsy, they may occur in patients with cerebrovascular disorder, syncope attacks, and psychiatric conditions (manic-depressive disorder). Some authors believe that they are nonspecific patterns, while others associate a moderate degree of epileptogenicity to them.

127. D. GPDs in CJD usually have a duration of 100 to 600 ms, and occur at a frequency of 0.5 to 2 Hz. They are present during wakefulness but tend to disappear during sleep, sedation, and stimulation. They are not necessarily time-locked to clinical myoclonus. As a rule, GPDs do not occur in variant CJD but exceptions to this rule have been described. GPDs may be localized to the occipital region in the Heidenhain variant of CJD. In the initial stages of the illness, the GPDs can be unilateral. GPDs have a sensitivity of 64%, specificity of 91%, positive predictive value of 95%, and negative predictive value of 49%.

128. B. The EEG demonstrates left temporal intermittent rhythmic delta activity (TIRDA), an interictal abnormality, which increases the risk of epileptic seizures. IRDA, especially frontal predominant (i.e., FIRDA) or occipital predominant (i.e., OIRDA), can attenuate with alertness or eye opening and accentuate with drowsiness, eye closure, and hyperventilation. IRDA is not seen in N2 and N3 sleep but can be seen in REM. The activity in this question has no evolution to suggest a seizure. No periodic discharges or breach rhythm is noted. No pulse artifact is noted, which typically shows up as slow waves that occur at the same frequency as the heart rate.

129. E. Intermittent rhythmic delta activity (IRDA) is commonly bilateral rather than unilateral or focal. Unilateral or focal IRDA can be epileptiform in certain situations. The predominance of bilateral IRDA appears to vary with age with a frontal predominance (i.e., FIRDA) in adults and with an occipital predominance (i.e., OIRDA) in children. FIRDA is most likely to be consistent with encephalopathy. FIRDA is more commonly associated with metabolic or other diffuse encephalopathies rather than a focal lesion. Historically, FIRDA was felt to result from high intracranial pressure or a deep-rooted midline or subcortial lesion. If FIRDA is due to an underlying lesion, the lesion tends to be frontal. In mild encephalopathy, FIRDA can be present with preserved background activity. However, in more severe encephalopathy, FIRDA is seen with more suppressed background activity. TIRDA is seen interictally in patients with temporal lobe epilepsy. OIRDA can be seen in those with absence seizures. Lateralized periodic discharges (LPDs) are associated with increased risk for focal seizures. A normal PDR of 8.5 Hz, although can be seen in mild encephalopathy, is not in itself suggestive of encephalopathy. SREDA is a normal variant, not associated with encephalopathy.

130. A. Lambda waves are seen in this awake EEG. All of the choices listed occur in the posterior head region. Lambda waves occur during wakefulness, and likely represent an evoked response to visual stimuli related to actively scanning (i.e., eye movements) a picture. Note the saccadic eye movements in the figure, which suggest active scanning. POSTS occur during light and moderate levels of sleep and should not be mistaken for epileptiform activity. Spike-wave discharges by the nature of their name have a sharply contoured wave less than 70 ms followed by an aftergoing slow wave, which is not seen here. Posterior slow waves of youth are sporadically occurring single delta-range waves that attenuate with eye opening and are seen in children and adolescents. Photic driving is not seen here. Photic driving consists of an occipital-dominant rhythm occurring at the flash frequency or harmonic thereof. Of note, patients with large lambda waves and POSTS tend to have large photic driving responses. Also of note, a response at a flash frequency <5 Hz is not considered photic driving but instead an evoked potential.

131. E. Although the entire background is slow with predominately theta range rhythms, there is no appreciable anterior to posterior gradient to suggest the presence of a PDR in this epoch. Furthermore, without additional information, it is not possible to determine the state in which the epoch was acquired, which in turn is necessary to evaluate the PDR. Therefore, it is not reasonable to infer about the PDR. There are generalized, anterior-predominant spike-and-slow wave discharges in the setting of generalized, predominately theta activity with intermittent polymorphic delta slowing. There is additional lateralized intermittent rhythmic delta activity, maximal over the right frontotemporal region.

132. E. Chloral hydrate can be used to induce sleep, which increases the yield of detecting epileptiform activity. It also improves EEG quality by decreasing muscle and movement artifacts. Chloral hydrate is considered to be conscious sedation and therefore requires special staffing in most laboratories, precluding widespread routine use. It induces fast EEG activity, although less prominently than barbiturates. It is rapidly metabolized so the side effects (e.g., paradoxical excitation and irrational behavior) are rare.

133. E. HV can induce focal slowing in a patient with a history of stroke (options B and E), but the ACNS guidelines suggest certain clinical scenarios should be contraindicated, including acute stroke, recent intracerebral hemorrhage, large-vessel stenosis, recent transient ischemic attack (TIA), moyamoya disease, severe cardiopulmonary disorders and sickle cell trait or disease. Therefore HV can be safely done in a patient with a chronic stroke (option B) and should not be done in a patient with moyamoya disease (option E). Of note in moyamoya disease, the buildup of slowing can recur 3 to 5 minutes after HV cessation. HV can trigger absence seizures (option A) in more than 80% of untreated children. HV can be used but is less helpful in diagnosing focal epilepsy (option D) because the induced epileptiform abnormalities are seen in less than 5% of cases. HV can sometimes trigger psychogenic nonepileptic seizures (option C).

134. B. Generalized spike-and-wave discharges may occur in patients with focal seizures, particularly in frontal lobe epilepsy due to secondary bilateral synchrony. They usually have anterior predominance. Although a frequency of 3 Hz in children is invariably associated with good prognosis, a frequency of less than 3 Hz is associated with poor prognosis. They are activated by both HV and photic stimulation. It can be more difficult to classify a generalized discharge as an interictal or ictal pattern compared to classifying focal discharges. Many times, a generalized discharge is considered ictal solely based on its duration and repetitive nature because the other characteristics of EEG evolution, suggestive of a typical ictal pattern, can be absent.

135. B. Sleep spindles usually appear around 2 to 3 months, being well formed in amplitude and duration by 3 months. They reach a frequency of 12 to 15 Hz by 2 to 3 years, with 14 Hz being most commonly encountered. Throughout infancy, spindles are maximal over the centro-parietal region with shifting asymmetry without a clear-cut midline (vertex) maximum until age 2 to 3 years. Spindle bursts reach duration of 10 seconds by 6 months but there is decreased duration of each spindle run with an increase in the overall number of runs. By 6 to 12 years, the spindle trains are usually less than 1 second with the individual waves more rounded in appearance. Extreme spindles, characterized by 6 to 18 Hz activity with paroxysmal traits, appearing even while the child is awake, is rare in normal children (approximately 0.05%) but the prevalence reaches 5% to 18% in children with mental retardation or cerebral palsy. When clearly separable from typical spindle activity, extreme spindles might represent a mild abnormality. Similarly, the fast spiky spindles are also rare, and they consist of 16 to 20 Hz spindle-like activity occurring in a widespread distribution over central, parietal, vertex, and mid-temporal regions. The fast spiky spindles are seen mainly in early childhood, around the age of 3 years; some investigators believe that they represent a mild abnormality in children, correlated with static or progressive brain dysfunction.

136. B. According to the ACNS guidelines (Guideline 6: Minimum Technical Standards for EEG Recording in Suspected Cerebral Death), impedance should be between 100 and 10K ohms so the potentials are not attenuated. Other criteria are correct.

137. D. Eyelid flutter, along with eye opening, occur more frequently in absence seizures than with HIHARS. Behavior arrest, staring, and automatisms (oral and manual) can be seen in both groups. On the other hand, fidgeting, smiling, and yawning occur more frequently with HIHARS.

138. C. Triphasic waves can be seen in metabolic encephalopathies (liver failure, renal failure, Hashimoto's encephalitis) or infections (herpes simplex encephalitis [HSE]). LPDs or bilateral independent LPDs, particularly in the temporal region, can be seen in association with herpes simplex virus (HSV) encephalitis or limbic encephalitis. FIRDA is associated with metabolic encephalopathy, increased intracranial pressure, thalamic lesion, or deep frontal white matter abnormality. GIRDA is a nonspecific finding that is associated with encephalopathy. Thus, all of the above abnormalities are somewhat nonspecific, and the conditions associated with them do not lead to rapidly progressive dementia and myoclonus. On the other hand, continuous, bisynchronous GPDs occurring at a frequency of 1 to 2 Hz, can be pathognomic of Creutzfeldt–Jakob disease (CJD). In the context of rapidly progressive dementia and myoclonic jerks, GPDs occurring in close temporal association with myoclonic jerks strongly suggest CJD.

139. B. REM sleep constitutes about 50% of sleep at birth, about 40% at 3 months, and 30% between 1 and 2 years. Occipital sharp transients intermixed delta and theta activity occur in the REM sleep of infants at a frequency of 2 Hz at 6 weeks and 2 to 4 Hz at 12 weeks of age. The REM latency gradually lengthens during the first year of life, with the longest latencies between noon and 4 p.m. and the shortest between 4 a.m. and 8 a.m. In normal infants in the first year of life, brief apneic episodes lasting 3 to 10 seconds may occur during sleep; these pauses are more common in REM sleep. By 6 to 12 years, REM sleep shows increasing desynchronization with mixed activities in the theta, alpha, and beta frequency range.

140. E. All these patterns can be associated with ictal onset and subsequent evolution.

141. B. At 3 months, a 3 Hz PDR is identifiable. Drowsiness is characterized by the appearance of hypnagogic hypersynchrony around age 6 to 8 months (not 3 months), consisting of rhythmic theta activity around 4 Hz. Sleep spindles usually appear around 2 to 3 months, being well formed in amplitude and duration by 3 months. Minimal photic driving response can be seen as early as 3 to 4 months.

142. D. The activity seen is consistent with frontal sharp transients, also known as encoches frontales, which is seen in quiet sleep and is a normal finding in neonates 28 to 42 weeks CA unless they are persistently unilateral, in which case it would be an abnormal finding. They typically have "check mark" morphology. Although artifacts can present in a variety of ways, they are unlikely as this patient was noted to be resting quietly.

143. D. Laplacian is a synthetic referential recording in which each channel represents the difference between an electrode and a weighted average of the surrounding electrodes, aimed to enhance detection of focal discharges. The other listed montages are bipolar in configuration. Note that the double banana montage is another name for the longitudinal bipolar montage.

144. C. The International 10 to 20 system was developed to ensure standardized reproducibility so that a subject's studies could be compared over time and subjects could be compared to each other. This system is based on the relationship between the location of an electrode and the underlying area of cerebral cortex. The "10" and "20" refer to the fact that the actual distances between the adjacent electrodes are either 10% or 20% of the total front-to-back or right-to-left distances of the skull.

Each site has a letter to identify the lobe and a number to identify the hemisphere location. The letters F, T, C, P, and O stand for frontal, temporal, central, parietal, and occipital lobes, respectively. Note that there is no central lobe; the "C" letter is used for identification purposes only. A "z" (zero) refers to an electrode placed on the midline. Even numbers (2, 4, 6, 8) refer to electrode positions over the right hemisphere whereas odd numbers (1, 3, 5, 7) refer to those over the left hemisphere. Two anatomical landmarks are used for the essential positioning of the EEG electrodes: Nasion is the point between the forehead and the nose; inion is the lowest point of the skull from the back of the head and is normally indicated by a prominent bump.

The other answers are incorrect. EEGs may be done with extra electrodes placed using the 10% division, which is halfway between those of the 10 to 20 system, resulting in the 10-10 system with MCN, which introduces new letter codes for the intermediate electrode placements (e.g., FT between F and T and TP between T and P). The new letter codes represent placement and do not necessarily refer to an area on the underlying cerebral cortex. There is even a higher electrode density nomenclature called the 10 to 5 system, where the electrodes are placed at 5% divisions.

145. C. Frontalis muscle twitching is most associated with the photomyogenic response (formerly known as photomyoclonic response), which is felt to be due to a heightened brainstem reflex and results in muscle twitching of the forehead (i.e., frontalis muscle) or eyelids (i.e., orbicularis oculi muscle) time-locked with the photic stimulus.

146. A. The normal variant seen is a small sharp spike (SSS), also known as benign epileptiform transient of sleep (BETS). This is seen typically in drowsiness, in the temporal regions with either unilateral or bilateral independent distribution. It rarely appears synchronously and often has a transverse oblique dipole. It is usually less than 50 μV and less than 50 ms. The morphology is distinct with a steep downslope unlike an epileptiform spike, which has a steep upslope and a gradual downslope.

147. C. The EEG in the question shows two bilaterally independent, lateralized periodic discharges over the left and right hemispheres. "Generalized" would not be the best term in this case because the activity, although bilateral over homologous head regions, is not synchronized at all times. Lateralized would not be the best descriptor because the activity is seen bilaterally.

148. A. The abrupt change in EEG amplitude is most likely the result of a generalized seizure discharge ending with postictal suppression. Prior to the attenuation, the EEG consisted of bilateral anterior-predominant spike-wave discharges suggestive of a generalized seizure. Suctioning the patient can lead to a change in EEG and even lead to rhythmic activity. It is unlikely that suctioning would cause such a prolonged generalized electrodecrement. Cerebral hypoperfusion can lead to generalized electrodecrements, although the EEG change would not be as abrupt and his vital signs and ICP are noted to be stable, making this an unlikely choice. Although high doses of propofol can lead to a low-voltage EEG, turning off propofol is unlikely to result in such an immediate, dramatic attenuation. The reference electrode helps to eliminate artifact from a signal and therefore a proper reference electrode should be distant and inactive relative to the other recording electrodes. It would be unlikely that all channels would have attenuation if the reference electrode fell off.

149. A. Although generalized burst suppression is usually associated with poor prognosis, the prognosis tends to be better if the coma is toxic-metabolic or drug-induced as opposed to hypoxic-ischemic or posttraumatic. Diffuse monomorphic nonreactive alpha activity can be associated with brainstem lesions or hypoxic-ischemic coma (alpha coma). Normal sleep features such as spindles may be seen with cyclic variability in comatose patients (spindle coma). A pattern of LVI activity alternating with high-voltage slowing may be seen in patients with Cheyne–Stokes breathing pattern. EEG reactivity, both spontaneous and stimulus-induced, is a feature important in understanding the extent of encephalopathy and coma. EEG may still be reactive despite there being no bedside clinical signs of reactivity (e.g., withdrawal or posturing) to the same external stimulus.

150. B. Lambda waves typically occur in the occipital regions bilaterally as positive waves. They are usually bilaterally synchronous but can have voltage asymmetry. Although they are mostly confined to the occipital leads, spreading to the parietal and posterior-temporal areas is common, and sometimes, the maximum may be found adjacent to the occipital region. They can be seen in any age group but are most common in children 3 to 12 years of age with an incidence of 82%. Some investigators believe that lambda waves are predictive of a prominent posterior dominant rhythm (PDR), but others doubt it. However, marked similarities between lambda waves and visual evoked responses have been reported.

151. C. The activity shown in the figure is the mu rhythm. This is commonly seen in young adults (20% of people less than 30 years), and represents the resting rhythm of the pre- and post-Rolandic cortex. It is seen in the central region with a frequency of 8 to 12 Hz. It has an arciform morphology, may appear asymmetrically, and occurs during times of relaxation and drowsiness. It is reactive to motor programming. Mu rhythm disappears with movement or the thought of movement of the contralateral arm (e.g., making a fist, wiping nose, etc.). Mu rhythm is a normal variant, not an ictal phenomenon.

152. E. Drowsiness is characterized by the appearance of hypnagogic hypersynchrony at age 3 months, consisting of rhythmic theta activity around 4 Hz with gradual increase to 6 Hz over the next few years; it becomes generalized with centro-parietal predominance before disappearing by age 6 years (it is only rarely seen until age 12 years). Dropout of PDR occurs by 2 to 3 years and is combined with the presence of mixed low-voltage slow and fast activity in older children. By adolescence, drowsiness is characterized by the mature pattern with gradual alpha dropout along with long stretches of diffuse low-voltage pattern with mixed slow and fast activity. During drowsiness, there is loss of the muscle and movement artifacts, reduction of eye blinks, and emergence of slow rolling eye movements with a frequency of 0.25 to 1.0 Hz.

153. A. NREM sleep stages are clearly defined with the development of V-waves, K-complexes, and sleep spindles. While V-waves and K-complexes may be apparent in a neonatal EEG, they are not well developed until 5 to 6 months of age. In contrast to adults, infant V-waves are higher in amplitude, have a spiky appearance, and often occur in spontaneous bursts or trains. V-waves are synchronous from birth, but may be asymmetric during early stages of sleep. The amplitude and incidence of V-waves and K-complexes decrease around 3 to 4 years of age until the adult waveforms are attained. K-complexes can be elicited with auditory stimulation

154. B. Sleep spindles appear as early as 46 to 48 weeks GA but become clearly expressed by 3 to 4 months of age, and are most abundant around 4 to 6 months. They occur in runs lasting 8 seconds or more. Sleep spindles in children under 2 years are asynchronous but should have shifting asymmetry. They are comb-shaped rather than sinusoidal, which is typical for adult spindles. Sleep spindles are fully developed, synchronous, and symmetrical by 2 years.

155. A. LPDs are seen in the left frontal/midline region. The activity is intermittent and rhythmic and has interdischarge intervals; therefore, it is not consistent with IRDA or sharply contoured polymorphic delta slowing. Sometimes, LPDs can be ictal, in which case, they tend to be more persistent and accompanied by clinical signs, such as active twitching or altered mental status. The prominent waveforms do not coincide with the QRS complexes on the EKG channel, and thus are not EKG artifact.

156. B. IRDA is activated by HV but attenuated by sleep and eye opening. It has posterior predominance in children (occipital intermittent rhythmic delta activity [OIRDA]) and anterior predominance in adults (frontal intermittent rhythmic delta activity [FIRDA]). Generalized IRDA (GIRDA) tends to be associated with enceophalopathy with a low risk of seizures. However, focal IRDA (e.g., temporal (TIRDA) and occipital (OIRDA)) are associated with an increased risk of seizures.

157. E. Compared to scalp electrodes, subdermal needle electrodes have a smaller contact area, higher input impedance, more susceptibility to noise, and less propensity to skin breakdown. Needle electrodes are short (12 to 13 mm in length) and thin (27 to 28 gauge). Their beveled edge makes them easy to insert with minimal patient discomfort. One advantage is that there is no need for abrasive skin prep, conductive paste, or adhesive use. Typical needle electrode impedances are 5 to 8K ohms, with interelectrode impedances being within 2K ohms.

158. B. IEDs may not be seen in certain forms of mesial temporal lobe epilepsy on scalp recordings. About 50% of patients with epilepsy show IEDs on the first routine EEG. Frequency of IEDs does not seem to correlate with seizure frequency. HV can activate both generalized and focal IEDs. Certain epileptic syndromes have dramatic increases in the abundance of IEDs in sleep, including LKS, continuous spike-wave pattern during slow-wave sleep (CSWS), and benign partial epilepsy of childhood with centrotemporal spikes (BECTS).

159. B. The term "sigma activity" has been used to refer to sleep spindles and to the activity in the 11 to 15 Hz range. The term "rho waves" has been used to refer to POSTS. The term "phi rhythm" has been used to refer to occipital intermittent rhythmic delta activity (OIRDA) in children. Activity above 70 Hz is generally considered as high-frequency oscillations, with the 80 to 200 Hz activity being referred to as ripples and 250 to 500 Hz activity referred to as fast ripples.

160. A. Ciganek rhythm consists of theta (typically 5 to 7 Hz) activity seen in the midline (vertex or Cz) but can be more broadly distributed. It has a notched or arciform morphology like the mu rhythm. The pattern waxes and wanes, and can react to eye opening or limb movement, although there is no strong correlation. The duration can be variable. It can be seen in wakefulness and drowsiness. It can be activated by mental task. Although once considered to be epileptiform, the pattern is now considered to be a normal variant.

161. E. The EEG shows rhythmic mid-temporal theta bursts of drowsiness (RMTD), which was previously known as psychomotor variant. Although historically it was associated with psychomotor seizures, this has not been proven and the pattern is now felt to be of unclear significance. Intermittent theta slowing has been associated with mild cerebral dysfunction, but in the setting of drowsiness, this can be a normal finding. Polymorphic theta activity can rarely be seen in temporal lobe seizures, but this is a nonspecific finding and the diagnosis cannot be made based on just that. A breach rhythm, which consists of frequent sharper and faster frequencies, is not seen.

162. C. Within 24 hours after a large middle cerebral artery (MCA) infarction, absence of delta activity and the presence of theta and fast beta frequencies within the infarcted region predict a benign course, whereas diffuse slowing in the ischemic hemisphere suggests predisposition to develop cerebral edema. Extensive infarcts causing cerebral edema and midline shift can be associated with slowing in the contralateral hemisphere and FIRDA. Epileptiform discharges and LPDs are associated with acute strokes, particularly the embolic type. Vertebrobasilar stroke with bilateral pontine infarct involving the tegmentum, manifesting with coma and bilateral motor deficits, can be associated with an alpha coma pattern (i.e., retained alpha activity nonreactive to stimuli) similar to the pattern seen after cardiac arrest and drug overdose.

163. A. Wicket spikes predominantly occur in adults older than 30 years, and have an incidence of 1% to 3%. They occur in wakefulness, light sleep, and REM sleep. They occur independently in the left and right temporal regions, typically with a midtemporal maximum. They tend to occur with a frequency of 6 to 11 Hz, either as single transients (wicket spikes) or in runs (wicket rhythm). They are commonly misinterpreted as sharp waves, especially when they occur as single sharp transients. Examining the context and determining whether they arise out of an ongoing rhythm without an after-going slow wave and without disruption of the underlying background are important in differentiating them from epileptiform discharges. They are considered to be a normal variant, not associated with underlying seizures.

164. A. Lambdoid waves, also known as positive occipital sharp transients of sleep (POSTS), are surface-positive waves that occur in the bilateral occipital region during light and deeper stages of sleep but not in REM sleep. They are similar if not identical to lambda waves in morphology and distribution and, therefore, are referred to as lambdoid waves. Unlike lambda waves, they are not seen during wakefulness. It is believed that POSTS might represent a "playback" of information to the visual cortex in order to reexamine visual material collected during the day. They are not triggered by scanning complex visual patterns, unlike lambda waves. They are relatively common, being seen in 50% to 80% of healthy adults.

165. D. EEG reactivity is present when stimulation causes the EEG to change in amplitude, frequency, and / or continuity. Some studies have shown reactivity to first appear as early as 30 to 32 weeks gestational age (GA). Note that stimulation can lead to changes in behavioral activity (e.g., movement, crying, change in breathing patterns), which may lead to artifacts mimicking EEG reactivity. In this scenario, the term infant's EEG may show diffuse flattening or a burst of slow activity in response to tactile or auditory stimuli. However, the occipital rhythmic activity noted in option D is likely artifact mimicking EEG reactivity.

166. C. Continuous focal rhythmic monomorphic slow activity suggests an underlying gray matter, not white matter, lesion. Continuous focal arrhythmic polymorphic delta activity can be seen in a brain tumor, during a migraine attack, or even in a focal seizure. On the other hand, intermittent focal rhythmic monomorphic delta activity, especially in the temporal region (i.e., temporal intermittent rhythmic delta activity [TIRDA]), can be seen interictally in temporal lobe epilepsy.

167. C. Rasmussen syndrome is a condition characterized by progressive neurologic deterioration associated with multiple seizure types with focal motor seizures (epilepsia partialis continua). In one-fifth of these children, the first seizure presents as partial or generalized convulsive status epilepticus. The EEG frequently shows persistent high-amplitude polymorphic delta activity over the affected hemisphere with interictal discharges occurring in the affected as well as the unaffected hemisphere.

168. B. The EEG shows generalized excessive beta activity, which is most likely a medication side effect, and can be seen in the setting of benzodiazepine (an anxiolytic) or barbiturate administration. The remaining choices may or may not affect the EEG; if they do, they would lead to diffuse slowing. Of note, some antipsychotic medications have led to the appearance of interictal epileptiform discharges.

169. E. As infants grow, a 3 to 4 Hz PDR may be first appreciable at 2 to 3 months. It becomes more regular and increases in frequency to 4 to 5 Hz at age 5 to 6 months and to 5 to 7 Hz by the end of the first year of life.

170. C. Sphenoidal electrodes are long and thin electrodes, typically made of stainless steel or platinum. They can be placed in a sterile manner at bedside (or under fluoroscopic guidance) such that the tip is lateral to the foramen ovale. They may be more sensitive to recording potentials from the anterior temporal lobe than surface electrodes; this view, however has been disputed. Similar potentials can be seen with use of FT9 and FT10 electrodes.

171. D. Slow transient precedes (not follows) the electrodecremental pattern in an infantile spasm. Other statements regarding the ictal correlate of generalized seizures are true. Note that tonic seizures may present either with a generalized polyspike pattern or an electrodecremental pattern.

172. B. The anterior slow activity is likely a sweat artifact. The EEG is compressed to show 30 seconds with slow frontal waves (less than 0.5 Hz) with superimposed normal activity. The large baseline sways are due to the sodium chloride and lactic acid in the sweat reacting with the electrode-gel complex. Lateral eye movements appear in the homologous anterior channels (i.e., FP1/FP2, F7/F8) with out-of-phase deflections due to the dipole effect of the eyeball (the cornea is relatively positive compared to the retina). The activity is too slow for 60-Hz artifact (or its subharmonics) or FIRDA. The morphology and distribution do not support glossokinetic artifact. Glossokinetic artifact is produced due to the polarity of the tongue, which has a negative tip and a positive root. With movement of the tongue, especially when the tongue touches the roof of the mouth or pharynx, single or rhythmic delta waves can be seen diffusely with a frontal predominance.

173. B. TIRDA is specific for seizure disorder. Other patterns are nonspecific and do not necessarily indicate potential epileptogenicity. However, recent reports suggest that GRDA may be associated with predisposition to seizures, especially in critically ill patients.

174. D. Generalized slowing and an increase in amplitude may depict onset of drowsiness. However, correlating the background with clinical observation is difficult at this age because infants may still have their eyes open when drowsy. Decrease in movement and muscle tone are also helpful in determining drowsiness. Temporal slowing can be a normal finding during drowsiness in the elderly.

175. D. In SSPE, the periodic complexes occur in the second stage and are specific to the illness. It is a very reliable and highly contributory diagnostic finding in this disease. The discharges in SSPE have generalized distribution with fronto-central predominance, more prominent in wakefulness, last 0.5 to 3 seconds, have mean amplitude of 500 μV, occur at an interval of 4 to 15 seconds (0.06–0.25 Hz), and may be accompanied by myoclonus. In HSE, the periodic discharges occur in the temporal region at 2- to 4-second intervals (0.25–0.5 Hz), last 70 to 150 ms and have 100 to 500 μV amplitude. In CJD, the periodic discharges may have triphasic morphology, last 100 to 300 ms, and occur at a frequency of 0.5 to 2 Hz; these discharges have a frontal predominance (may show occipital predominance in the Heidenhain variant), tend to disappear during sleep, and may be associated with myoclonus. Periodic lateralized epileptiform discharges (PLEDs) are most commonly seen after acute stroke but may also be associated with tumors, inflammatory disorders (HSE, infectious mononucleosis encephalitis), and seizures, especially status epilepticus. PLEDs typically have 100 to 300 μV amplitude and occur at a frequency of 0.2 to 3 Hz. The maximum is usually over the posterior–temporal region (boundary zone between middle and posterior cerebral territories). PLEDs can be associated with focal motor twitching on the contralateral side (face, extremities).

176. C. The standard paper speed of EEG recordings in the United States is 30 mm/sec, which on traditional digital displays results in displaying 10 seconds of EEG per page (i.e., screen). Faster paper speeds (e.g., 60 mm/sec), which result in reduced number of seconds per page (e.g., 5 sec/page), can be used to evaluate high-frequency or closely spaced activity. Slower paper speeds (e.g., 15 mm/sec), which result in an increased number of seconds per page (e.g., 20 sec/page), can be used to evaluate slower frequencies.

177. C. The EEG shows occipital interictal epileptiform discharges (IEDs). Therefore, partial (localization-related, focal) epilepsy with occipital potential epileptogenicity is the most likely diagnosis. Panayiotopoulos syndrome, the early-onset form of benign occipital epilepsy of childhood, could present with occipital discharges but typically presents at an average age of 5 years (typical range: 2–12 years). Although the background otherwise looks normal, the presence of interictal discharges makes a normal awake study incorrect. Idiopathic generalized epilepsy syndromes can present with bioccipital predominance; this is typically seen in children and not in adults, in whom a more anterior predominance is noted. Lennox–Gastaut syndrome is a symptomatic generalized epilepsy syndrome presenting with slow spike-wave discharges in the setting of background slowing, neither of which are not seen here.

178. B. In the EEG in the question, the eye blink deflection is seen on the right but not on the left. Among the choices, enucleation is the most likely reason. The eyeball acts as a dipole with the cornea being relatively positive compared to the retina. With eye closure, the eyeball rotates about its horizontal and vertical axes as it moves superior and lateral, respectively (referred to as the Bell phenomena). During REM sleep, fast horizontal movements can be seen which would result in waveforms of opposite, not absent, polarities in the frontal channels. Misplaced Fp1 electrode is not the likely answer because the eye blink artifact is not seen in F3–C3 (left) but is clearly seen in F4–C4 (right). Bell's palsy results in abnormal eyelid closure but not in abnormal eye movements; therefore, the EEG should appear normal. Sweat artifact appears as slow frontal waves (less than 0.5 Hz) with superimposed normal activity, which is not seen here.

179. B. At 3 months of age, the distinctive pattern of hypnagogic hypersynchrony appears, replacing the high amplitude 2 to 3 Hz rhythm seen during drowsiness. By 6 to 8 months, nearly 100% of normal infants display this drowsy pattern. It usually disappears by 6 years. It is only rarely (~10%) seen in children after age 6 years. This high-amplitude, synchronous, rhythmic 3 to 6 Hz activity can be paroxysmal or continuous for several minutes either at the beginning or at the end of the sleep cycle. When occurring at the end of sleep, the arousal transition is often referred to as hypnopompic hypersynchrony.

180. A. The background is usually abnormal in between LPDs because they represent a high degree of cortical irritability. They occur at a frequency of 0.05 to 2 Hz and have a biphasic or triphasic morphology. LPDs usually represent an interictal pattern associated with a high risk of seizures, but they fall on the ictal-interictal continuum, and therefore, they can be a manifestation of ictal activity. LPDs are difficult to suppress with antiseizure medications, but many will attenuate at the underlying brain pathology resolves. LPDs are usually unilateral but may have a field in the contralateral hemisphere. In addition, LPDs can occur bilaterally and independently, collectively referred to as bilateral periodic discharges (biPDs). When this occurs, the frequency, morphology, and distribution of each LPD is usually independent of each other. The occurrence of biPDs on EEG generally portends a worse prognosis than LPDs.

181. B. Hypnagogic hypersynchrony is a normal pattern in infants (as early as 3 months) and children. It is seen during transition from drowsiness (N1) to sleep (N2), but not after N2 sleep is reached. It consists of diffuse, anteriorly predominant, high-amplitude, paroxysmal, rhythmic bursts with a frequency of 3 to 5 Hz. The pattern can be continuous when seen in infancy and becomes more paroxysmal after infancy. It starts to disappear around age 6 years and typically rare after that age. It is not associated with sharp waves. Hypsarrhythmia, seen in West syndrome, is characterized by high-amplitude disorganized slowing intermixed with multifocal sharp waves. In children through young adults, hyperventilation may lead to buildup of high-amplitude or hypersynchronous background slowing.

182. C. The PDR (i.e., alpha rhythm) is usually found over occipital, parietal, and posterior-temporal regions but may extend into central regions. It is attenuated by visual stimuli (eye opening), and by auditory, tactile, and other somatosensory stimuli. It is also attenuated (not enhanced) by heightened mental activity (such as solving difficult arithmetical problems). However, the attenuation with eye opening tends to be more pronounced than the other stimuli. The menstrual cycle has been shown to affect the alpha rhythm: its frequency increases during preovulatory and premenstrual phases and decreases during postovulation (luteal) and menstrual phases. The PDR may also appear as a subharmonic, slow alpha variant, typically occurring at half of the patient's typical PDR. A fast, supraharmonic, variant can also be seen, typically occurring at double the patient's typical PDR.

183. B. By 3 months of age, the awake portion of the EEG shows a distinguishable 3 to 4 Hz PDR as well as a rhythmic centrally dominant 5 to 8 Hz background. Because the infant's eyes are usually open during the awake portion, central rhythmic activity is more identifiable than the PDR. However, if the technologist passively closes the infant's eyes for a few seconds, the PDR may become more apparent.

184. B. Ctenoids (also known as 14- and 6-Hz positive bursts) are comb-shaped in appearance, and consist of 14- or 6-Hz positive bursts. They appear around age 3 to 4 years, but are more commonly seen in children and adolescents, especially those aged 13 to 14 years. The reported incidence is 58% in normal teenagers and 12% in healthy adults. They are typically seen in the posterior–temporal regions, unilaterally or bilaterally, with shifting predominance. They are typically seen during drowsiness or light sleep. They occur in short trains of less than 2 seconds.

185. C. Solid tumors are not generally epileptogenic in themselves. Seizures are typically caused by the infiltrated or surrounding nontumor tissue except in developmental tumors such as hypothalamic hamartoma. Seizures are more common with low-grade than high-grade tumors, with up to 90% of patients with low-grade astrocytomas manifesting with seizures at some point. In up to one-third of patients, the seizure focus localizes to an area remote from the tumor site. EEG abnormalities in nondevelopmental tumors are usually due to displacement of normal tissue, alteration of neuronal circuitry or neurotransmitters, ischemia, or hemosiderin deposition. LPDs are signs of cortical irritability and can be seen in the setting of brain tumors.

186. C. Posterior slow waves of youth (also known as sail waves or posterior fused transients) are 2 to 4 Hz delta waves, seen bisynchronously with shifting asymmetry in the occipital region. They are considered part of the normal alpha rhythm although the voltages may be high compared to the background rhythm. They typically form a complex that consists of the slow delta component with superimposed and following alpha rhythm of the waking background, hence the term "fused." They are typically seen in adolescents 6 to 12 years old, and are rare before age 2 years or after 21 years. They are best seen with eyes closed in a relaxed wakefulness. They attenuate with eye opening, increase with hyperventilation (HV), and disappear in drowsiness. They occur as sporadic single waves or in bursts interspersed by one or several seconds or regular background activity.

187. A. In adults, HV for 3 to 5 minutes is commonly performed as an activation method. The technologist usually tries to double the base breathing rate, and to have the subject exhale more deeply than usual. This act causes the subject to exhale excessive amounts of CO_2, leading to a drop in $PaCO_2$ and hypocapnia. The hypocapnia can cause mild cerebral vasoconstriction and mild cerebral hypoxia. HV may bring out focal or generalized slowing in cases of structural disease or diffuse encephalopathic disorders. HV-induced diffuse slowing usually disappears rapidly after stopping HV, but it may persist for up to 30 seconds in normal adults; further persistence at any age, by itself, is not necessarily abnormal. HV-induced slowing is enhanced by an upright position as opposed to a recumbent position, probably as a result of relative cerebral anoxia. In adults, a low blood glucose level (less than 80 mg/dL) tends to enhance the slow waves, whereas a high level (greater than 120 mg/dL) tends to inhibit such an effect. HV can also bring out interictal epileptiform discharges (IEDs) or trigger more overt seizures. Although any seizure can be triggered during hyperventilation, those with primary idiopathic generalized epilepsy are more susceptible.

188. D. The EEG electrode nomenclature for the most part has remained unchanged over the years. In general, the even-numbered electrodes are placed over the right hemisphere while the odd-numbered electrodes are placed over the left hemisphere. The midline electrodes are followed by "z," the ear electrodes are labeled "A," and the mastoid electrodes are labeled "M." More recently, higher density arrays have been used such as the 10-10 system with modified combinatorial nomenclature (MCN), which introduces new letter codes for the intermediate electrode placements (e.g., FT between F and T and TP between T and P).

189. A. The resulting sensitivity is 5 μV/mm. The channel FP1–F3 equals –10 μV, which equals the 2 mm deflection; this would result in a sensitivity of 5 μV/mm [ABS (10/2)]. Sensitivity cannot be a negative number.

190. C. The EEG shows a 5 to 6 Hz rhythm in the bioccipital region. Although no clear state is discernible, one possibility is slow alpha variant, which is the posterior dominant rhythm (PDR) occurring at a subharmonic frequency. No event was noted on the EEG, so psychogenic nonepileptic event and scalp-negative epileptic seizure discharge are not correct. Of note, the diagnosis of a psychogenic nonepileptic event requires video and adequate patient testing. The lack of delta-range activity and the advanced patient age make OIRDA unlikely as well. POSTS have a biphasic (checkmark) morphology with initial positivity, can appear in trains up to 4 to 5 Hz, and are usually seen in light sleep appearing before the alpha rhythm completely disappears in drowsiness. This is not seen here. Therefore, slow alpha variant is the best answer among all the choices.

191. D. Myoclonic seizure is characterized by spike-and-wave or polyspike-and-wave discharge, not an electrodecremental pattern. Tonic, atonic, and spasms can be associated with an electrodecremental ictal EEG pattern.

192. E. The EEG in the question shows left temporal interictal epileptiform discharges and intermittent polymorphic delta activity, consistent with left temporal potential epileptogenicity. Accordingly, postictal nose wiping with the left hand can be seen in patients with left temporal onset seizures, and seems to be the most appropriate answer. Grunting and bilateral asymmetric posturing are more commonly seen in frontal lobe seizures. Dystonic posturing of the left hand would likely be seen in right temporal, not left temporal, seizures. RINCH movements typically occur in the hand contralateral to the seizure focus in temporal lobe epilepsy.

193. D. The EEG shows left parasagittal activity that evolves in frequency, morphology, and distribution consistent with a seizure (i.e., ictal) discharge. There are no periodic discharges. In addition, there is brief intermittent (not continuous) rhythmic delta activity. Although the patient has a skull defect, breach rhythm is not noted in the EEG. An asymmetric PDR can be seen with localized cerebral lesions and could be expected in this patient. However, in the epoch provided, a PDR cannot be appreciated and therefore, the extent of side-to-side symmetry cannot be determined.

194. C. An interpeak duration of 100 ms equates to about 10 Hz, which is within the normal PDR range for a 15-year-old child. 25 ms equates to about a 40 Hz frequency, 70 ms equates to about a 14 Hz frequency, 150 ms equates to about a 7 Hz frequency, and 200 ms equates to about a 5 Hz frequency, all of which would not be consistent with a normal PDR. This is calculated as follows: Frequency (Hz) = 1000 ms (1 second) / Interpeak duration (ms).

195. A. The EEG in the question shows lateralized sharply contoured activity over the left hemisphere, maximal in the temporal region. The most appropriate clinical scenario to explain that would be an acute left MCA stroke. Lithium overdose may present with diffuse periodic complexes. Those with early-onset Alzheimer's disease may have a normal EEG, but if abnormal, it may show mild cerebral dysfunction presenting as a slow posterior dominant rhythm (PDR) and/or intermittent diffuse theta or polymorphic delta activity. In patients with brainstem glioma, the EEG is more often abnormal in children than in adults and could show slowing, which can be posteriorly predominant and bilateral. Intermittent rhythmic delta activity (IRDA) may be observed, especially if hydrocephalus is present. Gangliogliomas are slow growing and rarely malignant tumors frequently found in the temporal lobe and can lead to seizures, making option E a possible answer choice. However, a 12 Hz PDR is noted in the latter half of the epoch which would unusual in a 1-year old child; PDR (typically, about 5 to 7 Hz at this age).

196. C. Elimination of visual fixation rather than darkness activates paroxysmal occipital activity in benign occipital epilepsy of childhood, which can be classified as early-onset (known as Panayiotopoulos type) and late-onset (known as Gastaut type). The early-onset type may present with autonomic features, behavioral disturbances, headache, vomiting, and change in awareness, whereas the late-onset type may present with visual hallucinations, ictal blindness, or feeling of ocular movement or pain. Although both types present with large-amplitude interictal epileptiform discharges (IEDs) resembling those seen in benign Rolandic epilepsy (BRE), extra-occipital spikes are more frequently seen in the early-onset type occurring in a unilateral, bilaterally independent, or bilaterally synchronous distribution. They can attenuate with eye opening and reoccur with eye closure. The early-onset type also has ictal discharges that present with rhythmic theta or delta activity vs the late-onset type, which presents with faster rhythms.

197. E. Reliable predictors of death or persistent vegetative state after cardiac arrest include absence of early cortical somatosensory evoked potentials, electrographic seizures, suppressed EEG (less than 5 μV amplitude), and burst-suppression pattern. Spindle coma pattern indicates relative integrity of the cerebral hemispheres; its prognostic significance depends on the underlying etiology with best outcomes reported when the coma is due to drugs, encephalopathy, or seizures. With posttraumatic coma, normal-looking sleep spindles carry a good prognosis. The absence of spindles after anoxia is associated with poor outcome, whereas its presence does not necessarily indicate a favorable prognosis.

198. B. ECI recordings need to be at least 30 minutes long to be in accordance with the ACNS guidelines (Guideline 6: Minimum Technical Standards for EEG Recording in Suspected Cerebral Death). Other guidelines include the use of a full set of conventional 10 to 20 scalp electrodes since the study may or may not be ECI; interelectrode impedances should be between 100 and 10K ohms; the integrity of the entire recording system should be tested (i.e., touching each electrode to create an artifact potential on the recording); interelectrode distances should be at least 10 cm; sensitivity must be increased to at least 2 μV/mm for at least 30 minutes of the recording with inclusion of appropriate calibrations (i.e., use a 2 or 5 μV calibration signal instead of a 50 μV signal); filter settings should be set such that the low-frequency filter is no higher than 1 Hz and the high-frequency filter is no lower than 30 Hz; additional signals can be monitored (e.g., EKG); if muscle artifact is significant, then the use of a short-acting neuromuscular blockade may be necessary; no reactivity to intense stimulation (e.g., auditory, visual, tactile); recordings should be done by a qualified technologist (of note, not mandated to be R.EEG.T. certified) working under the supervision of a qualified electroencephalographer; and repeat EEG should be done if there is any doubt of ECI. Of note, routine, non-ECI EEGs should be at least 20 minutes to be in accordance with the ACNS guidelines (Guideline 1: Minimum Technical Requirements for Performing Clinical EEG).

199. B. FAR is seen in the frontal region, more commonly in children. It has theta or alpha range frequency with a morphology that could be notched. The pattern can last as long as 20 seconds. It is typically seen during sleep-to-wake transitions but is not apparent during maximal arousal. This pattern is generally considered to be nonspecific, although association with cerebral dysfunction or seizures has been shown in case series.

200. C. The sharper and faster frequencies seen over the right temporal region are consistent with a breach rhythm, likely from the skull defect (see axial CT head image below showing the two skull defects on the right side of the head). There was no activity that appeared periodic without evolution to suggest LPDs. The faster frequencies were more persistent and not paroxysmal. There was no appreciable evolution to suggest a seizure. The activity did not appear to disrupt the background or have morphology suggestive of IEDs.

201. C. Neonatal seizures are never generalized, due to the premature interhemispheric connections, and thus are focal or multifocal. They typically start in the central or temporal region, and out of an abnormal EEG background. Seizures are not seen in neonates less than 34-week conceptual age.

202. D. The phantom spike-and-wave pattern is usually diffuse, bilaterally symmetric, and synchronous with predominance over the anterior or posterior head regions with a frequency of 5 to 7 Hz (usually 6 Hz). Two distinct subtypes of this pattern have been proposed: WHAM (wake, high amplitude, anterior location, male gender) and FOLD (female gender, occipital location, low amplitude, lrowsiness). It is further suggested that the WHAM pattern is more likely associated with seizures. Current consensus is that this EEG pattern is of unclear clinical significance; however, high amplitude of the spikes, frequency less than 6 Hz, and persistence of the discharges in deeper stages of sleep are more likely associated with seizures. It is felt that most of the 6-Hz spike-and-wave bursts are part of the 14- and 6-Hz positive bursts, and the transition between these two patterns may lead to occurrence of both patterns in the same person.

203. B. Using ipsilateral ear reference to evaluate changes in the temporal region may result in cancellation of desired waveforms, because the ipsilateral ear electrodes may be part of the electrical field. Increasing the interelectrode distance between the recording and reference electrodes tends to allow for better visualization of regional waveforms. Cz is a typical reference used to visualize temporal changes because the vertex is not typically affected, but may not be the best reference to use in sleep. Contralateral ear reference measures the difference across the head and allows for good visualization, but this montage may not be helpful if there is synchronous bitemporal activity because the ear electrodes can reflect the ipsilateral temporal activity and cancel desired waveforms. Average reference can be used in most cases because the majority of the electrodes that comprise the average reference tend to be unaffected. Each channel in the Laplacian montage is referenced to an average of the electrodes surrounding it, thereby eliminating widespread activity and emphasizing the localized waveforms.

204. C. Cerebral hypoperfusion is the most likely cause of the decreased EEG amplitude as there was bradycardia that progressed to asystole. The progression of his EEG from his baseline heart rate to asystole is illustrated in five successive EEG epochs (filter 1–70 Hz) below. Typically, as cerebral blood flow (CBF; measured as milliliters of blood per 100 g of brain tissue per minute) relates to the EEG changes as follows: normal (above 35); loss of beta frequencies (25–35); theta slowing (18–25); polymorphic delta slowing (12–18); suppression of all frequencies (less than 10). Of note, ischemia or reversible injury is felt to occur at CBF between 10 and 35, while infarct or irreversible injury is felt to occur at CBF less than 10. The EEG changes occurred in parallel with the decreasing heart rate, which was about 30 beats per minute at the beginning of the epoch and asystole by the end of the epoch. A generalized seizure discharge ending with postictal suppression would present with more of an abrupt change in EEG. Suctioning the patient can lead to a change in EEG and even lead to rhythmic activity. It is unlikely that suctioning would cause such a prolonged generalized electrodecrement. Although high doses of propofol can lead to a low-voltage EEG, starting propofol without a bolus is unlikely to do it. Salt bridges between two electrodes can result in a channel that is relatively isoelectric, but it would not result in diffuse attenuation as seen here.

205. C. Goodwin described this normal variant in 1947. The slow alpha variant is a subharmonic, typically occurring at half of the patient's typical PDR. The fast variant is a supraharmonic, typically occurring at double the patient's typical PDR. Both occur in the posterior head regions with eye closure. Sometimes, the alpha rhythm speeds up immediately after eye closure; this so-called alpha squeak should not be confused with the fast alpha variant.

206. B. In NCL, EEG background activity is attenuated, disorganized, or slow. Occipital spike-wave discharges in response to slow, 1 to 2 Hz photic stimulation is seen in late infantile NCL. Visual evoked potentials are usually abnormal or unrecordable, particularly in infantile NCL. Similarly, somatosensory evoked potentials also tend to be abnormal, either attenuated or of high amplitude (giant waveforms).

207. C. Wicket spikes occur in wakefulness, light sleep, and REM sleep, unlike epileptiform discharges that increase in deeper stages of sleep. They usually occur singly or in short runs with a frequency of 6 to 11 Hz (wicket rhythm). They typically occur in the temporal regions with shifting predominance. The morphology is sharp, monophasic, or arciform without an aftergoing slow wave, unlike epileptiform discharges, which have a more complex morphology, sometimes with an aftergoing slow wave. The amplitude of wickets may be high (up to 200 μV), but the transients arise out of an ongoing rhythm and do not stand out. Wicket spikes are commonly misinterpreted as sharp waves, especially when they occur as single transients. Examining the context and determining whether they arise out of an ongoing rhythm along with the presence of an aftergoing slow wave and disruption of the underlying background are important in differentiating them from epileptiform discharges. Among the choices, monophasic morphology is the only feature of wicket spikes that serves to differentiate them from epileptiform spikes.

208. D. This pattern is the least pathognomonic as it can be seen in acute stroke, tumor, infection, abscess, seizure disorders interictally, and recovery phase of status epilepticus. The first three patterns are specific for sporadic Creutzfeldt–Jakob disease (sCJD; option A), subacute sclerosing panencephalitis (SSPE; option B), and herpes simplex encephalitis (HSE; option C). Note that variant CJD does not typically present with generalized periodic discharges (GPDs). Option E is highly suggestive of a toxic-metabolic etiology. In one study evaluating patients with GPDs with triphasic morphology, 56% had hepatic encephalopathy and 20% had uremic encephalopathy. Although option E is not as specific as options A to C, it is more pathognomonic than option D.

209. A. Subdural strips and grids are discs embedded in a plastic or silicone sheet that are surgically placed to cover the cortex. They are not usually susceptible to motion or muscle artifacts, or signal filtering effects of the dura and scalp. In addition to measuring EEG activity, they can be used to stimulate and map the eloquent cortex. When used for epilepsy monitoring, they are typically implanted for up to 1 to 2 weeks. Associated morbidity from subdural grids includes cerebral edema, hemorrhage, and infection. They can be used in conjunction with stereotactically implanted depth electrodes.

210. A. Phantom spike-wave discharges occur at a frequency of 6 Hz. It is best seen in drowsiness. The spike component is rather small and tends to be positive. It is usually seen in adults. About 50% to 60% of the patients have a history of seizures while others have a history of syncope, posttraumatic states, or psychiatric conditions. This is an uncommon pattern with a prevalence of 0.5% to 1%. The 6-Hz phantom spike waves are divided into two types: WHAM (Wake, High-amplitude, Anterior, Male) and FOLD (Female, Occipital, Low-amplitude, Drowsy). It has been reported that patients with anterior (frontal) 6-Hz spike waves are more likely to have epileptic seizures, whereas those with posterior (occipital) discharges are more likely to have neuroautonomic disturbances. Rudimentary spike-wave discharges (pseudo petit mal discharges) consist of bursts of generalized high-voltage 3 to 4 Hz waves with a poorly developed spike in the positive trough between the slow waves, typically seen in drowsiness. This pattern is most prominent over parietal areas, and can be seen in infants and children with hypnagogic hypersynchrony. These bursts may contain small spikes (i.e., rudimentary spike waves). They are not believed to transition into the classic spike-wave patterns associated with seizures. Needlelike occipital spikes are seen in congenitally blind children. They are unrelated to seizure disorder, and probably represent functional deafferentation. These discharges disappear during childhood or adolescence.

211. A. Cone waves, also known as O waves, are surface-positive, monophasic or diphasic, high-amplitude, "cone-shaped" delta waves that are seen in the posterior head regions. They are commonly observed during light and deeper stages of sleep. They are interspersed with slow delta waves of sleep. They appear around 6 months of age when sleep patterns evolve from the QS patterns of neonates to the adult NREM patterns, and persist up to 5 years of age. Although the cone waves are sometimes mistaken for abnormal sharp-wave or slow-wave activity, they do not increase the risk for epileptic seizures.

212. D. In the longitudinal bipolar montage (left panel), the phase reversals are at C3 and T7. In the transverse bipolar montage (right panel), the phase reversals are at F7 and T7. Therefore, the maximal negative potential is at T7.

213. C. The frequency of the PDR is expected to be 8 Hz by 3 years and 10 Hz by 10 to 15 years. By adolescence, drowsiness is characterized by the mature pattern, with gradual alpha dropout along with long stretches of diffuse low-voltage pattern with mixed slow and fast activity. The photic driving response appears around 3 to 4 months. Driving is best seen below 8 Hz flash frequency in children 3 to 5 years of age, and at 6 to 16 Hz in children 6 to 12 years of age. Healthy adolescents may occasionally exhibit photomyoclonic as well as photoconvulsive responses with intermittent photic stimulation (IPS). Prolonged rhythmic sharp or spiky activity over the midline frontal region, called frontal arousal rhythm (FAR), is typically seen in children aged 2 to 4 years but not in adolescents.

214. C. $PaCO_2$ falls continuously during HV and begins to increase immediately after cessation of HV. On the other hand, PaO_2 increases during HV but falls to an average of 25 mmHg below baseline around 5 minutes after cessation of HV. Post-HV decline in PaO_2 has been felt to be related to hypocapnia-induced hypopnea. Thus, in patients with borderline cerebral perfusion, HV can be deleterious because of hypocapnia-induced vasoconstriction and shunting, post-HV hypoxia, or both. HV is contraindicated in patients with acute stroke, recent intracranial hemorrhage, transient ischemic attack (TIA), moyamoya disease, severe cardiopulmonary disease, and sickle cell disease or trait.

215. A. Neonatal seizures are never generalized, due to the premature interhemispheric connections, and thus are focal or multifocal, typically starting in the central or temporal regions. They are uncommon before 34 weeks of CA. The evolution of neonatal seizures can be highly variable, including onset in one hemisphere and termination in the opposite hemisphere. They can present as brief apneic periods.

216. D. SSS are also known as benign epileptiform transients of sleep (BETS). They are mainly seen in adults. They occur sporadically (not in trains) so they are also known as benign sporadic sleep spikes (BSSS). Their duration is usually less than 50 ms and the amplitude is less than 50 μV. They are relatively common, occurring in 25% of normal EEG records. They are not associated with epilepsy. However, they have been correlated with psychotic disorders.

217. E. FIRDA tends to have no interval between consecutive waveforms of monomorphic morphology. If intervals were present, then the pattern would be better classified as a periodic pattern, such as generalized periodic discharges (GPDs) that are anterior predominant. FIRDA can be a normal finding post-HV and during drowsiness in the elderly. It can also be an abnormal finding suggestive of encephalopathy in such clinical scenarios as sepsis and hydrocephalus.

218. E. Photosensitive response is not a specifically defined response during IPS. Photic stimulation can be traced back to ancient Greece using the potter's wheel to screen those with seizures. The use of IPS for EEG was reported around 1934. The responses that can be seen during IPS include photic driving, photomyogenic (photomyoclonic) response, photoparoxysmal (photoconvulsive) response, and photoelectric response. Photic driving response refers to activity in the posterior head regions time-locked to the photic stimulus and occurring at the same or harmonic frequency of the stimulus frequency. PMR refers to the appearance of brief repetitive muscle spikes over the anterior head regions. They often increase in amplitude as stimulation continues and stop promptly when the stimulus is withdrawn. PMR can be associated with eyelid flutter or discrete muscle twitches involving the face and head. PPR refers to the generalized, bisynchronous, spike-and-wave or polyspike-and-wave discharges that occur during IPS and typically outlast the stimulus by a few seconds. They may be accompanied by impairment of consciousness or brisk jerks involving predominantly the upper extremities and head. Photoelectric response is actually an artifact during IPS where each flash causes a photochemical reaction in the electrode with high impedance, resulting in brief spike-like transients in the electrode simultaneously with the flash. Photoelectric artifact disappears when the involved electrode is covered.

219. D. The EEG waveforms that occur after scanning a complex pattern in a brightly lit room are known as lambda waves. Typically, they are confined to the occipital leads but spread to the parietal and posterior–temporal areas is common. Sometimes, the maximum may be found adjacent to the occipital region. However, they are not seen in the frontal region. They are triangular, biphasic or triphasic waves with the most prominent phase being positive, which may be preceded and followed by a negative component. Typically, their amplitude is 20 to 50 μV and duration is 160 to 250 ms. They occur during wakefulness and are most evident when the subject scans a complex picture in a well-lit room; they are also time-locked to saccadic eye movements. Most lambda waves follow an exploratory eye movement with a mean latency of 78 ms. They tend to disappear with eye closure, removal of the visual stimuli, or turning off the lights. They cannot be triggered by hypnotic suggestion of a test picture. They are felt to represent an evoked response to a visual stimulus in association with scanning movements of the eyes. Lambda waves occur when reading and occasionally when watching TV. Their morphology and distribution are similar to positive occipital sharp transients of sleep (POSTS).

220. C. The EEG shows an asymmetric posterior dominant rhythm with a well-formed 10 Hz, 50 to 100 μV rhythm on the right, and a poorly formed, 10 to 25 μV, often difficult-to-recognize rhythm on the left. This is most suggestive of left hemispheric dysfunction. Although differences in the amplitude of the posterior dominant rhythm (PDR) alone may not be significant, asymmetries in frequency and regulation of the PDR are much more suggestive of a focal lesion as in this case. While the causative lesion may be at some distance from the occipital pole, the lesion is usually ipsilateral to the abnormal PDR, in this case the left. There is no clear evolution to suggest a seizure discharge. Although a breach rhythm can present with higher amplitude activity, there also tends to be superimposed faster and sharper activity that does not change with eye opening or closure. There is no temporal theta activity nor does it represent an interictal epileptiform abnormality.

221. A. Occasionally, one sees occipital positive sharp slow waves (lambda waves) in the record of a patient who is awake and actively reading or scanning the room. These waves tend to be asymmetric and raise the possibility of a focal abnormality. The lambda waves are identified by having the patient reproduce the maneuver that caused the waves to appear. Eye closure will block the normal lambda wave but usually not have an effect on the abnormal activity. The lambda waves can also be blocked by having the patient look at a plain piece of paper. Of note, lambda waves are not seen when doing mental tasks.

Refer to the following figure (filter 1–70 Hz; solid vertical lines are 1 second apart) for Questions 222 to 225.

222. A. The tracing represents an awake EEG depicting how the EEG changes with eyes open (Point 1) and eyes closed (Point 2). In general, the posterior dominant rhythm (PDR), which is typically greater than 8.5 Hz and seen over the parieto-occipital region, is more robust in the awake, restful state with the eyes closed, as shown at Point 2. The PDR attenuates with eye opening, as shown in Point 1. There is no clear attenuation of the PDR at Point 2 to suggest drowsiness. There are no rapid eye movements or changes in the background to suggest REM sleep.

223. D. At Point 2, posterior dominant rhythm (PDR) is seen. Normal PDR is typically between 8.5 and 12 Hz and follows a normal distribution, centering around 10.0 Hz. However, in less than 2% of people, no overt PDR is appreciable, and in less than 7% of people, a low-voltage PDR is seen. In such cases, increasing the interelectrode distances can increase the sensitivity of detecting a PDR. Normal PDR attenuates with eye opening. Varying CBF can vary the PDR by up to 2 Hz. Earlier studies have shown that the PDR may slow by 1 Hz every decade after the age of 50 years but the PDR does not appear to decrease beyond 8 to 8.5 Hz typically in healthy elderly controls. The frequency increases by approximately 0.3 Hz during the follicular phase of the menstrual cycle. Ambient light has no effect on PDR.

224. E. The activity seen at Point 2 is the posterior dominant rhythm (PDR), which is most prominent over the posterior head regions. In most people, the PDR is most prominent over the occipital region, although the PDR has a broader field in about a third of healthy adults. The PDR can be seen over the parietal and posterior–temporal head regions and may also extend into central regions. The PDR does not typically extend to the frontal region.

225. C. The activity seen at Point 2 is the posterior dominant rhythm (PDR). About 60% have a side-to-side amplitude asymmetry with the right side being higher except in some left-handed people. Up to 50% amplitude asymmetry is typically considered normal; however, given the right-sided amplitude predominance, asymmetry of 35% to 50% could be considered abnormal when the lower voltage is on the right. The amplitude of the PDR tends to decrease with age because of thickening of the skull, which attenuates the amplitude. In most people, the PDR amplitude decreases with eye opening and with mental effort, such as doing simple math.

226. E. A slow PDR even without generalized slowing may be the only finding in a patient with mild encephalopathy. EEG patterns in encephalopathy and coma are often nonspecific but in some cases suggest or narrow down potential etiologies. In agitated delirium, the agitation and the fluctuating nature of the mental status implies the presence of a reactive EEG. An increase in delta activity with stimulation is considered reactivity and does not portend a poor prognosis. When seen in a comatose patient, it can be considered a paradoxical arousal response. Patients that have encephalopathic EEG patterns can also have intermittent seizures, which can only be captured with continuous EEG. Therefore, in certain situations, some recommend continuous EEG monitoring for at least 12 to 24 to increase the yield of detecting nonconvulsive seizures.

227. B. Encephalopathy can be classified as mild, moderate, severe, and ECI. In general, mild encephalopathy refers to slowing of the posterior dominant rhythm (typically less than or equal to 8 Hz), more reactive theta than delta activity, preservation of some sleep architecture. Moderate encephalopathy has state changes, loss of the PDR, and increased amount of delta slowing. Severe encephalopathy has predominately delta slowing (but can have mixed faster frequencies), diffuse electrodecremental segments or background attenuation, and no reactivity or state changes. ECI has EEG activity less than two microvolts.

228. D. The EEG shows generalized triphasic waves (also known as generalized periodic discharges with triphasic morphology), which are associated with a number of different clinical scenarios including hypoxic ischemic insults, metabolic disarray (e.g., hepatic and uremic states; hypercalcemia; hyperthyroidism), status epilepticus, drug intoxication (e.g., baclofen and lithium toxicities), and neurodegenerative states (e.g., Creutzfeldt–Jakob disease [CJD]). Changes in potassium do not typically lead to EEG changes.

229. D. This EEG shows a slow posterior dominant rhythm (PDR) of 7 to 7.5 Hz, which is abnormal even given the advanced age. Even in centarians, a PDR is still greater than

8 Hz. The eye blink artifact indicates a wakeful, nondrowsy state. In addition, no sleep architecture is noted to suggest sleep.

230. A. The EEG in Huntington's disease has a characteristic low-voltage background (<10 microvolts), making hard it to appreciate the posterior dominant rhythm (PDR). Although about 10% of the normal population have a low-voltage EEG less than 20 microvolts, it is unusual for the voltages to be less than 10 microvolts. Hyperventilation can increase the PDR amplitude in normal individuals, but this is not seen in Huntington's disease. In addition, sleep architecture, including vertex sharp waves, sleep spindles, and K-complexes, have lower amplitudes. Amplitudes attenuation rather than latency delays are seen in visual-evoked potentials and median nerve somatosensory-evoked potentials.

231. B. The most likely statement of the listed choices is that the patient has had a stroke. The EEG shows right posterior quadrant lateralized periodic discharges (LPDs) with a frequency of about 1 Hz. LPDs are a maker of cortical irritability and can be seen in variety of clinical scenarios, including focal (not primary generalized) seizures, strokes, tumors, and infection. Although LPDs tend to represent interictal activity with respect to seizures, in rare situations, they can represent ictal activity. There is no evolution of the LPDs to suggest an ictal discharge or a tonic seizure in this patient. This patient is not likely comatose due to the movement artifact and the slow posterior dominant rhythm (PDR) seen over the left posterior quadrant. The right parietooccipital stroke is the reason for the asymmetric PDR.

232. E. Continuous EEG monitoring is commonly used to detect nonconvulsive seizures. However, it can also be used to monitor depth of coma, to monitor ischemia (e.g., vasospasm in subarachnoid hemorrhage), in prognostication (e.g., poststatus epilepticus or postcardiac arrest), or to diagnose conversion disorders (e.g., episodic loss of consciousness). The diagnosis of brain death is a clinical diagnosis. EEG is not required but can serve as an aid in the diagnosis. If used, there are specific criteria and guidelines (e.g., Guideline 6: Minimum Technical Standards for EEG Recording in Suspected Cerebral Death by the American Clinical Neurophysiology Society) that need to be followed. In the ACNS guideline, the minimum recommended duration of the EEG is 30 minutes. However, recording continuous EEG is not typically needed in most situations.

233. B. The patient is in a burst-suppression state with high amplitude bursts alternating with periods of suppression, which based solely on this epoch, has an interburst interval of around 12 seconds. Given the suppression length is longer than the burst length, the suppression ratio (suppression length/(suppression length + burst length)) is greater than 50%. Although hypothermia and sedation can lead to a burst-suppression pattern, a definitive conclusion cannot be made in this case without seeing the baseline pretherapy EEG. Although agitation artifact can lead to deflections on the EEG, the question stem mentioned that no movement has been noted thus far. Although the bursts have generalized spike wave discharges, which in some patients can correlate with myoclonic jerks, the patient cannot be considered to have myoclonic status epilepticus due to the lack of clinical myoclonus.

234. B. The EEG shows diffuse low voltage and is best described as severe cerebral dysfunction. The EKG channel does not show asystole, and therefore, lack of cerebral perfusion is unlikely. Brain death is a clinical diagnosis, and this EEG cannot support brain death as it was not done per the electrocerebral inactivity (ECI) protocol. In addition, the patient is on pentobarbital, which prevents the clinical diagnosis to be made. Despite the patient having recently been in status epilepticus, there is no evidence of continued seizure activity to suggest malignant status epilepticus, persisting despite anesthesia. When a low-voltage record is seen, care must be taken to ensure that the technical settings, including the filter and sensitivity settings, are appropriate. Setting the sensitivity too high would imply a low microvolt/mm setting, resulting in highly amplified waveforms. On the other hand, artificial suppression of the waveforms can result from setting the sensitivity too low.

235. A. Reduce the timebase. Treatment of refractory status epilepticus may require burst suppression with a varying interburst interval (IBI). If a burst is not visible on every screen, this implies that the IBI is longer than the number of seconds being displayed. This should trigger the EEG technologist to change some of the display parameters to be display more seconds on the screen in order to visualize at least one burst per page. This can be achieved by reducing the timebase (less mm/sec) or by reducing the paper speed (more seconds per page). Adjusting the sensitivity would change the amplitudes (y-axis) of the waveforms and would not adjust timebase (x-axis) of the display. Changing montages also affect how the waveforms on the display are visualized but will not affect the timebase.

236. D. SSPE is a chronic measles infection involving the cerebral cortex, white matter, and brainstem. The bursts in SSPE are typically high-voltage (300–1,500 microvolts) polyspike- and sharp- and slow-wave complexes (lasting 0.5–2 seconds in duration) occurring every 4 to 15 seconds. Of note, in earlier stages of this illness, external stimuli can evoke the complexes.

237. E. All of the listed clinical scenarios can present with unresponsiveness but still have a preserved and reactive posterior dominant rhythm. In general, EEG can help to differentiate coma from other types of unresponsiveness. Locked in syndrome occurs typically when ventral pontine lesions affect the descending motor pathways but spare the arousal systems. Catatonia and psychogenic coma are psychiatric conditions that do not affect the arousal pathways. Bithalamic strokes can occur due to an occlusion of the Artery of Percheron. In this scenario, the patient may be unresponsive but at times may have periods of wakefulness. Generalized periodic discharges with triphasic morphology have also been noted in these patients. Of note, the thalamus is part of the human arousal system with the medial thalamus being involved with sleep regulation. The EEG typically has normal awake and sleep features in psychogenic coma.

238. E. Specific EEG patterns have been associated with CJD, and the World Health Organization has included EEG into its diagnostic classification criteria of CJD. EEG patterns in sCJD change with the stage of the disease. Early stages are characterized by diffuse slowing and FIRDA, whereas middle and late stages present with PSWC. Preterminal stages can be characterized by alpha coma. PSWC are not seen in patients with vCJD.

239. B. PSWC occur in about two-thirds of patients with sporadic CJD (sCJD) and are not seen in variant CJD (vCJD). PSWC can be lateralized or generalized. They occur more commonly in patients with methionine homozygosity and methionine/valine heterozygosity but only rarely in patients with valine homozygosity at codon 129 of the prion protein gene. They tend to disappear during sleep and may be attenuated by sedative medication and external stimulation. Iatrogenic CJD presents with regional PSWC usually at the site of inoculation.

240. B. A diffusely suppressed EEG is consistent with severe cerebral dysfunction. Determination or support of brain death should not be made without having followed minimum technical standards for EEG recording in suspected cerebral death (e.g., American Clinical Neurophysiology Society [ACNS] Guideline 6; 2016). Care must be taken when commenting that the EEG is consistent with anesthesia when no sedatives are being currently administered, even though there is a possibility that prior sedatives may still be having a clinical effect.

241. D. Brain death is a clinical diagnosis, and at times ancillary tests are needed to make that determination. Examples of such tests include EEG, cerebral angiography, nuclear medicine brain scan, and transcranial doppler. Ancillary tests could be used to shorten the duration of the observation period. These tests can be used if parts of the neurological exam have uncertainty or are unreliable. They also can be used if the apnea test cannot be done. Note that ancillary tests cannot replace the neurologic examination. Care must be taken to understand the potential for false-positives of these tests, i.e., the ancillary tests suggest brain death when the clinical data do not. American Clinical Neurophysiology Society (ACNS) Guideline 6: Minimum Technical Standards for EEG Recording in Suspected Cerebral Death is one EEG technique when followed will help to reduce the false positives and provide a proper assessment of brain death.

5

Evoked Potentials and Intraoperative Monitoring

QUESTIONS

1. Intraoperative monitoring (IOM) of brainstem auditory evoked potentials (BAEPs) is least likely to be helpful in which of the following surgical procedures?
   A. Resection of acoustic neuroma
   B. Resection of cerebellopontine angle (CPA) meningioma
   C. Resection of superior temporal gyrus glioma
   D. Microvascular decompression for trigeminal neuralgia
   E. Resection of pontine glioma

2. Which of the following statements best describes the predictive value of multimodality evoked potentials (visual evoked potential [VEP], brainstem auditory evoked potentials [BAEPs], and somatosensory evoked potential [SSEP]) in multiple sclerosis (MS)?
   A. In patients with suspected MS and an evoked potential abnormality, one-third eventually develop definite MS
   B. In patients with suspected MS and normal evoked potentials, less than 0.1% eventually develop definite MS
   C. In patients with suspected MS, VEP abnormalities are more likely to be seen in those who eventually develop definite MS
   D. In patients with suspected MS, SSEP abnormalities are more likely to be seen in those who eventually develop definite MS
   E. In patients with suspected MS, BAEP abnormalities are more likely to be seen in those who eventually develop definite MS

ANSWERS TO THIS SECTION CAN BE FOUND ON PAGE 311

The figures in this chapter can be viewed in a larger size by accessing the digital version of this chapter found on Springer Publishing Company Connect™. Refer to the front of this book for access instructions.

3. In a 22-year-old male with right arm pain, a median somatosensory evoked potential (SSEP) with absent N9 and normal P14 and N20 potentials suggests:
   A. Brachial plexopathy
   B. Radiculopathy
   C. Root avulsion
   D. Median neuropathy at the wrist
   E. Normal study

4. All of the following statements regarding infant audiologic screening are true *except:*
   A. Initial infant screening should be done around 3 to 6 months of age
   B. Transient-evoked otoacoustic emissions (EOAE) test can be used instead of brainstem auditory evoked potentials (BAEPs)
   C. Infants failing the screening should be retested within 3 months
   D. A false positive failing screening test can occur because of middle ear infection
   E. A false positive failing screening test can occur if tested before 1 month of age

5. Which of the following brainstem auditory evoked potential (BAEP) findings makes the diagnosis of brain death doubtful?
   A. Intact Wave I unilaterally and bilateral absence of other waves
   B. Intact Wave I bilaterally and bilateral absence of other waves
   C. Intact Waves I and II unilaterally and bilateral absence of other waves
   D. Intact Waves I and II bilaterally and bilateral absence of other waves
   E. Absence of all waveforms bilaterally

6. Which of the following statements is true regarding the myogenic motor evoked potentials (mMEPs; M-waves) obtained by transcranial electrical stimulation (TES) during intraoperative monitoring (IOM)?
   A. They represent the compound muscle action potentials within the muscle
   B. They are recordable only by needle electrodes
   C. They are resistant to anesthetic effects
   D. They are resistant to any type of neuromuscular blockade
   E. All of the above

7. Which of the following statements is true about the pattern-reversal visual evoked potential (PRVEP)?
   A. Larger check size distorts P100 waveform
   B. Slower reversal rate distorts P100 waveform
   C. Higher luminance increases P100 latency
   D. Higher luminance decreases P100 amplitude
   E. All of the above

8. Which of the following methods is acceptable for measuring the peak waveform amplitude of the somatosensory evoked potentials (SSEPs) during intraoperative monitoring (IOM)?
   A. With respect to the following peak of opposite polarity
   B. With respect to the preceding peak of opposite polarity
   C. With respect to the baseline level of the waveform preceding the peak
   D. A and B
   E. A, B, and C

9. Which of the following represents the sequence of EEG changes during induction of anesthesia with intravenous (IV) propofol?
A. Widespread delta, loss of alpha, and widespread beta
B. Widespread theta, widespread delta, and widespread beta
C. Beta, loss of alpha, widespread beta, and frontally predominant delta
D. Loss of alpha, frontally predominant delta, widespread beta
E. Widespread delta and burst suppression

10. Pattern-reversal visual evoked potential (PRVEP) is most suitable in which of the following patients?
A. Comatose patients
B. Neonates
C. Patients with severe visual impairment
D. Patients with suspected psychogenic blindness
E. All of the above

11. Which of the following measurements of the interpeak interval (IPI) provide an estimate of the central conduction time (CCT)?
A. P14–N20
B. N13–N20
C. N22–P37
D. A and C
E. A, B, and C

12. Which of the following statements regarding the EEG changes observed after carotid cross-clamping during carotid endarterectomy is highly suggestive of cerebral ischemia?
A. EEG changes appearing after 60 seconds of cross-clamping
B. Appearance of anterior alpha and beta activity on the clamped side
C. Increase of delta amplitude on the clamped side
D. Bilateral EEG changes
E. All of the above

13. Which of the following is true in terms of recording D-waves and M-waves (myogenic motor evoked potentials [mMEPs]) with transcranial electrical stimulation (TES) during intraoperative monitoring (IOM)?
A. Both D-waves and M-waves are generated by the action potentials in the spinal cord
B. D-waves are more likely to be suppressed with inhalational anesthesia than M-waves
C. D-waves are more consistent across multiple runs than M-waves
D. D-waves are not affected by spinal cord pathology
E. D-waves show changes earlier than M-waves when motor tracts are compromised

14. Which of the following is a characteristic of the peripheral ascending volley of the median somatosensory evoked potential (SSEP)?
A. It is recorded from an electrode placed over the mid-sternum
B. It occurs about 9 ms after stimulation
C. It has monophasic morphology
D. It is best seen when the reference electrode is placed over the shoulder on the stimulated side
E. It can be affected by medullary tumors

15. A 56-year-old female presented with difficulty walking. On examination, she was found to have spastic paraplegia with a mid-thoracic sensory level. The cranial nerve and upper extremity exams were normal. Which of the following somatosensory evoked potential (SSEP) findings may be expected in this patient?
A. Normal N22 latency, normal N22–P37 interpeak interval (IPI), normal N9–N20 IPI
B. Normal N22 latency, abnormal N22–P37 IPI, abnormal N9–N20 IPI
C. Abnormal N22 latency, normal N22–P37 IPI, abnormal N9–N20 IPI
D. Abnormal N22 latency, abnormal N22–P37 IPI, normal N9–N20 IPI
E. Abnormal N22 latency, abnormal N22–P37 IPI, abnormal N9–N20 IPI

16. Which of the following statements is true regarding the effects of administration of anesthesia on the focal EEG abnormalities prior to carotid clamping during carotid endarterectomy?
A. Ipsilateral EEG abnormalities may be induced in over 90% of patients
B. EEG abnormalities consist of widespread high-amplitude delta activity
C. EEG abnormalities consist of increased amplitude of the anterior beta and alpha activity
D. EEG abnormalities can be unmasked or obscured by anesthesia
E. Anesthesia has no effect on EEG abnormalities

17. Flash visual evoked potential (VEP) is advantageous compared with pattern-reversal VEP (PRVEP) because
A. It has less latency variability
B. It is more sensitive to conduction defects
C. It assesses the entire visual pathway including the occipital cortex
D. The subject's eyes can remain closed
E. It ensures better visual fixation

18. A new clinical neurophysiology fellow was assisting the technologist during a brainstem auditory evoked response procedure. He noted that there was a fairly sudden increase in all of the absolute latencies. Which of the following could the fellow have noted in addition to the above change?
A. Decrease in all the interpeak latencies (IPL)
B. Increase in the amplitude of all waveforms
C. The knob for the click intensity was inadvertently decreased
D. The patient had fallen asleep
E. The patient became more awake

19. A demyelinating lesion in the pons is likely to show:
A. Prolonged N9 absolute latency
B. Prolonged N9–P14 interpeak latency (IPL)
C. Prolonged P14 absolute latency
D. Prolonged P14–N20 IPL
E. B and D

20. The overall utility of MRI and evoked potentials (EP) in multiple sclerosis (MS) can be summarized by all of the following statements *except:*
A. EP may be more efficient than MRI in detecting isolated optic neuritis
B. EP is useful in monitoring the disease course
C. EP is useful to confirm organic nature of subjective symptoms when MRI is normal

D. MRI shows diagnostic lesions in more than 80% of patients with MS
E. Multimodal EPs are abnormal in about 30% of presumptive MS patients with normal MRI

21. Compromise to which of the following blood vessels is likely to be detected by intraoperative monitoring of the somatosensory evoked potentials (SSEPs)?
A. Posterior inferior cerebellar artery
B. Anterior spinal artery
C. Posterior spinal artery
D. Medial lenticulostriate artery
E. None of the above

22. A 34-year-old male presents with new onset headache and bilateral upper and lower extremity numbness worse on the right side. Median somatosensory evoked potential (SSEP) shows intact potentials with prolonged N9–P14 interpeak latency (IPL) and normal P14–N20 IPL. Which of the following conditions is likely?
A. Parsonage–Turner syndrome
B. Guillain–Barré syndrome
C. Pontine glioma
D. Thalamic hemorrhage
E. Midbrain hemorrhage

23. An intact N13 with reduced or absent P14 and N20 potentials can be seen in:
A. Cervical syringomyelia
B. Medullary glioma
C. Wallenberg syndrome
D. Pontine hemorrhage
E. B and D

24. Bilateral absence of lumbar potentials (LPs) with normal P37 latencies after tibial nerve stimulation is seen in which of the following conditions?
A. Severe peripheral neuropathy
B. Bilateral cauda equina syndrome
C. Guillain–Barré syndrome
D. Technical problem with stimulation or recording
E. A, B, and C

25. Which of the following statements regarding the utility of somatosensory evoked potentials (SSEPs) during intraoperative monitoring (IOM) is true?
A. SSEPs are useful for monitoring during surgical lesioning of dorsal roots
B. Postoperative SSEP amplitude reduction correlates with relief of pain and spasticity
C. Pudendal nerve monitoring supplements median and tibial nerve monitoring
D. SSEPs are useful for monitoring dorsal rhizotomy
E. All of the above

26. Which of the following statements is true regarding the effect of rarefaction clicks on the brainstem auditory evoked potential (BAEP) waveforms?
A. Prolongation of Wave I latency
B. Prolongation of Wave V latency

C. Shortening of Waves I-III interpeak latency (IPL)
D. More distinct Waves IV and V
E. All of the above

27. Shortened Waves I-V interpeak latency (IPL) is seen in which of the following conditions?
A. Multiple sclerosis (MS) plaque in brainstem
B. Brainstem glioma
C. Cochlear hearing loss
D. Conductive hearing loss
E. Small cerebellopontine angle tumor

28. Which of the following agents is likely to cause a spike-wave pattern on the EEG at high doses?
A. Enflurane
B. Isoflurane
C. Halothane
D. Desflurane
E. Nitrous oxide

29. Which of the following EEG patterns is least likely to be seen when the level of inhalation anesthesia is below the minimal alveolar concentration (MAC)?
A. Widespread alpha and beta activity with anterior predominance
B. Widespread attenuation with short bursts of mixed frequency activity
C. Intermittent bursts of delta activity with anterior predominance
D. Widespread polymorphic slow waves
E. Diffuse alpha activity

30. Delayed N9, P14, and N20 potentials with normal interpeak latencies (IPLs) in the somatosensory evoked potential (SSEP) after stimulation of the right median nerve suggest:
A. Carpal tunnel syndrome
B. Pronator teres syndrome
C. Brachial plexopathy
D. Radiculopathy
E. Guillain–Barre syndrome

31. An 8-year-old boy was undergoing lumbar spine surgery for an injury sustained after a fall. Which of the following statements indicates proper placement of the pedicle screws based on the elicited EMG activity?
A. Absence of EMG activity with 10 V stimulation
B. Absence of EMG activity with 30 V of stimulation
C. Presence of EMG activity with 10 V of stimulation
D. Presence of EMG activity with 30 V stimulation
E. EMG monitoring is unreliable in pedicle screw sugery

32. The following tibial somatosensory evoked potentials (SSEPs) were recorded during intraoperative monitoring (IOM) from a patient undergoing resection of an intradural

extramedullary tumor in the lower thoracic region. The second, fourth, and sixth traces represent the baseline potentials; the first, third, and fifth traces represent traces obtained after decompression. Which of the following statements is most consistent with the findings shown in the figure?

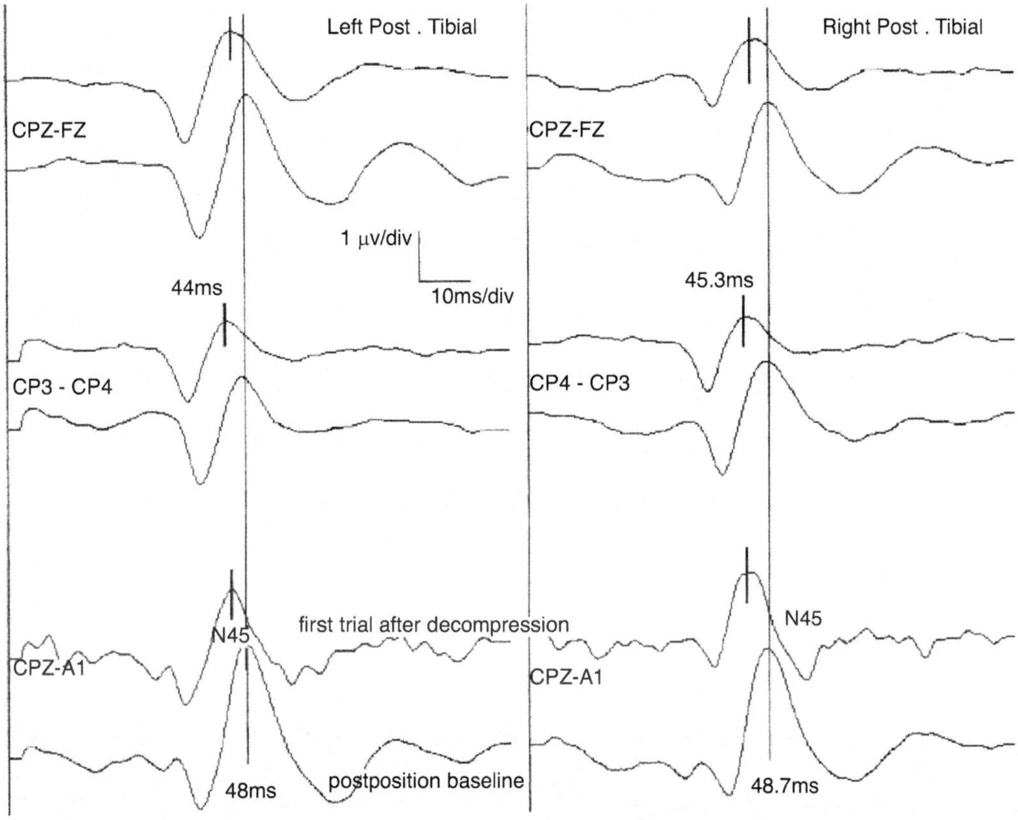

Source: Reprinted from Simon, M. *Intraoperative Neurophysiology: A Comprehensive Guide to Monitoring and Mapping.* New York, NY: Demos Medical Publishing; 2010.

A. The changes in latencies are due to the effect of decompression
B. The changes in amplitude are due to the effect of decompression
C. The changes in latencies and amplitudes are due to the effect of decompression
D. The changes in latencies are due to the effect of anesthesia
E. None of the above

33. Which of the following interpeak latencies (IPL) are commonly evaluated as part of brainstem auditory evoked potentials (BAEPs)?

A. I–III
B. III–V
C. V–VII
D. I–V
E. A, B and D

34. Which of the following regarding intraoperative monitoring (IOM) of brainstem auditory evoked potentials (BAEPs) is generally true?
A. Amplitude drop of 50% or higher of a waveform measured from the peak to the following trough is considered significant
B. Amplitude drop of 50% or higher of a waveform measured from the preceding trough to the peak is considered significant
C. Increase in absolute peak or interpeak latencies (IPLs) by greater than 2 ms is considered significant
D. Wave III is primarily followed during surgery
E. BAEPs are more sensitive to volatile anesthetics than to cold water irrigation

35. During facial nerve decompression, which of the following electromyography (EMG) findings is consistent with nerve manipulation?
A. Neurotonic discharges
B. Myotonic discharges
C. Neuromyotonia
D. Fibrillations
E. All of the above

36. Increasing the stimulation rate (click rate) beyond 30 Hz during brainstem auditory evoked potential (BAEP) recording can be associated with all of the following *except:*
A. Decreased amplitude
B. Dispersion of waveforms
C. Prolonged interpeak latencies (IPLs)
D. Decreased absolute latencies
E. Disappearance of the previously noted abnormality

37. Which of the following statements regarding pattern electroretinogram (PERG) is true?
A. Normal PERG accompanied by abnormal visual evoked potential (VEP) suggests optic nerve demyelination
B. PERG is a useful measure of both ganglion cell macular functions
C. Abnormal PERG after recent optic neuritis predicts poor visual recovery
D. Progressive decrease in PERG amplitude after recent optic neuritis correlates with development of optic nerve atrophy
E. All of the above

38. Which of the following is NOT an effect of the inhaled anesthetics on the evoked potentials?
A. Decreased latency
B. Increased latency
C. Decreased amplitude
D. Increased amplitude
E. None of the above (neither latency nor amplitude is affected)

39. Wave I of a brainstem auditory evoked potential (BAEP):
A. Arises in the cochlear nucleus
B. Is recorded as a near-field, positive potential around the stimulated ear
C. Is recorded as a far-field, positive potential at the vertex

D. Cannot be recorded with an electrode within the external auditory canal
E. May persist after proximal sectioning of the eighth nerve during surgery for acoustic neuroma

40. Which of the following technical considerations is applicable for motor evoked potential (MEP) recording by transcranial electrical stimulation (TES) during intraoperative monitoring (IOM)?
A. Signal averaging should be used for recording myogenic MEPs (M-waves) since the amplitude of M-waves are only in the tens of microvolts
B. Signal averaging should be used for recording myogenic MEPs (M-waves) since the subset of activated alpha motor neurons varies from run to run
C. Stimulus intensity should be kept low enough to produce the MEP waveforms in only one limb
D. A train of three to seven pulses is used to obtain D-waves
E. Limb movement is more likely while recording D-waves

41. The N13 component of the median somatosensory evoked potential (SSEP) is characterized by all of the following *except:*
A. It is generated by stimulation of large myelinated fibers in the dorsal horn
B. It is best seen as a negative potential over the C5–C7 spinous processes
C. It is preserved in brain death
D. It is abolished in cervical cord gray matter lesions involving the dorsal columns
E. It is abolished in cervicomedullary lesions

42. Which of the following waveforms encountered in the median somatosensory evoked potential (SSEP) is a far-field potential?
A. N9
B. N13
C. P14
D. N20
E. None of the above

43. Which of the following findings is least likely to be seen on a brainstem auditory evoked potential (BAEP) in a patient with an acoustic neuroma presenting with hearing difficulty?
A. Normal BAEP
B. Wave I–III interpeak latency (IPL) latency is prolonged ipsilateral to the lesion
C. Wave I–V IPL is prolonged contralateral to the lesion
D. Wave I is prolonged ipsilateral to the lesion
E. Absent Wave III and subsequent BAEP components ipsilateral to the lesion

44. A 35-year-old, previously healthy female with sudden onset of bilateral visual loss undergoes a visual evoked potential (VEP) study as shown below (left panel shows left eye stimulation, right panel shows right eye stimulation). The patient was cooperative and able to maintain fixation at the center of the screen. The findings on the VEP are least likely to occur in which of the following conditions?

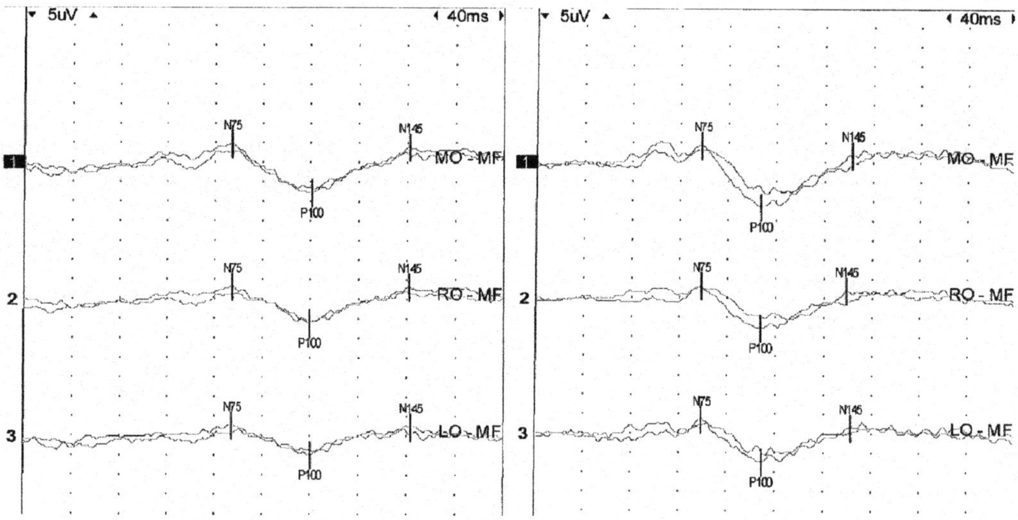

A. Pituitary tumor compressing the optic chiasm
B. Bilateral optic neuritis
C. Psychogenic blindness
D. Bilateral parieto-occipital metastatic tumors
E. Friedreich's ataxia

45. Studies on monitoring brainstem auditory evoked potentials (BAEPs) during intraoperative monitoring (IOM) suggest:
A. No role for BAEP monitoring as it does not improve postoperative neurologic outcome
B. Adverse neurologic outcome even after a transient loss of all BAEP waves
C. Potential for hearing impairment only when Wave V latency is delayed by greater than 2 ms
D. Preservation of functional hearing after acoustic neuroma resection if BAEP and electrocochleogram waves are present at the end of surgery
E. Abrupt loss of Wave I is usually technical in nature

46. Which of the following statements is true regarding the morphology of brainstem auditory evoked potential (BAEP) waveforms in the channel contralateral to the stimulated ear?
A. Wave I has a smaller amplitude in the contralateral ear channel
B. Wave III is absent in the contralateral ear channel
C. Wave IV latency is longer in the contralateral ear channel
D. Wave V latency is longer in the contralateral ear channel
E. A and D

47. Amplitude of somatosensory evoked potential (SSEP) waveforms can be increased in all of the following conditions *except:*
A. Nitrous oxide
B. Benzodiazepines
C. Etomidate
D. Certain focal epilepsy syndromes
E. Certain myoclonic epilepsy syndromes

48. Superior olive is the generator for which wave of the brainstem auditory evoked potential (BAEP) shown below?

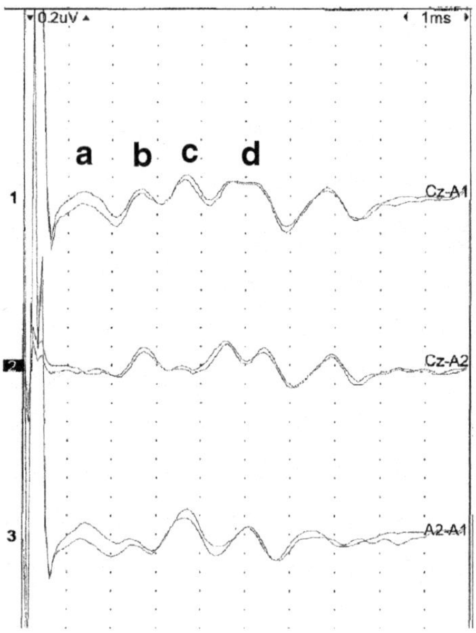

A. Wave I
B. Wave II
C. Wave III
D. Wave IV
E. None of the above

49. Which of the following statements is true about brainstem auditory evoked potentials (BAEPs)?
A. Wave I is seen only ipsilateral to the stimulated ear
B. Wave III is absent contralateral to the stimulated ear
C. Wave V is generated by structures located in the lower pons
D. Waveforms can be significantly affected by anesthetic agents
E. Waveforms can be affected by the level of consciousness

50. Which of the following is true regarding check size when performing visual evoked potentials?
A. Larger checks are more sensitive in detecting visual defects
B. Smaller checks stimulate peripheral vision better
C. Larger checks produce more consistent responses
D. Larger checks have better sensitivity to contrast in central vision
E. Larger checks can prolong P100 latency, especially when the stimulus field size is small

51. Which of the following waveforms is least likely to be reduced or abolished by a medullary tumor?
A. N13
B. P14
C. N18
D. P31
E. P38

52. The following median somatosensory evoked potentials (SSEPs) were recorded during intraoperative monitoring (IOM) from a patient before (A) and after (B) surgery. Which of the following statements is true regarding the findings shown in the figure?

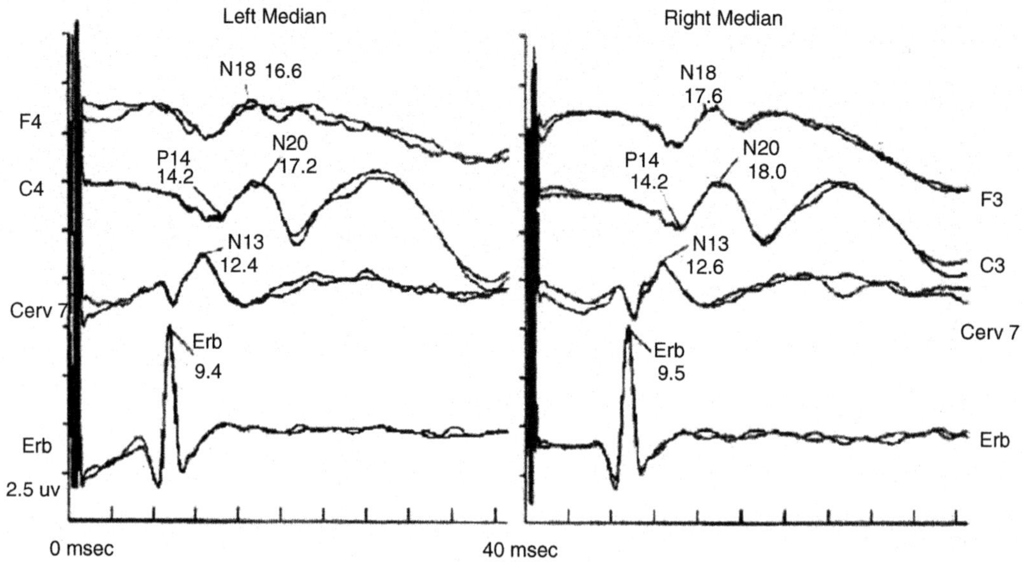

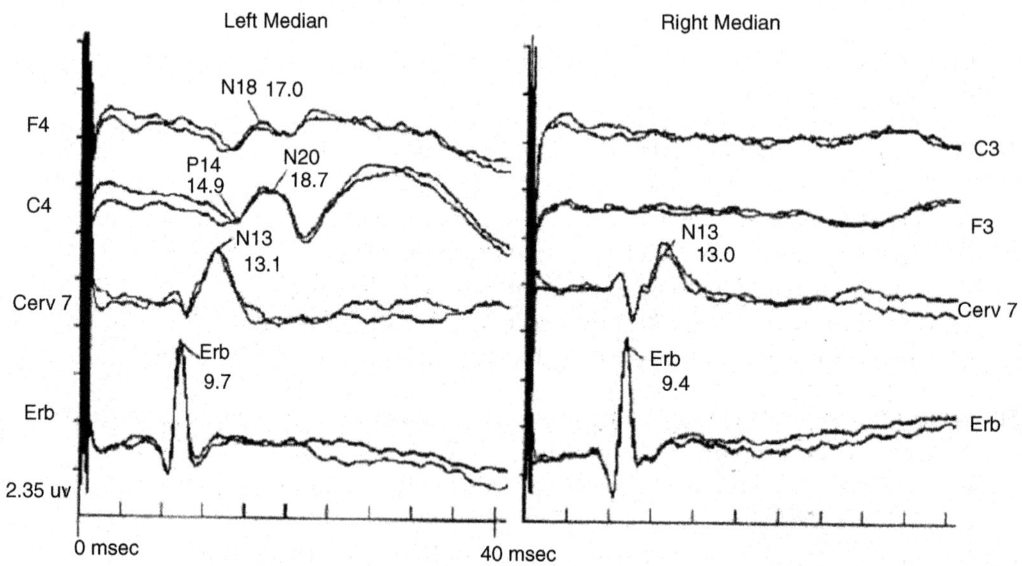

Source: Reprinted from Husain, AM. *A Practical Approach to Neurophysiologic Intraoperative Monitoring.* New York, NY: Demos Medical Publishing; 2008.

A. The changes may have occurred as a consequence of resection of a pontine glioma
B. The changes may have occurred as a consequence of resection of an intramedullary tumor at the cervicomedullary junction
C. The changes may have occurred as a consequence of resection of a parietal tumor
D. The patient can be expected to have impaired proprioception in the left arm postoperatively
E. The patient can be expected to have right arm weakness postoperatively

53. Which of the following statements is true regarding stimulus polarity during brainstem auditory evoked potential (BAEP) recording?
A. Rarefaction clicks are recommended for clinical BAEPs testing
B. Rarefaction clicks decrease the absolute latencies
C. Alternating stimulus polarity during the testing may help in reducing the artifacts
D. Alternating stimulus polarity may cause phase cancellation
E. All of the above

54. D-waves obtained by transcranial electrical stimulation (TES) during intraoperative monitoring (IOM) are characterized by all of the following *except:*
A. They reflect postsynaptic potentials generated by the pyramidal neurons
B. They are recorded by an epidural electrode
C. They are resistant to anesthetic effects
D. They may be attenuated due to desynchronization of the descending corticospinal volley in spinal cord pathology
E. All of the above

55. The following figure shows myogenic motor evoked potentials (mMEPs) from a patient undergoing abdominal aortic aneurysm repair. The top, middle, and bottom panels represent recordings obtained from the left abductor pollicis brevis (APB), left quadriceps, and left tibialis anterior, respectively. Within each panel, the traces from bottom to top represent 2 minutes before, 2 minutes after, 8 minutes after, and 22 minutes after aortic cross-clamping, respectively. Which of the following statements best describes the findings shown in the figure?
A. Both the upper and lower limbs are irreversibly affected by aortic cross-clamping
B. The upper limb is spared and the flat potentials in the lower limb are artifacts
C. Changes in lower limb potentials represent transient spinal cord ischemia corrected by an increase in mean arterial pressure
D. Changes in both the upper and lower limb potentials represent transient spinal cord ischemia corrected by an increase in mean arterial pressure
E. The mMEPs are uninterpretable without simultaneous somatosensory evoked potentials (SSEPs)

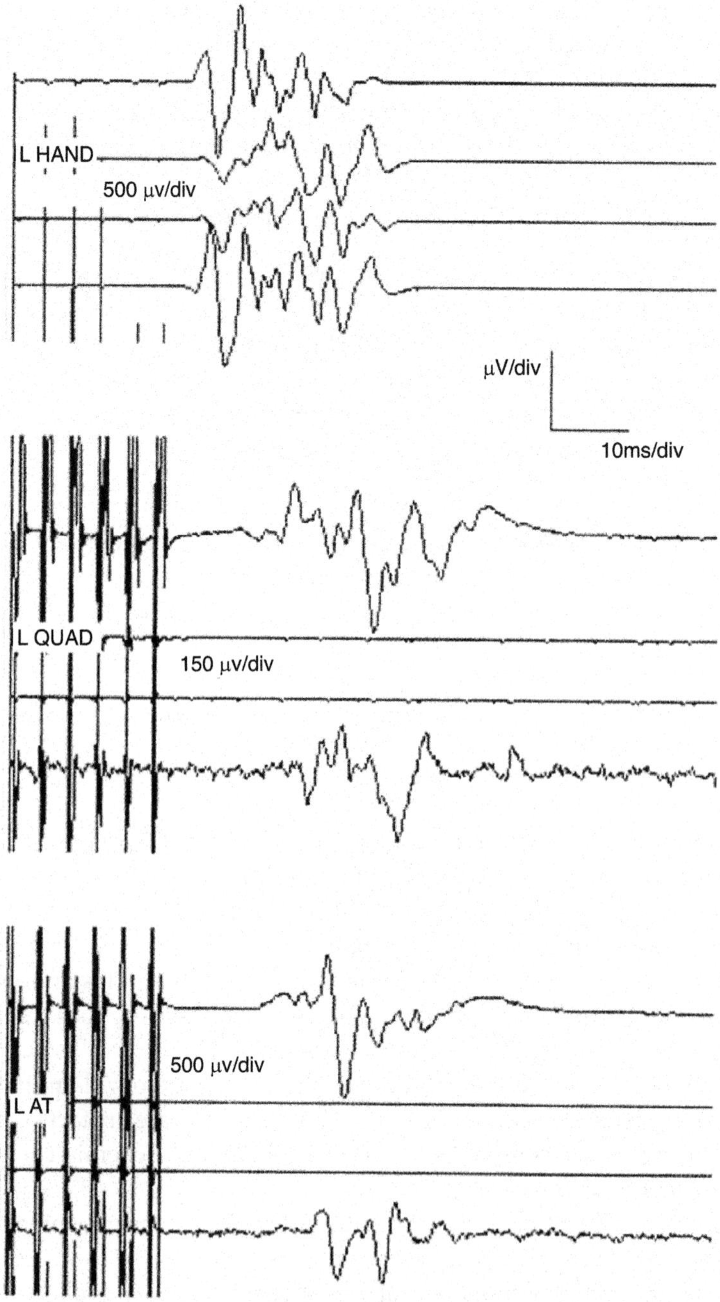

Source: Reprinted from Simon, M. *Intraoperative Neurophysiology: A Comprehensive Guide to Monitoring and Mapping.* New York, NY: D,emos Medical Publishing; 2010.

56. Prolongation of central conduction time (CCT; i.e., N22–P37 interpeak latency [IPL]) after tibial nerve stimulation can be seen in all of the following conditions *except:*

A. Barbiturate-induced anesthesia
B. Brainstem multiple sclerosis
C. Neuromyelitis optica
D. Adrenomyeloneuropathy
E. Pontine hemorrhage

57. Which of the following statements best describes the utility of somatosensory evoked potentials (SSEPs) in the evaluation of peripheral nervous system disorders?
   A. Intact N9 and absence of subsequent potentials suggest brachial plexus trunk lesion
   B. Absent popliteal fossa potential but intact lumbar potential (LP) is characteristically seen in Guillain–Barré syndrome
   C. SSEPs obtained by dermatomal stimulation are useful in the evaluation of radiculopathy
   D. SSEPs are always normal in Friedreich's ataxia despite abnormal nerve conduction studies
   E. All of the above

58. Which of the following statements is true regarding P100 latency?
   A. It tends to decrease with age
   B. It is shorter in men than women
   C. It is not affected by refractive errors
   D. It decreases with decrease in pupillary diameter
   E. It can be normal in the setting of visual disturbance

59. An appropriate montage for recording median somatosensory evoked potential (SSEP) includes all of the following channels *except:*
   A. CPc–CPi
   B. CPc–EPc
   C. CPi–EPc
   D. C5S–EPc
   E. EPi–EPc

60. Which of the following statements is true about visual evoked potential (VEP)?
   A. It is a short-latency near-field potential
   B. Bifid P100 waveform may be corrected by stimulation of the inferior visual fields
   C. Visual acuity does not affect P100 latency
   D. P100 potential is best seen over the contralateral occipital region after hemifield stimulation
   E. All of the above

61. Utility of median somatosensory evoked potential (SSEPs) in the prognosis of coma is reflected by all of the following *except:*
   A. Bilateral absence of N20 potentials is associated with death or persistent vegetative state (PVS) in 90% of patients
   B. Bilateral absence of N20 potentials predicts PVS more frequently in postanoxic coma than in posttraumatic coma
   C. Intact N9 and N13 potentials with absence of subsequent waveforms bilaterally is associated with death or PVS in 100% of postanoxic coma
   D. Intact N9 and N13 potentials with absence of subsequent waveforms bilaterally can be associated with good recovery in coma due to a primary brainstem lesion
   E. Presence of normal N20 potentials in the acute stage of coma predicts good recovery

62. Which of the following statements are true regarding giant somatosensory evoked potentials (SSEPs)?

A. Their peak-to-peak amplitude is usually more than 15 μV
B. They can be seen in pyramidal myoclonus
C. They reflect cortical hyperexcitability in area 3b
D. They can be preceded by an abnormal cortical spike, which is best seen with jerk-locked back-averaging of EEG
E. All of the above

63. The yield of somatosensory evoked potentials (SSEPs) in the diagnostic evaluation of multiple sclerosis (MS) is:

A. Excellent, because only 5% of patients with sensory symptoms or signs have normal SSEPs
B. Excellent in those with spinal cord lesions, because they frequently detect spinal cord pathology not observed with MRI scans
C. Unlikely to increase when all four limbs are tested
D. Likely to increase by 10% when upper limbs are tested after normal lower limb SSEPs
E. Likely to be similar between possible MS and definite MS

64. A median somatosensory evoked potential (SSEP) study was done on a 60-year-old male as shown below (left median stimulation on the left panel, right median stimulation on the right panel). What is the best interpretation?

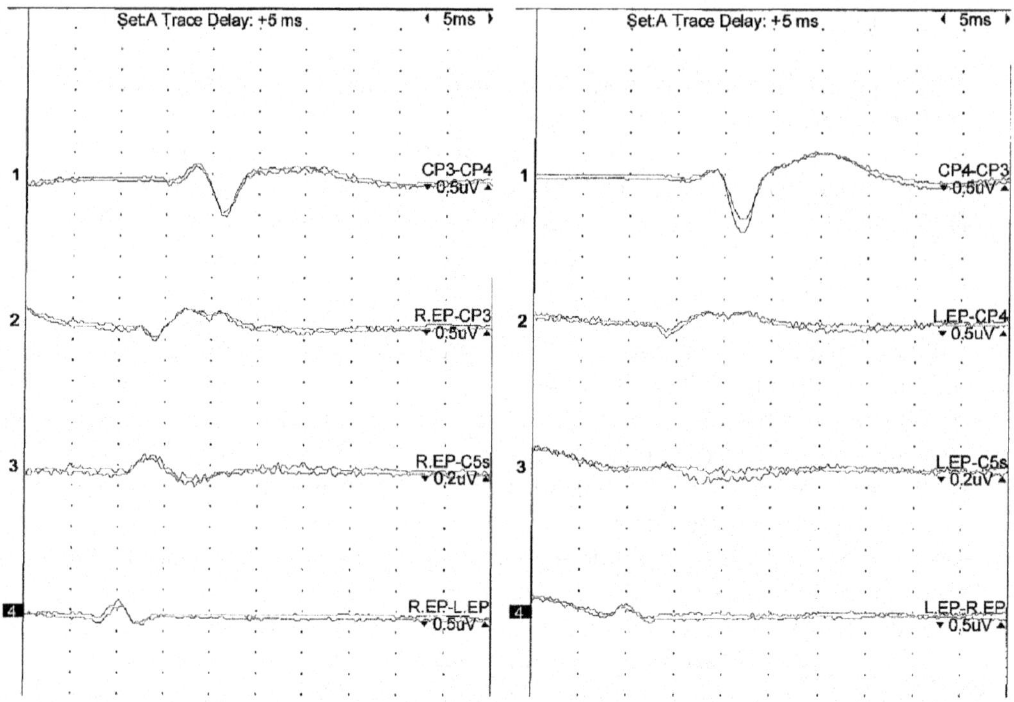

A. Pontine hemorrhage
B. Cervicomedullary lesion
C. Brain death
D. Guillain–Barré syndrome
E. Normal study

65. Which of the following statements regarding somatosensory evoked potentials (SSEPs) is true?
A. Up to 40% of patients with multiple sclerosis (MS) without sensory symptoms may have abnormal SSEPs
B. The N20 waveform may be abolished by anesthesia
C. Amplitude of cortical potentials may be increased in progressive myoclonus epilepsy syndromes
D. Amplitude drop greater than 50% and/or latency prolongation of 10% over baseline are common criteria to detect a change during neurophysiologic intraoperative monitoring (NIOM)
E. All of the above

66. Which of the following statements regarding the tibial somatosensory evoked potential (SSEP) is true?
A. N7 potential reflects the afferent volley in the cauda equina
B. N22 potential reflects activity in the lumbar cord
C. P37 potential reflects activity in the parietal cortex
D. A and B
E. B and C

67. The P100 waveform amplitude is decreased by which of the following?
A. Low contrast; low luminance
B. Low contrast; high luminance
C. High contrast; low luminance
D. High contrast; high luminance
E. None of the above

68. The P14 component of the median somatosensory evoked potential (SSEP) is:
A. A near-field potential
B. Best seen on the scalp with a cephalic reference
C. Generated by activity in the medial lemniscus
D. Preserved in cervicomedullary lesions
E. Abolished in thalamic lesions

69. All of the following statements are true regarding the cortical N20 and P22 potentials recorded with median somatosensory evoked potential (SSEP) *except:*
A. N20 is generated in the frontal cortex and P22 is generated in the parietal cortex
B. Dissociated loss of N20 and P22 can be seen in less than 10% of patients with focal hemispheric lesions
C. Loss of N20 is associated with astereognosis
D. Loss of N20 is associated with impaired elementary sensory modalities
E. Loss of P22 is associated with motor impairment with intact sensation

70. An intact P100 waveform after monocular stimulation in a person with visual impairment is most likely to indicate:
   A. Cataract
   B. Optic neuritis
   C. Cortical blindness
   D. Poor visual fixation
   E. None of the above

71. A 64-year-old man is undergoing continuous upper and lower somatosensory evoked potential (SSEP) monitoring during cervical decompression. The intraoperative monitoring (IOM) technologist annotated on the screen that the patient just received a bolus of pentobarbital. What significant change to the subcortical potentials is most likely?
   A. Increased amplitude
   B. Decreased amplitude
   C. Increased latency
   D. Decreased latency
   E. No change

72. Visual evoked potential (VEP) abnormalities in optic neuritis are characterized by all of the following *except:*
   A. Abnormal VEP to smaller check size is more common during the initial stages
   B. VEP latency can remain prolonged after recovery of vision in up to 50% of patients
   C. VEP can be abnormal in greater than 50% of multiple sclerosis (MS) patients with normal visual function and neuro-ophthalmologic examination
   D. Abnormalities in VEP are more common than abnormalities in optical coherence tomography
   E. P100 latencies are more affected than the amplitudes

73. Intraoperative monitoring (IOM) of somatosensory evoked potentials (SSEPs) is least likely to be helpful in detecting neural pathway compromise in which of the following surgical procedures?
   A. Total hip arthroplasty
   B. Carotid endarterectomy
   C. Resection of parietal glioma
   D. Reduction of pelvic fracture
   E. Cervical spinal cord decompression

74. Which of the following has *not* been shown to contribute to somatosensory evoked potentials (SSEPs)?
   A. Joint afferents after median nerve stimulation
   B. Joint afferents after tibial nerve stimulation
   C. Muscle afferents after median nerve stimulation
   D. Muscle afferents after tibial nerve stimulation
   E. Cutaneous afferents after median nerve stimulation

75. P100 waveform is characterized by which of the following statements?
   A. It can be preceded and followed by negative waveforms
   B. It can be "W-shaped" because of an active mid-frontal reference
   C. It can be "W-shaped" because of projections from different parts of the calcarine cortex

D. The true latency of distorted P100 waveforms can be determined by stimulation of inferior visual fields
E. All of the above

76. Unilateral P100 prolongation in a visual evoked potential (VEP) with full-field stimulation indicates:
A. Occipital lobe tumor
B. Thalamic hemorrhage
C. Compression at the optic chiasm
D. Contralateral demyelinating process anterior to the optic chiasm
E. Ipsilateral demyelinating process anterior to the optic chiasm

77. Which of the following agents can increase the amplitude of cortical waveforms?
A. Nitrous oxide
B. Etomidate
C. Barbiturates
D. Halothane
E. Isoflurane

78. Which of the following statements is true about the alternating polarity clicks used in recording brainstem auditory evoked potentials (BAEPs)?
A. They are recommended in routine clinical practice
B. They can cause artifacts making it difficult to identify the true waveforms
C. They can lead to phase cancellation
D. They decrease Wave I latency
E. They may cause Wave V to disappear

79. A 51-year-old male undergoes brainstem auditory evoked potential (BAEP) monitoring during resection of a right vestibular schwannoma. Which of the following changes is correct in terms of the adverse postoperative outcome that may occur?
A. Loss of Waves I, III, and V suggests damage to the internal auditory artery
B. Attenuation of Wave I with intact Waves III and V during bone drilling suggests permanent damage to the cochlea
C. Delay of Waves III and V but not Wave I suggests distal eighth nerve damage
D. Loss of Waves I, III and V suggests damage to the lower pons
E. Unilateral BAEP changes suggest brainstem abnormalities contralateral to the stimulated ear

80. The following figure shows serial brainstem auditory evoked potentials (BAEPs) from a patient undergoing microvascular decompression of the trigeminal nerve. The bottom trace is the earliest (11:51 a.m.) and the top trace is the latest (13:30 p.m.). All of the following statements are true based on the observed changes in BAEPs *except:*
A. Wave I is absent after 12:21 p.m.
B. Changes at 13:30 p.m. are consistent with cochlear infarction
C. Changes after 12:23 p.m. are consistent with increase in sevoflurane dose
D. Changes in Wave V until 12:05 p.m. are consistent with cerebellar traction
E. Changes in the waveforms are severe enough to cause postoperative hearing deficit

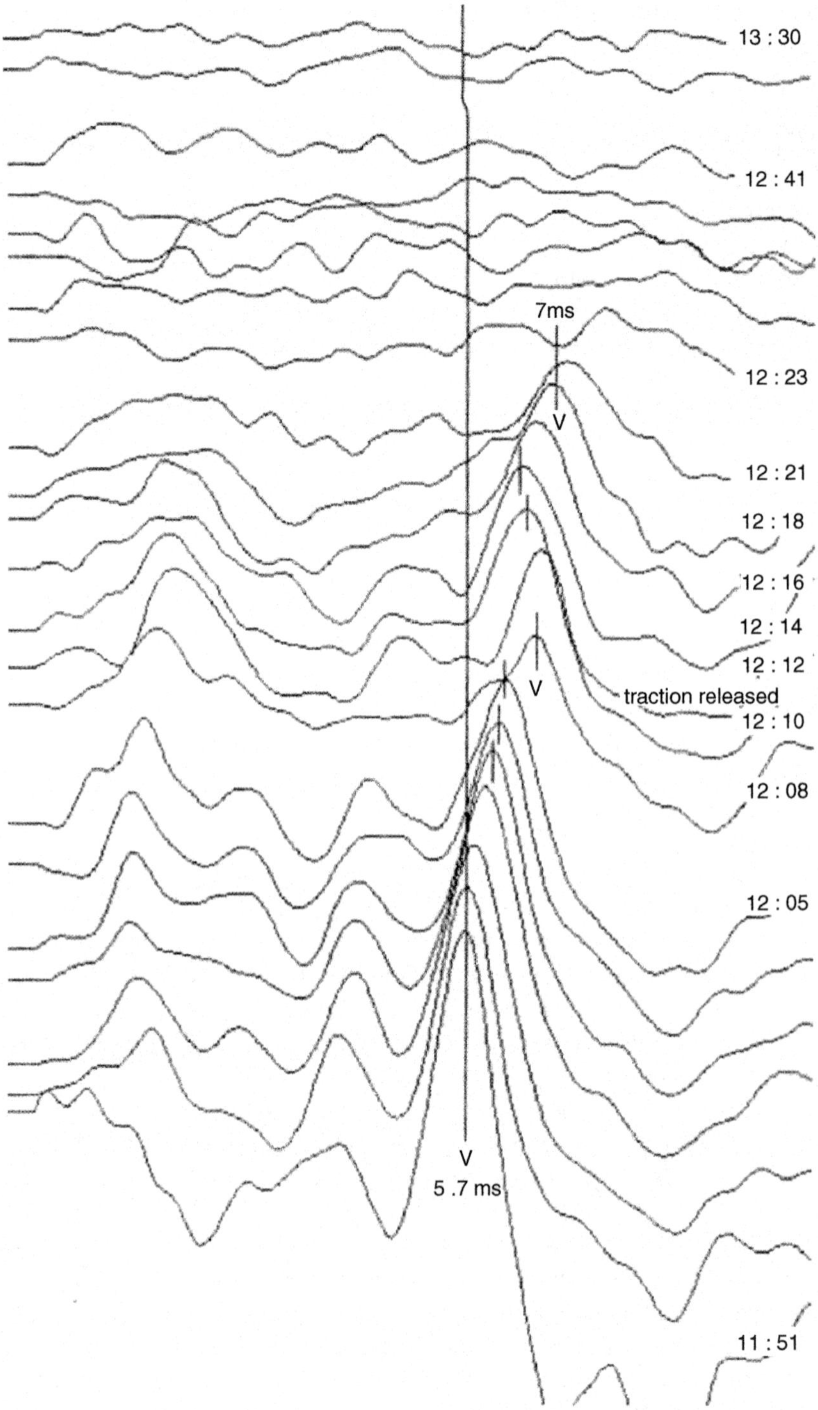

Source: Reprinted from Simon, M. *Intraoperative Neurophysiology: A Comprehensive Guide to Monitoring and Mapping.* New York, NY: Demos Medical Publishing; 2010.

81. Which of the following statements is true regarding the effect of age on visual evoked potential (VEP)?

A. P100 latencies reach adult values by age 6 months for larger check sizes

B. P100 latencies reach adult values by age 1 year for smaller check sizes

C. P100 latency may increase during adolescence
D. P100 latency increases after age 60 years
E. P100 latency prolongation with age has no relationship with check size

82. Which of the following conditions is least likely to be associated with giant somatosensory evoked potentials (SSEP)?
A. Lafora body disease
B. Conditions causing focal motor seizures
C. Creutzfeldt–Jakob disease (CJD)
D. Hemispheric hemorrhagic stroke
E. Juvenile myoclonic epilepsy

83. In brainstem auditory evoked potentials (BAEPs), absence of Wave I with intact Waves III and V is most commonly due to:
A. Cortical lesion
B. Mild peripheral hearing loss
C. Brain death
D. Inferior colliculus lesion
E. Severe peripheral hearing loss

84. In cervical spondylotic myelopathy:
A. Median somatosensory evoked potential (SSEP) is more sensitive than tibial SSEP in detecting abnormalities
B. Median SSEP abnormalities correlate with narrowing of cord diameter
C. Median SSEP abnormalities correlate with increased cord T2 signal
D. Either median or tibial SSEP is abnormal in more than 60% of patients with normal MRI
E. All of the above

85. Which of the following statements is true regarding the clinical significance of visual evoked potential (VEP)?
A. Abnormal VEP is seen in 25% of patients with suspected multiple sclerosis (MS) and normal MRI
B. Bilateral P100 prolongation almost always suggests chiasmal or retrochiasmal lesions
C. In suspected psychogenic blindness, a normal VEP essentially rules out blindness
D. Early cataract causes clinically significant prolongation of P100
E. P100 tends to be prolonged in early cataract

86. Which of the following statements regarding brainstem auditory evoked potentials (BAEPs) is true?
A. BAEP waveforms recorded at the vertex consist of both far-field and near-field potentials
B. BAEP waveforms are surface negative at the vertex
C. BAEP waveforms occur within 8 ms of the click
D. Clinically relevant BAEP waveforms measure conduction between caudal medulla and midbrain
E. Wave I recorded at the vertex is a far-field potential

87. A large posterior thalamic hemorrhage can be associated with:

A. Intact N9
B. Intact P14
C. Intact N18
D. Absent N20
E. All of the above

88. All of the following statements regarding the generators of median somatosensory evoked potential (SSEP) waveforms are true *except:*

A. N9 is a near-field potential reflecting the afferent volley in the brachial plexus
B. N10 is a far-field potential reflecting activity at Erb's point
C. N13 is a far-field potential reflecting activity in the dorsal columns of cervical cord
D. P14 is a far-field potential reflecting activity in the caudal medial lemniscus in the CPi–EPc derivation
E. N20 is a near-field potential reflecting activity in the parietal cortex

89. All of the following statements are true about the generators of the tibial somatosensory evoked potential (SSEP) waveforms *except:*

A. Lumbar potential (LP) is a near-field potential reflecting postsynaptic activity in the lumbar cord
B. N23 is a near-field potential reflecting activity in the conus medullaris
C. P31 is a far-field potential reflecting activity in the caudal medial lemniscus
D. N34 is a near-field potential reflecting activity in the brainstem and thalamus
E. P37 is a near-field potential reflecting activity in the parietal cortex recorded. ipsilateral to the stimulated side

90. What structure is the source of Wave I of the brainstem auditory evoked potential (BAEP)?

A. Organ of corti
B. Hair cells
C. Distal cochlear nerve
D. Proximal cochlear nerve
E. Cochlear nucleus

91. An EEG pattern resembling frontal intermittent rhythmic delta activity (FIRDA) can be seen in:

A. Induction with isoflurane
B. Steady-state anesthesia with isoflurane
C. Recovery from isoflurane anesthesia
D. Addition of nitrous oxide to isoflurane
E. A, B and C

92. During intraoperative monitoring (IOM) of somatosensory evoked potentials (SSEPs):

A. An electrode around the elbow can substitute for the Erb's point electrode for median SSEP
B. The spinal potentials, the median N13 and tibial N22, are crucial to record
C. The cervicomedullary potentials, the median P14 and tibial P31, are best recorded using a dorsal scalp to noncephalic linkage

D. Larger cortical potentials with median nerve stimulation are obtained using a CPc–CPi linkage
E. All of the above

93. Which of the following statements is true regarding the effect of recording parameters on the latencies of brainstem auditory evoked potentials (BAEPs)?
A. Click rates greater than 10 Hz decrease interpeak latencies (IPLs)
B. Click rates greater than 10 Hz increase waveform amplitudes
C. Higher click intensity decreases IPLs
D. Condensation clicks decrease Wave V latency
E. Rarefaction clicks decrease Wave I latency

94. Which of the following statements best describes the influence of physiologic factors on somatosensory evoked potential (SSEP)?
A. Children attain adult peak latency values by 5 to 6 years of age
B. Myelinogenesis and body growth have similar effects on the maturation of SSEPs
C. Hypothermia with core body temperature at 17°C abolishes all median SSEP waveforms
D. Sleep does not affect the latencies
E. Body height affects interpeak latencies (IPLs) less than the absolute latencies for tibial SSEPs

95. Which of the following technical considerations for intraoperative monitoring (IOM) of the eighth nerve using brainstem auditory evoked potential (BAEP) is recommended?
A. If Wave I is indistinct, repositioning of the ipsilateral earlobe electrode is helpful
B. Masking of the contralateral ear with white noise is strongly recommended
C. Shorter epoch length of less than 10 ms is recommended for averaging the signals
D. Stimulation with alternating click polarities is not recommended as it can cause artifacts
E. All of the above

96. Clamp-related EEG abnormalities during carotid endarterectomy:
A. Occur in about two-thirds of patients undergoing surgery
B. Are more likely in patients with an occluded contralateral carotid artery
C. Predict the need for shunt placement in 90% of patients with contralateral occlusion
D. Are more common in patients with diffuse abnormalities on the preoperative EEG
E. Are more common in patients with only ipsilateral abnormalities on the preoperative EEG

97. A median somatosensory evoked potential (SSEP) was performed in a 67-year-old male in coma who was originally found down after an altercation. The findings on the study included intact N9 and N13 but absent P14 and N20 bilaterally. Which of the following conditions is likely?
A. Brachial plexus injury
B. Traumatic cervical syrinx
C. Wallenberg syndrome
D. Pontine hemorrhage
E. Brain death

98. Which of the following statements is true regarding transcranial electrical stimulation (TES) to elicit motor evoked potentials (MEPs) during intraoperative monitoring (IOM)?
   A. Amplitude reduction of 50% or higher for myogenic motor evoked potentials (mMEPs; M-waves) and D-waves compared to baseline is considered significant for impending neural compromise
   B. During surgeries lasting several hours, thresholds required to elicit MEPs tend to increase
   C. M-waves are elicited predominantly in muscles contralateral to the cathode
   D. Anesthesia has less effect on M-waves than somatosensory evoked potentials (SSEPs)
   E. Latency prolongation of 50% or more for M waves compared to baseline is considered significant for impending neural compromise

99. All of the following statements are true about interpretation of brainstem auditory evoked potentials (BAEPs) *except:*
   A. Prolongation of Wave I absolute latency suggests peripheral hearing loss
   B. Absence of Wave I is diagnostic of cerebellopontine angle (CPA) tumor such as acoustic neuroma
   C. Prolongation of I-III interpeak latency (IPL) suggests an upper pontine lesion
   D. Prolongation of III-V interpeak latency (IPL) suggests an upper midbrain lesion
   E. Absence of Waves I, III and V suggests brain death

100. A 50-year-old male had intractable back pain and the diagnostic workup was significant for L3–L5 disc bulges. He underwent surgical decompression with intraoperative monitoring (IOM). All the baseline tibial somatosensory evoked potentials (SSEP) were within normal limits. During the procedure, the N34 and P37/38 potentials disappeared with preservation of the N22 potential. What is the most appropriate localization?
   A. Tibial nerve
   B. Cauda equina
   C. Lumbar anterior horn cells
   D. Cortex
   E. Lumbosacral plexus

101. The P100 waveform latency is increased by which of the following?
   A. Low contrast; low luminance
   B. Low contrast; high luminance
   C. High luminence
   D. High contrast; low luminance
   E. High contrast; high luminance

102. Visual evoked potentials (VEPs) may be successfully recorded in patients with visual field defects and impaired visual acuity by:
   A. Dilating the pupils
   B. Decreasing the check size
   C. Placing the recording electrodes more laterally
   D. Asking the patient to fixate at different points around the target
   E. Asking the patient to remove eyeglasses and squint

103. Tibial somatosensory evoked potential (SSEP) is preferred to common peroneal SSEP during intraoperative monitoring (IOM) because:

A. It allows recording of peripheral compound nerve action potential
B. It produces a larger cortical potential
C. Its abnormalities correlate better with adverse postoperative outcome
D. A and B
E. A, B and C

104. Which of the following strategies is NOT recommended in obtaining optimum somatosensory evoked potential (SSEP) waveforms during intraoperative monitoring (IOM)?

A. Use of higher stimulus intensities
B. Use of a stimulus rate of 7 Hz instead of 5 Hz or 6 Hz
C. Use of 60 Hz notch filter
D. Use of epoch duration of at least twice the latency of the longest component of interest for signal averaging
E. Use a bandpass filter of 30 to 3,000 Hz

105. During a left acoustic schwanomma surgery, the baseline brainstem auditory evoked potentials (BAEPs) demonstrated a low amplitude Wave I. Which of the following measures is least likely to enhance Wave I amplitude?

A. Increasing the stimulus intensity
B. Decreasing the stimulus intensity
C. Increasing the stimulus rate
D. Changing polarity from rarefaction to condensation
E. Using a supplementary electrode in the external canal

106. Which of the following is true regarding hemifield stimulation to obtain visual evoked potentials (VEPs)?

A. It is sensitive for detecting small retrochiasmal lesions
B. It requires stimulation of each field in each eye separately
C. P100 waveform is prominent in the contralateral occipital electrode as opposed to the mid-occipital electrode
D. It requires the use of smaller check sizes compared to full-field stimulation
E. The normal and abnormal potentials frequently change depending on the eye stimulated

107. Which of the following somatosensory evoked potential (SSEP) abnormalities is least likely to be seen in multiple sclerosis (MS)?

A. Reduced N9 amplitude
B. Prolonged or absent P37
C. Prolonged or absent P14
D. Prolonged or absent N20
E. Prolonged central conduction time

108. In evaluating a spinal cord lesion with somatosensory evoked potential (SSEP):

A. SSEP has no prognostic value regarding sensory recovery compared to clinical examination after acute spinal cord injury
B. Clinical improvement always precedes SSEP improvement after acute spinal cord injury
C. SSEP has no value in evaluation of cervical intramedullary tumors because the SSEP abnormalities are always accompanied by clinical symptoms
D. Prolonged central conduction time (CCT) with intact potentials suggests extramedullary tumor rather than an intramedullary tumor
E. Cervical syrinx is most typically associated with intact N13 and absent P14 and N20 potentials

109. Which of the following statements regarding clamp-related EEG abnormalities during carotid endarterectomy is true?

A. They occur in less than 30% of patients
B. They are associated with a low false positive rate for predicting postoperative stroke risk
C. They are associated with a low false negative rate for predicting postoperative stroke risk
D. They persist despite shunting in the majority of patients
E. They are sensitive in detecting both subcortical and cortical ischemia

110. Which of the following interventions is expected to contribute to the EEG abnormalities observed after carotid clamping during carotid endarterectomy?

A. Placement of shunt
B. Administration of vasopressors
C. Changing the level of anesthesia
D. Administration of intravenous (IV) fluids
E. All of the above

111. Which of the following conditions is least likely to be associated with widespread slow waves on the EEG?

A. Hypocarbia ($PaCO_2$ less than 40 mmHg)
B. Severe hypotension
C. Intravenous (IV) etomidate induction
D. IV propofol induction
E. Hypothermia at 20°C

112. Changes in somatosensory evoked potential (SSEP) waveforms during intraoperative monitoring (IOM) suggestive of neural pathway compromise include all of the following *except:*

A. Fifty percent or higher drop in waveform amplitude compared to baseline
B. Ten percent or higher increase in waveform latency compared to baseline
C. Sudden disappearance of both peripheral and central potentials
D. Disappearance of P14 and N20 waveforms with intact peripheral waveform
E. Disappearance of cortical waveform with intact subcortical and peripheral waveforms

113. Which of the following agents is likely to cause EEG suppression only at very high doses?

A. Enflurane
B. Isoflurane
C. Halothane
D. Desflurane
E. All of the above

114. Which of the following medications in therapeutic doses can cause abnormalities in brainstem auditory evoked potential (BAEP) waveforms?

A. Barbiturates
B. Benzodiazepines
C. Chloral hydrate
D. Halogenated anesthetics
E. Carbamazepine

115. A 41-year-old female with ataxia undergoes median somatosensory evoked potential (SSEP) study, which shows intact potentials with the only abnormality being prolonged P14–N20 interpeak latency (IPL). Which of the following conditions is least likely?

A. Neuromyelitis optica
B. Friedreich's ataxia
C. Midbrain tumor
D. Demyelination in the thalamocortical radiation
E. Multiple sclerosis

116. Which of the following conditions is least likely to cause symmetric bilateral prolongation of P100 latency?

A. Leber's hereditary optic neuropathy
B. Adrenoleukodystrophy
C. Pseudotumor cerebri
D. Friedreich's ataxia
E. Parkinson's disease

117. Which of the following set of findings is compatible with a diagnosis of brain death based on median somatosensory evoked potential (SSEP)?

A. Absent N9, N13, P14, N18, N20
B. Intact N9; absent N13, P14, N18, N20
C. Intact N9, N13, P14, N18; absent N20
D. Intact N9, N13, P14; absent N18, N20
E. Intact N9 and N13; absent P14, N18, N20

118. An appropriate montage for recording tibial somatosensory evoked potential (SSEP) includes all of the following channels *except:*

A. CPc–Fpz
B. CPi–Fpz
C. CPz–Fpz
D. Fpz–C5S
E. T12S–IC

119. Which of the following findings on a brainstem auditory evoked potential (BAEP) can be interpreted as normal?

A. Wave I is absent contralaterally
B. Wave I is absent ipsilaterally with normal Wave V having a peak latency of less than 6 ms
C. Waves II, VI, and VII are absent
D. Wave IV is indistinguishable from Wave V
E. All of the above

120. Which of the following is true regarding somatosensory evoked potential (SSEP) changes during intraoperative monitoring (IOM)?

A. Transient or persistent changes in central conduction time (CCT) compared to baseline occur in a small number of patients
B. Transient intraoperative SSEP changes can be associated with adverse postoperative clinical outcome in less than 25% of patients
C. Transient intraoperative SSEP changes do not predict postoperative SSEP deterioration
D. Persistence of SSEP changes at the end of surgery increases the risk of adverse postoperative clinical outcome
E. Postoperative deterioration of SSEPs can occur despite absence of SSEP abnormalities during surgery

121. Which of the following statements is true regarding the visual evoked potential (VEP)?

A. The most clinically relevant wavform is a large negative polarity wave
B. In pattern reversal VEP, both eyes are stimulated simultaneously
C. Hemifield stimulation allows identification of retrochiasmatic abnormalities
D. Waveform amplitude is more sensitive than latency in evaluating the integrity of the visual pathways
E. All of the above

122. Which of the following changes can be seen with decreasing click intensity during brainstem auditory evoked potential (BAEP) recording?

A. Prolongation of interpeak latencies (IPLs)
B. Increase in waveform amplitude
C. Shortening of absolute latencies
D. Change in the shape of Wave I
E. None of the above

123. A patient is undergoing descending thoracic aorta surgery. The neurophysiologic intraoperative monitoring (NIOM) consists of bilateral ulnar somatosensory evoked potential (SSEP), tibial SSEP, and upper and lower motor evoked potentials (MEPs). During the monitoring, loss of MEP responses from both lower extremities with preservation of both upper extremities is seen. In addition, there is loss of bilateral P37 responses with preserved bilateral PF, EP, and N20 responses. Which of the following provides the best possible interpretation of these findings?

A. Lower limb ischemia
B. Scalp edema

C. Spinal cord ischemia
D. Brachial plexus injury
E. Neuromuscular blocking agent

124. A 3-year-old girl was undergoing surgical resection of a laterally exophytic ganglioglioma arising from the lateral pons and medulla extending into the left cerebellopontine angle (CPA). What is the best interpretation and likely clinical correlation seen with brainstem auditory evoked potential (BAEP) monitoring this case?

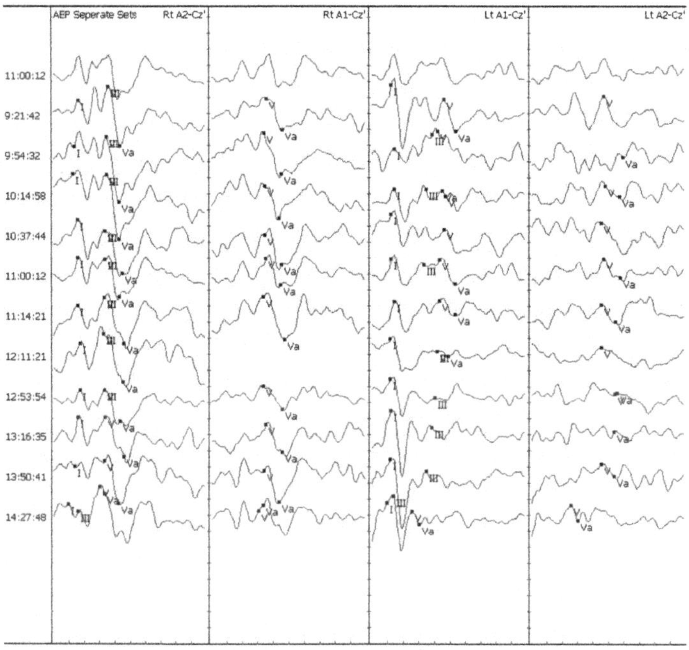

Source: Reproduced from Husain, AM. *A Practical Approach to Neurophysiologic Intraoperative Monitoring*. NewYork, NY: Demos Medical Publishing; 2008.

A. No significant change in brainstem auditory evoked potential (BAEP); hearing will be preserved
B. No significant change in BAEP; hearing will not be preserved
C. Drop in left BAEP amplitude; hearing will not be preserved
D. Drop in right BAEP amplitude; hearing will not be preserved
E. Increase in right BAEP latency; hearing will not be preserved

125. For detection of nerve root injury using neurophysiologic intraoperative monitoring (NIOM) during lumbosacral surgery, compared to sensory evoked potential (SEP), electromyography (EMG) has:
A. Low sensitivity and low specificity
B. High sensitivity and low specificity
C. High sensitivity and high specificity
D. Low sensitivity and high specificity
E. High positive predictive value

126. Which of the following statements regarding multifocal visual evoked potentials (mfVEP) is *true*?

A. It allows assessment of a larger cross-sectional area of the optic nerve
B. It is dependent on the central macula
C. It is prone to cancellation and distortion because it is a summed response of all stimulated neurons
D. Studies have shown no clear utility in glaucoma or optic neuritis
E. The results of mfVEP and full-field pattern-reversal VEP (PVEP) are the same

127. Which of the following statements regarding multifocal visual evoked potentials (mfVEP) is true?

A. A normal pattern-reversal VEP (PVEP) response can be present in the setting of an abnormal mfVEP response
B. An abnormal PVEP response can be present in the setting of a normal mfVEP response
C. The check sizes in mfVEP decrease in size from the center to the periphery
D. mfVEP and PVEP are equally effective in assessing peripheral visual fields
E. mfVEP has more intra-subject than inter-subject variability

ANSWERS

1. **C.** BAEPs can be used for IOM of surgeries on the ears, eighth nerves, and brainstem. They are not useful for monitoring the thalamus or the auditory pathways within the cerebrum, such as that seen during resection involving the auditory cortex. As such, the indications include surgery for acoustic neuromas, and tumors or vascular abnormalities within the posterior fossa. In addition, IOM of BAEPs is also useful in detecting excessive eighth nerve stretch, which can lead to postoperative hearing loss; this can occur from cerebellar retraction during surgery in the CPA and during microvascular decompression.

2. **C.** In patients with suspected MS and an evoked potential abnormality, 50% to 86% will be eventually reclassified as definite MS over a 3- to 6-year period. On the other hand, in patients with suspected MS and normal evoked potential, only about 4% will be reclassified as definite MS. In patients with suspected MS who eventually develop definite MS, the diagnostic EP abnormalities are 66% for VEPs, 23% for SSEPs, and 13% for BAEPs, indicating that VEPs are superior to other modalities in the diagnosis of the condition.

3. **E.** A median SSEP with absent N9 and normal P14 and N20 potentials is considered normal. This may be technical in nature. The presence of brainstem P14 and cortical N20 potentials indicates that the impulses are reaching the sensory cortex, and therefore, no conduction defect along the sensory pathway of the median nerve.

4. **A.** Initial infant screening should be done prior to postpartum discharge from the hospital or within 1 month of birth. BAEP or EOAE test can be used for audiologic screening. For infants who pass the test, no additional intervention is needed. Infants who fail the screening test should be retested within 3 months. It is recommended that definitive intervention to restore hearing should be performed within 6 months to prevent language delay. False positive results may occur because of occlusion of the ear canal, middle ear effusion, or middle ear infection.

5. **E.** BAEP findings in brain death may include intact Wave I or II unilaterally or bilaterally with absence of other waves. Preservation of Wave II in cases with postmortem confirmation of brainstem destruction suggests that Wave II may represent an action potential from the acoustic nerve as it enters the brainstem. Bilateral absence of Wave I is difficult to interpret as the integrity of the peripheral hearing mechanism cannot be inferred, for example, in patients with preexisting deafness. Although absence of all the BAEP waveforms is reported in brain death, this finding should therefore be interpreted with caution.

6. **A.** M-waves are the mMEPs obtained by TES. They reflect the compound motor action potentials elicited within the muscles. They can be recorded using surface or needle electrodes placed in or over the muscles of interest. They are sensitive to anesthetic effects at the anterior horn cell synapses. They can also be attenuated or abolished by neuromuscular blockade; however, they may be successfully recorded using partial neuromuscular blockade maintained by a continuous infusion of paralytic drug rather than by intermittent boluses.

7. **A.** P100 waveform can be distorted by larger check size and faster reversal rates. Higher luminance decreases P100 latency but increases its amplitude.

8. **E.** Depending on the configuration of the waveforms, and the degree to which the waveforms are contaminated by lower-frequency noise, the peak waveform amplitude of SSEPs during IOM can be measured in three ways: with respect to the following peak of the opposite polarity; with respect to the preceding peak of the opposite polarity; and with respect to the baseline level of the waveform preceding (not following) the peak.

9. **C.** Induction of anesthesia with IV propofol initially produces beta activity on the EEG with decrease in alpha. The beta activity rapidly becomes more widespread, with an increase in amplitude. The beta activity then slows into the alpha range, and is accompanied by a burst of high amplitude, frontal intermittent rhythmic delta activity (FIRDA) before a steady-state anesthetic pattern becomes established.

10. **D.** PRVEP is the typical stimulus for VEP and utilizes a checkerboard pattern where the black and white squares alternate at a frequency of 1 to 2 Hz. About 100 to 200 responses are averaged, and the trial is repeated for reproducibility. PRVEP requires adequate visual acuity and maintenance of visual fixation on the center of the patterned screen; therefore, it is not suitable for comatose patients, neonates, and those with severe visual impairment. Although the check size can be increased to allow for fixation in those with mild visual impairment, those with severe impairment may need to be done with flash stimuli. Patients with psychogenic blindness may be able to maintain visual fixation so PRVEP can be tried.

11. **D.** CCT refers to the transit time of the ascending volley in the central segments of the somatosensory pathways. This is typically estimated by measuring the IPIs of the somatosensory evoked potential waveforms. P14–N20 IPI measures the CCT between the brainstem and parietal cortex after median nerve stimulation. Similarly, N22–P37 estimates the CCT between the lumbar cord and parietal cortex after tibial nerve stimulation. In contrast, N13–N20 IPI measures the conduction time starting with the ascending volley in the dorsal columns and does not allow a strict assessment of CCT within the intraspinal and intracranial segments.

12. **C.** Carotid cross-clamping causes EEG changes to occur within the first minute in greater than 80% of patients, with nearly 69% showing changes within 20 seconds after clamping. During steady-state anesthesia, the EEG change is characterized by widespread anteriorly dominant rhythm (WAR pattern), consisting of alpha and beta activity. However, a decrease of this WAR pattern (rather than its appearance) on the clamped side is the most common and sensitive indicator of cerebral ischemia. Progression of ischemia is indicated by an increase in amplitude of delta or slower frequencies followed by "flattening" of the EEG on the clamped side. The EEG changes occur primarily on the side

of clamping, but bilateral changes may be seen. When bilateral EEG changes are seen, it is important to consider the possibility of occlusion or severe stenosis of the contralateral carotid artery resulting in hypoperfusion of the contralateral hemisphere, which is dependent on the collateral circulation from the ipsilateral hemisphere. However, it is worthwhile noting that bilateral changes can also be caused by other factors, such as change in anesthetic level, blood pressure, temperature, $PaCO_2$, or PaO_2. Bilateral EEG changes secondary to hypoperfusion usually consist of more "flattening" in the presence of delta activity with or without reduction of fast activity over the ipsilateral hemisphere.

13. **C.** D-waves are recorded from the spinal cord during TES. D-waves are generated by the propagating action potentials in the spinal cord, whereas the M-waves reflect the compound motor action potentials generated within the muscles. D-waves can be recorded using epidural electrodes or by electrodes placed close to the surgical field, whereas the M-waves can be recorded by needle or surface electrodes placed in or over the muscles. D-waves are resistant to anesthetic effects, and are more likely to be seen than M-waves when inhalational anesthesia is administered. D-waves are more consistent across multiple runs compared to M-waves because the latter are affected by the variable alpha motor neuron pool that is activated. D-waves may get attenuated in the presence of spinal cord pathology due to desynchronization of the descending corticospinal volley. D-waves show changes later than M-waves when motor tracts are compromised.

14. **B.** The peripheral ascending volley of the median SSEP is the N9 potential. It is recorded at the Erb's point in the supraclavicular fossa. It has triphasic morphology (positive–negative–positive), with the negative peak occurring about 9 ms after stimulation (i.e., N9). It is best seen with a noncephalic reference electrode placed over the shoulder on the nonstimulated side. As the N9 potential is generated by the brachial plexus, it will not be affected by proximal lesions such as medullary tumors.

15. **D.** The tibial and median SSEP findings in this patient are likely to show a normal or abnormal N22 latency depending on the extent and type of cord pathology. N22–P37 IPI can be expected to be abnormal given that the lesion is between the lumbrosacral and the lower cervical cord (mid-thoracic sensory level). N9–20 IPI is expected to be normal given the normal exam in the upper extremities and above.

16. **D.** After administration of anesthesia, about 30% to 40% of cases may show focal EEG abnormalities ipsilateral to the clamp side prior to clamping; this usually consists of reduced amplitude of the widespread anterior-dominant rhythm (WAR) pattern, which consists of beta and alpha activity; this may occur with or without polymorphic delta activity. Most focal EEG abnormalities that occur with anesthesia correlate with preoperative abnormalities found on waking EEG. Anesthesia may unmask an abnormality that was absent during the waking state; for example, in patients with a frontal lesion, anesthesia may bring out a reduction of the WAR pattern with decreased beta along with increased polymorphic delta. Similarly, preexisting intermittent rhythmic delta in the temporal region in the wake state may become more prominent and persistent, along with a reduction of the WAR pattern. Anesthesia may also obscure a focal abnormality that was apparent during the waking state; for example, asymmetry of the posterior dominant rhythm during wakefulness associated with an ipsilateral occipital lesion may disappear when the background is replaced by the WAR pattern after anesthesia.

17. **D.** VEP can be elicited by pattern reversal or light flashes. If light is used, then repetitive strobe sequence, alternating intensities, or alternative luminances could serve as stimuli. A flash VEP is typically used in subjects who cannot cooperate, and has the advantage over PRVEP in that visual fixation or eye opening is not required. The drawbacks of flash VEP compared to PRVEP include greater latency variability and less sensitivity to conduction defects. Flash VEP assesses the visual pathway at least through the lateral geniculate nucleus, whereas the PRVEP assesses up to the occipital cortex.

18. **C.** The relatively sudden increase in absolute latencies was likely associated with decreasing the click intensity, which could also lead to an increase in IPLs and decrease in amplitudes. Higher click intensities tend to decrease absolute latencies. To ensure maximal and consistent waveforms, the stimulus intensity is typically set to 65 decibels (dB) above the sensation or hearing levels, termed "dBSL" and "dBHL," respectively. Sleep does not usually significantly affect the brainstem auditory evoked responses; in fact, patients are encouraged to sleep to reduce the muscle artifact.

19. **D.** A demyelinating lesion in the pons is likely to show prolonged P14–N20 IPL because P14 is generated distal to pons and N20 is generated in the cortex. Neither N9 (generated at brachial plexus) nor P14 (generated at caudal medial lemniscus distal to pons) is likely to be prolonged.

20. **E.** With advancements in MRI technique, the utility of EP in the diagnosis of MS has decreased. However, EP can be used to evaluate the organic nature of the subjective symptoms in patients with normal MRI and to follow the clinical course of the disease after making the diagnosis. EP may be more efficient than MRI in isolated optic neuritis. Multimodal EPs tend to be abnormal in about 10% of presumptive MS patients with normal MRI. MRI reveals abnormal lesions in more than 80% of patients with MS.

21. **C.** SSEPs assess the somatosensory pathways carried in the dorsal columns to the parietal cortex, traversing the brainstem and ventral posterolateral (VPL) nucleus of the thalamus. Accordingly, compromise of the posterior spinal artery during surgery can affect the dorsal columns, resulting in changes that can be detected by SSEP monitoring. Anterior spinal artery compromise affects spinothalamic and corticospinal tracts; posterior inferior cerebellar artery compromise affects spinothalamic tracts (Wallenberg syndrome); medial lenticulostriate artery compromise affects motor fibers; therefore, none of these can be expected to cause abnormalities in the SSEPs.

22. **B.** Intact median SSEP potentials with prolonged N9–P14 IPL and normal P14–N20 IPL can be seen in Guillain–Barré syndrome when the affected segment is rostral to the brachial plexus, sparing the N9 potential. Median nerve compression will be caudal to the generation of N9, and is not expected to prolong N9–P14 IPL. Pontine glioma, midbrain hemorrhage, and thalamic hemorrhage affect pathways that are rostral to the generator of P14, and therefore not expected to prolong the N9–P14 IPL. Parsonage–Turner syndrome affects the brachial plexus and is not compatible with the clinical presentation or the SSEP findings.

23. **B.** N13 potential is generated by the postsynaptic activity in the large myelinated fibers in the dorsal horn caudal to the medulla, and is likely to be intact in medullary glioma; however, P14 and N20 potentials are generated rostral to the medulla, and are likely to be affected. In cervical syringomyelia, N13 potential is reduced or absent with normal

P14 and N20 potentials; this selective N13 abnormality reflects a global dysfunction of the dorsal horn in syringomyelia. Wallenberg syndrome is associated with interruption of the spinothalamic tract in the medulla, and it does not abolish P14 or N20 potentials. More than 50% of patients with a pontine lesion have reduced or absent N20, and in most of them, the N13, P14, and N18 potentials are normal.

24. **D.** Normal P37 latencies suggest that impulses are transmitted to the parietal cortex regardless of the underlying pathology. Among the listed conditions, severe peripheral neuropathy, bilateral cauda equina syndrome, and Guillain–Barré syndrome affect the dorsal roots and/or peripheral nerves, and can abolish the LP (N22) potentials; if that occurs, it is unlikely that a normal P37 will be recorded. A technical problem with stimulation or recording is most likely in this situation since LPs are sometimes difficult to obtain even in normal individuals.

25. **E.** SSEPs are useful for monitoring during functional posterior rhizotomy and microlesioning of the dorsal root entry zone. Both procedures aim at deafferenting or damaging enough dorsal horn cells to obtain relief of pain and spasticity, with sparing of large-diameter fibers subserving joint and touch sensation at and below the operated metameric levels, and preservation of perineal sensation and bladder tone at the sacral level. A 60% to 75% postoperative amplitude reduction in segmental potentials (median N13, pudendal N15, or tibial lumbar potential [LP]) correlates well with optimal results on pain and spasticity.

26. **D.** Rarefaction clicks result in decrease of Wave I latency, decrease of V latency, prolongation of Waves I–III IPL, and more distinct Waves IV and V.

27. **C.** In cochlear hearing loss, Wave I may be prolonged but Wave V typically has a normal latency, resulting in shortened Waves I–V IPL. In conductive hearing loss, the Waves I–V IPL is normal. Waves I–V IPL is prolonged in conditions affecting the brainstem, such as multiple sclerosis and glioma. Waves I–V IPL may be normal, but not shortened, in a small cerebellopontine angle tumor.

28. **A.** At levels above the minimal alveolar concentration (MAC) level, enflurane causes spike-wave discharges (at 1.5 MAC), a burst-suppression pattern with spike components, or frank seizures (at greater than 2 MAC). In contrast, isoflurane and desflurane tend to exert an antiepileptic effect, producing an intermittent suppression pattern at 1.5 MAC and continuous suppression at greater than 2 MAC. Halothane also has an antiepileptic effect but produces suppression at greater than 4 MAC. Adding nitrous oxide potentiates the EEG suppression caused by isoflurane and desflurane.

29. **B.** At the sub-MAC level of steady-state anesthesia with inhalation agents, a widespread anteriorly dominant rhythm (WAR) pattern, consisting of low beta and alpha frequencies, is seen. This anesthetic WAR pattern is similar in appearance to the alpha-coma pattern often seen after anoxic brain injury. In addition to the WAR pattern, anteriorly predominant intermittent slow (AIS) waves may appear. The AIS waves are usually biphasic, negative–positive waves, less than 1 second in duration, and occur singly or in bursts. Another pattern that can be seen is a widespread persistent slow (WPS) pattern, which consists of polymorphic slow waves, greater than 1 second in duration. With deepening of the anesthetic level, the WPS pattern becomes more prominent while the WAR

pattern becomes less obvious. Widespread attenuation with bursts of activity (burst-suppression), as indicated in option B, is not seen below the MAC level of anesthesia.

30. **B.** A median SSEP with delayed N9, P14, and N20 potentials with normal interpeak latencies (IPLs) indicates a conduction defect distal to the brachial plexus since N9 is generated by the brachial plexus. Because the median nerve is typically stimulated at the wrist, carpal tunnel syndrome is unlikely. Pronator teres syndrome, caused by entrapment of the median nerve between the two heads of pronator teres muscle at the elbow, is most likely. Guillain–Barre syndrome is more likely to result in bilateral abnormalities.

31. **B.** Pedicle screws are used as a point of fixation for spinal instrumentation. As many as 20% of screws were found to be misdirected in cadaver studies, which can lead to postoperative symptoms. Stimulus-triggered EMG has been shown to verify screw placement in real-time. If the screw is stimulated with a constant voltage of more than 30 V or a current intensity of 25 mA without eliciting EMG activity, then the screw placement is likely correct without broaching the vertebral cortex. A response to stimulation with less than 20 V or a current intensity of 4 to 6 mA suggests a low impedance pathway to the nerve root under the pedicle, likely from the pedicle screw broaching the vertebral cortex.

32. **A.** The changes in latencies represent an improvement due to the effect of decompression because they occur soon after the procedure. Changes in latency related to anesthetic effect are expected to occur gradually, toward the end of surgery, rather than immediately after decompression. On the other hand, the smaller amplitudes seen after decompression compared to baseline could be related to the effect of anesthesia.

33. **C.** BAEP consists of seven waveforms, labeled in order I-VII, which occur in response to an auditory stimulus, and are generated by specific areas along the auditory pathway. Absolute latencies are measured for each individual wave, and interpeak latencies (IPLs) are measured typically for the following intervals: I-III, III-V, and I-V, in order to localize dysfunction. Waves VI and VII have limited clinical application, and therefore IPLs involving these waves are not common.

34. **A.** The amplitude of BAEP component peaks is measured with respect to the trough that follows it; a 50% or higher drop in amplitude is considered significant to cause an "alarm." Similarly, typically a 1 ms increase in component latencies or in the IPLs is considered significant, although some consider a lower prolongation of 0.5 ms to be significant. Wave V is the most consistent and easily recognized component, and therefore Wave V is primarily followed during surgery. The observed latency or amplitude changes may have variable meaning depending on the clinical scenario, including the timing of the change in relation to surgical tasks and other biometric or neurophysiologic intraoperative monitoring (NIOM) signals. In general, BAEP are insensitive to anesthesia, including volatile anesthetics, but are sensitive to surgical tasks, including cold water irrigation and auditory nerve traction.

35. **A.** Nerve manipulations can lead to neurotonic discharges, which are high-frequency and irregular bursts of motor unit potentials with a characteristic sound and appearance. These are felt to result from mechanical stimulation of axonal nerve membranes. In addition to direct nerve manipulaton (e.g., nerve abrasions, stretching, and compression), neurotonic discharges can be triggered by saline irrigation and ischemia.

36. D. BAEP typical stimulation rates are 8 to 11 Hz but can be increased to faster rates of 70 to 100 Hz. Faster stimulation rates can affect waveform characteristics, including decreases in amplitude, dispersion of waveforms, prolongation of IPLs, and increase of absolute latencies. Increasing the stimulus rate, typically greater than 30 Hz, may worsen the appearance of the abnormality. In addition, an abnormality not noted at the typical rates may appear at the higher rates.

37. E. PERG is a retinal evoked potential generated by a high-contrast, patterned stimulus (e.g., alternating black and white checkerboards or stripes). In contrast to full-field ERG assessing the overall retinal function, PERG can record the central visual field. Following the reversal of the contrast, a positive wave is seen at 50 milliseconds (P50) and a negative wave at 95 milliseconds (N95). PERG provides a measure of macular function (P50) and ganglion cell function (N95). VEP can be abnormal in both macular dysfunction and optic nerve disease; the addition of PERG can add more insight and meaning to the VEP interpretation. In general, PERG is abnormal in maculopathy and normal in demyelinating optic nerve diseases. However, abnormal PERG accompanied by abnormal VEP suggests axonal involvement with retrograde degeneration of ganglion cells. Normal PERG accompanied by abnormal VEP suggests optic nerve demyelination. After recent optic neuritis, an abnormal PERG predicts poor visual recovery while a progressive decrease in PERG amplitude correlates with development of optic nerve atrophy.

38. A. Inhaled anesthetics (e.g., isoflurane, desflurane, enflurane, nitrous oxide, sevoflurane) do not decrease the latencies of evoked potentials (e.g., brainstem auditory evoked potentials [BAEP], somatosensory evoked potential [SSEP], and motor evoked potential [MEP]). Instead, they typically increase the latencies and decrease the amplitudes. Many agents do not appear to significantly change the amplitude of BAEP except for nitrous oxide, which decreases the amplitude. Nitrous oxide does not appear to significantly change the latencies of BAEP or SSEP but can increase latency of MEP. Of note, enflurane can increase the latency and amplitude of SSEP.

39. E. Wave I of BAEP reflects the action potential volley in the distal portion of the auditory nerve. It is recorded as a near-field, negative potential at the skin surface around the stimulated ear with very little presence at the vertex. This negativity is picked up in the Ai electrode and represented as an upgoing (i.e., positive) peak in the Cz-Ai recording based on the BAEP convention of displaying positive waveforms in G1 and negative waveforms in G2 as upward deflections. Because Wave I is recorded as a near-field potential around the stimulated ear, repositioning of the Ai/Mi recording electrode can substantially alter it. Wave I may be better seen with an electrode within the external auditory canal. Because Wave I is generated distally in the auditory nerve, it may persist after the nerve is sectioned more proximally during surgery for acoustic neuroma.

40. C. With each TES stimulus to obtain MEPs, only a small number of the alpha motor neuron pool is activated, and the subset of activated alpha motor neurons varies from run to run. This causes the mMEPs (M-waves) to vary substantially in morphology from trial to trial. Accordingly, signal averaging should not be used to record M-waves; besides, M-waves are large waveforms (hundreds of microvolts in amplitude) so no averaging is needed. However, D-waves are much smaller in amplitude, and signal averaging is needed to obtain clearer and more consistent waveforms. As the stimulus intensity is increased, more of the corticospinal axons away from the surface of the head get stimulated, sometimes as far caudally as the medulla. If the at-risk part of the nervous system that is being monitored is rostral to the caudal extent of the stimulated motor tracts, surgery-related abnormalities may not be detectable by high intensity stimulation. To avoid this, stimulus intensity should be kept low enough to produce the waveforms in only one limb but not in multiple limbs. M-waves are recorded by using a train of closely spaced stimuli to achieve temporal summation of the excitatory postsynaptic potentials (EPSPs) in order to activate the anterior horn cells. Usually, three to seven stimuli per train with an interpulse interval of 2 to 4 ms are used. In contrast, for recording D-waves, pulse train stimulation is not used because there is no intervening synapse; this also makes it less likely that the stimulation will cause undesirable limb movement.

41. E. The N13 component of the median SSEP is felt to be generated by stimulation of large myelinated fibers in the dorsal horn by the afferent volley. It is best seen as a negative potential over the C5–C7 spinous processes (it can be recorded as a positive potential over the anterior neck). It is preserved in brain death and cervicomedullary lesions; however, it is abolished in cervical cord gray matter lesions affecting the dorsal columns. The ascending limb of N13 may contain the N11 potential, which is felt to be generated by the ascending volley of action potentials in the dorsal columns of the cervical spinal cord. Therefore, the N13 can have two components, one generated in the dorsal columns and the other in the dorsal horn gray matter.

42. C. The P14 component of the median SSEP is a far-field potential, best seen on the scalp using a noncephalic reference; it is felt to be generated at the subthalamic level, most likely by the afferent volley in the medial lemniscus. In addition, N18 is also a subcortical far-field potential recorded over the ipsilateral centro-parietal region using a noncephalic reference; it is felt to reflect postsynaptic activity in the brainstem caudal to the thalamus generated by multiple sources (nucleus cuneatus, pretectal, and tectal nuclei). N9 is a near-field potential at Erb's point using a noncephalic reference, felt to be generated by the afferent volley in the brachial plexus. N13 is a near-field potential recorded at the C5–C7 spinous process using a noncephalic reference, felt to be generated by the postsynaptic activity in the large myelinated fibers in the dorsal horn. N20 is a near-field potential recorded in the contralateral centro-parietal region using a cephalic reference; it represents activity in the parietal cortex with a generator located in the posterior bank of the Rolandic fissure.

43. A. Although BAEP may be abnormal in the setting of normal imaging, a normal BAEP makes the presence of an acoustic neuroma unlikely. In acoustic neuromas, Wave I usually has prolonged latency or is absent. Compression of the auditory nerve and/or brainstem usually leads to delayed Wave I–III IPL, which is felt to be the most sensitive abnormality with acoustic neuromas. Of note, brainstem distortion can lead to delays in Wave I–III IPL and/or Wave I–V IPL both ipsilateral or contralateral to the lesion. If the tumor is large enough, absence of Wave III and subsequent BAEP components can occur. Normal preoperative BAEPs are associated with a higher probability of hearing preservation postoperatively.

44. **C.** The VEP in the question shows asymmetric bilateral P100 prolongation (approximately 240 ms on the left, approximately 185 ms on the right). This can be seen in chiasmal lesions, retrochiasmal lesions, bilateral optic nerve lesions, metabolic disorders, and degenerative diseases. Psychogenic blindness is not likely as there is marked prolongation of P100 latencies despite good cooperation and fixation. Note that an abnormal P100 could occur if a patient is uncooperative, does not focus on the checkerboard pattern, or maintain fixation at the center of the screen. Of note, although nearly two-thirds of patients with Friedreich's ataxia have abnormal VEPs, other types of spinocerebellar degeneration typically have normal VEPs.

45. **D.** BAEP monitoring has been shown to improve postoperative neurologic outcome. Transient complete disappearance of BAEPs can be compatible with complete neurologic recovery, but persistent loss of waveforms is usually associated with hearing loss and neurologic deficit. A delay in Wave V latency of 1 ms is felt to be critical, indicating potential permanent hearing loss. Intact BAEP and electrocochleogram waves at the end of acoustic neuroma resection have been associated with preservation of functional hearing postoperatively. Abrupt loss of Wave I is usually the result of compromise of the internal auditory artery.

46. **D.** Wave I is typically absent in the contralateral ear channel. Wave III has a smaller amplitude in the contralateral ear channel. Wave IV latency is shorter and Wave V latency is longer in the contralateral ear, allowing separation of the Wave IV to V complex in the contralateral channel.

47. **A.** Nitrous oxide can attenuate cortical SSEP waveforms. Benzodiazepines can decrease the waveform amplitude or increase it paradoxically. Etomidate is known to increase waveform amplitude. Progressive myoclonic epilepsies (PMEs) and certain focal epilepsies with focal motor seizures can be associated with giant SSEP potentials.

48. **C.** Wave I reflects activity at the distal end of the cochlear nerve. Wave II may represent the summation of more than one generator: postsynaptic potentials in the cochlear nucleus in the brainstem and action potential in the proximal portion of the auditory nerve. Wave III is thought to represent potentials evoked within the superior olivary complex and trapezoid body. Wave IV is felt to be generated in the lateral lemniscus (LL) but it is unclear whether Wave IV represents postsynaptic potentials in the LL, action potentials from lemniscal fibers, or a combination of the two. Wave IV is believed to originate in the inferior colliculus, although a contribution from LL is suggested. Sources of Waves VI and VII (data not shown) are even less clear: Wave VI is believed to originate in the medial geniculate body while Wave VII is believed to originate in the auditory radiation.

49. **A.** Wave I of BAEPs is seen only ipsilateral to the stimulated ear. Wave III has lower amplitude contralateral to the stimulated ear. Wave V is generated by lateral lemniscus or inferior colliculus located in the upper pons or lower midbrain. Most anesthetic agents do not significantly affect BAEP waveforms. The waveforms are not dependent on cognitive ability or level of consciousness, and thus can be used in infants and children.

50. E. The size of the check is based on the visual angle it subtends. A circle makes up 360°, and 1° consists of 60 minutes. The entire checkerboard usually has a visual angle of 8°, and each square typically has a visual angle of 30 minutes, but that depends on the check size. The smaller checks are more sensitive in detecting visual defects, produce more consistent responses, and have better sensitivity to contrast in central vision. Larger checks, on the other hand, stimulate the peripheral vision better. Larger checks can prolong P100 latency, especially when the stimulus field size is small.

51. A. N13 potential after median stimulation is felt to be generated by the postsynaptic activity in the large myelinated fibers in the dorsal horn caudal to the medulla; it is therefore likely to be preserved in medullary lesions. P14 and N18 potentials after median stimulation and P31 after tibial stimulation are generated close to the dorsal column nuclei in the medulla; P38 after tibial stimulation is generated in the primary sensory cortex. Therefore, these waveforms, which are cephalad to the medullary lesions, are likely to be affected.

52. B. The noted figure shows loss of P14, N18, and N20 potentials postoperatively with right median stimulation. This suggests compromise of the somatosensory pathways at or distal to the cervicomedullary junction but proximal to the brachial plexus. Such changes can be seen after midline myelotomy for resection of a cervical intramedullary tumor. Absence of cortical SSEPs after right median stimulation can be associated with impaired proprioception in the right arm, not the left arm. Because SSEPs reflect posterior column function, motor deficits, such as weakness, cannot be inferred from the SSEP abnormalities.

53. E. Condensation is the movement of the speaker membrane *toward* the eardrum, whereas rarefaction is the movement of the speaker membrane *away from* the eardrum. Rarefaction clicks are recommended for clinical BAEPs testing. Rarefaction clicks decrease Waves I and V latencies. At times, it may be difficult to assess artifact from true BAEP waveforms. In those cases, alternating the stimulus polarities during the test may help because artifact should reverse in polarity with the stimulus polarity change; however, the BAEP waveforms should maintain their polarities. Alternating stimulus polarity is not generally recommended because of phase cancellation, which tends to occur in patients with high-frequency hearing loss.

54. A. D-waves are recorded from the spinal cord during TES. They are generated by the propagating action potentials within the corticospinal tract. They are typically recorded using an epidural electrode inserted percutaneously via a Touhey needle or by electrodes placed within the surgical field close to the spinal cord. They are relatively resistant to anesthetic effects as there are no intervening synapses between the stimulation site in the brain and the recording site in the spinal cord. D-waves may get attenuated in the presence of spinal cord pathology due to desynchronization of the descending corticospinal volley. However, they may be normal in unilateral spinal cord abnormalities if the motor tracts in the brain are stimulated bilaterally.

55. C. The noted figure shows evidence of spinal cord ischemia in the left lower limb because of decreased blood flow in the segmental artery distal to the site of aortic cross-clamp. Increase in mean arterial pressure to improve collateral flow can correct such changes while grafting of the vessels is performed. mMEPs can show changes independently of SSEPs. Upper limb mMEPs are intact.

56. A. Intravenous barbiturate anesthesia depresses EEG activity and brainstem reflexes. However, short-latency somatosensory evoked potentials (SSEPs) are relatively resistant to barbiturate anesthesia, and remain within normal limits in this condition. Other listed conditions are associated with brainstem or spinal cord pathology, and can cause prolongation of CCT.

57. C. Despite dermatomal overlap between roots and inter-individual variations, dermatomal SSEPs have been found to be useful in the evaluation of radiculopathies, especially those causing only pain or sensory symptoms. Intact N9 and absence of subsequent potentials suggest a lesion proximal to the dorsal root ganglion (DRG) such as root avulsion (not brachial plexus lesion); however, absence of all the potentials including N9 suggests a lesion distal to DRG such as brachial plexopathy. Guillain–Barré syndrome is usually associated with absence of both popliteal fossa and lumbar potentials with tibial SSEP, and absent N9 and N13, or prolonged N9–N13 interpeak latency (IPL) with median SSEP. In Friedreich's ataxia, sensory nerve action potentials can be reduced or absent; in those with a long history, SSEPs tend to be absent as well.

58. E. P100 latency tends to increase with age, especially after age 45 years. P100 latency is shorter in women than men, and is felt to be related to differences in brain size and the related shorter pathways in females. As little as two diopters of refractive error can lead to delayed latency and decreased amplitude of P100, especially with the use of small checks and low contrast level. P100 latency increases with decrease in pupillary diameters, and is due to decreased retinal illuminance. The P100 latency may be normal even in the setting of visual disturbance.

59. B. The cortical potential, N20, is a near-field potential. As such, it is best seen in the CPc–CPi channel with the CPi cephalic reference, not the CPc–EPc channel with the EPc noncephalic reference. CPi–EPc is suitable for recording the far-field potentials P14 and N18; C5S–EPc is suitable for recording the near-field spinal potential, N13; EPi–EPc is suitable for recording near-field potential N9, representing the afferent volley in the brachial plexus at Erb's point.

60. B. VEP is a long-latency near-field potential. Bifid P100 waveform can be caused by projections from upper and lower visual fields or by phase-shifted activity at the mid-frontal reference electrode. Such a waveform may be corrected by stimulation of the inferior visual fields. Visual acuity affects P100 latency, with less than 20/200 vision increasing the P100 latency. Although the P100 potential is generated by the contralateral occipital cortex, it is best seen ipsilateral to the stimulated side after hemifield stimulation because of the orientation of the stimulated occipital neurons.

61. E. Presence of normal N20 potentials in the acute stage of coma does not necessarily predict good recovery because only two-thirds of such patients will have a good recovery, either complete or with minimal disability. In patients with coma due to head injury or vascular damage, bilateral absence of N20 potential is associated with death or PVS in 90%. In the same patient population, the rate of adverse outcome (i.e., death, PVS, or severe disability) is as follows: in 74% of cases when N20 is absent unilaterally; in 58% when the central conduction time (CCT) is increased; in 35% when cortical SSEPs are normal; and in 14% when all cortical SEPs including middle-latency and late-latency responses are preserved. Intact N9 and N13 potentials with absence of subsequent waveforms bilaterally to median nerve stimulation carries a prognosis of death or PVS in 90%

of coma due to primary hemispheric lesions identifiable on MRI, and in almost 100% of coma due to anoxia. Bilateral absence of N20 potentials is associated with PVS more frequently in coma due to anoxia than in coma due to head trauma or vascular lesions, particularly when brainstem auditory evoked potentials (BAEPs) are preserved. In contrast, in coma due to primary brainstem lesions, moderate disability or good recovery can occur, despite absence of cortical potentials on SSEP.

62. E. The peak-to-peak amplitude of giant SSEPs is usually greater than 15 μV, and can reach 50 μV or more. The P14 and N20 potentials in giant SSEPs have normal latency and amplitude in most patients with cortical myoclonus, suggesting that the sensory input to the cortex and the cortical response are essentially normal. It is believed that the giant SSEP results from an abnormal enhancement of other components of the SSEP such as the N24-P24 generator in area 3b. In conditions causing pyramidal myoclonus, giant SSEPs are preceded by an abnormal cortical spike, which is best seen with jerk-locked back-averaging of EEG; however, giant SSEPs can also occur in the absence of such abnormal spikes.

63. D. In MS, SSEPs have been shown to be abnormal in the absence of clinical sensory impairment as well as in those with chronic disease who have never experienced sensory symptoms. However, the yield of SSEPs is not considered excellent because of high false negative rate (i.e., they may be normal in nearly 25% of patients with sensory symptoms or signs). SSEPs may be abnormal in those with spinal cord lesions but are rarely abnormal in the setting of a normal MRI spine. The occurrence of abnormal SSEPs is maximal when all four limbs are tested. The diagnostic yield increases by about 10% by testing the upper limb when lower limb SSEPs are normal. A couple of studies have shown that the yield of abnormality varies depending on the stage of MS, with more frequent abnormalities being seen in definite MS compared with possible MS.

64. E. In the question, all the SSEP waveforms are preserved bilaterally (N9 in channel 4, N13 in channel 3, P14/N18 in channel 2, and N20/P22 in channel 1) with the exception of poorly formed N13 (channel 3) on the right side. There is no evidence of brain death as both N20 potentials are intact. Although the absolute and interpeak latencies (IPLs) are not specified, they appear grossly normal. Thus, this is likely a normal study. Of note, if all of the absolute latencies were prolonged, it would be suggestive of a peripheral process such as neuropathy or Guillain–Barré syndrome.

65. E. Nearly 40% of patients with MS without sensory symptoms may have abnormal SSEPs. Although the cortical potentials may be abolished by anesthesia, intravenous etomidate can increase the amplitude of cortical potentials. Amplitude of cortical potentials may be increased in progressive myoclonus epilepsy, resulting in "giant SSEPs." SSEPs are commonly used in NIOM since they can assess the neuroaxis at virtually all levels. Common criteria to detect a change during NIOM include an amplitude drop greater than 50% and/or latency prolongation of 10% over baseline. However, these criteria may need to be modified in certain cases, including alteration of anesthesia gases during the case, significant blood loss, and initial poor signal quality.

66. E. N7 is a near-field potential caused by activation of the tibial nerve fibers (not cauda equina), and is recorded in the popliteal fossa; it reflects a mixed response of motor and sensory fibers. N22 is a near-field potential reflecting postsynaptic activity in the dorsal horn neurons of the lumbar cord corresponding to S1 root; it is recorded over the T12 spinous process using a reference over the iliac crest. P31 is a far-field potential reflecting activity in the brainstem (likely, caudal medial lemniscus in the medulla), and is analogous to the P14 potential recorded from median SSEP; it is best recorded over the mid-frontal region (Fpz) using a noncephalic reference over C5–C6 spinous process. N34 is a near-field potential reflecting activity in the parietal cortex. P37 is also a near-field potential reflecting activity in the parietal cortex; it is best recorded in the midline (CPz) or ipsilateral central-parietal region (CPi) using a mid-frontal reference (Fpz). The most likely reason for the paradoxical lateralization of P37 to the side of stimulation relates to the somatotopic representation of the foot that is situated on the medial aspect of the hemisphere.

67. **A.** Luminance is the brightness, and contrast is related to the difference in luminance of the white and black checks. Low luminance and low contrast result in decreased amplitude and increased latency of the P100 waveform.

68. **C.** The P14 component of the median SSEP is a far-field potential, best seen on the scalp using a noncephalic reference. It is felt to be generated at the subthalamic level, most likely by the afferent volley in the medial lemniscus. It is preserved in thalamic lesions but abolished in cervicomedullary lesions and brain death. P14 is the only scalp far-field potential that is reduced by interfering stimulations (e.g., vibrations) applied to the hand on the stimulated side, suggesting that it is generated after the synaptic relay in the nucleus cuneatus.

69. **A.** N20 is generated in the parietal cortex while P22 is felt to be generated in the central or frontal cortex. Less than 10% of patients with focal cortical lesions present with dissociated abnormalities of N20 and P22 waveforms. This suggests that parietal and frontal potentials may have distinct generators activated by the thalamocortical pathways. When N20 is lost, patients exhibit astereognosis and sensory impairment to elementary modalities without motor deficit. Conversely, patients with absent P22 exhibit motor impairment with intact sensation.

70. **C.** Advanced cataract, severe optic neuritis and technical problems during the study (hardware defects, poor visual fixation, etc.) can cause an absent P100 waveform. Extensive bilateral occipital lesions can result in cortical blindness; however, in this condition, visual evoked potentials (VEPs) have been found to be present in most cases. There are two possible explanations for VEP preservation in cortical blindness: VEPs either originate in extrastriate areas (areas V2 and V3) via retinotectal cortical pathways, or they are generated by small islands of striate cortex that have survived the pathologic process, causing bilateral occipital damage.

71. **E.** In general, subcortical SSEP waveforms are more robust than the cortical waveforms in IOM and are unlikely to show significant changes. The cortical waveforms, such as N20 and P37/38, can be prolonged or diminished by sleep, sedation, and anesthesia, especially inhalation anesthetics. Decreased thalamocortical activity could account for the reduced cortical but preserved subcortical waveforms.

72. **B.** In optic neuritis, abnormal VEP to smaller check size is more common during the initial stages. VEP latency can remain prolonged after recovery of vision in up to 95% of

patients. Thus, VEP is a reliable indicator of resolved optic neuritis. VEP can be abnormal in 54% to 70% of MS patients with normal visual function and neuro-ophthalmologic examination. Thus, VEP has great sensitivity to detect subclinical optic nerve lesions. VEP is more sensitive than optical coherence tomography in detecting optic nerve dysfunction (81% vs 60%). In optic neuritis, the P100 latencies are characteristically prolonged. If both eyes are affected, the latency prolongation may be asymmetric. However, in optic neuritis, because it is mainly a demyelinating and not an axonal process, the amplitude and waveform morphology are typically preserved.

73. **A.** SSEPs can be used to monitor the condition of the central somatosensory pathways during surgery on the brain, brainstem, or spinal cord that places those structures at risk or during orthopedic surgery that poses a risk to the spinal cord or plexus. SSEP monitoring is useful for carotid endarterectomy to detect ischemia. Phase reversal of N20/P20 potentials across the central sulcus after median nerve stimulation can be used to localize the central sulcus during resection of a parietal glioma. Injury to the lumbar plexus can be detected during reduction of a pelvic fracture. However, SSEP monitoring has not been found useful for preventing sciatic nerve injury during total hip arthroplasty; electromyography (EMG) monitoring has been found to be useful in this procedure.

74. **C.** SSEPs from electrical stimulation of mixed nerves mostly reflect the activity of cutaneous and joint afferents. However, stimulation of muscle afferents was shown to elicit a cortical response after stimulation of the tibial nerve but not the median nerve; this activity peaks a few milliseconds earlier than that evoked by cutaneous afferents.

75. **E.** P100 is a positive waveform. It is preceded by N75 and followed by N145 peaks, both negative waveforms. It can be distorted, and may appear to have a "W-shape" because of an active mid-frontal reference or because of projections from different parts of the calcarine cortex. True latency of such distorted waveforms can be determined by stimulation of inferior visual fields or by finding the intersection of tangents drawn to the positive and negative slopes of the waveform. P100 is primarily generated in the visual (striate) cortex, although there is some indication that it may also be generated in the extrastriate cortex based on its preservation in cortical blindness.

76. **E.** Unilateral P100 prolongation is suggestive of a lesion in the anterior visual pathways on the side of stimulation. Such a prolongation is etiologically nonspecific, and can occur in demyelinating lesions, compressive lesions, and ischemic lesions. Retrochiasmatic lesions are not likely to cause unilateral P100 prolongation with full-field stimulation but can cause abnormalities in the affected visual field with half-field stimulation of each eye.

77. **B.** Etomidate increases the amplitude of cortical waveforms. The other listed agents can cause attenuation of cortical waveforms, which is more likely with halogenated anesthetic agents, such as halothane.

78. **C.** Alternating polarity clicks are not used routinely in clinical practice because of phase cancellation; rarefaction clicks are the most reliable and recommended in clinical practice. However, alternating polarity clicks can differentiate true waveforms from artifacts because true waveforms do not change polarity whereas artifacts do. Rarefaction clicks decrease Wave I latency. In some patients, Wave V may become visible only after the click polarity is reversed.

79. A. Sudden loss of Waves I, III, and V can occur as a result of damage to the internal auditory artery, causing cochlear ischemia or infarction. Loss or delay of Waves III and V with preservation of Wave I reflects compromise of the proximal part of the eighth nerve (not the distal part) or of the lower pons. If the BAEP changes are unilateral or asymmetrical, the predominant pathology is likely to be ipsilateral to the ear whose stimulation gives the most abnormal BAEPs. Drilling of bone can produce high noise levels in both ears via bone conduction, and cause alteration of the waveforms due to acoustic masking, which simulates cochlear dysfunction; this represents a false positive change with no real compromise of the auditory system. It is recommended that the BAEP recording be paused during bone drilling.

80. C. The figure shows the absence of all BAEP waveforms starting at 12:23 p.m., consistent with cochlear infarct, which is most likely from vasospasm. This is not due to changes in anesthesia because BAEPs are resistant to anesthetic effects, and no clinically significant changes are expected even with halogenated agents. The prolongation of Wave V latency from 11:51 a.m. to 12:05 p.m. can be attributed to cerebellar retraction with some improvement noted upon release of traction until 12:18 p.m. The noted changes in BAEPs are severe enough to cause postoperative hearing deficit.

81. D. P100 latency is less than adult values during infancy, and reaches typical adult values by age 1 year for the larger check sizes. P100 latency for smaller check sizes reaches normal adult values by age 5 years. There may be a subtle decrease in P100 latency in adolescence but the P100 latency can increase by 2 to 5 ms per decade after age 60. One study showed age-related linear increase in P100 latency with greater prolongation with smaller check size and lower-intensity stimulation.

82. E. Giant SSEPs are characteristically seen in progressive myoclonic epilepsies (PMEs), such as Lafora body disease. In some conditions causing focal motor seizures, giant SSEPs may be seen in the absence of stimulus-induced myoclonus. Giant SSEPs are not typically seen in juvenile myoclonic epilepsy or other nonprogressive isolated forms of myoclonus. However, they can be variably seen in Creutzfeldt–Jakob disease (CJD), postanoxic myoclonus, and over the affected hemisphere in patients with supratentorial tumors, posttraumatic cortical atrophy, and ischemic or hemorrhagic stroke. In PME, the giant SSEPs and myoclonus reflect cortical hyperexcitability to afferent impulses. In destructive hemispheric lesions (e.g., tumors, trauma, stroke), the enhancement of the cortical response tends to be less than that observed in PME; loss of inhibitory control and collateral sprouting of cortical afferents are felt to underlie giant SSEPs in these conditions.

83. B. Absence of Wave I with intact Waves III and V is most consistent with mild to moderate peripheral hearing loss. In severe hearing loss, all the waves are absent. In brain death, Wave I is present but the rest of the waves are absent. Absence of Wave V indicates a lesion above lower pons. Cortical lesion is not expected to produce abnormalities in Waves I, III, or V.

84. D. In cervical spondylotic myelopathy, lower limb stimulation is more sensitive than upper limb stimulation in detecting abnormalities of central conduction. Neither narrowing of the cord diameter nor increased cord T2 signal is associated with median SSEP abnormalities. The practical utility of median and tibial nerve SSEPs is in patients without

MRI evidence of a cervical cord abnormality; in more than 60% of patients with normal MRI, evidence of cervical cord dysfunction can be detected by SSEPs.

85. A. Abnormal VEP is seen in 25% of patients with suspected MS and normal MRI. Bilateral P100 prolongation does not always suggest chiasmal or retrochiasmal lesions as they can be seen in bilateral optic nerve lesions, metabolic disorders, and degenerative diseases. When psychogenic blindness is suspected, a normal VEP supports the diagnosis but it does not completely rule out blindness because cortical blindness can be present with an intact P100. P100 is prolonged in late (not early) cataract, causing severe visual impairment.

86. E. All BAEP waveforms are far-field potentials. Unlike near-field potentials that are generated near the surface electrodes, far-field potentials are thought to be generated by deep gray and/or white matter structures. That being said, theoretically certain dipole potentials can be recorded as near-field and far-field potentials. Wave I, for instance, recorded at Cz (which is what is done routinely), is a far-field potential but Wave I recorded at the ear (which is not done routinely) is a near-field potential. BAEP waveforms are surface positive at the vertex and are generated within 12 ms of the click. Clinically relevant BAEP waveforms measure conduction between rostral medulla (Wave I) and midbrain (Wave V).

87. E. Extensive thalamic lesions affecting the ventral posterolateral (VPL) nucleus are associated with loss of cortical potentials after median stimulation including N20 and P22. However, P14 and N18 are intact. In addition, all peripheral waveforms should be intact.

88. C. N13 is a near-field potential (not a far-field potential) reflecting activity in the dorsal columns of cervical cord. The other options are correct.

89. D. N34 is a subcortical far-field potential, not a near-field potential. The other options are correct. Note that the sensory representation for the lower leg is located on the medial aspect of the parietal cortex. As a result, it is believed that the evoked tangential dipoles result in the P37 waveform that is prominent ipsilateral to the stimulated side.

90. C. Wave I reflects activity at the distal end of the cochlear nerve in the region of the ganglion cells. Wave II is generated in the proximal portions of the cochlear nerve in the region of its entry into the brainstem. Wave III is generated in the region of the ipsilateral cochlear nucleus. Waves IV and V are generated bilaterally in the region of the midbrain tegmentum.

91. E. An EEG pattern resembling FIRDA can be seen during induction, steady-state anesthesia at sub-MAC (minimal alveolar concentration) level, and recovery from sub-MAC level anesthesia. Addition of nitrous oxide potentiates the EEG suppression caused by isoflurane such that suppression can be seen at lower MAC levels of isoflurane.

92. A. For extraoperative median SSEP, the afferent volley at the brachial plexus is recorded by an electrode at Erbs' point (i.e., N9); during IOM, however, the Erbs' point may be too close to the surgical field. In such cases, the afferent peripheral volley can be recorded by an electrode near the nerve around the elbow, referred to an electrode on the lateral or medial aspect of the arm at the same level. For tibial stimulation, the peripheral nerve volley can be recorded from a midline electrode behind the knee, referred to either the lateral or medial aspect of that knee. The spinal potentials following median (N13) and tibial (N22) stimulation are of limited utility during IOM because they are often small, difficult to record, generated caudal to the brainstem that the IOM is intended to safeguard, and require placement of recording electrodes too close to the surgical field. During IOM, it is important to record the cervicomedullary potentials, following median (P14) and tibial (P31) stimulation. Although these components are typically recorded between the dorsal scalp and a noncephalic electrode, such a long interelectrode distance recording during IOM can result in an unacceptable amount of noise. To avoid this, a forehead-to-inion or a forehead-to-earlobe recording can be used. Cortical potentials with median nerve stimulation (N20) tend to be smaller but clearer with a CPc-CPi linkage because of the cancellation of the subcortical N18 component, which has a wide symmetrical distribution over the vertex. However, if the SSEPs are being used to monitor spinal cord function, a forehead reference instead of CPi will provide a larger waveform, which is a composite of N18 and N20 that would still be acceptable because both the waveforms are expected to be affected by spinal cord compromise.

93. E. BAEPs are short-latency, far-field potentials. Waveform amplitudes decrease and IPLs increase with click rates greater than 10 Hz. Higher click intensity decreases absolute latencies but the click intensity does not affect IPLs. Click polarity affects the latencies with rarefaction clicks, not condensation clicks, decreasing the latencies of Waves I and V. In some cases, an absent Wave V may be made visible by reversing the click polarity.

94. E. Maturation of SSEPs from birth to adult life is influenced by two phenomena with opposing effects: myelinogenesis causes an increase in conduction velocities and synchronization of potentials, whereas body growth causes prolongation of latencies and desynchronization. Spinal cord conduction in lower limb fibers reaches adult values by 5 to 6 years, with the peak latencies reaching adult values by the age of 15 to 17 years. Hypothermia with core body temperature down to 17°C abolishes N20 and P14 potentials but not N9 and N13. Stage II sleep is associated with prolongation of N20 latency by about 0.4 ms compared to wakefulness, and a shortening of N20 latency by about 0.3 ms compared to REM sleep. Although body height affects both absolute and IPLs for tibial SSEPs, the effect is less pronounced on IPLs, and hence the latter are used to calculate the central conduction time (CCT).

95. A. Wave I is recorded as a near-field potential close to the ear; therefore, it is subject to alteration based on the location of the ipsilateral electrode (Ai). Thus, if Wave I is indistinct, repositioning of the ipsilateral earlobe electrode can help make it clearer. Masking of the contralateral ear with white noise to prevent acoustic crosstalk is not feasible during IOM if the stimuli are interleaved (i.e., auditory stimuli are delivered alternately to the left and right ears); furthermore, lack of masking will not interfere with recognition of new auditory pathway compromise when a functioning ear is stimulated. Unlike extraoperative BAEP recording, longer epoch length of about 15 ms is recommended during IOM because the latencies of component waveforms can be prolonged by preexisting pathology, hypothermia, or intraoperative compromise of the auditory system. Stimulation with alternating click polarities and averaging the responses together can be helpful to cancel large stimulus artifacts.

96. B. The incidence of clamp-related EEG abnormalities is estimated to be about 10% to 30%. The incidence is higher in patients with occluded versus patent contralateral carotid artery (39% vs 16%). Furthermore, the higher incidence of clamp-related EEG abnormalities is associated with greater than 90% stenosis rather than less than 50% stenosis of the contralateral carotid artery. It is estimated that 30% to 40% of the patients with contralateral occlusion require shunt based on EEG findings. Clamp-related EEG changes are more common in patients with contralateral abnormalities on the preoperative awake EEG than in patients with only ipsilateral or diffuse abnormalities.

97. E. In brain death, the pattern of abnormalities on median SSEP consists of intact peripheral N9 and spinal N13 but absent P14, N18, and N20 responses. It is important to note that the above pattern may also be seen in lesions affecting the cervicomedullary junction; however, this is not one of the options listed. With brachial plexus injuries, there is decreased peripheral conduction with normal central conduction times. This may present with a delayed or absent N9 with absent or delayed N13 and N20 potentials. In cervical syringomyelia, N13 potential is reduced or absent with normal P14 and N20 potentials; this selective N13 abnormality reflects a global dysfunction of the dorsal horn in syringomyelia. Wallenberg syndrome is associated with interruption of the spinothalamic tract in the medulla, and it does not abolish P14 or N20 potentials. More than 50% of patients with a pontine lesion have reduced or absent N20, and in most of them, the N13, P14, and N18 potentials are normal.

98. B. Since D-waves are highly consistent across repeated trials, a 50% or higher decrease in amplitude or a 10% or higher increase in latency would constitute a significant change indicating impending neural compromise. On the other hand, M-waves vary substantially across repeated trials; therefore, a rigid 50% amplitude drop criterion would lead to too many false alarms. To avoid this, complete disappearance of M-waves or a 75% to 90% amplitude drop may be more reasonable. During surgeries lasting several hours, MEP amplitudes tend to decrease while thresholds required to elicit MEPs tend to increase ("anesthetic fade"); this may require reestablishment of the MEP baseline. Since TES preferentially stimulates the brain under the anode, M-waves are predominantly elicited in muscles contralateral to the anode. However, M-waves may also be present in muscles contralateral to the cathode, but these cathodal stimulation-elicited MEPs may disappear from anesthetic effects rather than corticospinal tract compromise. Furthermore, anesthesia is likely to attenuate M-waves more so than SSEPs.

99. A. Most CPA tumors spare Wave I. Absence of Wave I with intact Waves III and V is suggestive of mild to moderate peripheral hearing loss. Presence of Wave I and absence of subsequent waveforms can be seen in severe brainstem dysfunction such as brain death. Prolongation of IPL I–III suggests an ipsilateral lower brainstem lesion between the acoustic nerve and lower pons. Prolongation of IPL III–V suggests upper brainstem dysfunction between the lower pons and midbrain, such as with demyelination.

100. D. The lesion is proximal to the lumbar spine. Thus, localization to the cortex is the best option. Given normal N22 potential, the peripheral nerve, lumboscaral plexus, cauda equina, and lumbar anterior horn cells are not likely to be involved.

101. A. Luminance is the brightness, and contrast is related to the difference in luminance of the white and black checks. Low luminance and low contrast result in decreased amplitude and increased latency of the P100 waveform.

102. C. Dilating the pupils will increase luminance but this is not recommended to ensure test standardization. Increasing the check size will be beneficial in patients with poor visual acuity. Usual eyeglasses should be used. In patients with field defects, P100 may be distorted; in such cases, recording from more laterally placed electrodes may be helpful. It is important to make sure that the patient fixates vision on the target at all times; inability to achieve visual fixation can cause prolonged latency and distorted waveforms.

103. D. Both tibial and common peroneal SSEPs during IOM have similar correlation with postoperative outcome. However, the tibial nerve tends to be the most frequently used. It is the largest sensory nerve of the leg with the greatest representation in the somatosensory cortex. Stimulation of the tibial nerve behind the medial malleolus allows recording of the tibial nerve compound action potential (CAP) in the popliteal fossa (N7). The presence of N7 confirms delivery of the stimulus as intended, and therefore aids in the interpretation of changes in the more rostral waveforms. In contrast, the common peroneal nerve is stimulated at the knee behind the fibula, and there is no easy way to record the peroneal CAP. Tibial stimulation produces a larger waveform than peroneal stimulation. Tibial nerve stimulation causes less patient movement than peroneal nerve stimulation. Tibial nerve stimulating electrodes at the ankle are usually easier to reach and replace in a draped patient during surgery if they are dislodged as opposed to the peroneal stimulating electrodes at the knee.

104. C. In contrast to extraoperative recording, higher stimulus intensities are recommended for SSEP recording during IOM to ensure adequate stimulation in case there are technical problems, such as the development of edema. Stimulus rates of 2 to 8 Hz are used, although exact submultiples of the line frequency (e.g., 5 or 6 Hz) should be avoided because signal averaging in such cases would not effectively eliminate the line-frequency artifact. Typical filter settings include 5 to 30 Hz for the low-frequency filter and 1,000 to 3,000 Hz for the high-frequency filter. The 60 Hz notch filter should be avoided because it can cause a "ringing" oscillatory artifact. It is recommended that the epoch duration used for signal averaging be at least twice the latency of the longest SSEP component that is of interest (50 ms for upper limb and 80–100 ms for lower limb SSEP). Usually, 200 to 1,000 sweeps are averaged.

105. C. Decreasing the stimulus rate, not increasing, may enhance Wave I. Other employable techniques include increasing the stimulus intensity if the waves are of low amplitude and poorly defined; decreasing the stimulus intensity if there are too many or poorly defined waves; changing the click polarity from rarefaction to condensation; using a supplementary electrode in the external canal; and using sedatives to decrease the muscle artifact.

106. B. Visual hemifield stimulation requires stimulation of each field (nasal and temporal) in each eye separately. Even with hemifield stimulation, VEPs are sensitive for detecting only large retrochiasmal lesions. Such lesions usually produce clinically detectable field cuts. The normal and abnormal potentials should not change depending on the eye stimulated. Although the P100 waveform is generated in the contralateral occipital cortex, it is paradoxically more prominent in the occipital electrode ipsilateral to the stimulated field because of the orientation of the stimulated occipital neurons. For hemifield stimulation, larger check sizes are typically used to stimulate more of the peripheral retina.

107. A. The most frequent SSEP abnormality in MS is prolongation or absence of the P37 component after tibial nerve stimulation. Other common abnormalities include prolonged or absent P14 and N20 potentials after median nerve stimulation. Latency abnormalities are also associated with prolonged interpeak latencies or central conduction time. However, peripheral potentials (e.g., N9 generated by the afferent volley in the brachial plexus) are normal in central demyelination.

108. D. It has been shown that after acute spinal cord injury, SSEPs predict the sensory recovery better than clinical examination and that SSEP improvement may precede clinical improvement. In cervical intramedullary tumors, median SSEPs show abnormalities in up to 86% of patients; more than one-third of these abnormalities tend to be clinically silent, that is, not associated with sensory deficit or abnormal reflexes. Prolonged CCT with intact potentials is more likely to occur from extrinsic compression of the spinal cord from an extramedullary tumor. In cervical syringomyelia, 83% have reduction or absence of N13 potential; this is associated with normal P14 and N20 potentials in 75% of cases. This selective N13 abnormality reflects a global dysfunction of the dorsal horn in syringomyelia.

109. A. EEG monitoring during carotid endarterectomy shows clamp-related EEG abnormalities in up to 25% of patients. Out of these patients with clamp-related EEG changes, only 8% to 9% develop postoperative stroke even when no shunting is performed. Thus, there is a high rate of false positive clamp-related EEG changes. However, postoperative stroke incidence is lower in those who undergo selective shunting based on EEG abnormalities in contrast to those who do not have EEG monitoring and shunting (0.3% vs. 2.2%). About 20% to 66% of patients who have postoperative stroke do not show EEG abnormalities (false negative EEG). When clamp-related EEG changes are seen, they tend to resolve with shunt placement or raising blood pressure. Possible reasons for false negative EEG include lack of sensitivity of EEG to show changes related to subcortical, capsular, or small cortical ischemia on visual inspection, and occurrence of embolic stroke during postoperative recovery after EEG monitoring has ended.

110. E. EEG abnormalities observed postclamping can be reversed with shunt placement. After the shunt is placed, the EEG can gradually return to the preclamp state over several minutes in the majority of patients. It appears that a longer clamp time prior to shunting correlates with slower recovery. In the minority of patients in whom the EEG does not return fully to the preclamp state, the postoperative neurologic deficit tends to be minor or transient. In some patients, transient and focal EEG abnormalities may appear long after clamping due to the asymmetrical effect of changing the level of anesthesia, decreased blood pressure, or resurgence of preexisting focal abnormality. Such transient changes usually have no neurologic consequence. Slight reduction of systemic blood pressure may result in focal areas of ischemia that bring out the EEG abnormalities, especially when the blood pressure at the time of clamping is close to the threshold level. Raising the blood pressure by administration of IV fluids or vasopressors usually corrects these EEG abnormalities.

111. E. Widespread slow waves on the EEG can be seen in hypocarbia ($PaCO_2$ less than 40 mmHg); severe hypotension; and IV induction with etomidate, propofol, and thiopental. Although mild hypothermia can cause widespread slowing, severe hypothermia at 20°C to 25°C causes EEG suppression.

112. C. In general, the criteria for potential neural pathway compromise are 50% or higher drop in waveform amplitude or a 10% or higher increase in waveform latency compared to baseline. If the peripheral nerve compound action potential (CAP) persists but the rostral waveforms (e.g., P14 and N20) disappear, it is most likely due to compromise of the afferent pathways from surgical manipulation. Unilateral cortical loss with preserved subcortical and peripheral waveforms is suggestive of cerebral ischemia, which can be seen during carotid retraction. On the other hand, if both peripheral and central potentials disappear, it is most likely due to technical factors leading to inadequate stimulation of the peripheral nerve; however, one needs to be cognizant of the rare possibility of a mechanical or ischemic compromise of the peripheral nerve in the limb.

113. C. Halothane has an antiepileptic effect and produces EEG suppression at a greater than 4 MAC (minimal alveolar concentration) level. Isoflurane and desflurane tend to exert an antiepileptic effect, producing an intermittent suppression pattern at 1.5 MAC and continuous suppression at greater than 2 MAC. Adding nitrous oxide potentiates the EEG suppression caused by isoflurane and desflurane. At supra-MAC level, enflurane causes spike-wave discharges, a burst-suppression pattern with spike components or frank seizures.

114. E. Barbiturates, benzodiazepines, chloral hydrate, and most anesthetics do not cause significant abnormalities in BAEPs except in extreme doses. Aminoglycosides and salicylates cause prolonged Wave I latency and reduced BAEP amplitudes, which are usually reversible with discontinuation of the medication. Platinum-containing chemotherapeutic agents, antiepileptic drugs (phenytoin, carbamazepine, and valproate), and ethanol intoxication can prolong the latencies.

115. A. Intact median SSEP potentials with prolonged P14–N20 IPL suggest an abnormality in the somatosensory pathways rostral to the lower medulla. Neuromyelitis optica is characterized by demyelination in the spinal cord along with optic neuritis but no lesions in the brain; it is therefore unlikely to result in the above abnormality. However, this pattern can be seen due to multiple sclerosis plaques. Friedreich's ataxia of long-standing duration can abolish all SSEP waveforms; however, in the early stages when P14 is present, N9–P14 IPL will be normal but P14–N20 IPL may be prolonged. Both midbrain tumor and thalamocortical demyelination are rostral to the generator of P14 potential, and can be expected to prolong the P14–N20 IPL.

116. C. Conditions associated with symmetric bilateral prolongation of P100 include Leber's hereditary optic neuropathy, adrenoleukodystrophy, Friedreich's ataxia, spinocerebellar degeneration, Parkinson's disease, Alzheimer's disease, chiasmal lesions, and bilateral retrochiasmal lesions. P100 latency is usually not affected by pseudotumor cerebri. Asymmetric bilateral prolongation of P100 suggests demyelinating optic neuritis such as that seen in multiple sclerosis.

117. E. For practical purposes, brain death equates to brainstem death. In that context, the pattern of abnormalities on median SSEP consists of intact peripheral N9 and spinal N13 but absent P14, N18, and N20 responses. A similar pattern can occur with lesions at the cervicomedullary junction, which must be excluded prior to concluding brain death.

118. A. The cortical potential, P37, is a near-field potential. It is relatively large and restricted to the ipsilateral parietal region, and as such, a CPi–Fpz montage (not CPc–Fpz) would be optimal. CPz–Fpz is also suitable for recording the near-field cortical potential; Fpz–C5S is suitable for recording the subcortical far-field spinal potential, N34; T12S–IC is suitable for recording the spinal lumbar potential, N22.

119. E. Although amplitudes of BAEP are variable and generally have no clear clinical relevance, the contralateral Wave III often has reduced amplitude. The contralateral Wave I is always absent. If the ipsilateral Wave I is absent, the study is still considered normal if there is a normal Wave V with a peak latency of less than 6 ms. Waves II, VI, and VII are often absent. Wave IV tends to be buried within and indistinguishable from Wave V.

120. D. IOM of SSEPs during spinal surgery reveals transient or persistent changes in CCT in 71% of patients. These changes have a good correlation with postoperative clinical and SSEP outcome. Transient intraoperative SSEP abnormalities are associated with postoperative clinical or SSEP deterioration in 70% or 40% of patients, respectively. The risk of postoperative adverse outcome increases to 85% when SSEP changes do not return to baseline values at the end of surgery. Conversely, no postoperative deterioration of SSEPs are expected when no SSEP abnormalities are seen during surgery.

121. C. The VEP typically has a large positive polarity wave, the P100, which is a measure of conduction time (the primary measure of pathway integrity) between the retina and the occipital cortex. With the commonly used full-field stimulation with only one eye stimulated at a time, only conclusions about the optic nerve anterior to the optic chiasm can reliably be made. However, with hemifield stimulation, pathology posterior to the optic chiasm could be identified in some cases. Although most evoked potentials have small amplitude, the large P100 waveform is many times seen on routine EEGs, usually during photic driving.

122. D. Decreasing click intensity does not substantially affect IPLs because the latencies of all BAEP waves shift nearly in parallel. However, decreasing click intensity reduces amplitudes and increase latencies (roughly linear with 0.3 ms per 10 dB decrease in intensity). Shape of Wave I is determined by differential activation of two neuronal populations that depends on click intensity. Hearing thresholds are determined for the specific ear being tested. The stimulus intensity is usually set for 65 dB above the decibel sensation level (dBSL) or decibel hearing level (dBHL).

123. C. Spinal cord ischemia is the best possible interpretation. There are a variety of patterns that can be seen during aortic surgeries. The table below summarizes some explanations of various permutations.

"Interpretation of Changes in NIOM During Descending Thoracic Aortic Surgery" from Husain 2E (Prod Code 00150)

	SEP				MEP	
	Ulnar		Tibial		Upper	Lower
	EP	N20	PF	P37		
Technical	–	–	–	–	–	–
Cerebral ischemia	+	–	+	–	–	–
Hypotension	+	–	+	–	–	–
Inhalational anesthetics	+	–	+	–	–	–
Neuromuscular blocking agents	+	+	+	+	–	–
Spinal cord ischemia	+	+	+	–	+	–
Lower limb ischemia	+	+	–	–	+	±
Upper limb ischemia	–	–	+	+	±	+
Brachial plexus injury	–	–	+	+	–	+
Scalp edema	+	+	+	+	–	–

Note: MEP, motor evoked potential; NIOM, neurophysiologic intraoperative monitoring; SEP, sensory evoked potential.

Source: Reproduced from Husain, AM. *A Practical Approach to Neurophysiologic Intraoperative Monitoring.* 2nd ed. New York, NY: Demos Medical Publishing; 2014.

124. C. The figure shows BAEPs changes with left ear stimulation. On the waterfall, note that there was an initial loss of amplitude of wave V, triggering an alert to the surgeon. However, by the end of the case, there was no wave V. If wave V is present at the end of a surgical case, this is a very good indicator that hearing will be preserved.

125. B. Compared to SEP monitoring, EMG monitoring has a high sensitivity for detecting mechanical nerve root manipulation but a lower specificity and positive predicitive value for postoperative nerve root injury. EMG activity occurs in 80% of cases, but less than 10% develop a persistent postoperative deficit. As it is more valuable to detect nerve root irritation prior to any potential irreversible injury, in general for NIOM, sensitivity is preferable to specificity.

126. A. mfVEP allows for simultaneous recording from multiple visual field regions, leading to an assessment of a much larger cross-sectional area of the optic nerve. This provides a more accurate functional evaluation of the visual pathway compared to PVEP. The mfVEP has been used in assessing glaucoma and optic neuritis. On the other hand, conventional full-field PVEP is a summation response of all neuronal elements stimulated and is therefore prone to cancellation and distortion. PVEP is greatly dependent on central macula function and is less dependent on the peripheral visual fields.

127. A. A normal PVEP response can be present in the setting of an abnormal mfVEP response. A normal PVEP response can occur when central vision is preserved even if there is significant peripheral visual field defect. The check size typically used for PVEP is optimal for central visual fields but not for the peripheral retina. On the other hand, mfVEP uses a dartboard pattern consisting of 58 segments of 4 × 4 checks cortically scaled to increase in size from the center to the periphery, which allows for greater resolution of the peripheral visual field. mfVEP has inter-subject variability due to differences anatomical differences between the location of primary visual cortex in relation to the electrodes. Intra-subject variability is reduced as there is no anatomical difference between the responses in the same individual.

6

Polysomnography and Other Sleep Studies

QUESTIONS

1. A 54-year-old man is being evaluated for loud snoring. A 30-second epoch of his overnight polysomnogram (PSG) is shown below. Which of the following statements best describes the findings on this epoch?

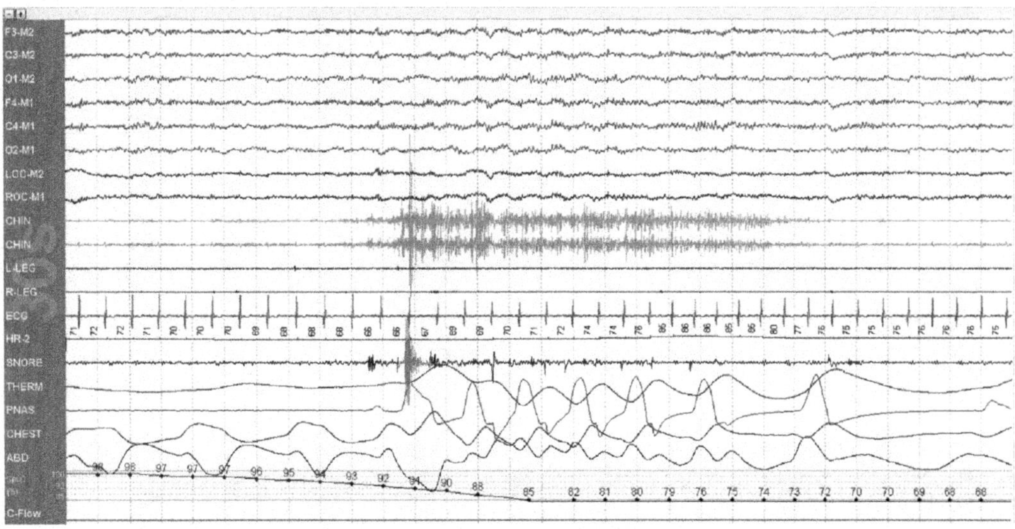

ANSWERS TO THIS SECTION CAN BE FOUND ON PAGE 352

The figures in this chapter can be viewed in a larger size by accessing the digital version of this chapter found on Springer Publishing Company Connect™. Refer to the front of this book for access instructions.

A. Sleep stage is N3
B. There is a hypopnea
C. There is an apnea
D. There is an apnea with arousal
E. There is elevated chin electromyography (EMG) suggestive of REM behavior disorder

2. Which of the following patterns has been associated with chronic fatigue/pain conditions?
A. Alpha intrusion
B. Alpha–beta sleep
C. Monomorphic spindle-like activity
D. Absence of REM sleep
E. A and B

3. Which of the following statements is true regarding the maintenance of wakefulness test (MWT)?
A. A preceding full-night polysomnogram (PSG) is required prior to the test
B. Four trials lasting 30 minutes each are performed at 2-hour intervals during daytime
C. The room is lit with bright light
D. Subjects are instructed to stay awake during the trial
E. Trial ends when the subject achieves one epoch of any stage sleep

4. A 30-second epoch of a polysomnogram (PSG) is shown below. What sleep stage is it?

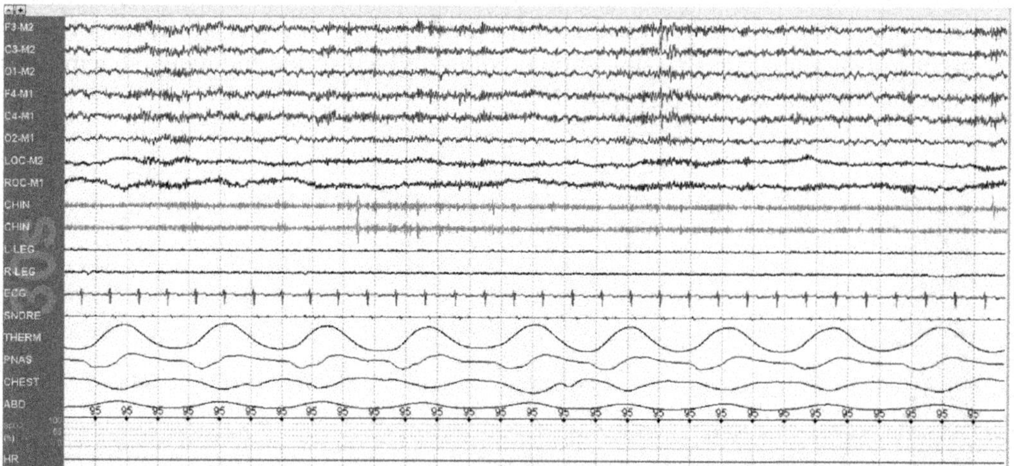

A. Wake
B. N1
C. N2
D. N3
E. REM

5. A 72-year-old male with congestive heart failure and excessive daytime sleepiness is being evaluated for sleep apnea. A 30-second epoch of his polysomnogram (PSG) is shown below. Which of the following findings is seen?

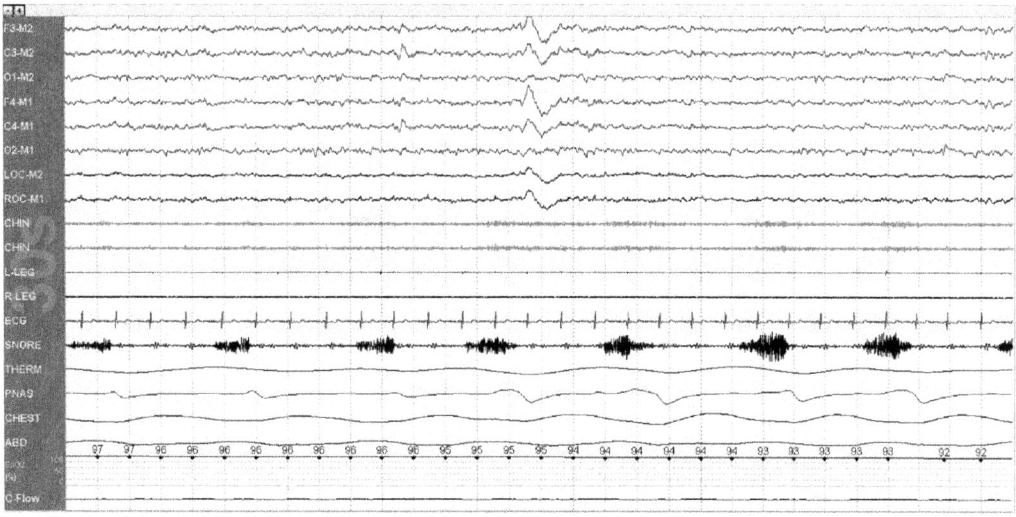

A. Snoring
B. Apnea
C. Hypopnea
D. A and B
E. A and C

6. A 40-year-old, obese male is being evaluated for snoring, witnessed apneas, and excessive daytime sleepiness. Which of the following statements is true about the 30-second epoch of his polysomnogram (PSG) shown below?

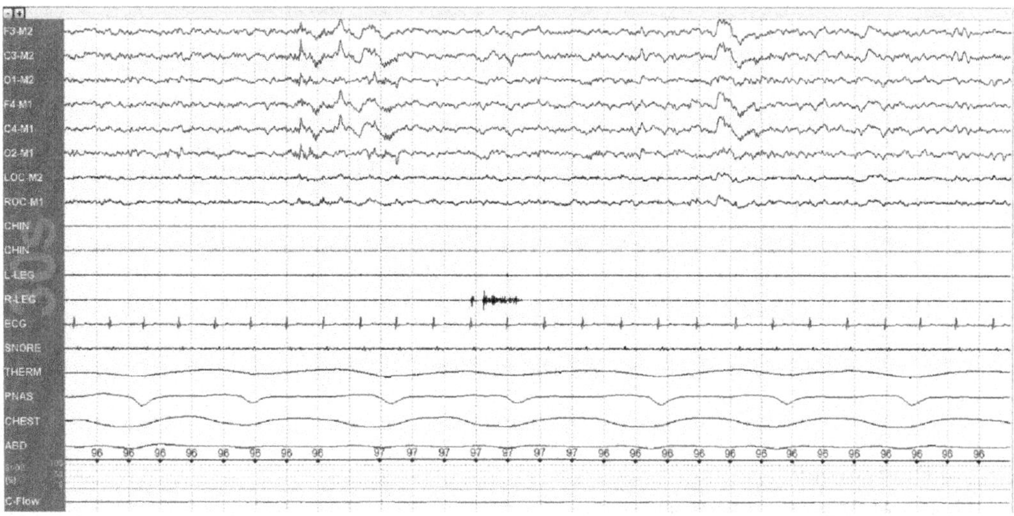

A. It shows Stage N1
B. There is a periodic limb movement of sleep (PLMS)
C. There are generalized epileptiform discharges
D. Nasal pressure channel (marked PNAS) is uninterpretable because of artifact
E. It shows REM sleep

7. A 54-year-old male with obstructive sleep apnea (OSA) undergoes an overnight sleep study for biphasic positive airway pressure (BiPAP) titration. His hypnogram is shown below. Which of the following interpretations is least likely?

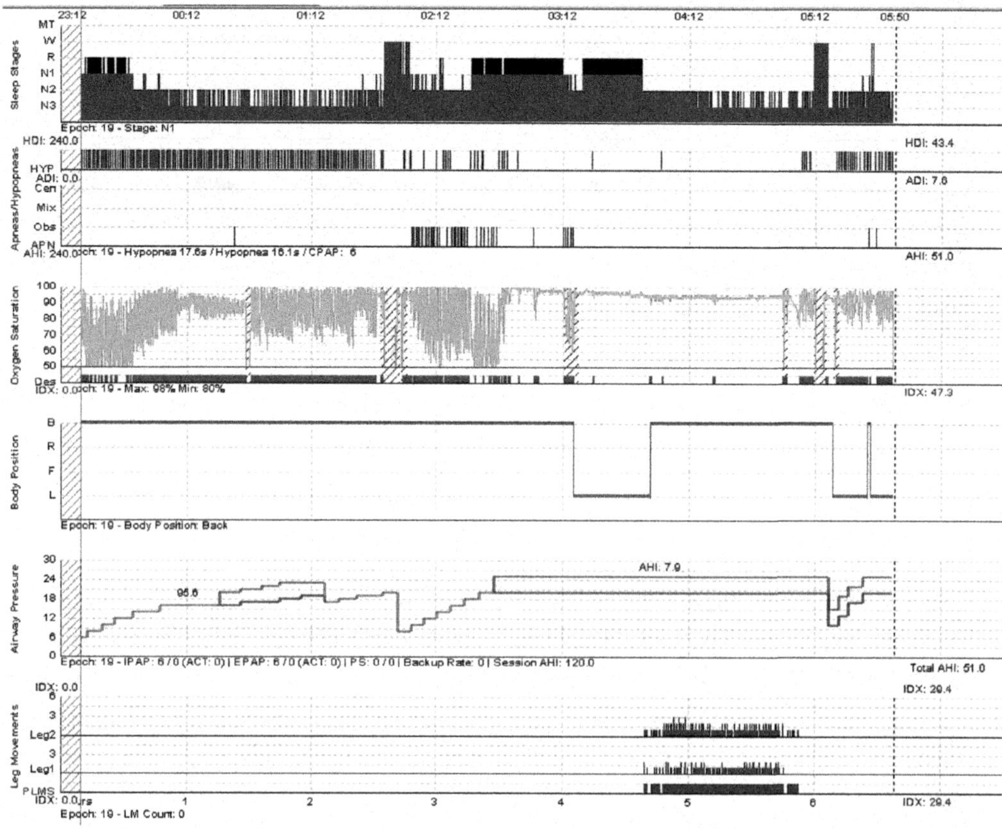

A. There is evidence of significant hypoxemia in REM sleep despite BiPAP
B. BiPAP therapy is partially successful
C. There is evidence of coexistent periodic limb movement disorder
D. There is evidence of positional variation of sleep apnea
E. There is evidence of poor sleep efficiency

8. What is the gold standard for measuring airflow?
A. Pneumotachograph
B. Thermistor
C. Thermocouple
D. Nasal pressure transducer
E. Respiratory inductance plethysmograph

9. In a 60-year-old female, which of the following findings on polysomnography is least likely to be associated with nonrestorative sleep?
A. Alpha intrusion
B. REM sleep without atonia
C. Sleep efficiency of 88%

D. Periodic limb movement arousal index of 10
E. Apnea-hypopnea index (AHI) of 15

10. Which of the following sleep disorders is known to predominantly manifest in the sleep stage depicted in the 30-second epoch below?

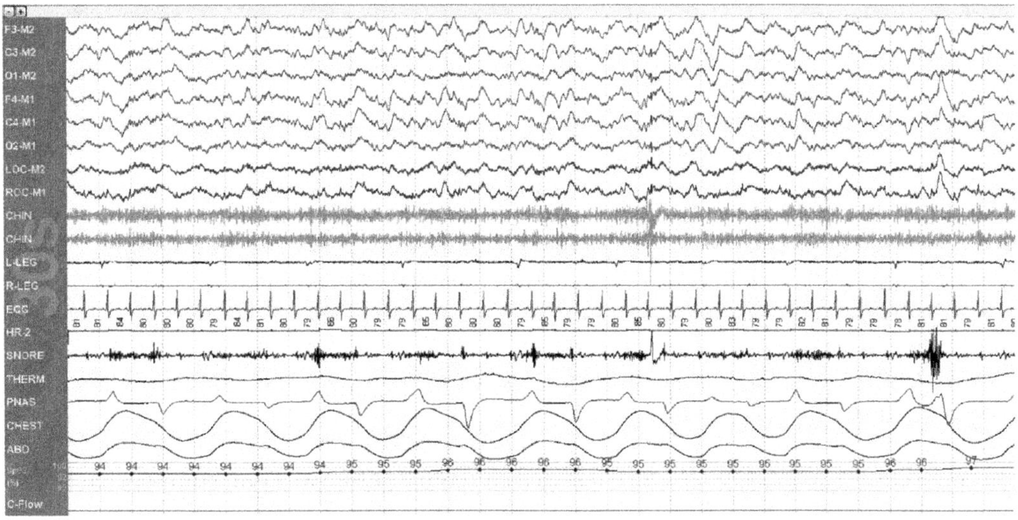

A. Bruxism
B. Sleep-related rhythmic movement disorder (head banging)
C. Sleep terror
D. Hypnic jerks
E. All of the above

11. Which of the following statements best describes the sleep stages?
A. Stage N1 is characterized by increased theta frequencies
B. Stage N2 is characterized by frontocentral sleep spindles
C. Stage N3 is characterized by delta activity occupying at least 10% of the epoch
D. A and B
E. A, B, and C

12. A 65-year-old female presented to a neurologist for possible seizure workup. Her husband mentioned that while she is sleeping, she kicks him, appears restless, and talks in her sleep. If he wakes her up, she is noted to be confused but able to recount her event as a dream that corresponds to the observed behavior. What is the most likely diagnosis?
A. Restless leg syndrome (RLS)
B. REM behavior disorder
C. Periodic limb movement disorder (PLMD)
D. Frontal lobe seizure
E. Temporal lobe seizure

13. The slow waves seen in Stage N3 sleep have which of the following characteristics?
A. 0.5–3 Hz, greater than 100 μV
B. 0.5–3 Hz, greater than 75 μV

C. 0.5–2 Hz, greater than 75 μV
D. 0.5–2 Hz, greater than 50 μV
E. 0.5–2 Hz, greater than 30 μV

14. Which of the following conditions is least likely to be associated with sleep-onset REM periods (SOREMPs)?
A. Narcolepsy
B. Recent sleep deprivation
C. Phenobarbital administration
D. Phenobarbital withdrawal
E. Circadian rhythm disorders

15. Which of the following statements regarding sleep stages is true?
A. N1 (Stage I) is characterized by the attenuation of posterior alpha activity
B. N2 (Stage II) is defined by the presence of vertex sharp transients
C. N3 (Stages III and IV) is defined by the presence of theta and delta waves in at least 10% of the epoch
D. REM is characterized by low-voltage theta background
E. All of the above

16. Which of the following signals is needed to score apneas on a polysomnogram (PSG)?
A. EEG
B. Electrooculogram (EOG)
C. Electromyography (EMG)
D. Thermistor
E. EKG

17. Scoring of a respiratory effort-related arousal (RERA) requires that:
A. The respiratory event last at least 10 seconds
B. There is at least 4% oxygen desaturation
C. There is stable respiratory effort
D. There is flattening of the expiratory portion of the nasal pressure
E. Absence of arousal

18. Which of the following statements is most consistent with the definition of sleep-onset REM period (SOREMP) in a multiple sleep latency test (MSLT)?
A. The occurrence of REM sleep at the onset of the nap
B. The occurrence of REM sleep within the first 2 minutes of the nap
C. The occurrence of REM sleep within the first 10 minutes of the nap
D. The occurrence of REM sleep within the first 15 minutes of the nap
E. The occurrence of REM sleep at any time during the nap

19. Which of the following features best describe the sawtooth waves?
A. They are notched waveforms
B. They typically occur after a burst of eye movements
C. They are seen in the occipital region
D. They are in the alpha frequency range
E. All of the above

20. Which of the following conditions is considered to be present or worsen during REM sleep?
    A. Sleepwalking
    B. Epileptic seizures
    C. Obstructive sleep apnea
    D. Periodic limb movement disorder
    E. Confusional arousals

21. How often is REM sleep thought to occur in adults?
    A. Every 30 minutes
    B. Every 50 minutes
    C. Every 60 minutes
    D. Every 90 minutes
    E. Every 120 minutes

22. A 42-year-old, obese female is being evaluated for suspected obstructive sleep apnea (OSA) based on excessive daytime sleepiness, fatigue, and snoring. Her hypnogram after an overnight polysomnogram (PSG) is shown below. Which of the following management strategies for her condition is least likely to be beneficial?

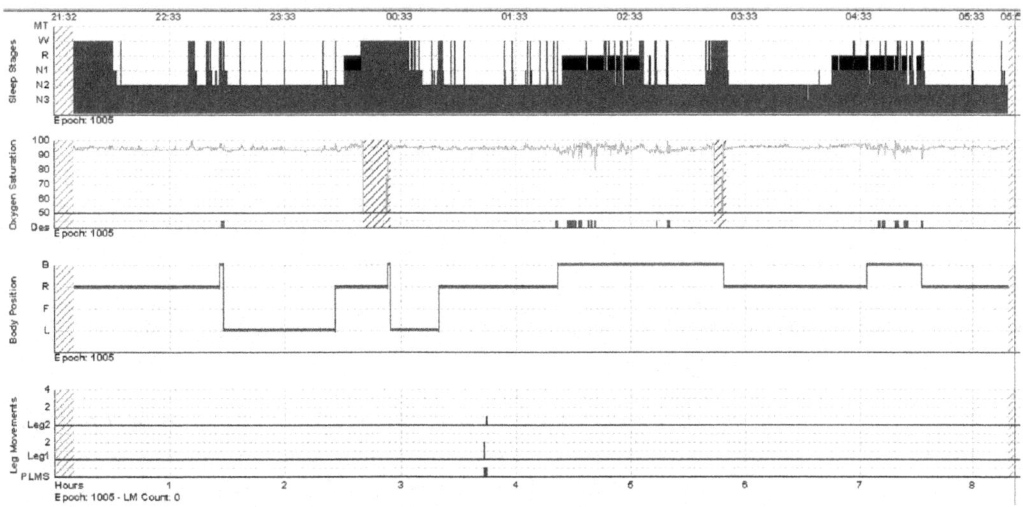

    A. Repeat overnight polysomnogram because of poor sleep efficiency
    B. Repeat overnight polysomnogram for continuous positive airway pressure (CPAP) titration
    C. Positional therapy
    D. Oxygen supplementation at night
    E. Weight loss

23. Which of the following criteria is required to classify periodic leg movement sequences?
    A. Amplitude of at least 10% above the resting electromyography (EMG)
    B. Sequence of at least three consecutive leg movements
    C. The interval between leg movements should be 5 to 60 seconds

D. Leg movements separated by 2 seconds or less in the two legs are counted as one movement
E. If the leg movement is associated with an arousal, the arousal must occur within 3 seconds of the leg movement

24. A 69-year-old woman is being evaluated for excessive daytime sleepiness. Four consecutive 30-second epochs (#153–#156, labeled at the top) of her polysomnogram (PSG) are shown below. Which of the following findings is correct?

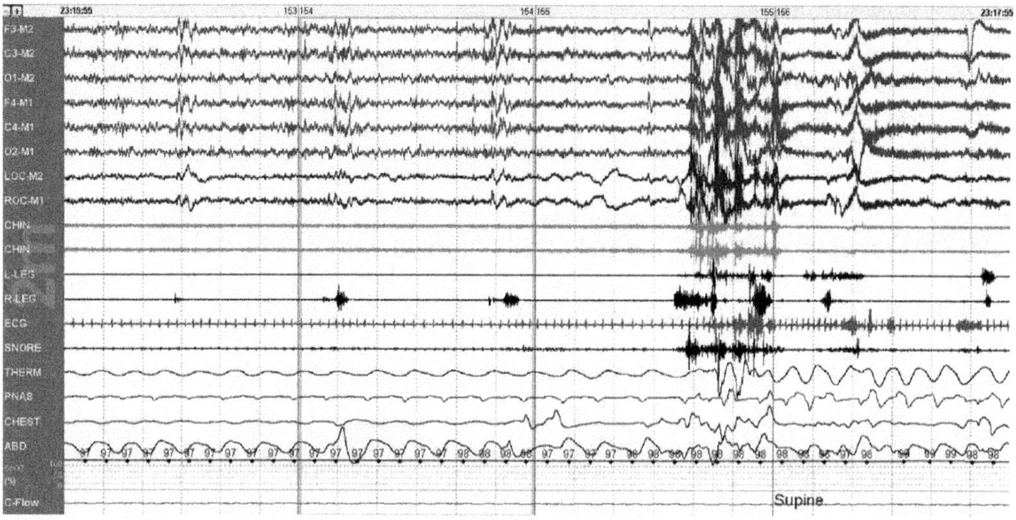

A. Only epochs #154 and #155 can be scored as periodic limb movement of sleep (PLMS)
B. Only epochs #154, #155, and #156 can be scored as PLMS
C. Only epochs #155 and #156 can be scored as PLMS
D. Only epoch #154 can be scored as PLMS
E. All four epochs can be scored as PLMS

25. A 42-year-old mother of three was evaluated for excessive daytime sleepiness, and found to have a normal overnight polysomnogram (PSG). On the following day, she had a multiple sleep latency test (MSLT) with a mean sleep latency of 4 minutes and one sleep-onset REM period (SOREMP) during the first two naps. What is the most likely diagnosis?
A. Narcolepsy
B. Idiopathic hypersomnia
C. Insomnia
D. Circadian rhythm disorder
E. Inadequate study

26. An obese 30-year-old male with excessive daytime sleepiness was evaluated. An overnight polysomnogram (PSG) showed sleep-onset latency of 20 minutes, sleep efficiency of 90%, periodic limb movement of sleep (PLMS) index of 10, and an apnea hypopnea index (AHI) of four. A multiple sleep latency test (MSLT) performed the following morning was not diagnostic for narcolepsy. Which of the following is the most likely cause of his excessive daytime sleepiness?

A. Apneas
B. Hypopneas
C. Periodic limb movements of sleep
D. Respiratory effort-related arousals (RERAs)
E. Insomnia

27. A 65-year-old female with a history of congestive heart failure complicated by stroke reported frequent awakenings with shortness of breath and excessive daytime sleepiness. A Cheyne–Stokes breathing pattern was noted on the polysomnogram (PSG). Which of the following physiological features can be expected in this patient?

A. Accentuation of the abnormal breathing pattern during REM sleep
B. $PaCO_2$ greater than 45 mmHg
C. Oxygen desaturation below 70%
D. Sleep fragmentation
E. Arousal at the beginning of apnea

28. What is the best interpretation of the hypnogram shown below?

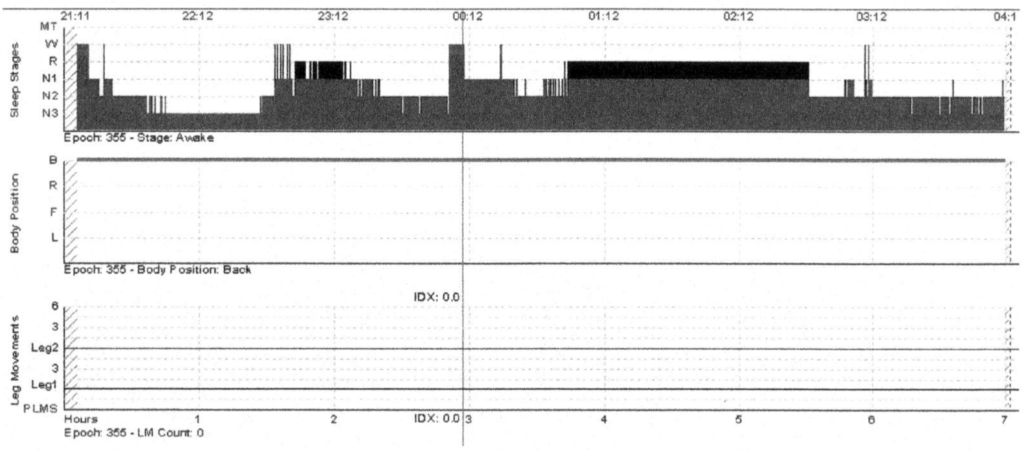

A. Poor sleep efficiency
B. REM rebound after continuous positive airway pressure (CPAP) therapy
C. Narcolepsy
D. Idiopathic hypersomnia
E. REM sleep behavior disorder (RBD)

29. A 56-year-old male is being evaluated for obstructive sleep apnea (OSA) with split-night polysomnogram (PSG). His hypnogram, including continuous positive airway pressure (CPAP) titration (labeled as "Airway Pressure"), is shown below. What would be the most appropriate CPAP pressure recommendation for this patient based on the information provided in the figure?

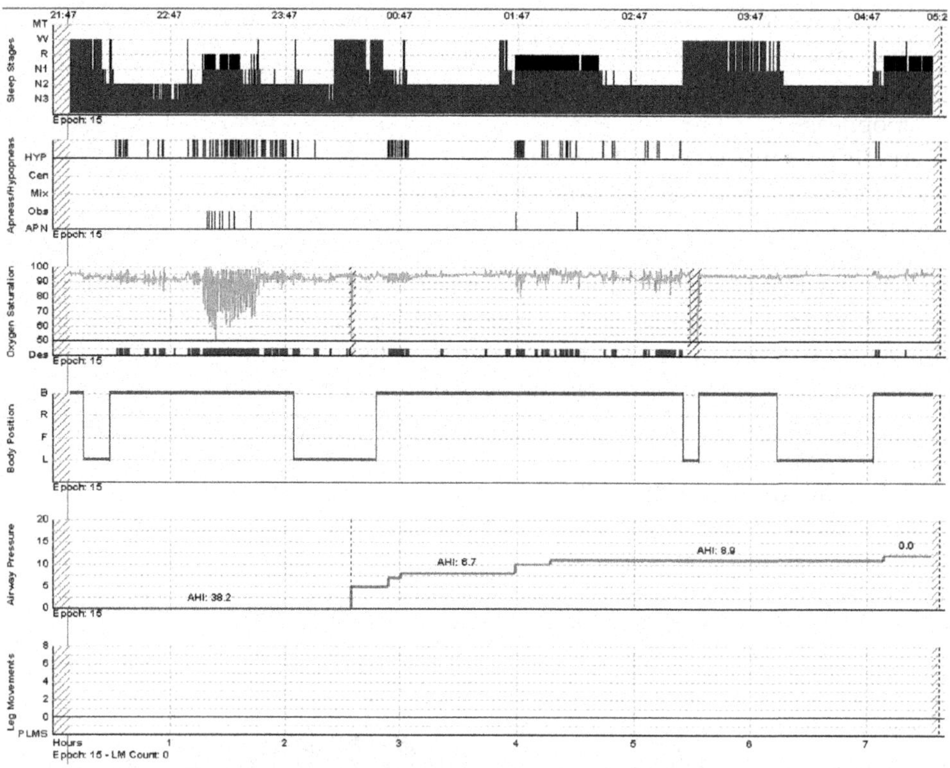

A. 8 cm water
B. 10 cm water
C. 11 cm water
D. 12 cm water
E. Cannot be determined

30. A 61-year-old man is undergoing continuous positive airway pressure (CPAP) titration study for obstructive sleep apnea (OSA). A 30-second epoch of REM sleep during CPAP titration is shown below. The stage of sleep shown in the epoch is associated with all of the following except:

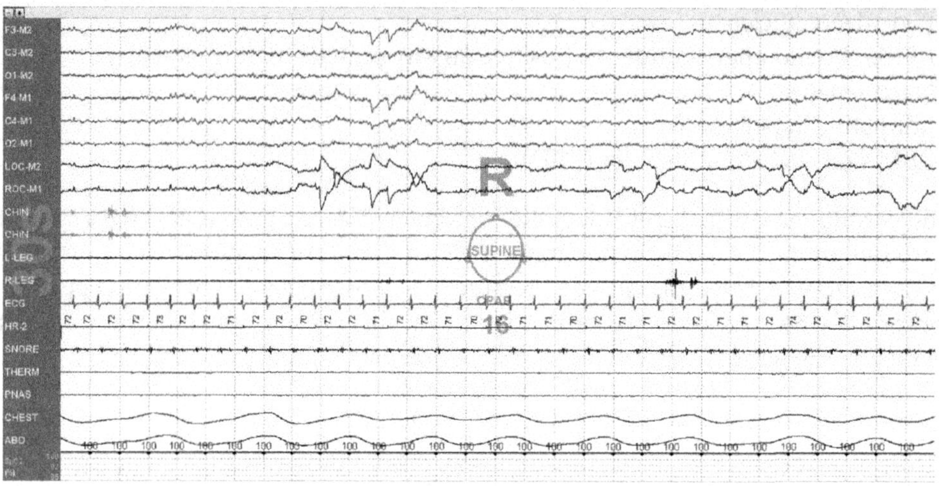

A. Rapid eye movements
B. Ponto-geniculo-occipital (PGO) waves in animals
C. Dream imagery
D. Regular heart rate
E. Irregular respiration

31. The use of traditional EEG filter settings in polysomnogram (PSG) studies would result in which of the following?
A. Underscoring of N3 sleep
B. Overscoring of N3 sleep
C. Underscoring of the posterior dominant rhythm
D. Underscoring of REM sleep
E. None of the above

32. Which of the following promotes sleep?
A. Ingesting an adenosine antagonist
B. A lesion in the ventrolateral preoptic nucleus of the hypothalamus
C. Low levels of orexin
D. High levels of hypocretin-1
E. None of the above

33. Which of the following is NOT and indication for polysomnography (PSG)?
A. Sleep-related breathing disorders
B. Intractable violent sleep-related behaviors
C. Sleep-related movement disorders
D. Narcolepsy in conjunction with a maintenance of wakefulness test (MWT)
E. Narcolepsy in conjunction with a multiple sleep latency test (MSLT)

34. A 34-year-old obese male presented to his neurologist with excessive daytime sleepiness and falling. Narcolepsy with cataplexy was suspected and a multiple sleep latency test (MSLT) was done. His sleep latencies for the five naps were as follows: 5 minutes; 7 minutes; 6 minutes; 5 minutes; and 7 minutes. He was also found to have two sleep-onset REM periods (SOREMPs). His cerebrospinal fluid (CSF) hypocretin-1 level was 90 pg/mL. A polysomnogram (PSG), done the night before, showed a sleep efficiency of 70% and an apnea hypopnea index (AHI) of four. What else is needed to confirm the diagnosis of narcolepsy with cataplexy?
A. Sleep log documentation
B. Repeat PSG and MSLT because MSLT results are nondiagnostic
C. Human leukocyte antigen (HLA) typing
D. Maintenance of wakefulness test (MWT)
E. Nothing more is needed

35. A 30-second epoch of a polysomnogram (PSG) is shown in the following figure. What sleep stage is it?
A. Wake
B. N1
C. N2
D. N3
E. REM

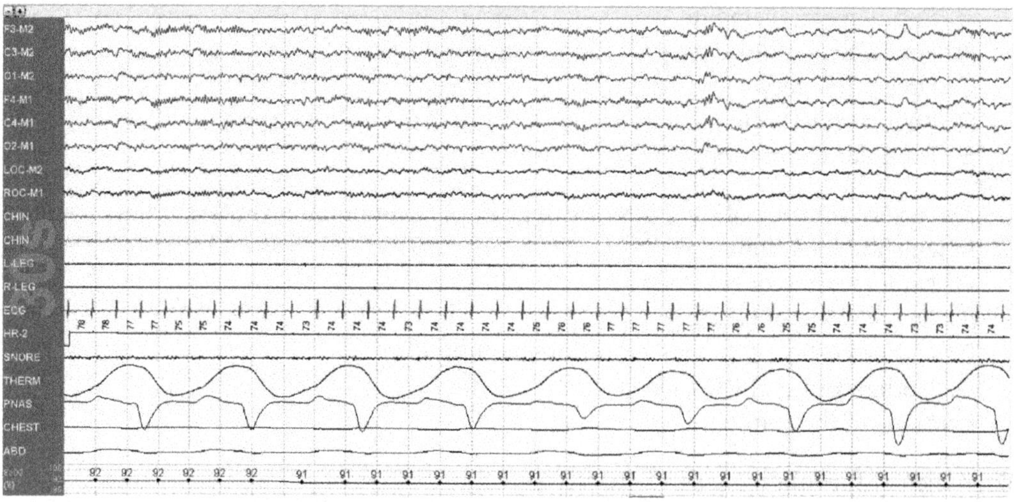

36. Which of the following statements regarding REM sleep is true?
   A. The first REM period tends to be long, lasting about 30 minutes
   B. The first REM occurs about 120 minutes after sleep onset
   C. REM sleep gets shorter toward the latter part of the night
   D. Newborns can spend up to 80% of sleep in REM sleep
   E. Adults typically have four to six REM cycles per night

37. A few hours after going to sleep, an 8-year-old boy woke up screaming. He was inconsolable, confused, and amnestic for the event. This event most likely occurred in which stage of sleep?
   A. N1
   B. N2
   C. N3
   D. REM
   E. Any of the above

38. Which of the following physiological changes is NOT a characteristic of REM sleep?
   A. Atonia
   B. Impaired thermoregulation
   C. Reduction in ventilatory chemosensitivity
   D. Decreased cerebral blood flow
   E. Increased intracranial pressure

39. A 30-second epoch of a polysomnogram (PSG) from a 30-year-old woman with insomnia is shown in the following figure. This is most consistent with:
   A. Normal wake epoch
   B. Normal N2 epoch
   C. Hypopnea
   D. Apnea
   E. Periodic limb movement disorder (PLMD)

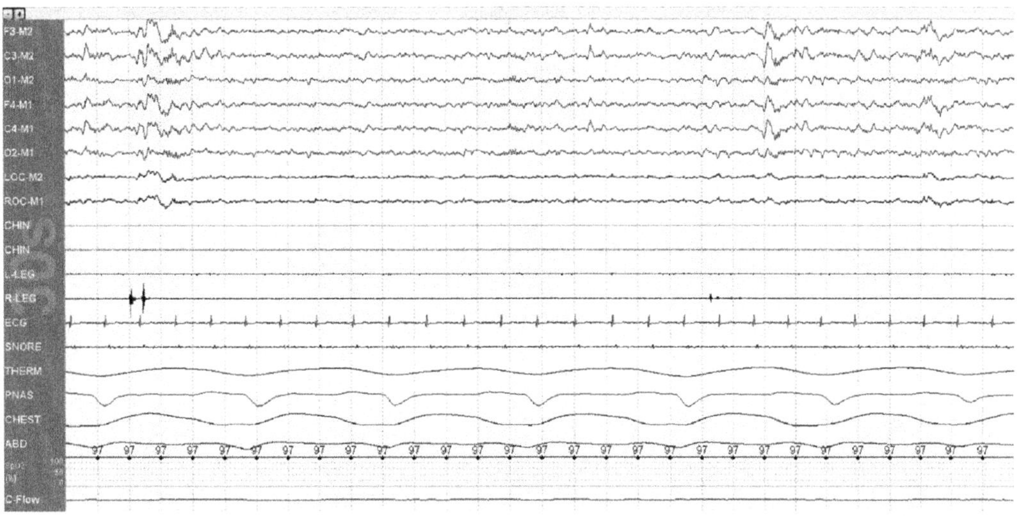

40. Which of the following statements is true regarding maintenance of wakefulness test (MWT)?

A. Staying awake for all the trials does not necessarily indicate that the subject can maintain wakefulness in all environments
B. Mean sleep latency of less than 8 minutes during the trials indicates an abnormality
C. Mean sleep latency between 8 and 40 minutes has an unclear clinical significance
D. MWT and multiple sleep latency test (MSLT) can be discordant in a significant number of patients
E. All of the above

41. The American Academy of Sleep Medicine (AASM) recommended parameters to be reported in a routine polysomnogram (PSG) include all of the following except:

A. Body position
B. Electrooculogram (EOG)
C. Leg electromyography (EMG)
D. Snoring monitor
E. Chin EMG

42. Which of the following statements is true regarding the multiple sleep latency test (MSLT)?

A. It is designed to distinguish between narcolepsy and idiopathic hypersomnia without the need for a preceding full-night polysomnogram
B. Occipital scalp EEG electrodes are used during the test
C. The patient has four opportunities to nap at 2-hour intervals
D. Medications affecting sleep need to be stopped the night prior to the study
E. The subject is instructed to stay awake during the study done in a dark, quiet room

43. A 43-year-old male was evaluated for excessive daytime fatigue. Otherwise, he is asymptomatic. He underwent a polysomnogram (PSG), which showed an apnea hypopnea index (AHI) of three. His hypnogram is shown below. Which of the following conditions is least likely in this patient?

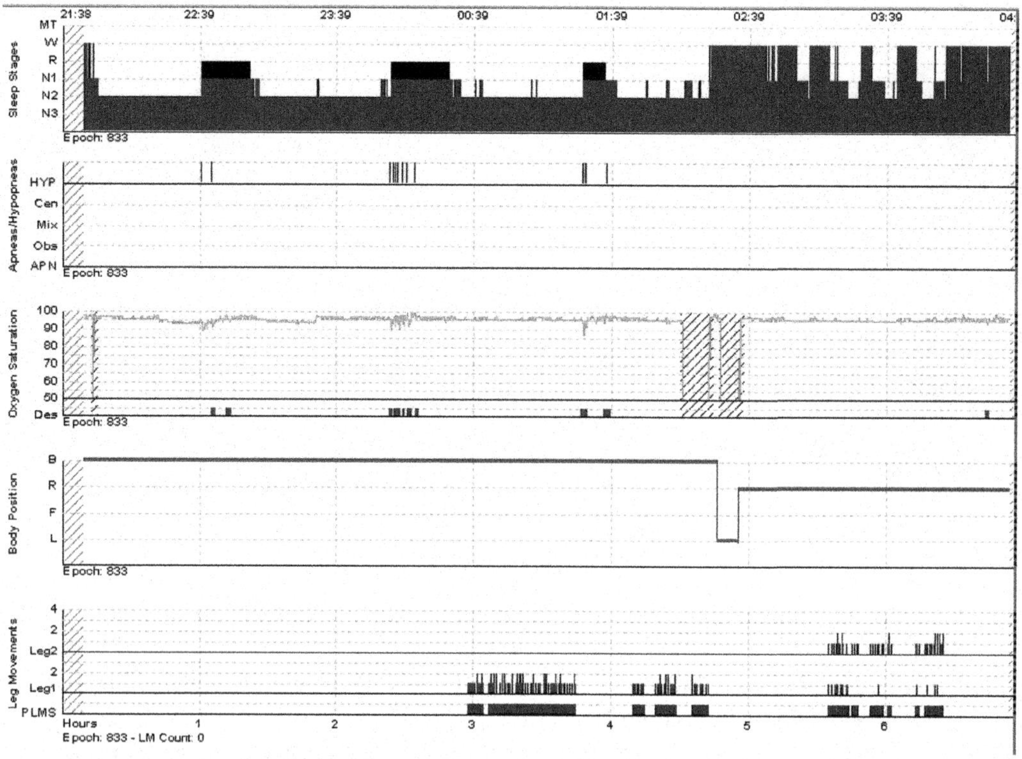

A. Obstructive sleep apnea
B. Restless legs syndrome (RLS)
C. Periodic limb movement disorder (PLMD)
D. Narcolepsy
E. Idiopathic hypersomnia

44. How many leg movements can be scored as periodic limb movements of sleep (PLMS) in the two consecutive 30-second epochs of a polysomnogram (PSG) shown below? Note that the thick vertical line separates the two epochs.

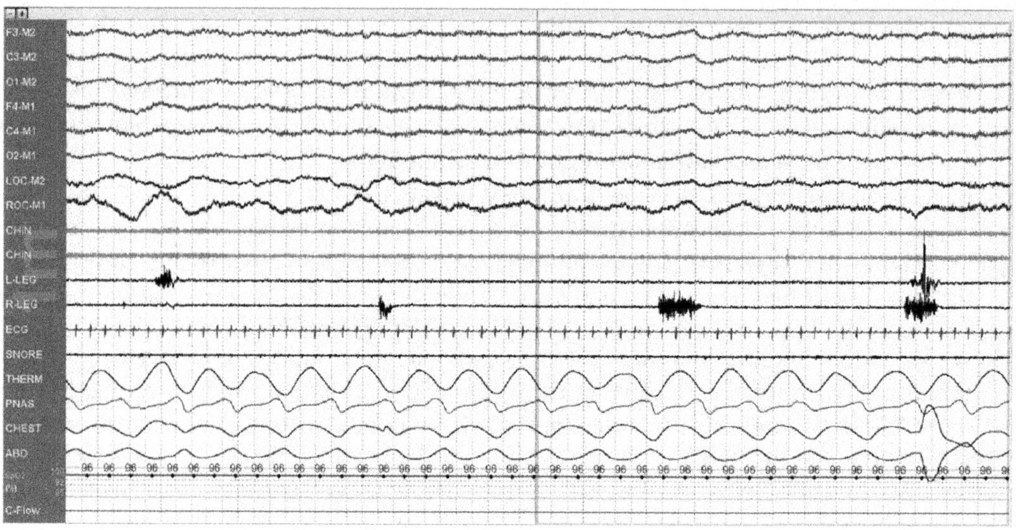

A. Two
B. Three
C. Four
D. Five
E. None because there is no arousal

45. Which of the following features is characteristic of normal REM sleep?
A. Low-voltage theta activity on the EEG
B. Trains of sharply contoured, notched waves in the occipital region
C. Occasional nonarousal-associated K-complexes
D. Short irregular bursts of electromyography (EMG) activity on chin EMG
E. High signal in the leg EMG lead

46. Which of the following statements is true regarding the homeostatic and circadian sleep drives?
A. The homeostatic drive increases with wakefulness
B. The circadian drive is controlled by the suprachiasmatic nucleus of the hypothalamus
C. The ventrolateral preoptic nucleus of the hypothalamus promotes sleep
D. The ventrolateral preoptic nucleus of the hypothalamus is inhibited by the wake-promoting areas
E. All of the above

47. A polysomnogram (PSG) is being scored. The technologist labeled an epoch as Stage N2 when he noticed a K-complex. During the next 2-minute period, there are no spindles or K-complexes, but the EEG background consists of low-voltage mixed-frequencies. At the end of the 2 minutes, there is an arousal; after the arousal, the background continues to show medium-voltage mixed-frequencies. What is the correct sleep staging for the epoch following the arousal?
A. Stage N1
B. Stage N2
C. Stage N3
D. Stage W
E. Stage R

48. To score an epoch as REM, changes in which of the following are required?
A. Electromyography (EMG) and EEG
B. EMG and electrooculogram (EOG)
C. EEG and EOG
D. EMG, EEG, and EOG
E. EMG, EEG, EOG, and EKG

49. Which of the following criteria are required for scoring an arousal?
A. Presence of stable sleep for at least 5 seconds before the arousal
B. A sudden shift in EEG frequencies lasting at least 3 seconds
C. Elevation of chin electromyography (EMG) signal for at least 3 seconds to score an arousal during REM sleep
D. Elevation of leg EMG for at least 5 seconds
E. All of the above

50. A 30-second epoch of polysomnogram (PSG) in a patient with a history of excessive daytime sleepiness is shown below. Which of the following conditions is least likely to cause the most significant finding noted in the figure?

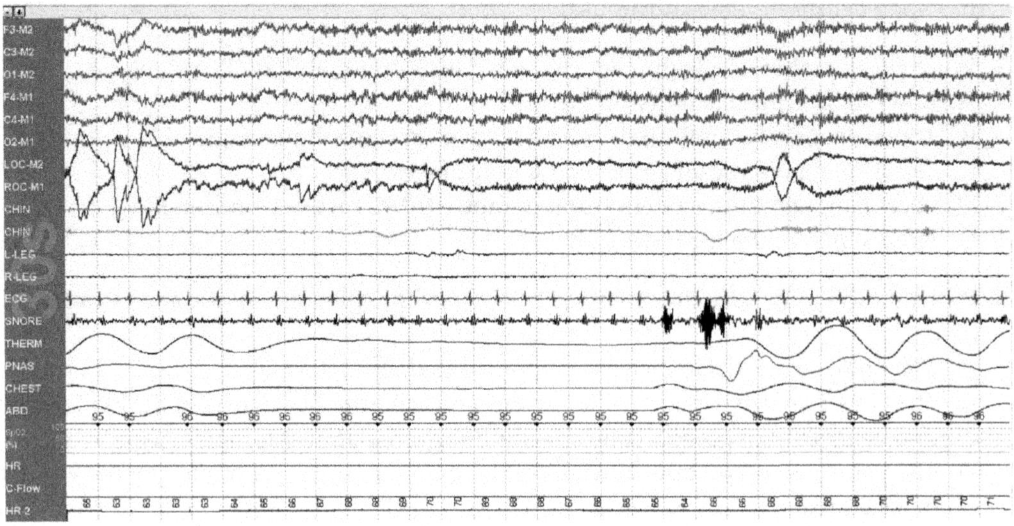

A. Postarousal
B. Stroke
C. Acetazolamide treatment
D. High altitude
E. Pregnancy

51. Which of the following sensors are routinely placed as part of a standard overnight polysomnogram (PSG) study?
A. C4–A1 EEG channel
B. C3–A2 EEG channel
C. O2–A1 EEG channel
D. Nasal thermistor
E. Electrooculogram (EOG)

52. Which of the following statements is true regarding sleep-related events that affect cardiac function?
A. Respiratory obstruction can cause tachycardia
B. Arousals can lead to bradycardia
C. REM sleep can be associated with autonomic changes
D. A and B
E. A, B and C

53. A 40-year-old obese female with hypertension, hypothyroidism, and excessive daytime sleepiness undergoes an overnight polysomnogram (PSG). Two consecutive 30-second epochs are shown below. Which of the following statements best describes the sleep stage? Note that the thick vertical line separates the two epochs.

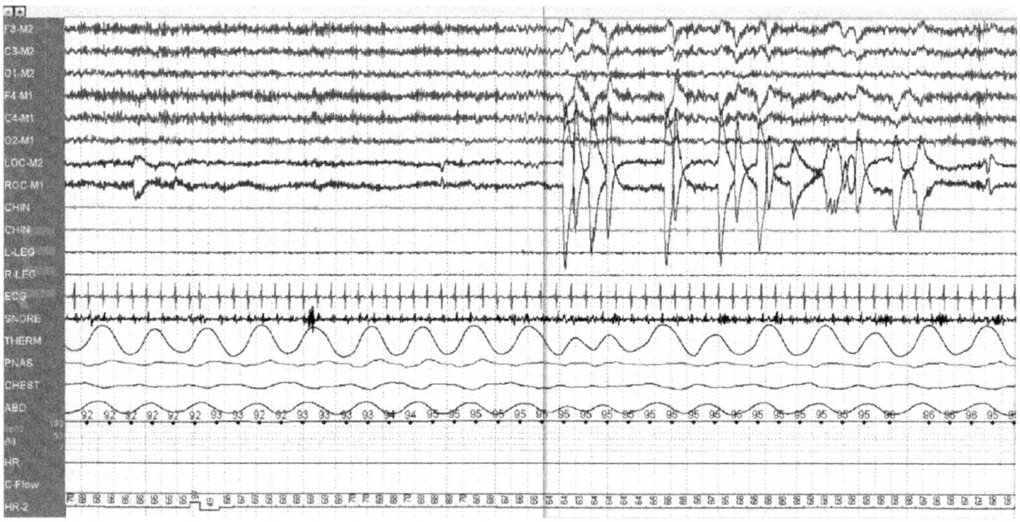

A. First epoch is Stage N2, second epoch is Stage REM
B. First epoch is Stage N2, second epoch is Stage W
C. First epoch is Stage REM, second epoch is Stage REM
D. First epoch is Stage N1, second epoch is Stage REM
E. First epoch is Stage REM, second epoch is Stage W

54. Which of the following statements is true regarding the relationship between age and the sleep stages?
A. Sleep latency tends to decrease with age
B. N1 decreases with age
C. N3 increases with age
D. REM tends to decrease with age
E. Sleep cycles tend to be longer in children than adults

55. Which of the following anticonvulsants decreases both slow-wave sleep and REM?
A. Carbamazepine
B. Gabapentin
C. Phenytoin
D. Barbiturates
E. None of the above

56. Which of the following physiological changes occurs in NREM sleep?
A. Secretion of thyroid stimulating hormone (TSH)
B. Secretion of growth hormone
C. Increased respiratory rate
D. Increased cardiac output
E. Increased blood pressure

ANSWERS

1. **D.** The epoch in the question shows low-voltage, mixed-frequency activity and low chin EMG signal. These findings suggest that it is REM although no clear eye movements are seen in the epoch. There is an obstructive apnea (not hypopnea) at the beginning of the epoch, resulting in significant oxygen desaturation, arousal, and elevation of the chin EMG signal. The occurrence of elevated chin EMG in the context of arousal from an apnea is not suggestive of REM behavior disorder.

2. **A.** Alpha wave intrusion occurs in some patients with chronic fatigue/pain. Alpha waves appear with NREM sleep when delta activity is expected. It is sometimes termed alpha–delta, not alpha–beta, sleep. Monomorphic spindle-like activity (i.e., spindle coma) occurs in patients with head trauma, hypoxic insults, or brainstem lesions, not in patients with chronic fatigue/pain. Patients with chronic fatigue will continue to have REM sleep.

3. **D.** The MWT assesses the ability to stay awake during multiple daytime naps. The setup is similar to the multiple sleep latency test (MSLT) but the subjects are instructed to stay awake instead of falling asleep. The room is lit with 0.1 to 0.13 lux or a 7.5-watt night light placed behind the patient's head. The test consists of four trials lasting up to 40 minutes each done at 2-hour intervals. The trial ends when the subject has unequivocal sleep, defined as having three continuous epochs of Stage N1 sleep or one epoch of any other sleep stage or at 40 minutes if there is no sleep. If no sleep is achieved during a trial, then the recorded latency for that trial is 40 minutes. The MWT does not require a preceding full-night PSG to be done.

4. **B.** Slow rolling eye movements are seen. Chin electromyography (EMG) is elevated. There is dropout of posterior alpha. No spindles or K-complexes are seen. These are consistent with Stage N1.

5. **E.** In the beginning of this PSG epoch, there is a hypopnea (not apnea), characterized by approximately 50% reduction in nasal pressure (PNAS channel) lasting about 13 seconds. The PNAS signal reverts to baseline toward the end of the epoch. The respiratory effort (Chest and Abd channels) is preserved throughout. This is accompanied by a 5% oxygen desaturation. Snoring is also noted.

6. **B.** The epoch in the question shows spindles and K-complexes with low chin electromyography (EMG) signal consistent with Stage N2. There is a PLMS in the right leg EMG lead (greater than 10 seconds in duration, clearly standing out from the background). There are no epileptiform abnormalities; the sharply contoured activity is most likely the result of

superimposition of spindles on K-complexes. The nasal pressure channel shows appropriate oscillations without any artifacts or abnormalities.

7. **E.** This hypnogram shows evidence of significant hypoxemia in REM sleep despite BiPAP although the oxygen saturation improves upon assuming the left lateral position. BiPAP therapy can be considered partially successful because apneas and hypopneas are essentially eliminated without significant hypoxemia in the last REM period in the left lateral position (in contrast to supine position). There is evidence of coexistent periodic limb movement disorder (PLMD) because of significant leg movements in NREM sleep (periodic limb movement [PLM] index: 29.4). Most of the hypnogram shows sleep except for very brief periods of wakefulness; therefore, it is not consistent with poor sleep efficiency.

8. **A.** Pneumotachograph is the gold standard for measuring airflow; it measures airflow across a resistor by using a differential manometer. Because the setup is cumbersome, they are typically used in the research setting. In the clinical setting, thermistors or thermocouples, placed at the nose and mouth, are commonly used to measure airflow. These devices base their measurements on the temperature difference of inspired and expired air. However, they cannot measure airflow volumes and they overestimate airflow and underestimate abnormalities.

9. **C.** Among the options given, a sleep efficiency of 88% is not likely to cause nonrestorative sleep. Alpha intrusion (e.g., as seen in fibromyalgia), REM sleep without atonia (e.g., REM behavior disorder), periodic limb movement (PLM) arousal index of 10, and an AHI of 15 can all be potentially associated with nonrestorative sleep and lead to excessive daytime sleepiness.

10. **C.** In the figure, the chin electromyography (EMG) appears noisy but there is no posterior alpha. Rare spindles and K-complexes are seen but not enough to be considered as N2. The background is predominantly made up of delta activity, consistent with Stage N3 (slow-wave sleep). Although bruxism can occur in any stage of sleep, greater than 80% of episodes occur in Stages N1 or N2. Sleep-related rhythmic movement disorder (head banging or jactatio capitis nocturna) occurs in children, and consists of repeated forcible banging of the head on the pillow or mattress; it is typically seen in N2 sleep but rarely in N3 or REM sleep. Sleep terror (night terror) is an NREM parasomnia causing feelings of terror or dread, and typically occurs in the first few hours of sleep during slow-wave sleep (N3). Hypnic jerks (sleep starts) are associated with brief body contractions that occur at sleep onset, usually at the time of transition from wakefulness to sleep; sometimes, they are associated with a sensation of falling, a sensory flash, or a dream.

11. **D.** NREM sleep is subdivided into three stages, N1 to N3. Stage N1 sleep is characterized by the gradual disappearance of the alpha rhythm of quiet wakefulness, which is replaced by theta activity and some fast activity. Vertex sharp waves can be seen in the frontocentral region. Stage N2 sleep is characterized by frontocentral sleep spindles and K-complexes. Stage N3 sleep is defined by the presence of high-voltage (greater than 75 μV) slow activity occupying at least 20% of the epoch. On the other hand, REM sleep is characterized by a background similar to wakefulness or Stage N1 sleep with REM and lack of muscle activity on the chin electromyography (EMG) with or without sawtooth waves seen in the frontal or vertex regions.

12. B. This is most consistent with a REM behavior disorder. The supporting evidence includes advanced age, hyperactive behavior during sleep, and ability to recount dreams. RLS is characterized by uncomfortable sensations along with the urge to move, typically in the legs. It is usually relieved by voluntary movements and tends to be worse in the evening time. It is not associated with dreams. Similarly, PLMD is unlikely because the leg movements are not the only feature in her presentation. Frontal lobe seizure is possible given nocturnal occurrence and hyperkinetic behavior, but the ability to recount the event as a dream is unusual in either frontal lobe or temporal lobe seizures.

13. C. Stage N3 sleep, referred to as slow-wave sleep or delta sleep, is characterized by high-voltage (greater than 75 μV), slow (0.5–2 Hz) activity occupying at least 20% of the epoch. Of note, a delta wave in sleep terminology is 2 Hz or less vs 4 Hz or less in EEG terminology.

14. C. Although SOREMPs are nonspecific, they are typically associated with narcolepsy. Other situations associated with SOREMPs include sleep deprivation, circadian rhythm disorders, medications, and medication withdrawal. Phenobarbital administration leads to decreased REM sleep and therefore is least likely to lead to a SOREMP. Withdrawal of phenobarbital, on the other hand, can lead to REM rebound and could lead to a SOREMP.

15. A. N1, which correlates with drowsiness, is characterized by attenuation of the posterior dominant rhythm (PDR), appearance of slow rolling eye movements, increase in frontocentral beta activity, and high-amplitude, symmetrical vertex sharp transients. N2 is defined by the appearance of frontocentral sleep spindles and high-amplitude K-complexes. N3 is characterized by the presence of diffuse polymorphic delta activity occupying more than 20% of the epoch. REM sleep is characterized by rapid eye movements and an EEG background consisting of low-voltage mixed-frequencies (not just theta waves) similar to wakefulness, which is why REM sleep is sometimes referred to as paradoxical sleep. However, trains of sharply contoured or triangular, 2 to 6 Hz, often serrated waves (sawtooth waves) can be seen in the central region in REM sleep.

16. D. A thermistor signal is needed to score apneas. EEG, EOG, and EMG signals are needed to score the sleep stages (NREM, REM, and wake states). EKG signal is not needed to score either apneas or sleep stages, although certain changes in that signal can be diagnostic (e.g., asystole during an apnea).

17. A. A respiratory event is scored as a RERA if the sequence of breaths lasts greater than or equal to 10 seconds. It is characterized by increasing respiratory effort or by flattening of the inspiratory portion of the nasal pressure (diagnostic study) or positive airway pressure (PAP) device flow (titration study) waveform, leading to arousal from sleep when the sequence of breaths does not meet criteria for an apnea or hypopnea. RERA refers to a scenario in which airway resistance increases, leading to an increased respiratory effort and an arousal. Given that oxygen desaturation and tidal volume may not be affected significantly, the situation does not technically reach the classification of an apnea or hypopnea. However, the event disturbs sleep. As RERAs are not included in the calculation of the apnea hypopnea index (AHI), it is possible that a patient with excessive daytime sleepiness could have a relatively normal AHI (and hence does not meet the requirements for obstructive sleep apnea [OSA]) but has many RERAs, which could be causing the symptoms. The respiratory disturbance index (RDI) is an index that incorporates RERAs.

18. **E.** Sleep-onset REM period (SOREMP) is the occurrence of REM sleep at any time during the nap. SOREMPs are an abnormal finding because stage REM sleep typically occurs about 90 minutes after sleep onset. Although SOREMPs are nonspecific, occurrence of two SOREMPs with a mean sleep latency of less than 8 minutes is consistent with narcolepsy.

19. **A.** Sawtooth waves are notched, theta-frequency waveforms best appreciated in the central head regions. They often but not always precede a burst of eye movements. Although sawtooth waves are specific for stage REM sleep, they are not required or sufficient for scoring stage REM sleep.

20. **C.** The diffuse atonia (except eye movements and respiration) and reduction in respiratory chemosensitivity associated with REM sleep worsen obstructive sleep apnea (OSA). Sleepwalking is seen with an arousal from Stage N3 sleep. Epileptic seizures may worsen during NREM sleep. Periodic limb movement disorder is seen in NREM sleep. Confusional arousals occur in NREM sleep, but are not associated with sleepwalking or sleep terrors.

21. **D.** REM sleep is felt to alternate with NREM sleep in cycles of 90 minutes in adults, whereas it tends to cycle every 50 to 60 minutes in children.

22. **A.** The hypnogram shows oxygen desaturation, which is worse in the supine position during REM sleep. Although the respiratory events are not shown in the hypnogram, one can predict an abnormally elevated apnea hypopnea index (AHI) based on history and hypoxemia. Thus, positional therapy and oxygen supplementation along with weight loss would be appropriate to consider in this case. It would be reasonable to repeat the PSG for CPAP titration given significant clinical symptoms. There is enough information in the hypnogram so repeating a PSG because of poor sleep efficiency alone is not really necessary.

23. **E.** According to the AASM scoring manual, a periodic leg movement sequence is defined as at least four consecutive leg movements separated by 5 to 90 seconds based on the EMG activity at least 25% higher than the baseline in the tibialis anterior lead. Leg movements between two legs separated by 5 seconds or less are counted as a single movement. If the leg movement is associated with an arousal, the arousal must occur within 3 seconds of the onset of the leg movements. If the sequence is seen during wakefulness, it is suggestive of restless legs syndrome (RLS), which is a clinical diagnosis. These movements correlate with periodic limb movements disorder (PLMD). Of note, PLMD should not be confused with RLS. RLS occurs while awake as well as when asleep, and when awake, there is a voluntary response to an uncomfortable feeling in the legs. PLMD, on the other hand, is involuntary, and the patient is often unaware of these movements altogether.

24. **A.** In the figure, the first three epochs (#153–#155) constitute N2, whereas Epoch #156 is scored as W. Although all four epochs contain leg movements, only two can be scored as PLMS. To score a leg movement as a PLMS, it should occur after sleep onset, have a duration of 0.5 to 10 seconds, and have an amplitude increase of at least 8 μV above the resting electromyography (EMG) baseline. Arousal and PLMS should be considered associated with each other when there is less than 0.5 seconds between the end of one event and onset of the other event regardless of which is first. Based on these rules, leg movement in Epoch #153 is too short (less than 0.5 second) to be scored as a PLMS; leg movement in

Epoch #154 can be scored as PLMS; leg movement in Epoch #155 can be scored as PLMS with arousal; leg movement in Epoch #156 (which is W) cannot be scored as PLMS.

25. **B.** The patient likely has idiopathic hypersomnia. She does not meet the criteria for narcolepsy, which requires two or more SOREMPs with a mean sleep latency of less than 8 minutes. Although SOREMPs are a nonspecific abnormality typically associated with narcolepsy, they can be seen in other situations, including sleep deprivation, circadian rhythm disorders, medications, and medication withdrawal. Given that she had a normal overnight PSG, insomnia, circadian rhythm disorder, and inadequate study are also less likely.

26. **D.** In this case, the sleep-onset latency, sleep efficiency, PLMS index, and AHI are all within normal limits, suggesting that insomnia, periodic limb movements of sleep, and apneas are unlikely to be causing his symptoms. Although other medical, neurological, and psychiatric assessments should be done, the possibility of RERAs, particularly in an obese individual with excess daytime sleepiness, should be considered. RERAs are scored when the respiratory events do not qualify as apneas or hypopneas and are calculated as part of the respiratory disturbance index (RDI). RERAs indicate a sleep-related breathing disorder.

27. **D.** There are many disorders causing central sleep apnea (CSA), including primary CSA, high-altitude periodic breathing, drug-induced apnea, and Cheyne–Stokes breathing. Cheyne–Stokes breathing is a periodic form of breathing with a crescendo–decrescendo breathing pattern. It is seen at transition from wakefulness to NREM sleep. It is prominent during N1 and N2 sleep but attenuates during slow-wave sleep and REM sleep. Typically, a central apnea hypopnea index (AHI) of at least 10 is seen in Cheyne–Stokes breathing. Arousals occur at the end of apnea, usually during the crescendo phase. Other physiological features noted include moderate oxygen desaturation but not below 80%, a $PaCO_2$ less than 45 mmHg (which distinguishes it from hypoventilation syndrome), attenuation of the periodic breathing pattern, and sleep fragmentation. This disorder is typically seen in those with severe medical conditions such as congestive heart failure, renal failure, and stroke.

28. **B.** The hypnogram shows a long period of continuous REM sleep after a short period in the beginning. Most likely, this could have occurred as a result of CPAP initiation, although that information is not provided in the hypnogram. There are very few wake periods, so poor sleep efficiency is unlikely. Although narcolepsy can be entertained, it is unlikely because there is no sleep-onset REM period (SOREMP) and the awakenings are infrequent. Besides, narcolepsy cannot be inferred on the basis of an overnight polysomnogram (PSG); it requires a multiple sleep latency test (MSLT) study. Idiopathic hypersomnia is a possibility, but an MSLT is needed to confirm the diagnosis. RBD is characterized by increased electromyography (EMG) activity and phasic twitches on the chin or extremity leads during PSG. Absence of such elevated EMG activity in the leg leads argues against RBD in the noted hypnogram.

29. **D.** The initial diagnostic part of the study shows significant hypopneas and apneas along with hypoxemia, which is worse in REM sleep. With initiation of CPAP titration at 5 cm water, the respiratory events and hypoxemia improve gradually. Toward the

end of the study, at CPAP of 12 cm water, REM sleep is noted in the supine position with only a few respiratory events and minimal hypoxemia; thus, a prescription of 12 m water pressure would be most appropriate from the data given. Note that at 11 cm water pressure, significant respiratory events and hypoxemia are noted both during NREM and REM sleep.

30. **D.** The epoch in the question shows phasic REM sleep characterized by rapid eye movements; low-voltage, mixed-frequency EEG background; and fine bursts of electromyography (EMG) activity in the chin and leg leads. This is different from tonic REM, which is characterized by atonia and eye movements. Phasic REM is associated with PGO waves in animals, dream imagery in humans, and irregular (not regular) heart rate and respiration.

31. **A.** Traditionally, the low-frequency filter setting of the EEG component of sleep studies is set at 0.3 Hz rather than the usual 1 Hz on routine scalp EEG studies in order to maximize the recognition of low-frequency components. By increasing the filter setting from 0.3 Hz to 1 Hz, the amplitude of signals below 1 Hz signal will be attenuated and therefore N3 sleep will be underscored. In routine PSG studies, the posterior dominant rhythm (PDR) can be appreciated despite the active electrodes being over the central head region rather than the posterior quadrant. However, increasing the low filter to 1 Hz has no significant effect on the scoring of PDR or REM sleep.

32. **C.** Decreased level of hypocretin-1 (orexin) due to loss of cells producing them promotes sleep and can lead to narcolepsy. Caffeine antagonizes adenosine and promotes wakefulness. A lesion in the ventrolateral preoptic nucleus of the hypothalamus causes insomnia.

33. **D.** The indications for PSG include suspicion of sleep-related breathing disorders; treatment and follow-up of sleep-related breathing disorders; combination with the MSLT for suspected narcolepsy; evaluation of sleep-related behaviors that are violent, potentially injurious, or do not respond to conventional therapy; assisting in the diagnosis of paroxysmal arousals that are suggestive of seizure disorder (with additional video and EEG); or evaluation of sleep-related movement disorders. Note that polysomnography is not indicated in conjunction with MWT for evaluation of narcolepsy.

34. **E.** The patient has a mean sleep latency of 6 minutes with two SOREMPs. There is no evidence of other sleep disorders (e.g., obstructive sleep apnea [OSA]) on the preceding PSG that could account for his symptoms. Cataplexy, especially with low CSF hypocretin-1 levels of less than 110 pg/mL, is highly specific for narcolepsy. All of these findings are consistent with narcolepsy and no other test is needed to confirm it. HLA typing in narcolepsy is almost always positive for HLA-DQB1*0602 and is not diagnostic for narcolepsy; this test is useful to exclude narcolepsy in selected cases. MWT may be needed to evaluate response to therapy for narcolepsy, but not for its diagnosis.

35. **C.** Chin EMG is low. There is no posterior alpha. Spindles and K-complexes are seen. These features are consistent with N2.

36. **E.** The first REM period tends to be short, approximately 10 minutes. It tends to occur about 60 to 90 minutes after sleep onset, while N3 sleep tends to occur 30 to 40 minutes after sleep onset. During the latter part of the night, the REM periods get progressively longer. Adults tend to experience four to six sleep cycles per night. Newborns tend to

spend close to 50% of sleep in REM, whereas adolescents and adults spend 20% to 25% of their sleep in REM.

37. C. The description is most consistent with sleep terror (night terror), which is a NREM parasomnia causing feelings of terror or dread. It typically occurs in the first few hours of sleep during slow-wave sleep (N3). It is commonly seen in children 3 to 12 years of age and in adults 20 to 30 years of age.

38. D. There are tonic and phasic changes seen in REM sleep. Tonic changes include diffuse atonia (except for eye movements), impaired thermoregulation, reduction in ventilatory chemosensitivity, hypotension, bradycardia, increased cerebral blood flow, increased intracranial pressure, increased respiratory rate, and penile erection. On the other hand, phasic changes include vasoconstriction, increased blood pressure, tachycardia, increased cerebral blood flow, and increased respiratory rate.

39. B. In the PSG epoch, the chin electromyography (EMG) is low. There is no posterior alpha. Spindles and K-complexes are seen. These features are consistent with N2. There is no evidence of hypopnea or apnea. A couple of bursts of EMG activity are seen in the initial part of the epoch and another, low-amplitude burst later, but they do not meet the criteria to be scored as periodic limb movements. Furthermore, a diagnosis of PLMD can be entertained only after looking at the entire PSG, not just a single epoch.

40. E. Although the MWT is difficult to interpret given its wide range of normal values, maintaining wakefulness for all four trials is considered strong evidence that the subject can maintain wakefulness in similar nonstimulating environments, but no conclusion can be made if the environmental conditions are changed. Mean sleep latency of less than 8 minutes during MWT is abnormal. Latencies between 8 and 40 minutes have an unclear significance. Of note, a sleep latency of 40 minutes is still assigned to a trial in which no sleep was achieved. MWT is a measure of the patient's ability to stay awake, whereas MSLT is a measure of the patient's tendency to fall asleep during normal waking hours; as such, the results of the two tests can be discordant in a significant number of patients.

41. D. According to the AASM scoring manual, the recommended parameters to be reported in a routine PSG include EEG (C4–A1 and/or C3–A2), eye movement recording EOG, EMG of chin, respiratory effort (chest and abdomen), airflow (nasal/oral), oxygen saturation (pulse oximetry), EKG, EMG of anterior tibialis muscle, and body position. Monitoring for snoring is commonly used but is not one of the recommended parameters.

42. B. An MSLT can help distinguish between narcolepsy and idiopathic hypersomnia but a full-night polysomnogram (PSG) on the preceding night is required to ensure adequate sleep of at least 6 hours. In contrast to the typical EEG setup for PSG, the MSLT requires the addition of occipital scalp EEG electrodes to better identify the posterior dominant rhythm attenuation seen with sleep onset. A standard MSLT consists of five nap opportunities offered at 2-hour intervals. The study is done in a dark and quiet room, and the subject is instructed to close his or her eyes and try to sleep. To maintain test validity, medications influencing sleep should be stopped, if possible, prior to the study for an interval of at least five half-lives of the longest metabolite.

43. A. The hypnogram shows periodic leg movements during sleep. A diagnosis of RLS can be suspected based on an elevated periodic limb movement (PLM) index, but the diagnosis is not made based on a PSG. RLS should not be confused with PLMD; with RLS, the patient has an uncomfortable feeling associated with voluntary movement of the legs during wakefulness and/or sleep, whereas with PLMD, the patient is often unaware of involuntary movement of the upper and/or lower limbs. The patient's bed partner may notice the movements more. Diagnosis of PLMD requires clinical sleep disturbance or daytime fatigue, with an elevated PLM index of 15/hr or more in adults. Even though the PLM index is not specified, PLMD is the most appropriate diagnosis to consider in this case. Obstructive sleep apnea (OSA) is not likely because the AHI is within the normal range (AHI should be five or more to entertain a diagnosis of OSA). The patient could possibly have narcolepsy or idiopathic hypersomnia, which can be definitively diagnosed based on a multiple sleep latency test (MSLT).

44. C. To score a leg movement as a PLMS, it should occur after sleep onset, have a duration of 0.5 to 10 seconds, and have an amplitude increase of at least 8 μV above the resting electromyography (EMG) baseline. Leg movements on two different legs separated by less than 5 seconds between movement onsets are counted as a single leg movement. Thus, four leg movements (two in the first epoch and two in the second epoch) can be scored as PLMS in the figure. Note that the difference between the onsets of leg movements in the left and right leg channels in the second epoch is less than 5 seconds, and therefore, the near-simultaneous movements in the two legs count as a single movement. Arousals are not necessary to score PLMS.

45. D. Normal REM sleep is characterized by low-voltage mixed-frequency (not theta) EEG background. Trains of sharply contoured or triangular, 2 to 6 Hz, often serrated waves (sawtooth waves) are seen in the central (not occipital) region. Chin and leg EMG signals remain low because of atonia. However, short irregular bursts of EMG activity (less than 0.25 seconds), superimposed on low EMG tone, are often seen in the chin or anterior tibial leads or EEG or electrooculogram (EOG) deviations. Nonarousal-associated K-complexes are not considered characteristic of REM sleep.

46. E. Although it is still not clearly understood, the current thought is that there are two sleep drives: homeostatic, which increases with wakefulness; and circadian, which is modulated by the suprachiasmatic nucleus of the hypothalamus. Specifically, the inhibitory neurons in the ventrolateral preoptic nucleus of the hypothalamus promote sleep and innervate wake-promoting regions, including the hypocretin (orexin)-containing neurons of the posterolateral hypothalamus, histaminergic neurons of the tuberomammillary nucleus, the serotonergic dorsal raphe, norepinephrine-containing neurons of the locus coeruleus, and the cholinergic neurons of the dorsal midbrain and pons. In turn, there is reciprocal inhibition from the wake-promoting areas on the ventrolateral preoptic nucleus, resulting in stable periods of sleep and wake.

47. A. Stage N2 sleep is defined by the appearance of frontocentral 12 to 14 Hz sleep spindles and K-complexes with each lasting at least 0.5 seconds in the absence of a significant slowing, as seen in Stage N3 sleep. Stage N2 ends once arousal occurs. The subsequent epoch, after the arousal, should be scored as Stage N1 until another spindle or nonarousal K-complex appears. Therefore, the answer is Stage N1.

48. D. Scoring REM sleep requires characteristic changes in EMG (lack of chin activity), EEG (low-voltage mixed-frequency), and EOG (episodic REMs). Note that although sawtooth waves are specific for Stage REM sleep, they are not required or sufficient for scoring Stage REM sleep. EKG is not required for scoring REM.

49. B. According to the American Academy of Sleep Medicine (AASM) scoring manual, an arousal is scored if there is an abrupt shift of EEG frequency, including alpha, theta, and/or frequencies greater than 16 Hz (but not spindles), that lasts at least 3 seconds, with at least 10 seconds of stable sleep preceding the change. Scoring of arousal during REM requires a concurrent increase in chin EMG lasting at least 1 second. Leg EMG changes are not needed for scoring arousal.

50. C. This PSG shows central sleep apnea (CSA), characterized by absence of both airflow and effort. This is noted in REM sleep and there is no evidence of significant oxygen desaturation associated with the event. CSA is most commonly seen in congestive heart failure. Other conditions causing CSA include postarousal state, high altitude, stroke, neuromuscular disorders, and pregnancy. Although certain medications can lead to CSA, acetazolamide is used to treat CSA; acetazolamide causes metabolic acidosis, which in turn leads to secondary respiratory alkalosis and abolition of CSA.

51. C. Although scalp EEG is part of a routine PSG, only two channels (C4–A1 and C3–A2) are routinely placed. Other sensors are used as part of a routine PSG to measure eye movement (electrooculogram [EOG]), respiratory effort (chest and abdomen), oxygen saturation (pulse oximetry), leg movements (electromyography [EMG] on the anterior tibialis muscle), and body position.

52. C. REM sleep has been associated with autonomic changes seen in the rhythm strip. Respiratory obstruction can cause bradycardia mediated by the vagal nerve with subsequent tachycardia during arousals due to increased sympathetic tone.

53. C. This PSG shows two consecutive epochs of REM sleep. Rapid eye movements are noted in both epochs and the chin electromyography (EMG) signal remains low throughout. EEG shows a mixture of different frequencies but there is no identifiable posterior alpha activity. No sleep spindles or K-complexes are seen.

54. D. N1 tends to increase with age, and older adults are felt to be "light sleepers." Sleep cycles, composed of REM and NREM sleep, last for about 50 to 60 minutes in children and 90 minutes in adults. In general, infants and children spend the majority of sleep in Stage N3, which declines in early adulthood. Older adults typically have relatively shorter and fewer periods of N3 sleep, and in general, their sleep is lighter and more fragmented with brief arousals or longer awakenings throughout the night. REM also decreases with age. It takes longer for adults to fall asleep than children, leading to a longer sleep latency.

55. D. Barbiturates decrease both slow-wave sleep and REM but increase spindle activity. The remaining choices listed increase slow-wave sleep and have differing effects on REM. Carbamazepine decreases REM, gabapentin does not change it, and the effect of phenytoin is unclear.

56. B. During NREM sleep, there is secretion of growth hormone, not TSH. There is also decreased blood pressure, heart rate, respiratory rates, and cardiac output.

7

Advanced Topics

QUESTIONS

1. While performing single-fiber electromyography (SFEMG), which of the following measures should be undertaken?
   A. Lower the high-frequency filter to 200 Hz
   B. Raise the high-frequency filter to 500 Hz
   C. Raise the low-frequency filter to 200 Hz
   D. Raise the low-frequency filter to 500 Hz
   E. Lower the low frequency filter to 0.5 Hz

2. Which of the following statements about single-fiber electromyography (SFEMG) is true?
   A. Normal SFEMG in a weak muscle is consistent with myasthenia gravis
   B. SFEMG is the most sensitive test for neuromuscular junction (NMJ) dysfunction
   C. SFEMG is the most specific test for NMJ dysfunction
   D. Jitter values remain constant with aging
   E. Blocking seen during SFEMG is inconsistent with NMJ dysfunction

3. Which of the following statements regarding single-fiber electromyography (SFEMG) is correct?
   A. Abnormal SFEMG always means there is an underlying neuromuscular junction (NMJ) disorder
   B. Normal SFEMG in a weak muscle makes a NMJ dysfunction less likely
   C. SFEMG is a very specific but not very sensitive test for NMJ dysfunction
   D. With increasing age, jitter remains the same but blocking increases
   E. Blocking can be seen in normal muscles

ANSWERS TO THIS SECTION CAN BE FOUND ON PAGE 381

The figures in this chapter can be viewed in a larger size by accessing the digital version of this chapter found on Springer Publishing Company Connect™. Refer to the front of this book for access instructions.

4. A blink study was performed in a 58-year-old man with facial symptoms. The results are summarized in the following table. What does this study suggest?

Side and Site of Stimulation	Ipsilateral R1	Ipsilateral R2	Contralateral R2
Right V1	Normal	Normal	Absent
Left V1	Absent	Absent	Normal

A. Right trigeminal neuropathy
B. Left trigeminal neuropathy
C. Right facial neuropathy
D. Left facial neuropathy
E. Left midbrain lesion

5. While performing a blink reflex study with right trigeminal stimulation, ipsilateral R1, ipsilateral R2, and contralateral R2 responses were absent. A focal lesion in which of the following locations could lead to these findings?
A. Right facial nerve or nucleus
B. Right trigeminal nerve or nucleus
C. Right oculomotor nerve or nucleus
D. Right abducens nerve or nucleus
E. Right medullary lesion

6. Which of the following statements about blink reflex study is true?
A. It is a monosynaptic reflex
B. Efferent and afferent fibers travel through different cranial nerves
C. R2 responses are seen bilaterally with the same latencies
D. R1 responses are seen bilaterally
E. All of the above

7. The figure below shows waveforms obtained after a normal Valsalva testing in a patient. Which phase of Valsalva does the arrow point to?

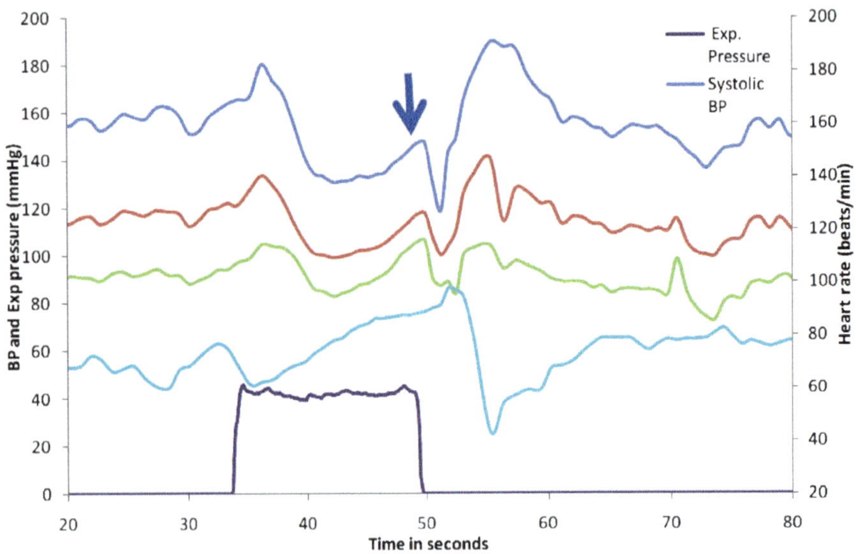

A. Phase III
B. Phase II Late
C. Phase IV
D. Phase I
E. Phase II Early

8. A 45-year-old male with syncope had autonomic testing. His heart rate deep breathing range was assessed based on the waveform shown below. The likely heart rate deep breathing range is

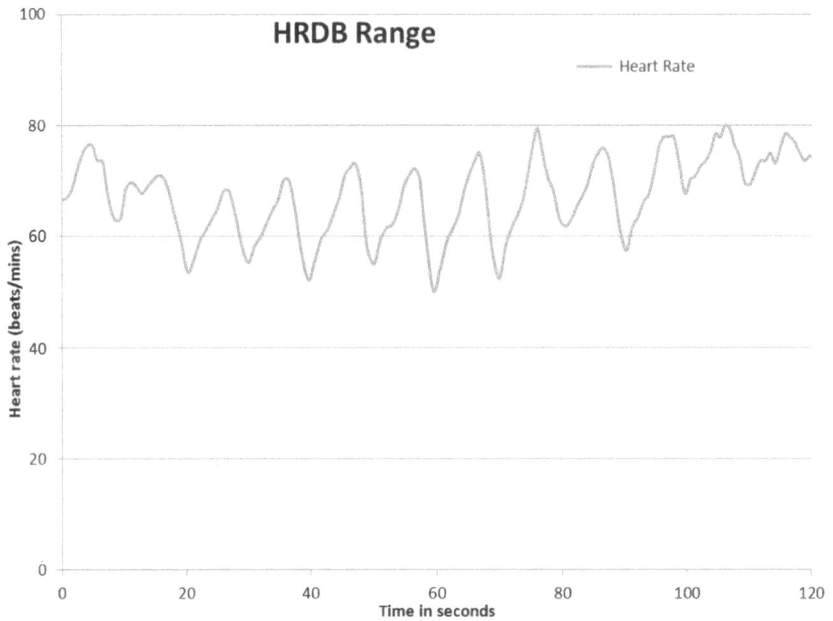

A. 8
B. 2
C. 18
D. 40
E. 60

9. A 70-year-old man with erectile dysfunction, difficulty walking, and imbalance undergoes Valsalva testing as part of his autonomic study. On tilt table testing, he had more than 50 mmHg drop in systolic blood pressure at 3 minutes. Valsalva waveforms are shown below (from top to bottom, the waveforms indicate systolic blood pressure [BP], mean BP, diastolic BP, and heart rate changes, respectively). What does this study suggest?

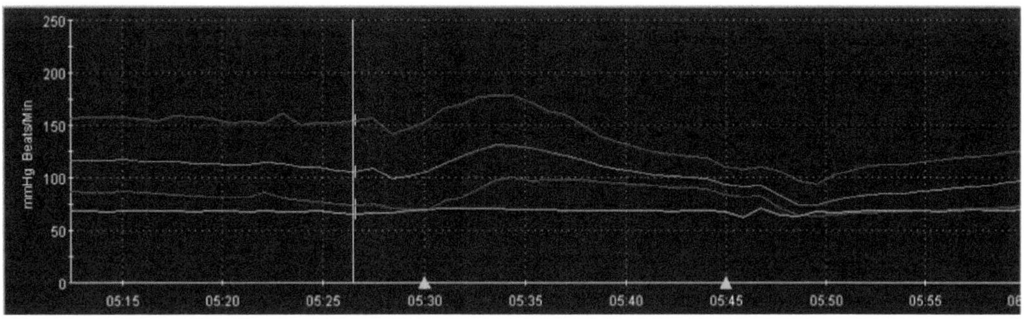

A. Normal adrenergic function
B. Severe adrenergic failure
C. Severe sudomotor failure
D. Mild adrenergic failure
E. Normal valsalva ratio

10. Which of the following neurotransmitters is released by the sympathetic neurons innervating sweat glands?
A. Epinephrine
B. Norepinephrine
C. Acetylcholine
D. Serotonin
E. Both epinephrine and norepinephrine depending on location

11. A 45-year-old woman presented with progressive orthostatic symptoms, constipation, and decreased sweating. Currently, she is unable to stand for more than a few minutes because of lightheadedness. Her tilt table test results with systolic, mean, and diastolic blood pressure and heart rate (green trace) are shown below. What is the most likely interpretation?

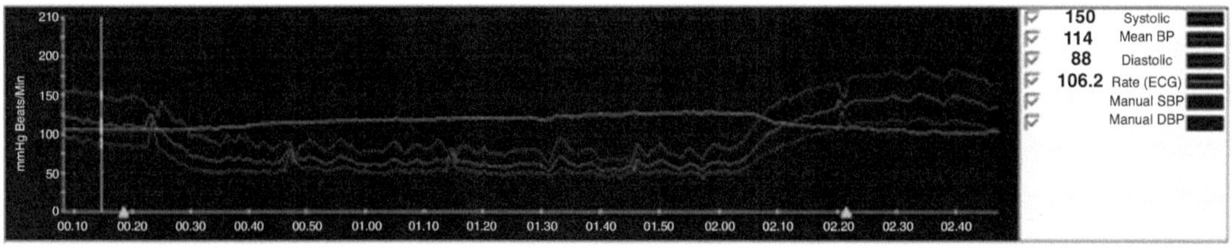

A. Postural orthostatic tachycardia syndrome (POTS)
B. Normal variant
C. Mild orthostatic hypotension
D. Severe orthostatic hypotension
E. Severe dehydration

12. Which of the following is the best test to differentiate Parkinson's disease with autonomic failure from multiple system atrophy (MSA)?
A. Degree of orthostatic hypotension
B. Heart rate (HR) variability
C. Cardiac sympathetic imaging
D. Valsalva ratio
E. Adrenergic index on Valsalva testing

13. Which of the following studies provides information regarding cardiovagal function?
A. Phase IV part of the Valsalva waveform
B. Phase II Late part of the Valsalva waveform
C. Quantitative sudomotor axon reflex test (QSART) testing
D. Heart rate deep breathing range
E. Phase I part of Vaslava waveform

14. Which of the following patterns of change in systolic blood pressure (SBP) and heart rate (HR) during tilt table study is suggestive of neurogenic orthostatic hypotension?

A. Drop in SBP of more than 20 mmHg and increase in HR of more than 30 beats/min
B. Drop in SBP of more than 20 mmHg and increase in HR of less than 15 beats/min
C. Drop in SBP of more than 25 mmHg and increase in HR of more than 40 beats/min
D. No change in SBP and increase in HR of more than 30 beats/min
E. Increase SBP of more than 20 mmHg and no change in HR

15. Which among the following neuromuscular disorders is also associated with autonomic dysfunction?

A. Muscle-specific kinase antibody (MuSK) myasthenia
B. Lambert–Eaton myasthenic syndrome (LEMS)
C. Pompe disease
D. Primary lateral sclerosis
E. Spinobulbar muscular atrophy

16. A 50-year-old man with chronically poorly controlled blood glucose levels because of poor compliance with oral agents was admitted to hospital with multiple complications and very high HbA1c. During the hospital stay he was started on insulin therapy and discharged home on insulin. Over the next 4 weeks, his glycemic control dramatically improves, but he develops burning pain in his feet, and also paresthesias in his limbs. Additionally, he is noted to orthostatic hypotension. What is best next step?

A. Stop insulin therapy
B. Start oral hypoglycemic agents
C. Continue excellent glycemic control and treat symptomatically
D. Start oral or intravenous (IV) prednisone
E. Start Intravenous immunoglobulin therapy

17. Mutation in which of the following genes can cause small fiber neuropathy?

A. Chloride channel
B. Sodium channel
C. Potassium channel
D. Calcium channel
E. Magnesium channel

18. Which of the following conditions is least likely to present with significant autonomic neuropathy manifestations in addition to somatic neuropathy?

A. Transthyretin (TTR) amyloidosis
B. Diabetic neuropathy
C. Guillain–Barré syndrome (GBS)
D. Chronic inflammatory demyelinating polyneuropathy (CIDP)
E. Sjogrens syndrome

19. A 45-year-old woman presents with recent history of burning pain in her feet which is worse at night and impairs her ability to fall asleep. She denies any weakness. On examination, she has normal strength and all her deep tendon reflexes are normal. Vibration and joint position sense in her toes are normal. She has reduced pinprick sensation in her feet. Gait is normal. Which of the following noninvasive tests can help confirm the diagnosis?

A. Skin biopsy from multiple sites
B. Quantitative sudomotor axon reflex test (QSART) for sweat volume output
C. Routine nerve conduction study including plantar responses
D. Somatosensory evoked potentials (SSEP)
E. Sleep study to assess nocturnal sleep disturbance

20. Which of the following statements are true regarding neurophysiological monitoring during spinal cord surgery?
A. Monitoring can reduce the likelihood of postoperative complications
B. Monitoring may be affected by type and depth of anesthesia
C. Monitoring may be affected by hypothermia
D. Monitoring may be affected by hypotension
E. All of the above

21. Which of the following methods provides the highest diagnostic yield in the assessment of small fiber neuropathy?
A. Quantitative sudomotor axon reflex test (QSART)
B. Quantitative sensory test (QST)
C. Quantitative direct and indirect axonal reflex test (QDIRT)
D. Skin biopsy for epidermal nerve fiber density
E. Confocal microscopy

22. Which of the following statements is true regarding quantitative EEG (qEEG)?
A. It allows for rapid detection of seizures compared to review of raw EEG
B. It can provide a quick overview of seizure location, frequency, and duration
C. It can be used to assess response to therapy
D. It allows for rapid assessment of the trend of depth of coma
E. All of the above

23. A 55-year-old female was transferred from an outside hospital with a right proximal middle cerebral artery (MCA) aneurysmal subarachnoid hemorrhage (SAH) 2 days ago and is lethargic on exam. The critical care attending physician calls to find out the utility of doing continuous video-EEG (cEEG) monitoring in this patient. Which of the following statements is correct?
A. cEEG monitoring is helpful in detecting nonconvulsive seizures that are not clinically apparent
B. cEEG monitoring is helpful in detecting delayed cerebral ischemia (DCI)
C. Decreasing relative alpha variability (RAV) would indicate impaired perfusion to areas of ischemia
D. Decreasing alpha–delta ratio (ADR) would indicate increasing perfusion to underlying cortex
E. A, B and C

24. A 46-year-old male was found down and intubated at the scene. He was taken to the nearest facility, and the patient was too unstable to get head imaging. Continuous video-EEG monitoring was started. From top to bottom: fast Fourier transform (FFT) of left hemisphere, FFT of right hemisphere, amplitude-integrated EEG (aEEG), and peak envelope trend. Color bar indicates the power, black being the lowest and white being the highest. What is the correct interpretation of the following quantitative EEG (qEEG) panels at the blue vertical line just past time marker 17:26?

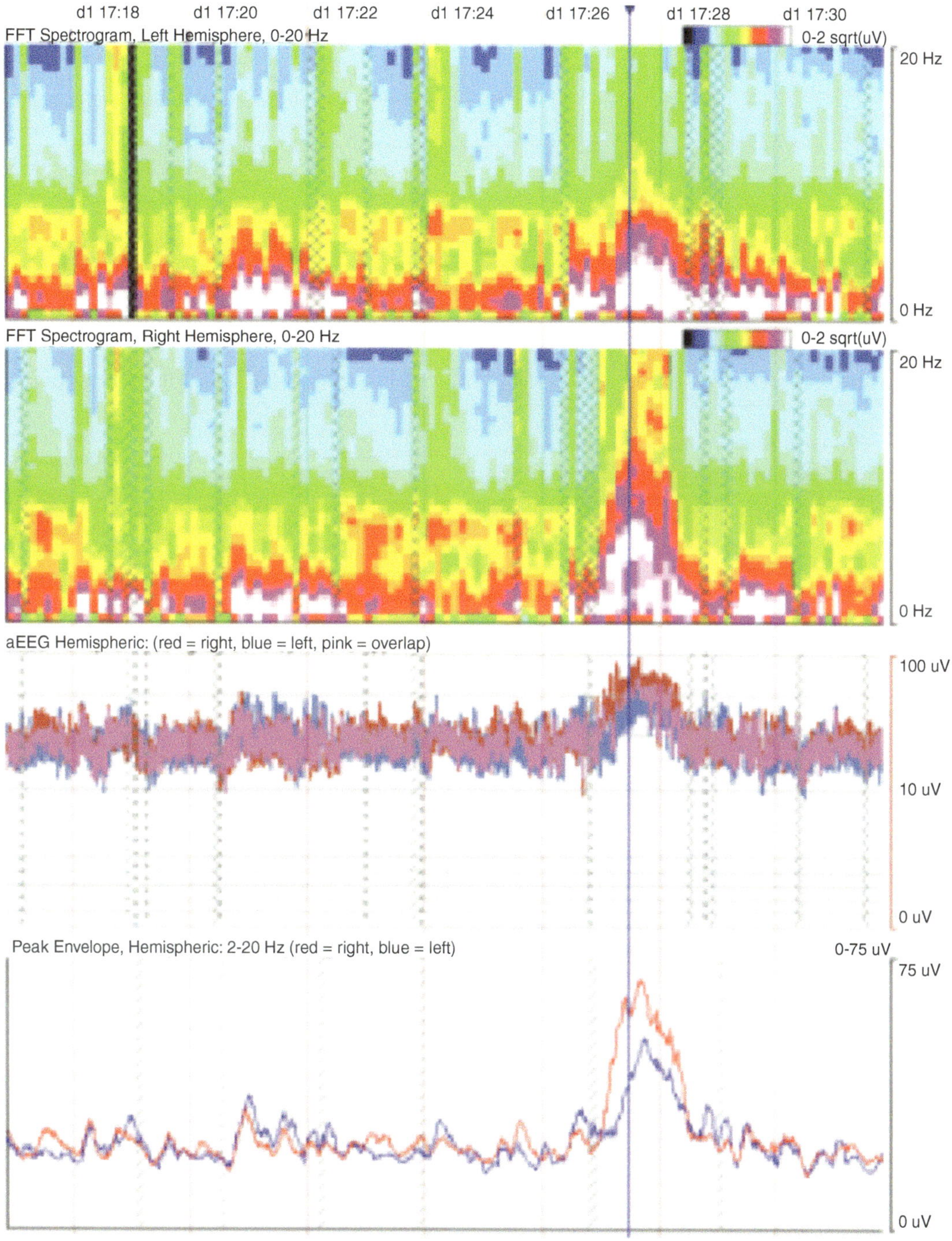

A. The increase in the peak envelope trend correlates with bihemispheric asymmetry, right more than left, indicating relative ischemia
B. The increase in the fast FFT spectrogram indicates that there is increasing higher power at the higher frequencies, indicating a state change from sleep to wakefulness
C. The deflection of the aEEG is most likely indicative of a burst of activity in the background of relative suppression
D. The deflection in the FFT spectrogram indicates that there is overall higher power, indicating a period of severe agitation in the patient
E. The color spectrogram indicates that the activity, in this case likely a seizure discharge, is involving the right hemisphere more than the left hemisphere

25. A 35-year-old male was admitted to the neurological ICU after a severe traumatic brain injury. He was found to have fluctuating mental status in the setting of a subarachnoid hemorrhage (SAH). Continuous video-EEG (cEEG) monitoring and head imaging were ordered. The EEG technician, a recent graduate, called the neurophysiology fellow to learn more about EEG electrode considerations with various imaging modalities. Which of the following statements is true?
A. Metal electrodes lead to a "starburst" effect on CT images due to the absorption of x-rays
B. All metal electrodes cause susceptibility artifact on MRI
C. Long leads and ferrous metals can lead to skin heating and burning during acquisition of MRI
D. Short-lead, silver, subdermal wire electrodes lead to significant artifact on both MRI and CT images
E. Plastic electrodes lead to significant artifact on CT but not MRI images

26. In which of the following clinical situations is continuous video-EEG monitoring (cEEG) in the ICU least likely to be helpful?
A. To characterize jerking events
B. To monitor for seizures when no seizures were identified in the first 24 hours of monitoring in a comatose patient
C. Prognostication after subarachnoid hemorrhage (SAH)
D. To monitor a patient with a witnessed generalized tonic–clonic seizure, felt to be due to hypoglycemia, who is back to his baseline mental state (Glasgow Coma Scale (GCS) 15)
E. To monitor the depth of coma in a patient with high intracranial pressure (ICP) placed in drug-induced burst suppression

27. The following fast Fourier transform (FFT) spectrograms from a 50-year-old male show 0 to 20 Hz activity from the left hemisphere (top panel) and right hemisphere (bottom panel); the color bar indicates the power, black being the lowest and white being the highest. All of the following interpretations is least likely to be correct at the time marker indicated by the blue vertical line?

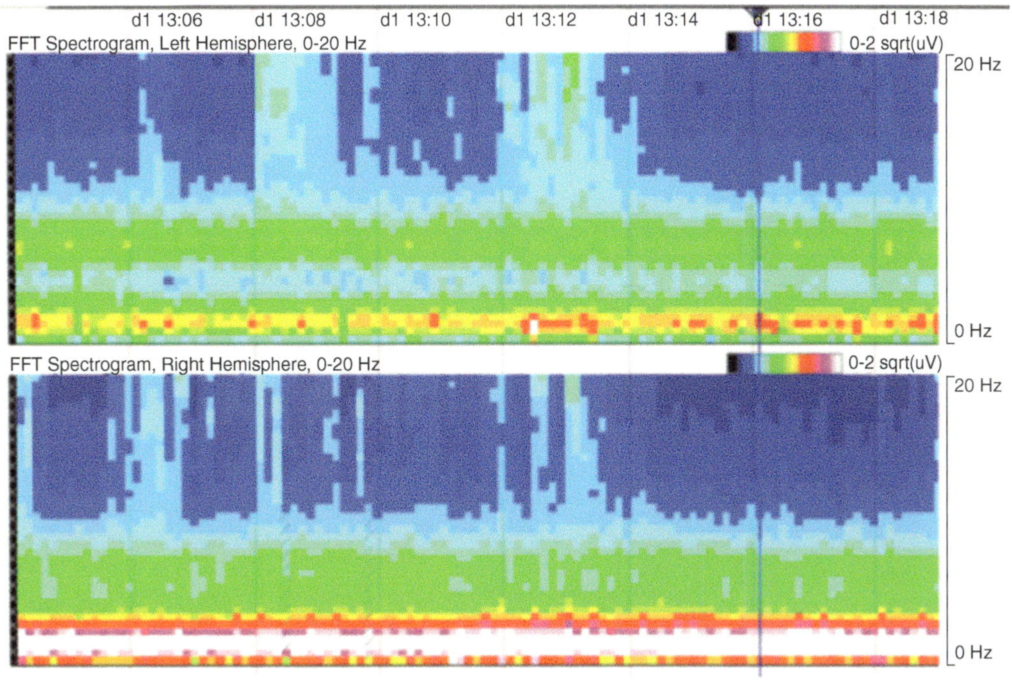

A. There is a symmetric posterior dominant rhythm (PDR)
B. The left hemisphere has more power in the alpha and beta frequencies than the right hemisphere
C. There is continuous high-amplitude delta slowing over the right hemisphere
D. There is continuous delta and theta activity over the left hemisphere
E. The right hemisphere has more power in the delta frequencies than the left hemisphere

28. The following quantitative EEG (qEEG) fast Fourier transform (FFT) spectrograms show 0 to 20 Hz activity from the left and right hemispheres (top two panels), amplitude-integrated EEG (aEEG), and peak envelope; the color bar indicates the power, black being the lowest and white being the highest. Note that the red vertical lines represent 2-minute intervals; for illustrative purposes, three different time periods are spliced together. What is the best explanation for the changes seen after the blue vertical line indicator?

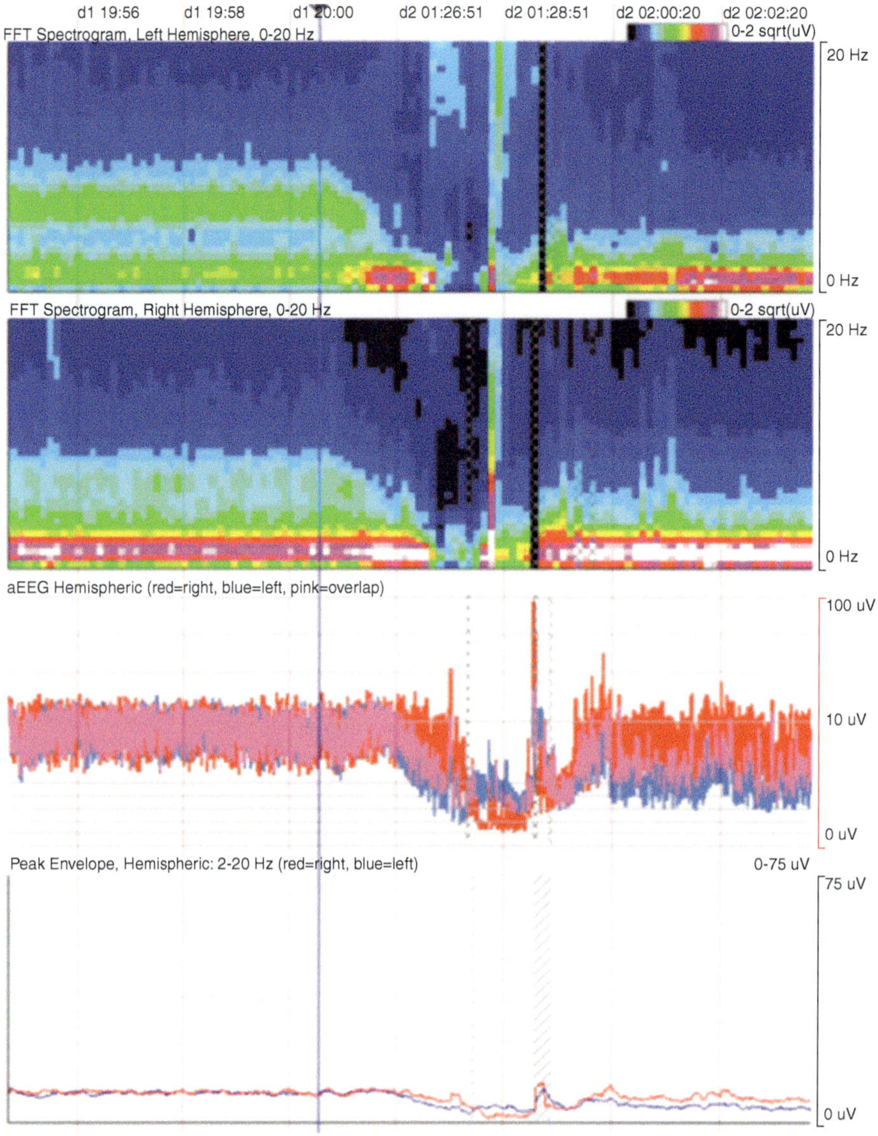

A. The patient had a seizure with postictal slowing afterward
B. The patient had diffuse cerebral ischemia due to cardiac arrest with subsequent infarction
C. The patient was disconnected from continuous video-EEG (cEEG) monitoring temporarily to be taken to CT scan without any significant interim clinical event
D. The patient transitioned from a wakeful state to deeper stages of normal sleep
E. The patient's sedation was lowered and then increased back to the previous level

29. A 35-year-old woman was found down and was placed on continuous video-EEG (cEEG) monitoring in the ICU. A clinical neurophysiology fellow was making rounds in the evening and saw the following quantitative EEG (qEEG panels), from top to bottom: fast Fourier transform (FFT) of left hemisphere, FFT of right hemisphere, amplitude-integrated EEG (aEEG), and peak envelope trend. Color bar indicates the power, black being the lowest and white being the highest. Which of the following is the most appropriate interpretation?

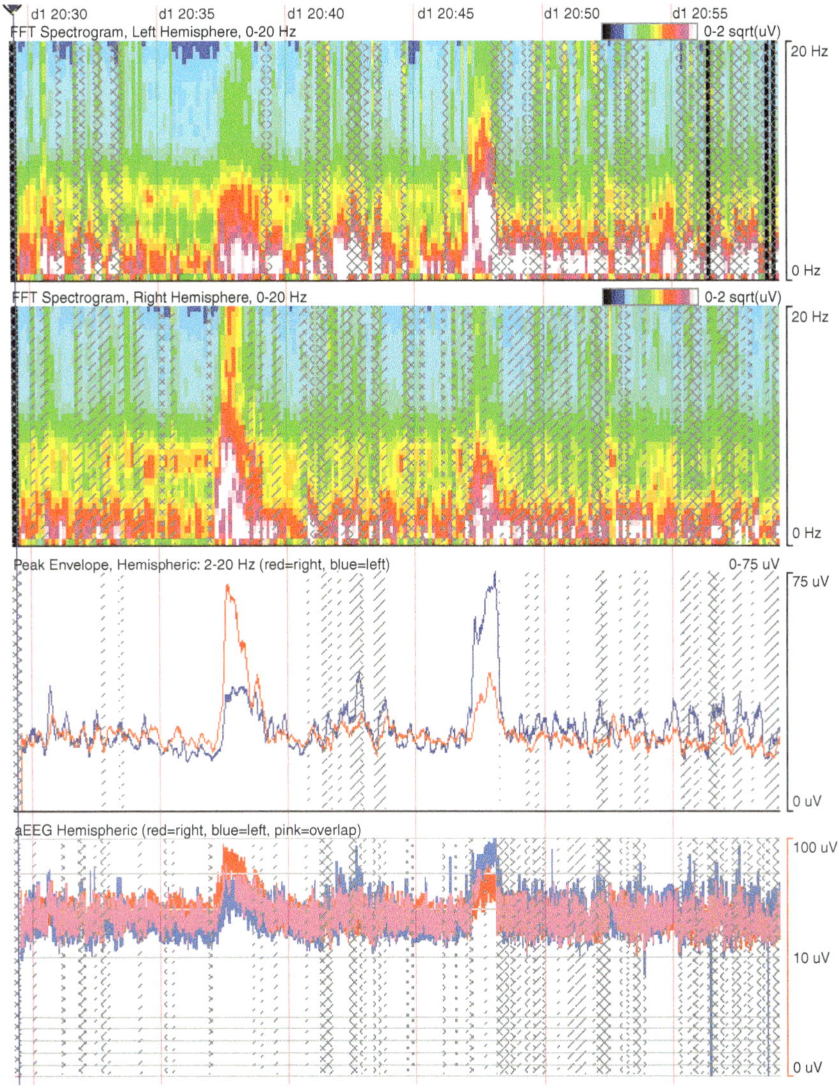

A. The patient has had two seizures, the first from the left hemisphere and the second from the right hemisphere
B. The patient has had two seizures, the first from the right hemisphere and the second from the left hemisphere
C. The patient has had three seizures, the first from the right hemisphere and the last two from the right hemisphere
D. The patient has had two primary generalized seizures
E. The patient has had three primary generalized seizures

30. A term infant was born by emergent cesarean section due to decreased fetal movements; the child arrived nonvigorous without respiratory effort and required intubation. The infant was placed on the hypothermia protocol and a high-frequency oscillatory ventilator (HFOV). Seizures were noted on continuous video-EEG (cEEG) monitoring, and the baby was placed on phenobarbital and midazolam infusions. Top: fast Fourier transform

(FFT) of left hemisphere; bottom: FFT of right hemisphere. Color bar indicates the power, black being the lowest and white being the highest. Which of the following is most likely seen on the following quantitative EEG (qEEG) panel?

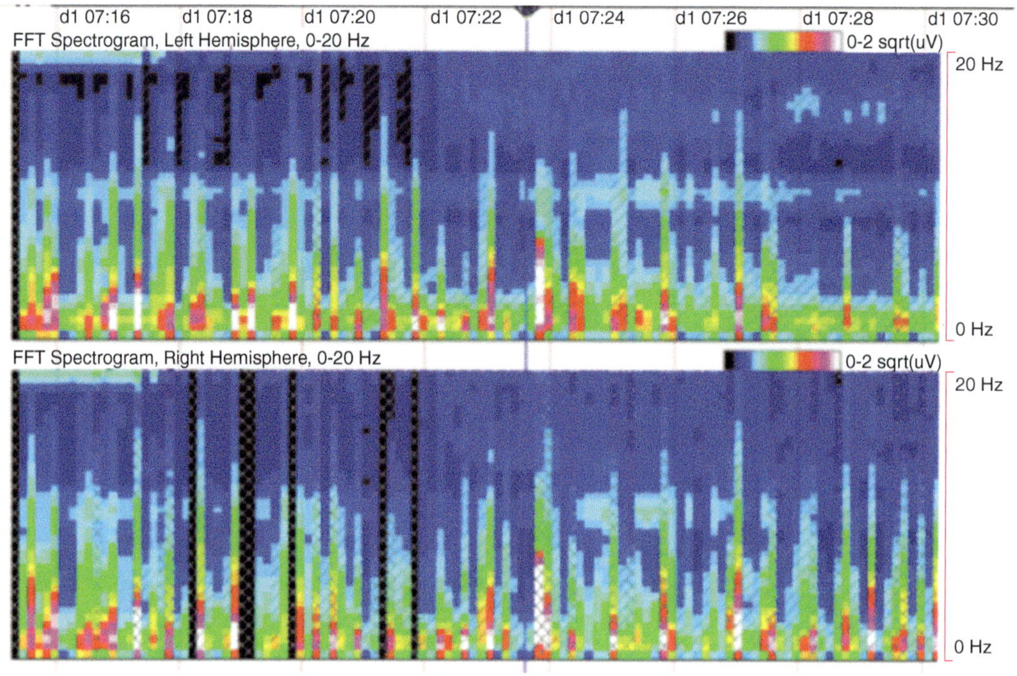

A. Periodic seizures
B. Burst-suppression-like pattern
C. Multiple sleep–wake cycles
D. HFOV artifact
E. Multiple periods of sedation vacation

31. Which of the following is true regarding the Main Term one of the American Clinical Neurophysiology Society's established standardized critical care EEG terminology?
A. Generalized (G) refers to bilateral activity that can be symmetric or asymmetric
B. Lateralized (L) refers to strictly unilateral hemispheric or focal patterns
C. Bilateral independent (BI) refers to bilateral activity that is asynchronous
D. Multifocal (Mf) refers to patterns occupying at least two brain regions and involving both hemispheres
E. All of the above

32. Which of the following is *true* regarding the Main Term two of the American Clinical Neurophysiology Society's established standardized critical care EEG terminology?
A. Periodic discharges (PDs) apply only to single discharges lasting less than 0.5 seconds to bursts lasting less than 1 second
B. The interval duration between PDs can have up to a 100% variation from one cycle to the next as long as the morphology is relatively uniform
C. Both rhythmic delta activity (RDA) and periodic discharges have an interval between consecutive waveforms

D. RDA is repetition of a waveform with either monomorphic or polymorphic morphology
E. Spike wave (SW) consistently follows the pattern of a spike or sharp wave followed by a slow wave

33. Which of the following is *true* regarding the modifiers of the American Clinical Neurophysiology Society's established standardized critical care EEG terminology?
A. Amplitude refers to the absolute height of a pattern and should be measured in a standard longitudinal bipolar montage (10–20 system) from peak to trough (not to baseline)
B. Prevalence refers to the percentage of the record occupied by a pattern and is classified as continuous if it occupies more than 90% of the record / epoch
C. Duration refers to the typical duration of a single occurrence of the pattern and is classified as brief if it is between 10 and 59 seconds
D. Sharpness applies only to periodic discharges (PDs) and spike wave (SW) and not rhythmic delta activity (RDA)
E. All of the above

34. Classify the following pattern using the American Clinical Neurophysiology Society's established standardized critical care EEG terminology.

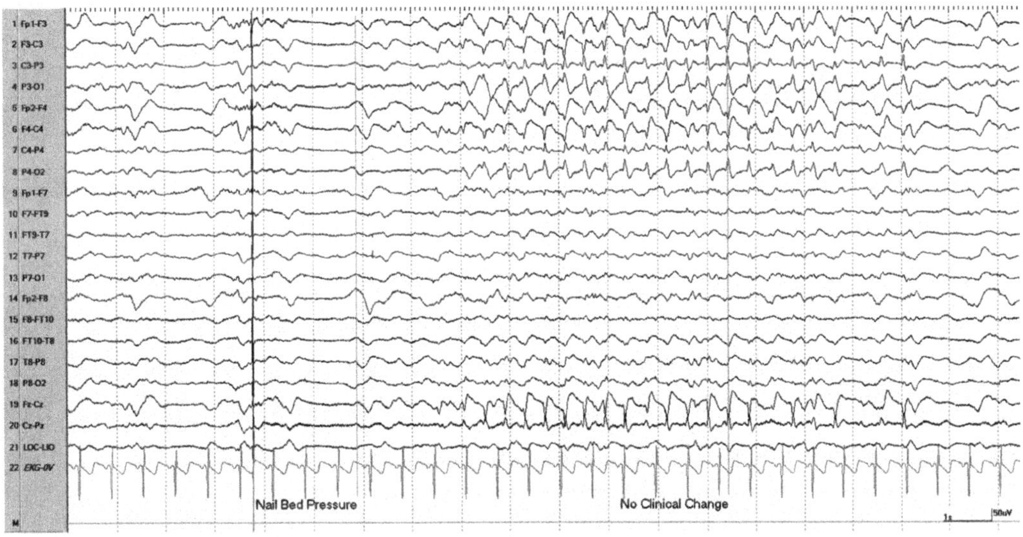

A. Stimulus-induced generalized rhythmic delta activity (SI-GRDA)
B. Lateralized spike wave (LSW)
C. Bilateral independent rhythmic delta activity (BIRDA)
D. Stimulus-induced generalized spike wave (SI-GSW)
E. Stimulus-induced lateralized spike wave (SI-LSW)

35. Which of the following EEG patterns is least likely to be associated with status epilepticus (SE)?
A. Recurrent 5 to 7 Hz rhythmic temporal activity
B. Generalized periodic discharges occurring at a frequency of 2 to 3 Hz
C. Normal scalp EEG
D. Intermittent temporal polymorphic delta activity
E. Lateralized periodic discharges occurring at a frequency of 2 to 3 Hz

36. Many types of artifacts exist in the ICU setting of physiological and nonphysiological origin. Which of the following is NOT a typical description of the EEG pattern associated with the listed artifact?
   A. Extracorporeal membrane oxygenation (ECMO) is associated with a 1 to 3 Hz square wave activity
   B. Ventilators can cause artifact that varies widely in morphology, amplitude, and polarity, but can be associated with a faster frequency artifact due to charged water molecules in the ventilator tubing that can be improved by suctioning
   C. Mechanical chest percussion device can cause rhythmic 5 to 6 Hz activity in a single electrode
   D. Cardiopulmonary resuscitation (CPR) can lead to high-amplitude, rhythmic 1 to 2 Hz activity that is due to movement and is not cerebral activity
   E. Continuous renal replacement therapy (CRRT) can lead to rhythmic 5 to 12 Hz activity in multiple electrodes with a sharp or sawtooth morphology

37. Which of the following EEG patterns is least likely to be independent predictor of poor outcome (modified Rankin Scale greater than 4) for patients with subarachnoid hemorrhage (SAH)?
   A. Presence of sleep spindles
   B. Bilateral independent lateralized periodic discharges
   C. Generalized periodic discharges
   D. Nonreactive EEG background
   E. Nonconvulsive status epilepticus

38. All of the following meet the minimum requirement for recording high-frequency oscillations (HFOs) except:
   A. Microelectrodes
   B. Depth electrodes
   C. Subdural electrodes
   D. Sampling rate of 1,000 Hz
   E. Sampling rate of 500 Hz

39. In patients with epilepsy, the high-frequency oscillations (HFOs) are:
   A. Absent outside the hippocampus and entorhinal cortex
   B. Recorded interictally and ictally
   C. Helpful in localizing the seizure onset zone when recorded interictally
   D. Considered pathologic if the frequency is greater than 250 Hz
   E. Present only within the seizure focus

40. Which of the following statements regarding the direct current (DC) shifts seen at seizure onset is true?
   A. DC shifts can only be recorded using dedicated DC-coupled amplifiers
   B. DC shifts can be recorded using an amplifier with a short-time constant
   C. DC shifts are better seen by increasing the low-frequency filter
   D. DC shifts at seizure onset are useful in localizing the seizure onset zone
   E. DC shifts are only seen on intracranial recordings

41. Advantages of magnetoencephalography (MEG) over EEG include all of the following *except:*
   A. Good spatial resolution
   B. Selectivity to activity in the Sylvian fissure
   C. Relative insensitivity to the properties of extracerebral tissue
   D. Selectivity to radial currents
   E. Reference free recording

42. In a spherical head model, magnetoencephalography (MEG) is least likely to detect which of the following signals?
   A. Those tangential to the cortical surface
   B. Those perpendicular to the cortical surface
   C. Those tilted 10 to 20 degrees from radial orientation to the cortical surface
   D. Those within the cortical fissures
   E. Those within the superficial cortex

43. Which of the following statements best describes the utility of magnetoencephalography (MEG) in epilepsy?
   A. Unlike EEG, MEG can differentiate between ictal and interictal spikes
   B. MEG is not suitable for evaluation of epileptic foci in the cerebral convexity
   C. MEG can identify time lags to differentiate between primary and mirror foci
   D. MEG studies have shown significant epileptiform activity in the motor speech area in Landau–Kleffner syndrome
   E. MEG is not useful for the study of neocortical epilepsy

44. A single electrical stimulus applied to the motor cortex during transcranial electrical stimulation (TES):
   A. Produces a single volley in the descending motor tracts
   B. Produces D-waves in the pyramidal axons
   C. Produces I-waves in the anterior horn cells
   D. Produces M-waves in the pyramidal neurons
   E. Produces an initial volley (I-wave), which is followed by subsequent volleys (D-waves)

45. Myogenic motor evoked potentials (MEPs) recorded with transcranial electrical stimulation (TES) are:
   A. Produced by summated D-waves
   B. Best recorded using trains of high-intensity stimuli with an interstimulus interval of 50 to 100 ms
   C. Consistent across multiple trials
   D. Unaffected by inhalation anesthesia
   E. Highly likely to be suppressed by a combination of propofol and opioid total intravenous anesthesia

46. Which of the following statements regarding the stimulating parameters used for transcranial electrical stimulation (TES) is true?
   A. Fz/Cz electrode pair stimulates corticospinal tracts to the legs
   B. C3/C4 electrode pair stimulates corticospinal tracts to both arms and legs
   C. C1/C2 electrode pair stimulates corticospinal tracts to arms

D. Laterally placed electrode pair selectively stimulates the corticospinal tracts contralateral to the anode
E. All of the above

47. Motor evoked potentials (MEPs) during scalp transcranial electrical stimulation (TES) are generated by:
A. Action potentials that are initiated at the axon hillocks of the cortical pyramidal neurons
B. Action potentials that are initiated in the cell bodies of the cortical pyramidal neurons
C. The outward inhibitory transmembrane current under the anode
D. The inward excitatory transmembrane current under the anode
E. None of the above

48. Which of the following statements regarding motor evoked potentials (MEPs) elicited by transcranial electrical stimulation (TES) is true?
A. D-waves are generated by action potentials in pyramidal cell axons
B. I-waves are generated by inhibitory synaptic activity
C. Myogenic waves are recorded ipsilateral to the anode
D. D-waves are suppressed by anesthesia
E. All of the above

49. Transcranial magnetic stimulation (TMS):
A. Is limited to stimulation of the motor cortex
B. Produces the strongest currents close to the inner table of the skull
C. Consistently activates brainstem
D. Is more likely to produce motor evoked potentials consisting of D-waves
E. Activates scalp pain fibers stronger than does transcranial electrical stimulation (TES)

50. Transcranial magnetic stimulation (TMS) is unsuitable for intraoperative monitoring of motor evoked potentials (MEPs) because:
A. It does not effectively activate the motor cortex
B. It produces waveforms that likely to be suppressed by anesthesia
C. It produces waveforms that can change dramatically depending on the orientation of the stimulating coil
D. B and C
E. A, B and C

51. All of the following statements are true regarding the utility of transcranial magnetic stimulation (TMS) *except:*
A. It is useful in the diagnosis of lesions involving corticobulbar tracts
B. It is useful in the diagnosis of lesions involving corticospinal tracts
C. It is useful in monitoring spinal surgeries under general anesthesia
D. It has therapeutic benefit in epilepsy
E. It has therapeutic benefit in major depression

52. In terms of neuropsychiatric effects, repetitive transcranial magnetic stimulation (rTMS) can:
A. Alter mood in nondepressed subjects
B. Improve mood in depressed patients
C. Induce mania
D. Improve or worsen neuropsychological function
E. All of the above

53. Stereo-EEG (SEEG) depth electrode study alone is LEAST likely to be helpful in the evaluation of suspected seizure onset in which of the following structures?
   A. Left posterior temporal lobe
   B. Bilateral hippocampus
   C. Left cingulate gyrus
   D. Right amygdala
   E. Right insula

54. Which of the following is an important consideration in planning a stereo-EEG (SEEG) implantation?
   A. Accurate localization of seizure onset by scalp video-EEG
   B. Determination of vascular anatomy
   C. Adherence to electrode nomenclature based on the targeted structure
   D. Symmetrical implantation with same number of electrodes in both hemispheres
   E. All of the above

55. Sampling of which of the following structures is LEAST desirable in a stereo-EEG (SEEG) evaluation of left anterior temporal cavernoma?
   A. Wernicke's area
   B. Left amygdala
   C. Left hippocampus
   D. Left orbitofrontal cortex
   E. Left temporal pole

56. Which of the following features is suggestive of the epileptogenic zone (EZ) in a stereo-EEG (SEEG) recording?
   A. Rhythmic faster frequency waveforms
   B. Repetitive spikes
   C. High-amplitude slow waves with superimposed faster frequency waveforms
   D. Rhythmic synchronous waveforms in multiple electrodes with or without a minor time lag between the electrodes
   E. All of the above

57. The rate of major complications attributed to stereo-EEG (SEEG) is:
   A. Less than 1%
   B. 2% to 3%
   C. 4% to 5%
   D. 6% to 8%
   E. 9% to 10%

58. The figure shows a 30-second epoch of an electrocorticogram (ECoG) recording from a patient with a responsive neurostimulator (RNS) device. Contacts LHip1-4 are located in the left hippocampus, whereas the contacts RIT1-4 are located over the right inferior temporal region. Markers "B1" and "B2" indicate the detections made by the device; marker "Tx" indicates the delivery of stimulation by the device; and marker "XTx" indicates the end of stimulations delivered by the device. Which of the following statements is true regarding this epoch?

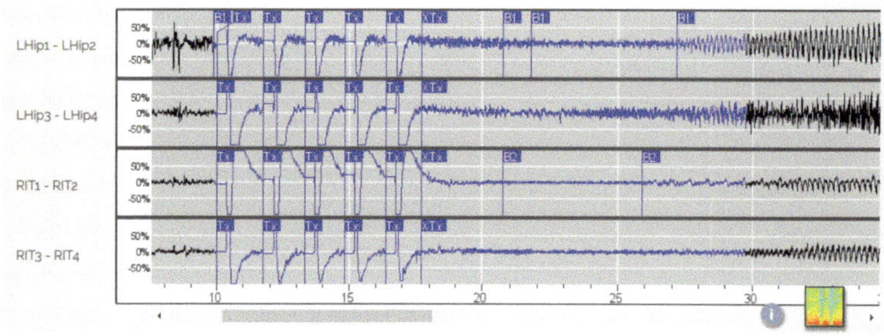

A. The patient has a left temporal lobe focal seizure with impaired awareness
B. The patient has a left temporal lobe seizure which is successfully terminated by the device
C. The patient has a left temporal lobe seizure which spreads to the right temporal lobe
D. A and B
E. A, B, and C

59. The figure shows a 30-second epoch of an electrocorticogram (ECoG) recording from a patient with a responsive neurostimulator (RNS) device. Contacts LIns1-4 are located in the left insula, whereas the contacts LTP1-4 are located over the left temporoparietal convexity. Marker "A1" indicates the detection made by the device; marker "Tx" indicates the delivery of stimulation by the device; marker "XTx" indicates the end of stimulations delivered by the device; and marker "LE" indicates a long episode. Which of the following features is LEAST likely to be seen as part of the patient's seizure semiology?

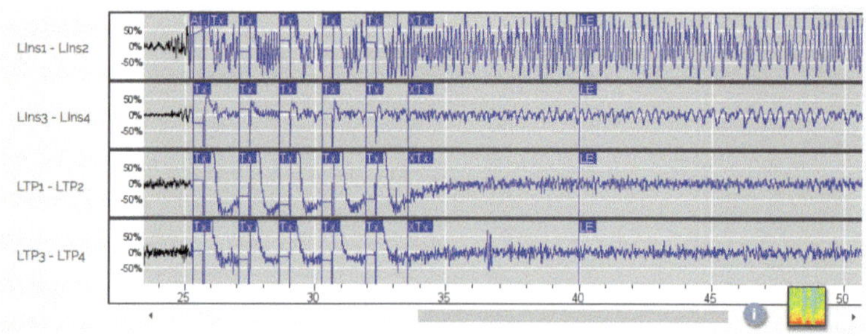

A. Impaired awareness
B. Choking sensation
C. Lip smacking
D. Light flashes in the right visual field
E. Right facial twitching

60. A 48-year-old male with MRI-negative, nonlateralized temporal lobe epilepsy undergoes stereo-EEG (SEEG) evaluation. The EEG recording (low frequency filter 1.6 Hz, high-frequency filter 300 Hz) shows one of his typical seizures involving the most relevant electrodes implanted in the right hemisphere (as labeled). The electrodes were implanted orthogonally into the temporal pole, amygdala, and hippocampus; obliquely into the anterior insula through the parietal cortex; and vertically into the orbitofrontal regions through the prefrontal cortex. As such, the lower-numbered contacts were in the targeted structures and the higher-numbered contacts were in the convexity. Which of the following features is most likely to be seen as part of his seizure semiology?

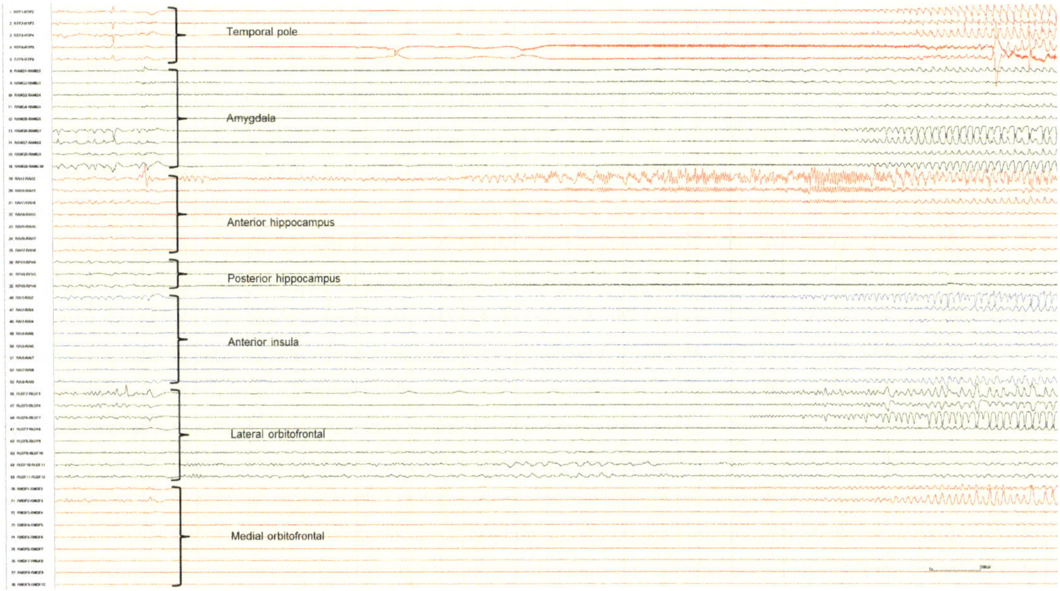

A. Left facial twitching, left hand clonic movements, and left head version
B. Loss of vision in the left visual field, throat spasm, and loss of awareness
C. Lip smacking, fumbling with right hand, and repetitive left hand opening and closing movements
D. Bicycling movements, agitation, and screaming for help
E. Staring, right hand dystonic posturing, and throat spasm

61. A 22-year-old female with left-sided periventricular nodular heterotopia undergoes stereo-EEG (SEEG) evaluation for seizure localization. The EEG recording (low frequency filter 1.6 Hz, high-frequency filter 300 Hz) shows two awake interictal epochs 15 minutes apart separated by the solid line in the middle. Which of the following electrodes are most likely to be located within or close to the heterotopic lesions?

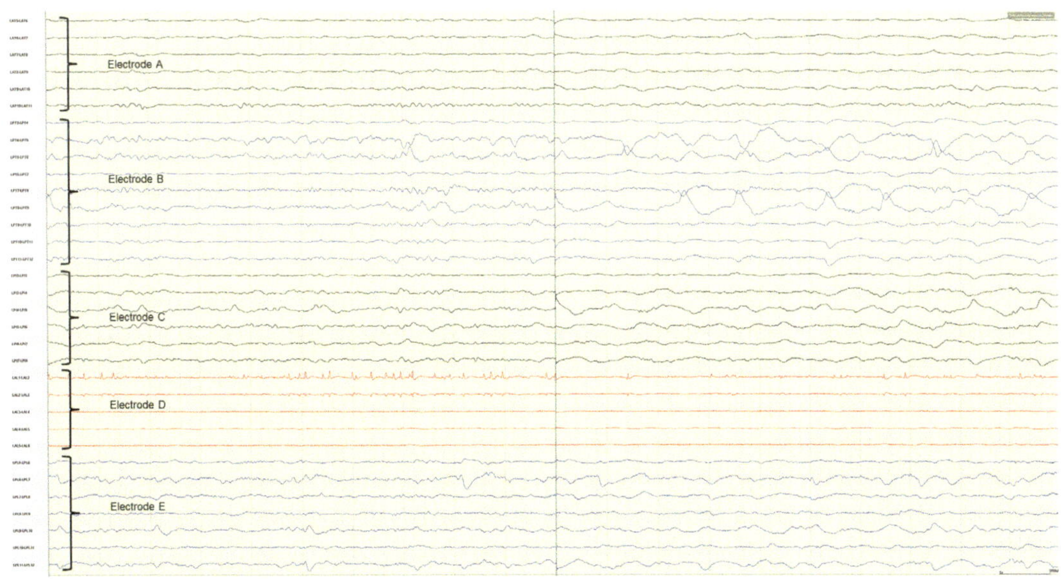

A. Electrodes A, B, and C
B. Electrodes A, B, and D
C. Electrodes A and E
D. Electrodes B, C, D, and E
E. Electrodes A, B, C, D, and E

62. In which of the following patients is subdural grid evaluation preferred over stereo-EEG (SEEG) evaluation?

A. A 19-year-old male with nonlateralized, bifrontal ictal discharges on scalp EEG and normal MRI
B. A 30-year-old female with left temporal ictal discharges on scalp EEG and bilateral periventricular nodular heterotopias and left mesial temporal sclerosis on MRI
C. A 22-year-old male with hyperkinetic focal seizures, uninterpretable ictal discharges on scalp EEG, and normal MRI
D. A 40-year-old male with right frontotemporal ictal discharges on scalp EEG and right inferior frontal cavernoma on MRI
E. A 38-year-old female with left temporoparietal ictal discharges on scalp EEG and left parietal encephalomalacia from prior arteriovenous malformation (AVM) resection on MRI

ANSWERS

1. **D.** While performing SFEMG, the low-frequency filter should be raised to 500 Hz so that distant low-frequency waveforms are not recorded. This allows the SFEMG needle to record only from a few muscle fibers close to the needle tip. Even though SFEMG can be performed with concentric needle, it is not the same as a routine needle EMG study and filter setting changes are required.

2. **B.** SFEMG is not specific for NMJ diseases, and can be abnormal in neurogenic conditions. SFEMG is the most sensitive test for NMJ disorders and a normal SFEMG in a weak muscle is not consistent with myasthenia gravis. Jitter value increases with age and varies by muscles. Blocking is suggestive of NMJ dysfunction.

3. **B.** A normal SFEMG in a weak muscle makes a NMJ dysfunction as the underlying cause of the weakness very unlikely. Abnormal SFEMG does not always mean NMJ disorder as this can be seen with neurogenic conditions as well. SFEMG is a sensitive but not very specific test for NMJ disorder. With increasing age, normal upper limit of jitter increases. Blocking is generally considered to be abnormal irrespective of the age.

4. **B.** On right-sided stimulation, ipsilateral R1 and R2 responses are normal, suggestive of normal right trigeminal and facial nerves and rest of the reflex arc. However, the contralateral R2 is absent. On left-sided stimulation, ipsilateral R1 and R2 are absent but contralateral R2 is normal, suggestive of normal left trigeminal nerve function. Because only the motor responses on the left side are absent with normal afferent pathways, this study is suggestive of left facial neuropathy. A midbrain lesion is not expected to lead to these findings as cranial nerve VII is not in the midbrain.

5. **B.** A lesion in the right trigeminal nerve or nucleus leads to absence of ipsilateral R1, ipsilateral R2, and contralateral R2 responses with right trigeminal stimulation. When all the responses are absent, the likely lesion is in the afferent loop, such as the trigeminal nerve or nucleus. Unilateral facial nerve or nucleus lesion should not cause deficits on both sides. Oculomotor and abducens nerves do not have any role to play with blink reflexes.

6. **B.** Blink reflex study is a polysynaptic study. The afferent fibers are in the fifth cranial nerve and efferent fibers are in the seventh cranial nerve, similar to the corneal blink reflex. After stimulation, R1 response is seen only unilaterally whereas R2 responses are seen bilaterally. However, ipsilateral and contralateral R2 responses have different latencies.

7. **B.** The arrow points to Phase II Late. During the Valsalva maneuver, phases I, II Early, and III are secondary to changes in intrathoracic pressure, whereas phases II Late and IV are considered reflex responses. In patients with adrenergic failure, phase II Late and IV responses are impaired. Generally, Phase IV becomes blunted followed by loss of Phase II Late response.

8. **C.** The heart rate deep breathing range is one of the parasympathetic markers of autonomic function. It is the mean change in heart rate over five respiratory cycles. In the waveform in the question, the maximum mean change over the five cycles is close to 18 to 20. One should pay attention to the Y-axis, which provides the magnitude of heart rate change.

9. **B.** Close observation of the Valsalva waveforms reveals absent Phase II Late and Phase IV, which suggests severe adrenergic failure, especially with the severe drop in the blood pressure on tilt table testing. Sudomotor function is normally measured by a quantitative sudomotor axon reflex test (QSART) or other forms of sweat testing. Valsalva ratio is defined as maximum heart rate divided by minimum heart rate during Valsalva maneuver. In this case, there is very minimal change in heart rate during the Valsalva maneuver and the ratio is significantly reduced.

10. **C.** Acetylcholine is the neurotransmitter for most parasympathetic postganglionic fibers and norepinephrine is the neurotransmitter for most sympathetic postganglionic fibers. However, sympathetic fibers innervating sweat glands are cholinergic fibers.

11. **D.** The waveforms reveal severe orthostatic hypotension with drop in systolic blood pressure of more than 50 mmHg within 1 minute of standing (1st arrowhead on the x-axis). Her blood pressure returns to baseline after she is bought back to the supine state (2nd arrowhead on the x-axis). This study was stopped before 3 minutes. These features are suggestive of severe orthostatic hypotension. This study is not consistent with POTS as there is a clear dramatic drop in blood pressure. In POTS, there is a profound increase in heart rate without a significant drop in blood pressure.

12. **C.** Cardiac sympathetic imaging is the best technique to differentiate Parkinson's disease with autonomic function from MSA. This distinction is important to make as the overall prognosis is significantly worse in MSA. Degree of drop in blood pressure on standing or tilt table does not help differentiate these two conditions. Cardiovagal markers such as HR variability or Valsalva ratio also do not help differentiate these two conditions.

13. **D.** Cardiovagal function is typically deduced from the heart rate deep breathing range and Valsalva ratio. Phase II Late and Phase IV of the Valsalva waveforms provide information regarding the adrenergic function. Sudomotor function measures postganglionic sweat fiber function and is normally assessed with QSART testing.

14. **B.** The definition of neurogenic orthostatic hypotension is a drop in SBP of more than 20 mmHg with less than 15 beats/min increase in HR during tilt table testing. Nonneurogenic causes of orthostatic hypotension are usually associated with >15 beats/min increase in HR along with >20 mmHg drop in BP. If there is no change in BP, but HR increase is more than 30 beats/min, it might reflect postural orthostatic tachycardia syndrome. Increase in BP during tilt table may be seen with orthostatic hypertension, a rare disorder.

15. **B.** Some rare neuromuscular disorders also have autonomic dysfunction. Autonomic dysfunction is classically noted in LEMS with dry mouth, erectile dysfunction, and orthostatic symptoms.

16. **C.** Rapid improvement in glycemic control in poorly controlled patients, especially after initiating insulin therapy, may lead to new neuropathic manifestations including neuropathic pain and autonomic symptoms. This is called treatment induced diabetic neuropathy or "insulin neuritis." Most patients have gradual improvement in overall symptom burden with time. There is no need for immunotherapy. Optimal glycemic control should be continued.

17. **B.** Mutation in sodium channel can cause small fiber neuropathy and genetic testing for SCN9A, SCN10A can be performed if there is no evidence of an acquired cause of small fiber neuropathy.

18. **D.** CIDP is not typically associated with significant autonomic neuropathy or failure. All other conditions including TTR amyloidosis, diabetic neuropathies, GBS, and Sjogens syndrome can cause both somatic and autonomic neuropathies.

19. **B.** This clinical picture is suggestive of small fiber neuropathy. Among the noninvasive choices, QSART testing to assess sudomotor function is the best diagnostic test for small fiber neuropathy. Routine nerve conduction studies are normal in small fiber neuropathy. SSEP are also normal in small fiber neuropathy. Sleep studies do not help with diagnosis of small fiber neuropathy. Skin biopsy, which is easy to perform and has the high diagnostic yield for small fiber neuropathy, is an invasive study.

20. **E.** Neurophysiological monitoring during spinal surgery is useful and can reduce the likelihood of postoperative complications related to spinal or nerve injury. However, monitoring is affected by multiple parameters during the surgery including anesthesia, body temperature, and hypotension.

21. **D.** Skin biopsy to assess epidermal nerve fiber density has the higher diagnostic yield for the assessment of small fiber neuropathy. Other measures of sudomotor function such as QSART are helpful and noninvasive, but sensitivity and specificity are not as high as skin biopsy. QDIRT is mostly a research methodology and is not widely used. Confocal microscopy has been shown to be very helpful in the diagnosis of diabetic neuropathy but has not been proven in nondiabetic neuropathies. QST, a standardized assessment of different sensory modalities, can help with the diagnosis of small fiber neuropathy, but sensitivity and specificity are much lower than epidermal nerve fiber sensory assessment with skin biopsy.

22. **E.** qEEG can provide a number of advantages over review of raw EEG, including allowing for rapid detection of seizures or depth of coma (a single qEEG screen typically consists of 1 to 4 hours vs 10 to 15 seconds of raw EEG per screen with conventional review); quick overview of seizure location, frequency, and duration; and assessment of response to therapy (e.g., treatment of seizures or burst-suppression for management of high intracranial pressure). There are some limitations, including false positive seizure detections due to high-amplitude, rhythmic artifacts commonly seen in the ICU (e.g., cardiopulmonary resuscitation [CPR], suctioning, ventilator, extracorporeal membrane

oxygenation [ECMO]) and false negatives due to missing brief, focal, low-amplitude seizures. Therefore, qEEG cannot replace expert review of raw EEG.

23. **E.** There has been increasing evidence that cEEG monitoring can be of utility in monitoring patients with SAH. In addition to detecting nonconvulsive seizures, which are difficult to detect clinically in patients with altered mental status as in this case, quantitative EEG (qEEG) measures could be used to detect for DCI, or infarction due to vasospasm that can typically occur 5 to 12 days (range: 3–21 days) after SAH. Normally, healthy individuals have high alpha variability, which fluctuates with sleep–wake cycles, eye opening/closure, and so on. When this variability decreases in the right setting, this could correlate with impaired thalamocortical pacemaker activity. In the setting of SAH, this could indicate ischemia. ADR is a measure of the percentage of alpha activity compared to the percentage of delta activity for a given time period. With decreasing cerebral blood flow (CBF), the amount of alpha activity will decrease and the amount of delta activity will increase. Thus, a decreasing ADR would indicate decreasing perfusion and likely ischemia or infarction. RAV is a measure of the theta-alpha power (6–14 Hz) to total power (1–20 Hz) and in retrospective analyses, has show good sensitivity and moderate specificity for detecting DCI. In general, decreasing RAV correlates with impaired perfusion, which can be an indicator of vasospasm.

24. **E.** The quantitative EEG (qEEG) panels displayed are consistent with a seizure discharge lasting about 2 minutes, originating over the right hemisphere and spreading to the contralateral side. The FFT spectrogram is a frequency-based qEEG trend that displays a three-dimensional representation of EEG power (which is proportional to the square of the amplitude) over time with respect to the various frequencies. Seizures are represented by increasing power that usually evolves from lower to higher frequencies. On the FFT spectrogram, increase in the color toward the red end of the color spectrum over both hemispheres indicates an increase in power at those frequencies. In this case, there appears to be an increase in power across many frequencies, right greater than left, which also supports a seizure discharge involving the right hemisphere greater than left hemisphere. Many artifacts (e.g., muscle or electrode) typically present with increased power on the FFT spectrogram as well but the increase is more abrupt without evolution. aEEG is an amplitude-based qEEG trend that displays the minimum and maximum amplitude of the EEG background over a preset time interval (typically 1–2 seconds). On the aEEG, the increase in baseline amplitude and the narrowing of the aEEG band suggest a seizure discharge. The higher amplitude of the red band suggests that the seizure discharge may be asymmetric and higher in the right hemisphere. Many other changes on aEEG are nonspecific and often represent artifact. The peak envelope trend is an amplitude-based qEEG trend that displays the median amplitude of the EEG background over a preset time interval (typically 10–20 seconds). On the peak envelope trend, the upward deflection of the red tracing represents an increase in median amplitude over the right hemisphere, corresponding to a seizure. The delayed upward deflection of the blue tracing represents contralateral spread of the seizure discharge. Peak envelop trend may be more specific than aEEG but can miss seizures that are brief in duration. In general, qEEG trends draw attention to the time of the recording where more detailed analysis is needed but they cannot replace expert review of raw EEG.

25. **C.** Long leads and ferrous metals can lead to skin heating and burning during acquisition of MRI. Moreover, the electrodes themselves may physically move, contributing to the incompatibility of these materials with MRI. Nonferrous metals, such as noble metals (e.g., silver, gold, copper, and platinum) lead to less artifact and are more conducive to being used in MRI. Metal electrodes lead to a "star-burst" effect on CT images due to deflection, not absorption, of x-rays. Conductive plastic electrodes (coated with a thin silver layer) and many subdermal wire electrodes (e.g., silver) do not lead to significant artifact, and can be used for both MRI and CT images. However, short-lead wires are preferred because the risk of coiling is less which minimizes MRI artifacts (the wires act less like an antenna); and risk to the patient is less (less current and heating). Unlike patients in the epilepsy monitoring unit (EMU), cEEG patients in the ICU may require frequent and/or urgent head imaging (e.g., CT, MRI, angiography), and a more educated decision regarding electrode choice can lead to lower risk and cost while increasing efficiency (by not having to adjust or redo the electrode setup).

26. **D.** In general, in about half of all studies, the first seizure is captured within the first hour of recording, and the longer the monitoring lasts, the higher the yield of capturing electrographic seizures. Although there may be little benefit of monitoring beyond 24 hours in noncomatose patients, there is some evidence to suggest that extending the monitoring at least another 24 hours in comatose patients may increase the yield about 10%. However, the actual length of cEEG monitoring in practice varies from center to center, and can deviate from what might be desired due to other constraints, including resource limitations. Many types of events are seen in the ICU setting (e.g., tremor, focal twitching or jerking, aphasia), which are sometimes difficult to characterize solely on a clinical basis. cEEG monitoring can assist in characterizing if these events are ictal, and in some cases help narrow down the origin in cases where the events are not epileptic. cEEG monitoring can help with prognostication in such insults as SAH, intracranial hemorrhage, and postcardiac arrest. Although cEEG monitoring can greatly assist in detecting nonconvulsive seizures, it may not provide any substantial benefit in situations in which there was a clinically apparent seizure (for eg, generalized tonic-clonic seizure) due to a known cause (for eg, hypoglycemia) with the patient's mental state back to baseline. cEEG can also help in monitoring the depth of coma, especially with the use of quantitative EEG panels assessing suppression ratios.

27. **A.** The FFT spectrograms in the question evaluate each hemisphere separately. In general, the two panels should appear similar, but that is not the case. The left hemisphere appears to have higher power than the right hemisphere in the alpha range frequencies. As an approximation, around 8 to 10 Hz, the left hemisphere is green while the right hemisphere is light blue, indicating lower power. In addition, around 10 to 12 Hz, the left hemisphere has light blue color while the right hemisphere has darker blue color, suggestive of an asymmetry of the posterior dominant rhythm. In addition, the beta frequencies appear to have equal or higher power in the left hemisphere. There is a thick band of bright white power in the delta range frequencies over the right hemisphere, suggestive of high-amplitude delta slowing. The fact that the band remains white for the entire duration suggests that the slowing is continuous. Similarly, the left hemisphere has bands of continuous slowing in the delta and theta range, although the slowing is at a lower power.

28. B. The most likely scenario is that the patient had diffuse ischemia with subsequent infarction due to decreased cerebral blood flow that occurred in the setting of cardiac arrest. From the FFT spectrogram panels, power in the alpha range diminished while the power in the theta range increased temporarily before diminishing itself with resultant higher delta power. This is synonymous with a lower or decreasing alpha–delta ratio (ADR; not shown). This occurred when the patient experienced bradycardia. This would be consistent with changes that would be expected when cerebral blood flow is reduced. Of note, there appears to be higher delta power in the right hemisphere (due to a prior right hemispheric tumor resection 20 years earlier). At about 01:27, there was an overall drop in power in both hemispheres as can be seen in the FFT, aEEG, and peak envelope panels. This suggests decreased or absent blood flow to the brain, which occurred when the patient was in asystole. The patient remained asystolic for just over a minute before spontaneously reverting to sinus rhythm, at which point there is an incomplete reversal in the qEEG trends. After the event, there was overall decreased power but an increase in delta activity, which lasted more than 30 minutes without any subsequent significant improvement, consistent with diffuse infarction. Although seizures can present with decreasing or increasing frequency power over time, the overall power tends to increase; however, that is not the case here. An exception may be in a case of ictal bradycardia or asystole, which would likely present with an overall increase in power prior to fairly rapid decrease in power correlating to the decrease in cerebral blood flow, which is not seen here. In addition, disconnecting a patient from cEEG monitoring leads to an overall decrease in EEG power, although the changes due to disconnecting and reconnecting would more likely occur abruptly rather than over several minutes. In addition, the predisconnection and postdisconnection trends would likely be similar (unless that patient had a clinical event while off cEEG monitoring). Sleep transitions can cause qEEG changes (e.g., decreasing alpha power and increasing delta power), but they would not typically lead to overall suppression in power as seen here. Lowering a patient's sedation would likely lead to higher power at higher frequencies which is not seen here.

29. B. The quantitative EEG (qEEG) panels show two seizures, the first (around 20:37) from the right hemisphere and the second (around 20:47) from the left hemisphere. There is a third area of increased power (around 20:43), which is fairly lateralized to the left hemisphere. Although from the FFT, this could potentially represent an ictal discharge, the peak envelope and aEEG do not support this. In this case, there was an electrode artifact at O1, which is likely contributing to the changes seen. This supports the notion that qEEG trends help to focus where more detailed analysis is needed but they cannot replace expert review of raw EEG. Although there is increased power over both hemispheres, there is earlier onset in the hemisphere that ultimately has the higher power. The presence of higher power in the contralateral hemisphere later in time likely represents seizure spread.

30. B. A burst-suppression-like pattern is most likely seen. Note the time divisions of 2 minutes. This would correspond to an interburst interval of about 20 seconds. The times of overall low power, presenting with darker blue hues at the majority of frequencies, represent periods of relative suppression, while the vertical bars consisting of various colors in the delta to alpha frequencies represent the burst of activity consisting of mixed frequencies. Associated amplitude-integrated EEG (aEEG; not shown) would be expected to present with a bottom margin (i.e., minimum voltage) in the range typically of 0 to 2 mV as well as a low upper margin (i.e., maximum voltage), resulting in a small bandwidth (i.e., thin band) during periods of suppression and higher margins and bandwidth (i.e., thicker band) during the EEG epochs containing the bursts. The associated peak envelope trend (not shown) would be expected to present with alternating high and low peaks, resulting in a wave-like appearance with peaks and valleys. Although periodic seizures could occur as frequently as every 20 seconds, there would likely be a buildup or ramp down of power over a period of time, which is not seen here. In addition, the frequency makeup of the seizures would likely be relatively stereotyped between the ictal events. Hence, the corresponding vertical lines of green, red, and white colors would all be very similar if not the same, which is not the case here. Sleep transitions can cause quantitative EEG (qEEG) changes. In normal term infants, periods of continuous activity (i.e., wakefulness) would transition to periods of alternating activity and periods of relative suppression (i.e., tracé alternant). The pattern present in the qEEG panel would be too quick for sleep transitions and too slow for a tracé alternant or tracé discontinu pattern. HFOV artifact, if present, could produce a more continuous, high-frequency (faster than the 3–5 Hz seen in the example in the question) artifact in both hemispheres. Sedation vacation is used in the ICU to clinically assess a patient, and during these periods the overall EEG power, especially at higher frequencies, may increase. However, if this were the case here, the sedation vacation would be occurring multiple times a minute, which is unlikely.

31. C. The American Clinical Neurophysiology Society established standardized critical care EEG terminology to create an objective EEG classification scheme using descriptive terms for frequently encountered EEG patterns in critically ill patients that are not biased regarding the clinical significance of a given pattern. Standardization allows for comparison of results between centers. Main Term one has four classifications. G refers to bilateral activity that is both synchronous and symmetric. If the activity is synchronous and asymmetric, then it falls under the term L, which also includes unilateral hemispheric or focal patterns. If the activity is asynchronous, then it falls under the term BI, and the activity can be hemispheric or more focal. Mf refers to patterns occupying at least three distinct brain regions and involving both hemispheres.

32. E. The American Clinical Neurophysiology Society established standardized critical care EEG terminology to create an objective EEG classification scheme. Main Term two has three classifications. PDs apply only to single discharges with relative uniform morphology lasting less than 0.5 seconds and do not apply to bursts. There is a quantifiable interval between the discharges that have less than 50% variation from one cycle to the next. RDA is repetition of a waveform with relatively uniform morphology and duration; it can be distinguished from periodic discharges in that RDA does not have an interval between consecutive waveforms. SW consistently follows the pattern of alternating spike or sharp wave followed by a slow wave.

33. E. The American Clinical Neurophysiology Society established standardized critical care EEG terminology to create an objective EEG classification scheme. Modifiers provide further descriptive information and include frequency, amplitude, prevalence, duration, sharpness, polarity, stimulus-induced, and plus (+) modifiers. They can be added to Main Terms one and two, but the plus (+) modifiers, with the exception of sharpness, can only be used with PDs or RDA, not with SW. Amplitude refers to the absolute height of a pattern and should be measured in a standard longitudinal bipolar 10 to 20 system montage (not referential montage), from peak to trough (not to baseline). Prevalence refers to the percentage of the record occupied by a pattern and is classified as follows: less than 1% of the record/epoch (rare), 1% to 9% (occasional), 10% to 49% (frequent), 50% to 89% (abundant), and greater than 90% (continuous). Duration refers to the typical duration of a single occurrence of the pattern and is classified as follows: less than 10 seconds (very brief), 10 to 59 seconds (brief), 1 to 4.9 minutes (intermediate), 5 to 59 minutes (long), and more than 1 hour (very long). Sharpness applies only to PDs and SW and not RDA and is classified as follows: spiky (200 msec) and blunt.

34. **D.** The best classification using the American Clinical Neurophysiology Society's established standardized critical care EEG terminology is SI-GSW. The activity is bilateral, symmetric, and synchronous, consistent with the Main Term one for generalized (G). If the activity were to be asymmetric, then lateralized (L) would be the most appropriate term. If the activity were to be asynchronous, then bilateral independent (BI) would be the best term. In addition, the pattern noted consists of a regularly repeating pattern of spike wave followed by a slow wave, consistent with the Main Term two for spike wave (SW). Although initially the activity appears to be rhythmic delta activity (RDA), this is not persistent but instead quickly evolves into SW. Periodic discharges (PD) are not correct since there is no interval between consecutive waveforms. The changes appeared to occur after external stimulation, making this consistent with the modifier stimulus induced (SI). Therefore, the terminology would be SI-GSW. This would also be consistent with the former term of stimulus-induced rhythmic, periodic, or ictal discharges (SIRPIDs) that was described in critically ill patients, which lies within the ictal–interictal continuum (i.e., depending on the clinical scenario, may or may not represent an ictal pattern). In this case, the pattern lasts less than 10 seconds, was without any clinical change, and was reproducible with stimulation, making it less likely to be ictal. That being said, the definition of an ictal EEG pattern in critically ill patients still remains elusive.

35. **D.** Intermittent temporal polymorphic delta activity is least likely to be associated with SE. SE can be divided into convulsive SE (CSE) and nonconvulsive SE (NCSE) as well as generalized SE (GSE) or partial SE (PSE). PSE can be divided into simple PSE (SPSE) and complex PSE (CPSE). Recurrent 5 to 7 Hz rhythmic temporal activity and lateralized periodic discharges at 2 to 3 Hz can be seen in CPSE. Generalized periodic discharges at 2 to 3 Hz can be seen in GSE. Given that simple partial seizures can frequently present with scalp negative ictal EEG, it is feasible that SPSE could present with a normal EEG, especially if the focus is small or far from the scalp. Although continuous rhythmic delta activity may be seen in SE, particularly NCSE, intermittent polymorphic delta activity will be unlikely; the latter is typically a nonspecific finding in a variety of underlying conditions.

36. **C.** A mechanical chest percussion device can cause rhythmic 5 to 6 Hz activity in multiple (not just 1) electrodes. ECMO is associated with a 1 to 3 Hz square wave artifact. Ventilators can cause artifact that varies widely in morphology, amplitude, and polarity, but can be associated with a faster frequency artifact due to charged water molecules in the ventilator tubing that can be improved by suctioning. CPR can lead to high-amplitude, rhythmic 1 to 2 Hz activity that is due to movement, not cerebral activity. Of note, if CPR is being done, there is a high likelihood that the EKG channel will be affected as well. The difficulty in identifying artifact solely by EEG analysis can be reduced significantly by simultaneous

video monitoring. The rotation of the motor used in CRRT leads to rhythmic 5 to 12 Hz activity in multiple electrodes with a sharp or sawtooth morphology.

37. **A.** Absence (not presence) of normal sleep architecture and the presence of bilateral independent lateralized or generalized periodic (epileptiform) discharges, nonreactive background, and nonconvulsive status epilepticus are all independent predictors of poor outcome (modified Rankin Scale greater than 4) in SAH.

38. **E.** The term HFOs refers to EEG activity greater than 70 Hz (30–70 Hz band activity is usually considered as gamma). The 80 to 200 Hz activity is often referred to as ripples, whereas the 250 to 500 Hz activity is referred to as fast ripples. The sampling rate determines the recording of high frequencies. Theoretically, the maximum frequency of the oscillations that can be evaluated corresponds to one-half of the sampling rate. However, due to the limitations of the amplifiers used in the EEG systems, the maximum frequency that can be clearly evaluated tends to be roughly one-third of the sampling rate, such that a sampling rate of 1,000 Hz allows evaluation of activity up to 333 Hz. Accordingly, a sampling rate of 1,000 Hz (preferably 2,000 Hz) is recommended for recording HFOs. Although initial studies recorded HFOs using microelectrodes, more recent studies have shown that HFOs can be recorded using clinical depth and subdural electrodes.

39. **B.** In patients with epilepsy, HFOs have been recorded from mesial temporal as well as neocortical structures. Although the initial studies focused on interictal HFOs, recent studies have shown that HFOs occur at seizure onset, and such ictal HFOs can be helpful in localizing the seizure onset zone. Interictal HFOs generally tend to be prominent within the seizure focus (seizure onset zone) but they are shown to occur outside, and even at a remote distance from the seizure focus. Initial studies using microelectrodes in rodents showed that only fast ripples (250–500 Hz) were pathologic, indicating epileptogenicity; however, several recent studies suggest that ripples (80–200 Hz) are pathologic as well in patients with epilepsy.

40. D. The term DC EEG refers to a frequency response of the EEG with a minimum at 0 Hz. Although this is typically recorded using dedicated DC-coupled amplifiers, the routine alternating current (AC) amplifiers with long-time constants (e.g., 10 seconds) can adequately record the DC shifts as well. Since DC shifts are ultraslow fluctuations of the EEG signal, they are best seen by decreasing the low-frequency filter (high-pass filter) to significantly low values (e.g., 0.016 Hz). Several studies have shown that DC shifts are useful in localizing the seizure onset zone, particularly on intracranial recordings that are relatively artifact free, unlike scalp recordings.

41. **D.** MEG has better spatial resolution than EEG in localizing the cortical events. MEG is sensitive to activity within the fissural cortex. In contrast to EEG, MEG signals are sensitive to the properties of the brain but insensitive to the properties of the skull and other extracerebral tissues. The MEG signals outside the head are less distorted than the EEG signals on the scalp. The MEG recording is reference free, whereas the recording of EEG signals depends on the location of the reference electrode. MEG has selectivity to tangential (not radial) currents in the presence of several simultaneous sources.

42. **B.** In a spherical model, only currents that are tangential to the surface will produce a magnetic field that can be detected by MEG. However, in reality, signals from the

convexity may also be detected when the currents are closer to the detector. Due to the decay of magnetic fields as a function of distance, MEG is more sensitive to superficial cortical activity, which makes it useful for the study of neocortical epilepsy. Currents that are perpendicular to the cortical surface cannot be theoretically detected by MEG. However, current sources that deviate from the radial orientation by only 10 to 20 degrees can be detected. MEG can also detect current sources within the cortical fissures.

43. C. MEG cannot differentiate between ictal and interictal spikes. However, one can position an electrode array over the area of interictal MEG activity, calculate the forward solution, and monitor the ictal activity during EEG to ascertain whether the MEG interictal focus is responsible for the ictal activity as well. Due to the decay of magnetic fields as a function of distance, MEG is more sensitive to superficial cortical activity, which makes it useful for the study of neocortical epilepsy. MEG is suitable for identifying the seizure foci in the convexity and can be used to guide placement of intracranial electrodes. In presurgical evaluation, it is important to know whether the interictal epileptic discharges are focal or multifocal, and whether the foci show any time lags. MEG current dipole analysis can identify such time lags and can be useful in differentiating between the primary and secondary (mirror) foci. MEG studies in patients with Landau–Kleffner syndrome have shown that the spike-and-wave discharges are indeed generated in the auditory cortex (not motor speech area); these continuous discharges are felt to explain the speech impairment in this disorder.

44. B. A single electrical stimulus applied to the motor cortex produces multiple (not single) volleys within the descending motor tracts, giving rise to D-waves and I-waves. The first volley (called a "D-wave") reflects direct stimulation of the pyramidal axons that comprise the corticobulbar and corticospinal tracts. Subsequent volleys (called "I-waves") reflect activation of the pyramidal neurons via excitatory synaptic input from other cortical neurons that were activated either directly or indirectly by the applied stimulus. The delay from the applied stimulus to an I-wave reflects the time required for the intervening synaptic transmission and represents an integral sum of the number of cortical synaptic transmission delays. This accounts for the relatively consistent intervals between the D-wave and the first I-wave and between successive I-waves. M-waves refer to myogenic motor evoked potentials (MEPs) recorded from the muscles (not pyramidal neurons) upon cortical stimulation.

45. A. A train of multiple TES stimuli produce multiple D-waves that can summate in the lower motor neurons to cause muscle contractions that elicit the myogenic MEPs (M-waves). Such repetitive stimuli applied to the cortex may also produce I-waves, which provide further excitatory drive to the anterior horn cells. If the interstimulus interval (ISI) between the stimuli in a train is too short, stimuli after the first may not effectively stimulate the corticospinal tract axons due to their refractory periods. On the other hand, if the ISI is too long, the excitatory postsynaptic potentials within the alpha motor neurons will decay during the long intervals between successive stimuli without resulting in temporal summation. An ISI of 2 to 3 ms has been shown to be useful for intraoperative monitoring of MEPs. Even with high-intensity train of stimuli, only a small fraction of the motor neuron pool is activated each time. With each trial, a different subset of the motor neuron pool gets activated, resulting in successive M-wave recordings with differing morphology. Due to this variability, signal averaging should not be applied to M-waves. Anesthesia, especially the use of halogenated inhalational agents with or without nitrous oxide, suppresses the myogenic MEPs; however, total intravenous anesthesia with propofol and opioid infusions seems to have less influence on them.

46. **A.** The electrical stimuli for TES can be given by a pair of electrodes (anode/cathode) inserted into the scalp. The Fz/Cz electrode pair predominantly stimulates the corticospinal tracts to the legs; C3/C4 preferentially stimulates the corticospinal tracts to the arms; and C1/C2 stimulates corticospinal tracts to both upper and lower extremities. A more laterally placed electrode pair can selectively stimulate the hemisphere ipsilateral to the anode, allowing recording of motor evoked potentials (MEPs) in the muscles contralateral to the anode. Stimulation can be adjusted to clear suprathreshold responses of all targeted muscles or set to the threshold of the last recruited muscle.

47. **A.** Upon stimulation of the cerebral cortex with an anode–cathode pair, current flow under the anode results in an inward, inhibitory transmembrane current in the superficial portion of the pyramidal neurons and an outward, excitatory current at the axon hillocks that produces the MEPs (i.e., D-waves). Current flow under the cathode is in the opposite direction (toward it), caused by excitation of the superficial portion of the pyramidal neurons as well as the interneurons; this current flow results in hyperpolarization at the axon hillocks that blocks the initiation or propagation of action potentials that would give rise to D-waves. Under anesthesia, when I-waves are suppressed and the MEPs consist of D-waves, the myogenic MEPs elicited by TES are predominantly recorded from muscles contralateral to the anode.

48. **A.** MEPs elicited by TES consist of D-waves that reflect direct stimulation of the pyramidal axons, which comprise the corticobulbar and corticospinal tracts, and I-waves, which reflect activation of the pyramidal neurons by excitatory synaptic activity. With inhibition of synaptic transmission under anesthesia, I-waves are suppressed but not the D-waves. In this case, the myogenic MEPs are predominantly recorded from muscles contralateral to the anode since the inward current flow under the anode comes out of the axon hillocks and blocks the generation of D-waves under the cathode. Thus, the myogenic MEPs are generated in the contralateral muscles innervated by the corticospinal tracts ipsilateral to the anode.

49. **B.** TMS does not activate scalp pain fibers as strongly as TES, and is therefore useful for assessing central motor pathways in conscious subjects. However, TMS can also be applied to nonmotor regions in the brain convexity. TMS induces current flow in a toroidal manner through the brain tissue underneath the coil. The strongest currents are encountered closest to the inner table of the skull where they will be predominantly tangential to the cortical surface. Activation of deeper structures (e.g., brainstem) is not likely as the magnetic field strength decreases with the square of the distance. Pyramidal cell axons are most effectively stimulated by radial currents flowing perpendicular to the cortical surface. However, depending on the position and orientation of the coil, TMS may induce predominantly tangential currents, which preferentially stimulate the horizontally coursing neurites within the cortex rather than the axon hillocks of the pyramidal neurons. Thus, motor evoked potentials (MEPs) produced by TMS may consist predominantly of I-waves rather than D-waves.

50. **D.** Because TMS activates motor cortex without activating scalp pain fibers as strongly as transcranial electrical stimulation (TES), it is extremely useful for assessing central motor pathways, especially in conscious subjects. TMS often induces tangential currents depending on the orientation and position of the coil, resulting in MEPs consisting of I-waves rather than D-waves. Since the I-waves are suppressed by surgical anesthesia, MEPs elicited by TMS are not suitable for intraoperative monitoring (IOM). Any minor change in the position and orientation of the stimulating coil may produce dramatic changes in MEPs; thus, in surgeries lasting several hours, it is difficult to maintain the coil in the same exact position relative to the patient's head. The magnetic field–pulse induced by TMS can interfere with the functioning of other equipment in the operating room, necessitating extra shielding of the equipment.

51. **C.** TMS is useful for eliciting motor evoked potentials (MEPs), which are useful in the diagnosis of dysfunction involving corticospinal and corticobulbar tracts. Repetitive TMS (rTMS)–induced changes in cortical excitability outlast the stimulation, and resemble those of long-term potentiation (LTP) and long-term depression (LTD) that are induced by repetitive electrical stimulation of the cortex or hippocampus. The ability of TMS to produce such lasting and focal changes in cortical excitability forms the basis of its therapeutic effect in major depression, chronic pain, and epilepsy. TMS is not useful for intraoperative monitoring since the MEPs (i.e., I-waves) generated by it are attenuated by anesthesia.

52. **E.** rTMS has been shown to alter mood in nondepressed subjects, have a greater impact on mood in depressed patients (although generally in a positive direction), induce mania or a hypomanic state in some subjects, and improve or worsen neuropsychological function with no consistent overall changes.

53. **A.** SEEG allows placement of depth electrodes stereotactically, often assisted by a robot, into intracerebral structures that are not easily accessible for recording using subdural electrodes. Examples of such structures include amygdala, hippocampus, insula, and cingulate gyrus. One disadvantage of SEEG is undersampling unless multiple electrodes are placed into the same structure. Also, functional cortical mapping with SEEG electrodes can be difficult to interpret. The larger spatial separation between the SEEG electrodes may allow confirmation that the area implanted by the electrode is eloquent, but does not allow determination of the boundaries of the eloquent area. Given these considerations, exclusive SEEG evaluation of the left posterior temporal lobe, which is adjacent to the Wernicke's area, is least likely to be helpful among the options provided; instead, a subdural evaluation or an SEEG combined with subdural evaluation would be more helpful.

54. **B.** Determination of the vascular anatomy of the brain is an important consideration in planning an SEEG implantation strategy to ensure safe trajectory of the electrodes to the intended targets. Although this was accomplished with catheter angiography in the past, most centers now use MR angiography for that purpose. Accurate localization of seizure onset by scalp video-EEG is not necessary because inconclusive localization is one of the main indications for SEEG. Adherence to electrode nomenclature based on the targeted structure is preferred by some, while others use alphabet letters to designate the electrodes. Symmetrical implantation of electrodes in both hemispheres may be needed to determine seizure lateralization (e.g., in bitemporal nonlateralized seizure onsets), but not necessary in all cases.

55. A. The goal of SEEG is to provide a three-dimensional view of the epileptic network, which means mapping not only the origin of seizures, but also the propagation pathways. In a case of left anterior temporal cavernoma, the preimplant hypothesis would include the left temporal and frontal regions. Although the Wernicke's area is located in the posterior aspect of the temporal lobe, sampling of this structure can be avoided, if necessary, as the epileptic network is most likely to involve the anterior temporal and frontal areas.

56. E. EZ is the presumed area of the brain, removal of which is necessary and sufficient to achieve seizure freedom. It is most commonly defined by the region of the brain that is primarily involved in generating the seizures. In an SEEG evaluation, the EZ is characterized by the presence of rhythmic faster frequency waveforms, repetitive spikes, high-amplitude slow waves with superimposed faster frequency waveforms, or rhythmic synchronous waveforms in multiple electrodes that occur with or without a minor time lag between the electrodes.

57. A. In a review of SEEG methodology across multiple centers in Europe and North America, it was found that the SEEG was a safe procedure with low morbidity and mortality. Four deaths were reported after SEEG: three associated with large intracranial hemorrhages and one with severe hyponatremia in a 3-year-old child. Other complications included nonfatal intracranial hemorrhages, intracranial infections, broken electrodes, hydrocephalus, status epilepticus, internal carotid artery dissection, and neurologic deficits. Overall, 35 major complications (including four deaths) were reported in approximately 4,000 patients implanted with approximately 33,000 electrodes, with a rate of 0.8%.

58. C. The ECoG epoch from the RNS device shows a focal seizure detected by the device (marker "B1") around 10 seconds. The device delivers consecutive stimulations, but fails to terminate the seizure. The persistent ictal pattern is redetected in the left temporal contacts around 21 seconds ("B1") and subsequently in the right temporal contacts ("B2"). The RNS device only provides data regarding the presence or absence of electrical activity indicative of seizures, and therefore, it is not possible to conclude about the clinical manifestations (e.g., impairment of awareness).

59. D. The ECoG epoch from the RNS device shows a focal seizure predominantly in the left insula with some involvement of the left temporoparietal region. The device delivers consecutive stimulations, but fails to terminate the seizure. It is possible that the seizure originated outside the insula, for example, in the left temporal or frontal lobes, and then spread to the insula. Therefore, features of insular seizures (e.g., choking sensation), temporal lobe seizures (e.g., impaired awareness and lip smacking), or frontal lobe seizures (e.g., facial twitching) can be expected as part of the seizure semiology. It is unlikely that the seizure originated in the left occipital lobe as the temporoparietal contacts are only minimally involved in the seizure; therefore, elementary visual hallucinations (e.g., light flashes), which suggest occipital lobe seizures, are least likely to be seen as part of the patient's seizure semiology.

60. C. The figure shows seizure onset in the right anterior hippocampus (lower-numbered contacts of the anterior hippocampal electrode) with subsequent spread to the right amygdala and temporal pole followed by the insula and orbitofrontal regions. Based on this onset and propagation, one can expect lip smacking, right hand automatisms (e.g., fumbling), and left hand RINCH (rhythmic ictal nonclonic hand motions, e.g., repetitive left hand opening and closing) as part of his semiology. Left facial twitching, left hand clonic movements, and left head version suggest right frontal onset, which is not seen (higher-numbered contacts of the orbitofrontal electrodes are not involved). Loss of vision in the left visual field, throat spasm, and loss of awareness suggest right occipital onset (which cannot be inferred from the given data) with spread to insula. Bicycling movements, agitation, and screaming for help suggest medial frontal onset, which is not the case here. Staring, right hand dystonic posturing, and throat spasm suggest left temporal onset, as dystonic posturing is usually contralateral, which cannot be inferred from the given data.

61. **D.** In an SEEG recording, the lesional zone is characterized by continuous slow activity; the irritative zone is characterized by waveforms with variable and complex morphology; and the epileptogenic zone is characterized by rhythmic waveforms of similar frequency, repetitive spikes, or high-amplitude slow waves with superimposed faster frequencies. In periventricular nodular heterotopia, both the lesions and the overlying cortex are known to be epileptogenic. As such, the electrodes located in the heterotopic lesions can be expected to show the characteristics of lesional, irritative, and epileptogenic zones. In the figure, electrode A shows normal waveforms; electrodes B and C show near-continuous or intermittent slowing; electrode D shows spikes with varying and complex morphology; and electrode E shows low voltage, slow activity. Thus, it is reasonable to conclude that the electrodes B, C, D, and E are most likely to be located within or in close proximity to the heterotopic lesions, whereas electrode A is located within normal tissue.

62. **D.** In patient D, it is important to determine not only the boundaries of the seizure onset zone but also its relationship with the motor strip given the location of the cavernoma. Functional cortical stimulation and mapping is best accomplished with subdural grids rather than SEEG as the latter requires multiple trajectories through eloquent cortex, increasing the risk of hemorrhagic complications. In patient A, SEEG would be preferred because the seizure onset is nonlateralized and diffuse; although bilateral subdural strips can be considered, it will not provide easy access to the medial frontal regions and deeper structures such as the cingulate gyrus. In patient B, SEEG would be preferred as it is important to sample the heterotopic lesions on both sides as well as the left hippocampus. In patient C, it is possible that the seizures arise from the bottom of the sulci or the orbitofrontal cortex, which can be best accessed with SEEG electrodes. In patient E, it would be ideal to pursue a subdural evaluation, which allows mapping of the Wernicke's area; however, given the history of prior resection and the possibility of dural adhesions, implantation of a large subdural grid may pose risks, making SEEG the preferred initial choice.

8

Ethics and Safety

QUESTIONS

1. Which of the following is an absolute contraindication to proximal stimulation with nerve conduction studies?
   A. Regular on-demand pacemaker
   B. External pacer wires
   C. Increased bleeding tendency
   D. Mechanically ventilated patient
   E. All of the above

2. Needle electromyography (EMG) of which of the following muscles is least likely to result in pneumothorax?
   A. Diaphragm
   B. Serratus anterior
   C. Rhomboids
   D. Teres minor
   E. Supraspinatus

3. Potential safety concerns with transcranial magnetic stimulation (TMS) can include all of the following *except:*
   A. Seizures
   B. Transient headache
   C. Hearing loss
   D. Malfunctioning of vagus nerve stimulator
   E. Malfunctioning of implanted cochlear prostheses

ANSWERS TO THIS SECTION CAN BE FOUND ON PAGE 402

The figures in this chapter can be viewed in a larger size by accessing the digital version of this chapter found on Springer Publishing Company Connect™. Refer to the front of this book for access instructions.

4. Which of the following situations the needle electromyography (EMG) should not be performed after nerve conduction studies are completed?
   A. If motor nerve conduction studies are normal
   B. If the patient does not have insurance
   C. If the patient requests that needle EMG not be performed
   D. If the patient is on anticoagulation medication and his international normalized ratio (INR) is greater than 1.5
   E. If the results will not change clinical outcome but may help with prognosis

5. A 55-year-old man is referred to the electrodiagnostic lab to find a neuromuscular cause for increasing shortness of breath. His routine nerve conduction study is normal. Needle electromyography (EMG) of the proximal and distal muscles, as well as the thoracic paraspinal muscles, is also normal. The patient requests you to perform a diaphragmatic EMG even though you are not trained in diaphragmatic EMG. The patient really would like to have the study performed right away as he does not want to come back on another day for the study. The best action is:
   A. Perform the study as this is convenient for the patient
   B. Request a colleague who is experienced in diaphragmatic EMG to perform the study
   C. Use an ultrasound machine to guide you with needle EMG even though you have not used the ultrasound machine before
   D. Perform phrenic motor studies and explain to the patient that this will provide as much information as needle EMG of the diaphragm muscle
   E. Tell the patient that you have run out of the special diaphragmatic needles

6. Hyperventilation (HV) during an EEG is considered safe in which of the following situations?
   A. In a patient with 2-day-old subdural hematoma
   B. In a patient with congestive heart failure and mild pulmonary edema
   C. In a patient with sickle cell anemia
   D. In a patient with moyamoya disease
   E. In a diabetic patient prone to hypoglycemic episodes

7. To ensure patient safety, which of the following measures should be followed?
   A. The ground electrode should always be placed on the patient's feet if possible
   B. The ground electrode should be connected to the earth ground
   C. The recording device plugged into the wall jack should have a second, direct earth ground connection
   D. The patient should not be connected to multiple recording devices simultaneously because of the risk of forming ground loops
   E. All of the above

8. Which of the following statements is true about electrical shock?
   A. A current of 100 mA or higher applied to the skin can cause ventricular fibrillation in a patient
   B. A current of 10 μA applied directly to the heart can cause ventricular fibrillation in a patient
   C. Using three-hole electrical receptacles eliminates risk of electrical shock to the patient
   D. Human susceptibility to electrical shock is maximal at 70 Hz
   E. Indwelling catheters do not pose additional risk for electrical shock

9. While performing needle electromyography (EMG) studies, which of the following measures can potentially cause serious injury to the examiner?
   A. Unwrapping a covered needle
   B. Recapping the needle after studying the first muscle
   C. Attaching a sheathed needle to cable
   D. Performing laryngeal EMG
   E. Performing a one-handed technique for needle recapping

10. As part of nocturnal polysomnogram, a three-channel EEG and a two-channel electromyography (EMG) are recorded. The appropriate way to bill for this procedure is:
    A. Bill for the polysomnogram, the routine EEG, and the surface EMG
    B. Bill for the polysomnogram and the routine EEG
    C. Bill for the polysomnogram and the surface EMG
    D. Bill for the polysomnogram only regardless of the number of additional parameters
    E. Bill for the polysomnogram with the appropriate number of additional parameters

11. A 42-year-old woman underwent right anterior temporal lobectomy 6 months ago, and has remained seizure-free since the surgery on lamotrigine monotherapy. She wants to drive as she satisfies the local law of 6 months of seizure freedom to be able to drive. Her neurologic examination is normal. An EEG shows rare right temporal sharp waves. The most appropriate recommendation would be to:
    A. Continue the driving restriction and repeat another routine EEG in 6 months
    B. Remove the driving restriction if she continues to take lamotrigine as prescribed
    C. Obtain inpatient video-EEG monitoring for 3 days while on lamotrigine to see if seizures occur spontaneously
    D. Obtain inpatient video-EEG monitoring after stopping lamotrigine to see if seizures can be induced
    E. Taper lamotrigine and immediately allow her to drive

12. A 55-year-old patient with extensive cardiac history has been in the ICU for more than 6 weeks because of multiple infections, sepsis, and severe heart failure. He also has an external cardiac pacemaker. The intensive care team has noticed that within the last few weeks he was not able to move his limbs and is concerned about a critical illness disease. An electrodiagnostic study is requested. Just before starting the study, the external pacemaker wires are noted. Which of the following options is the best course to take?
    A. Perform nerve conduction studies in the lower limbs only
    B. Perform nerve conduction studies in the upper limbs only
    C. Perform needle electromyography (EMG) only
    D. Perform repetitive stimulation of the ulnar nerve only
    E. Do not perform any part of the electrodiagnostic study due to safety concerns

13. The leakage current from a medical instrument should be:
    A. Less than 1 μA
    B. Less than 10 μA
    C. Less than 100 μA
    D. Less than 1 mA
    E. Less than 10 mA

14. A 40-year-old man presents with a history of two generalized convulsions over a period of 3 days after sustaining a closed head injury. Since then, he has remained seizure-free for 2 years on phenytoin monotherapy, and wants to discontinue the medication. His neurologic examination is normal. An appropriate recommendation would be to:
A. Obtain a routine EEG prior to stopping phenytoin
B. Stop phenytoin in the epilepsy-monitoring unit and obtain video-EEG monitoring for 1 week
C. Taper off phenytoin without obtaining an EEG
D. Change phenytoin to levetiracetam as it is better tolerated
E. Continue lifelong anti-seizure medication given the history of two seizures soon after a head injury

15. Which of the following is NOT considered to be a significant safety issue with transcranial electrical stimulation (TES)?
A. Malfunctioning of deep brain stimulator
B. Brain tissue heating
C. Excitotoxicity in brain tissue
D. Forceful jaw closure
E. Scalp burns

16. A 55-year-old man is referred to the electrodiagnostic lab for evaluation of large fiber polyneuropathy by his primary care physician. However, based on the history and examination, you suspect there is an underlying diffuse neurogenic process. Nerve conduction study reveals decreased motor amplitudes with normal sensory responses. Needle electromyography (EMG) revealed diffuse active denervation in multiple myotomes. Based on this, you suspect that the patient has a form of motor neuron disease. Which of the following is the most appropriate next step?
A. Tell the patient that he has amyotrophic lateral sclerosis (ALS)
B. Mention ALS in the report, but tell the patient that he has nerve damage
C. Call the referring physician to explain your findings and concerns for motor neuron disease
D. Refer the patient to the local ALS clinic
E. Schedule the patient as a new consult as soon as possible in your own clinic to discuss the testing results and for a more in-depth history and physical examination

17. Which of the following statements is true about the three-hole electrical receptacle encountered in North America?
A. The short slot is "neutral "
B. The long slot is "hot"
C. The D-shaped slot is the "true ground"
D. The three wires together constitute the "true ground"
E. Black wire is hot; white wire is neutral; green wire is ground

18. Which of the following recommendations is considered safe when needle electromyography (EMG) is required in patients on anticoagulation?
   A. It is safe to test superficial muscles only
   B. It is safe to test deep muscles, as bleeding is unlikely in deep muscles
   C. The gauge of the needle is not typically a consideration
   D. It is safe to test the paraspinal muscles, as they are superficial
   E. It is safe to test the gluteal muscle, as the risk for nerve compression is low if a hematoma develops

19. A ground loop occurs when:
   A. An extremely long EEG ground wire is spiraled multiple times
   B. A broken electrical receptacle causes connection between the "neutral" and "ground" wires
   C. Two grounds are connected, causing accidental current flow that often moves through the patient
   D. The electric bed and the EEG machine are connected to the same cluster of electrical receptacles on the wall
   E. The EEG ground and reference electrodes are shorted with a salt bridge

20. During a routine 30-minute EEG in the neurodiagnostic lab, the technologist records video to show the occasional leg movements that the patient exhibited. The neurologist should code this as:
   A. A routine EEG
   B. A routine EEG plus modified video recording
   C. Video-EEG monitoring
   D. Video-EEG monitoring with a modifier for reduced service
   E. Any of the above as they are all appropriate

21. A 33-year-old woman is being seen for a 1-month history of spells consisting of fall, impaired responsiveness, and shaking. Each spell lasts 2 to 3 minutes, and they occur multiple times daily. Prior routine EEG was normal. She is currently on carbamazepine. The most appropriate next step would be to:
   A. Repeat another routine EEG
   B. Stop carbamazepine
   C. Obtain inpatient video-EEG monitoring
   D. Add levetiracetam
   E. Refer to psychology

22. Which of the follow statements is true about neurophysiologic intraoperative monitoring (NIOM)?
   A. Abiding by monitoring practice standards prohibits lawsuits from occurring
   B. When done correctly, monitoring has been shown to not only reduce the incidence of but also eliminate all neurological injury
   C. Proper monitoring requires either a well-trained technologist or remote physician reader
   D. Communication with the surgeon regarding the monitoring is only necessary if there is a possibility of neurological injury
   E. The monitoring flow sheet maintained during the case should include summarizing the status of the peaks and all comments to the surgeons

23. A 22-year-old patient has new-onset generalized convulsions and presents to the emergency department (ED). She has a history of dropping things, especially in the morning. While the EEG technologist is running a routine EEG study, she sees the epoch shown below, and texts you a picture of it. She asks you, the reading physician, to see if activation procedures, such as hyperventilation or photic stimulation, are needed. What is the most appropriate answer?

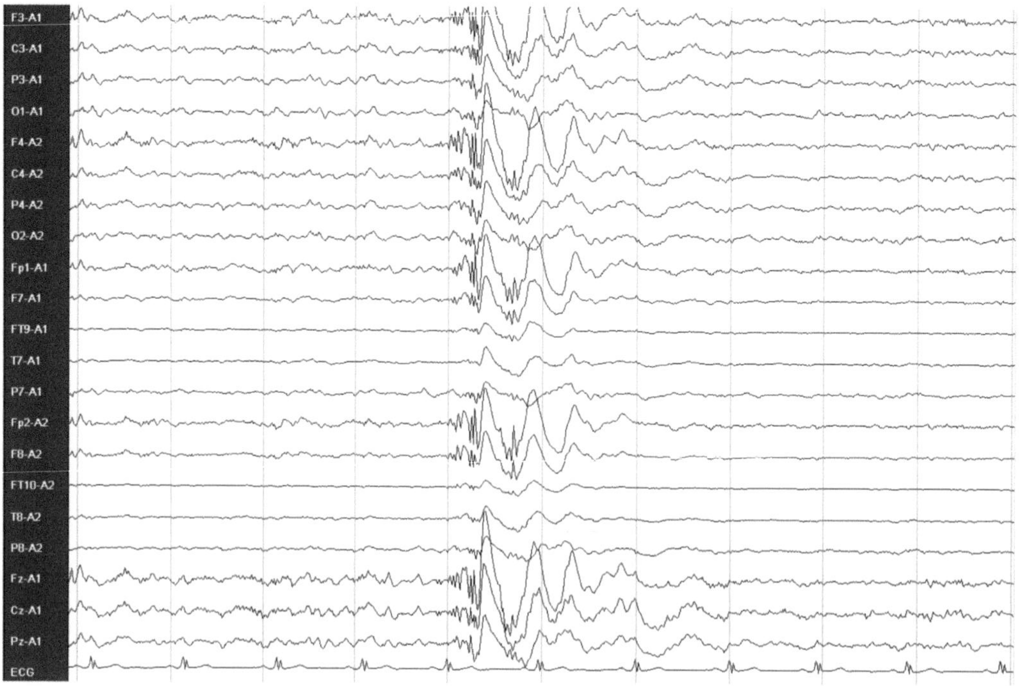

A. Activation procedures should be done on all patients
B. Ask the patient what they would prefer
C. It depends on how many minutes of EEG recording have already passed
D. Hyperventilation can be canceled, but photic stimulation should be done
E. No activation procedures are needed

24. On Saturday night at 11 p.m., a patient on continuous EEG (cEEG) monitoring in the ICU goes into nonconvulsive status epilepticus. The EEG-monitoring technologist is currently monitoring six patients and is getting concerned about his ability to safely monitor all the patients. He calls you, the interpreting physician, for advice. Which of the following measures would be the most appropriate immediate next step to safely monitor the patients?
A. Call in on-call technologist from home for backup help
B. Open up quantitative EEG (qEEG) panels
C. Call hospital administration to approve another EEG tech job
D. Transfer some of the patients to a different hospital that provides monitoring service
E. Let the least acute patients go unmonitored

25. A 67-year-old was admitted after cardiopulmonary resuscitation in the field. He is undergoing therapeutic hypothermia during which the EEG is "flat." Per the ICU team, no brainstem reflexes were noted on examination and the head CT showed evidence of hypoxic-ischemic injury. The ICU team was concerned and wanted to convey to the family that the patient was brain dead. As the EEG reader, what is the most appropriate clinical correlation to provide to the ICU team?

A. Agree that the patient is brain dead and that the EEG supports it
B. Agree that the patient is brain dead, but that the EEG cannot support it
C. Disagree, but state that there is severe irreversible brain dysfunction
D. Disagree, and state that there are therapies being done that could be contributing to the EEG findings
E. Refer the ICU team to the hospital ethics board

26. A 27-year-old woman with intractable epilepsy presents to the emergency department (ED) for terminated status epilepticus. Her head CT shows right temporal pole encephalomalacia. Her routine EEG shows left temporal intermittent rhythmic delta activity and frequent right anterior temporal spikes. Collateral information is obtained from her parents that the patient has had epilepsy for 11 years starting after a bike accident. She has failed at least six anti-seizure medications. Today, her parents witnessed her to have motionless staring, right hand posturing, and quick head and eye movement to the right before crying out and jerking. They said that her seizures have presented this way at least for the past year. She was worked up 2 years ago for surgical resection, but the patient lost insurance and could not get the planned right anterior mesial temporal lobectomy. She now has insurance and is scheduled for resection next month. The parents ask for your advice. What is the most appropriate response?

A. Support their decision to proceed with the surgery as the workup has already been done
B. Support their decision to proceed with the surgery as the epileptiform abnormalities on EEG are in the region of proposed resection
C. Politely tell them that you do not have enough information to provide any advice
D. Cancel the surgery, as the patient just had status epilepticus
E. Cancel the surgery and repeat the workup due to discordant information

ANSWERS

1. **B.** Patients with external pacemaker wires should not have nerve conduction studies with proximal stimulation because of the risk of electrical injury. A regular internalized pacemaker, increased bleeding tendency, and mechanical ventilation are not absolute contraindications for nerve conduction studies.

2. **D.** Needle EMG of the diaphragm is most likely to lead to pneumothorax. However, needle EMG of the other muscles except for teres minor can also lead to pneumothorax; therefore, the examiner should be cautious. Serratus anterior, rhomboids, and the supraspinatus are all periscapular or chest wall muscles; if anatomical guidelines are not followed carefully, needle EMG of these muscles may result in pneumothorax.

3. **D.** Energy delivery to brain tissue and tissue heating seem to be negligible with TMS. Seizures have occurred with TMS, although they are more common after repetitive TMS (rTMS); seizures have occurred in patients with and without a history of epilepsy. Transient headache has been reported with rTMS. TMS can affect implanted cochlear prostheses and deep brain stimulators, but not the extracranial stimulators such as a vagus nerve stimulator. The high-intensity and rapidly varying magnetic field associated with rTMS can cause transient deformations of the stimulating coil, producing an audible click; this can lead to transient increases in the hearing threshold and permanent hearing loss if no ear protection is used. High magnetic fields (~2T) can be produced during TMS, resulting in displacement of nearby metallic objects; however, forces on small objects such as aneurysm clips and titanium skull plates and screws are too small to be of clinical concern.

4. **C.** Electrodiagnostic testing should always stop if the patient requests that no further testing be done. Normal motor nerve conduction studies are seen in many neuromuscular studies, so not performing needle EMG based on this is incorrect. One should always attempt to complete the study to find the underlying cause of the patient's presentation, and not decide on the testing protocol purely based on the insurance status. INR greater than 1.5 is not an absolute contraindication and needle EMG can be performed in selected muscles without complications. Even if neurodiagnostic testing does not lead to a change in clinical outcome, it may help to further define prognosis, which may help define future expectations. Thus, it would still be appropriate to perform needle EMG.

5. **B.** If a physician is not very well trained in a particular procedure, especially one that can lead to complications such as pneumothorax, it is not appropriate to perform the study. The best response is to request a colleague with more experience to perform the study. One must be trained to even use an ultrasound machine. Phrenic nerve conduction study could potentially reveal decreased compound muscle action potential (CMAP) amplitudes, but this study does not replace needle EMG of the diaphragm. As a general rule of thumb, one should never lie to patients. Being forthcoming and explaining the situation and potential risks of having an inexperienced person performing the procedure will likely lead to a change in the patient's request.

6. **E.** HV-induced slowing may become more prominent during hypoglycemia (blood glucose less than 80 mg/dL) but a predisposition to hypoglycemia is not a contraindication to performing HV. However, HV is contraindicated in patients with recent intracranial hemorrhage, significant cardiopulmonary disease, large vessel stenosis, moyamoya disease, and sickle cell disease or trait. A patient's inability or unwillingness to cooperate with the procedure is a relative contraindication.

7. **C.** The ground electrode is commonly placed on the patient's head and it does not present a safety issue. When an electrical device is plugged into the wall jack, the current flows from the "hot" wire of the power line to the "neutral" wire at earth ground. If patients are also connected to the earth ground, any stray currents could flow through them. In modern devices, a third wire, which represents a second, more direct earth ground connection, is required. This additional ground increases safety in some situations but can constitute a risk if the patient is also connected to it. Therefore, modern safety standards require that the recording ground on the patient cannot form a direct connection to the power line ground. Ground loops may be formed when the patient is connected to more than one ground electrode through multiple medical devices. Theoretically, currents flowing through the power line ground could place the different components of the system at somewhat different voltages, in which case the voltages would attempt to equalize through the patient's body. However, with the requirement that the recording ground on the patient must never be connected to earth ground, it is rare that ground loops present a safety risk in modern systems. The disadvantage is that the ground loops may contribute substantially to electrical noise.

8. **A.** A current of 100 mA or higher applied to the skin can cause ventricular fibrillation in humans. By comparison, a current of 180 μA applied directly to the heart can cause ventricular fibrillation. Using a three-hole electrical receptacle does not completely eliminate the risk of electrical shock because powerline faults can cause excess leakage current to flow through the patient. Human susceptibility to electrical shock is maximal at 60 Hz, which is the same as the powerline frequency. Indwelling catheters pose a risk for electrical shock as they can provide direct paths to the heart for the passage of current.

9. **B.** Recapping the needle can be potentially dangerous, and can cause needle stick injury to the examiner. If it is necessary, performing a one-handed technique for needle recapping will reduce the chance for injury. Unwrapping or attaching a sheathed needle to cable is relatively safe. Performing laryngeal EMG might be technically difficult and can lead to potential complications, but it is not considered high risk for the performing physician.

10. **E.** Current procedural terminology (CPT) guidelines indicate that the parameters measured as part of a nocturnal polysomnogram include a three-lead EEG, submental EMG, and electrooculogram (EOG). Additional parameters that are typically required include ECG, airflow, respiratory effort, oxygen saturation, and leg movements. Depending upon the number of additional parameters monitored, only polysomnography should be billed using codes 95808 (polysomnography with one to three additional parameters) or 95810 (polysomnography with four or more additional parameters); neither EEG nor EMG component should be billed separately.

11. **B.** Persistent interictal epileptiform discharges can be seen after surgical resection. This finding does not carry any more risk than such a finding in a nonsurgical patient. As the patient satisfies the local driving laws, it would be appropriate to remove the driving restriction, particularly if she is willing to take the existing medication as prescribed. Inpatient video-EEG monitoring, with or without medication withdrawal, will not be necessary to make a decision regarding driving. It is not appropriate to allow someone to drive while tapering seizure medications.

12. **C.** It is safe to perform needle EMG even in patients with external cardiac pacemaker defibrillator wires since no electrical current is applied. Any kind of nerve conduction study is not recommended in patients with external cardiac pacemaker or defibrillator wires.

13. **C.** As established by the Underwriters Laboratories in the United States, the chassis leakage current for medical instruments should be less than 100 μA, although less than 10 μA is the goal.

14. **A.** Because the seizures occurred within 1 week of head trauma, it would be reasonable to consider tapering off antiepileptic medication therapy. Two years of seizure freedom and normal neurologic examination favor seizure remission with discontinuation of antiepileptic medication. A normal routine EEG would further support the possibility of seizure remission. Changing phenytoin to levetiracetam would be appropriate if a decision is made to continue antiepileptic therapy for any reason.

15. **B.** TES can affect implanted cochlear prostheses and deep brain stimulators and is contraindicated in patients with these devices. TES can cause scalp burns due to edge effects at the border of the electrodes. However, energy delivery to brain tissue and tissue heating are negligible. TES can cause neuronal damage due to excitotoxicity, although the total charge and total charge density produced in the brain are less than those produced by direct cortical stimulation and by electroconvulsive therapy. Seizures have also been produced by TES. TES can deliver high current levels to the scalp, causing strong contractions of the temporalis muscle and forceful jaw closure. This can result in mouth injury, tongue or lip lacerations, and even mandibular fracture.

16. **C.** The best response is to call the referring doctor and explain the findings and diagnosis. Mentioning the diagnosis of motor neuron disease in the report might not be enough because the diagnosis would be unexpected for the referring physician, and could delay care to the patient. It is inappropriate to tell the patient that he has ALS or refer him to an ALS clinic without discussing the findings first with the referring doctor, evaluating other tests, and thoroughly examining the patient. It is also inappropriate to self-refer a patient sent to you for a test to see you in clinic.

17. E. The three-hole electrical receptacle consists of a short slot (black wire, "hot"), a long slot (white wire, "neutral"), and a D-shaped slot (green wire, "ground"). The green wire (of the D-shaped slot) is not the "true" ground; it provides a path to the "true" ground; in other words, at some distance from the patient room, the white and green wires are bonded to a "true" ground that provides a low-resistance connection to the earth.

18. A. It is relatively safe to do EMG of the superficial muscles. Deep muscles are just as likely to develop hematomas as superficial muscles, but these sites cannot be manually compressed. The smallest gauge needle should always be used. EMG of paraspinal and gluteal muscles should be avoided because the risk of nerve compression (spinal or sciatic nerves, respectively) is higher if a hematoma develops. Ideally, EMG should be performed after the anticoagulation is stopped or reversed, but the risks of stopping anticoagulation should be discussed with the patient and the referring physician before this step is undertaken.

19. C. A ground loop occurs when there is a galvanic connection between two different grounds such that a current accidentally introduced into one ground completes the circuit by flowing through the other ground. Often, the circuit between the two grounds at different potentials is carried by the patient. The "neutral" and "ground" wires from an electrical receptacle are combined together away from the patient's room and eventually connected to the earth ground. To avoid ground loops, it is important to connect all medical instruments to the same cluster of power receptacles with a common power source.

20. A. This should be coded as a routine EEG only. The video recording is for clinical correlation purposes, and there is no separate code for the video. Video-EEG monitoring codes are reserved for procedures when simultaneous video and EEG are recorded to evaluate well-defined clinical questions, and they are not appropriate in the noted context.

21. C. From the description, it appears that nonepileptic seizures are a strong possibility. Prior routine EEG was normal and the patient is currently being treated with an antiepileptic medication. Yield of another routine EEG would be low. At this time, it is important to establish a definitive diagnosis; therefore, inpatient video-EEG monitoring would be appropriate. Without a definitive diagnosis, the benefit of adding another antiepileptic medication remains doubtful. Also without a definitive diagnosis of psychogenic, nonepileptic spells, referral to psychology would be inappropriate.

22. E. Documentation is central for billing as well as protection in any potential lawsuits and should include the patient's name, time of the tracings, and a flow sheet summarizing the status of the peaks and all the comments to the surgeon. Lawsuits can occur even if monitoring practice standards are followed. Monitoring has been shown to reduce the incidence of, but not eliminate, neurological injury. Therefore, in general, it is more valuable to have high sensitivity than specificity in NIOM. This requires well-trained staff, including the technologist in the operating room as well as the physician reader, who may be remote. Communication with the surgeon is necessary when there is a possibility of neurological injury, if the waveforms are poor quality and cannot be trusted, and even if the waveforms are not changing.

23. **E.** The EEG shows fast, generalized polyspike and wave discharges in the setting of a relatively normal background. This, along with the young-adult age of onset and clinical semiology of likely myoclonic jerks and generalized convulsions, suggests that the patient has a primary generalized epilepsy syndrome, such as juvenile myoclonic epilepsy (JME). Activation procedures are used to bring out epileptiform abnormalities, which are already seen in this study. If there are contraindications or if the patient is unable to tolerate the procedures, then activations procedures should be not be done. In certain syndromes, such as JME, activation procedures, especially photic stimulation, may lead to photoparoxysmal responses and clinical seizures. Triggering such an event should not be the goal of a routine EEG study done in the ED. If triggering a seizure is desired, then doing so in a more controlled, safe environment, such as an epilepsy-monitoring unit, should be considered.

24. **B.** Suggesting to use qEEG panels would provide the most immediate relief to monitor the patients. qEEG panels can help to observe trends and help to identify recent events that may have been missed while the EEG technologists eyes are off the patient. Although the monitored patients could be prioritized in terms of their acuity, it is not advisable to leave any patient unmonitored. The remaining answer choices, although each could be done, would not provide the most immediate help on a weekend night. It may take the on-call technologist up to 2 hours to provide assistance. Getting approval from hospital administration for increased staffing would not provide immediate help. Transferring patients out of the hospital does not bring immediate relief, and monitored patients may be too unstable for transfer.

25. **D.** Brain death is a clinical decision, but sometimes ancillary tests, such as EEG, are needed to assist in making the diagnosis. The patient in question is currently undergoing therapeutic hypothermia, which has been shown to lead to a low voltage EEG. Until, this therapy is completed (which typically also involves administering anesthetic sedation and paralytics), no conclusion about brain death or the reversibility of cerebral dysfunction should be made. As the EEG reader without having examined the patient, it is not advisable to make conclusions about the clinical exam or brain death. There is no reason for the hospital ethics board to get involved at this time.

26. **E.** The patient in question has evidence supportive of right temporal seizures, including an abnormal head CT and epileptiform discharges in the same region. The prior workup may have supported having a right anterior mesial temporal lobectomy. However, 2 years have passed and the patient's epilepsy may have evolved. The patient's semiology that brought her to the ED is suggestive of left hemispheric ictal onset with left temporal lobe involvement. In addition, the presence of left temporal intermittent rhythmic delta activity also is suggestive of localized cerebral dysfunction with increased risk for left temporal seizures. Thus, the most appropriate response is to cancel the surgery and repeat the workup.

9

Pearls for Passing

This chapter is a compilation of key facts to review for each section of the book and to serve as a quick refresher prior to an examination. Please keep in mind that reviewing these facts does not replace the time and effort needed to comprehend the larger concepts or principles they intend to summarize.

Nerve Conduction Studies and Electromyography

1. The rate of axonal regrowth is generally less than 1 mm/day.
2. Unmyelinated fibers predominantly convey autonomic, temperature, and pain modalities. These fibers have a very slow conduction velocity of 1 to 2 m/sec.
3. Conduction velocity of a nerve fiber is directly proportional to its diameter.
4. In motor and sensory nerve conduction studies, latency and nerve conduction velocity represent the fastest conducting fibers only. Amplitude and area reflect all the nerve fibers, whereas duration is a reflection of the synchrony of all the nerve fibers.
5. Small myelinated and unmyelinated fibers cannot be tested with routine nerve conduction studies; for this reason, routine conduction studies tend to be normal in patients with only small fiber neuropathy.
6. Motor unit action potentials (MUAPs), sensory nerve action potentials (SNAPs), and compound muscle action potentials (CMAPs) are all volume-conducted near-field potentials.
7. Stimulus artifact seen during nerve conduction studies is a far-field potential. Most evoked potentials are far-field potentials.
8. With appropriate placement of electrodes, the very first deflection from baseline is negative in CMAP recordings. In SNAPs, the very first deflection may be positive with triphasic morphology.

9. Stimulation should always be supramaximal while performing routine motor and sensory nerve conduction studies. During H-reflex testing, submaximal stimulation is used.

10. In sensory nerve conduction studies, both onset and peak latencies may be used. Onset latency is a reflection of the fastest conducting fibers. However, peak latency may be easier to identify in small amplitude responses or when there is significant background noise or stimulus artifact.

11. Antidromic SNAP amplitude is usually larger than orthrodromic SNAP amplitude.

12. SNAPs are normal in patients with radiculopathy, as the lesion is proximal to dorsal root ganglia. SNAPs are also normal in patients with spinal cord lesions. In contrast, motor nerve conduction studies may be abnormal in both radiculopathy and in spinal cord lesions.

13. Mixed nerve conduction velocities are faster than routine motor or sensory nerve conduction velocities as these include Ia fibers.

14. Reduced motor or sensory amplitude is the primary abnormality seen with axonal lesions. Mild slowing of conduction velocity or prolongation of latency may also be seen with primary axonal lesions.

15. Conduction block and abnormal temporal dispersion (not at the compressive site) are features of acquired demyelinating disorders.

16. Decreased motor amplitudes may be seen with myopathy, neuromuscular junction (NMJ) disorders (e.g., Lambert–Eaton myasthenic syndrome [LEMS]), neuropathies, radiculopathies, and motor neuronopathies.

17. In F-response testing, the afferent and efferent signals pass through the motor fibers only. However, in H-reflex testing, afferent signals go through Ia muscle spindle fibers and efferent signals go through the motor fibers.

18. Axon reflex is a late potential that typically occurs between the F and M responses. The latency and amplitude of an axon reflex remain identical and this response usually indicates reinnervation.

19. In blink reflex testing, afferent impulse is transmitted by the fifth cranial nerve, whereas the efferent impulse is transmitted by the seventh cranial nerve. Blink reflex is a polysynaptic reflex.

20. In blink reflex testing, ipsilateral R1 and R2 are seen along with a contralateral R2 response.

21. CMAP decrement is diminished in patients with NMJ disorders if the limb temperature is decreased.

22. The two common anomalous innervations are Martin–Gruber anastomosis in the upper limb and accessory peroneal nerve in the lower limb.

23. With decreased temperature, CMAP and SNAP conduction velocities are decreased; latency, amplitude, and duration are increased.

24. Conduction velocity decreases by 1.5 to 2.5 m/sec and distal latency increases by 0.2 m/sec for every 1°C drop in temperature.

25. Onset latency is affected by sweep speed and sensitivity, whereas peak latency is not affected by these factors.

26. Stimulus artifact can be reduced by increasing the distance between the stimulator and recording electrodes, and ensuring that the electrodes do not overlap.

27. SNAPs help to differentiate between plexopathy and radiculopathy. SNAPs are abnormal or absent in plexopathy and preserved in radiculopathy.

28. Wallerian degeneration starts around 3 to 5 days for motor fibers and around 6 to 10 days for sensory fibers.

29. Time to the onset of the active denervation is directly proportional to the distance between the site of the nerve lesion and the muscle tested.

30. In severe demyelinating neuropathies, conduction block correlates with distal weakness and distal sensory loss.

31. In demyelinating neuropathy with conduction block, distal muscle EMG may only reveal reduced recruitment patterns with normal motor unit potentials. No active denervation changes are seen.

32. Typically, no active denervation changes are seen in patients with NMJ disorders except in botulism.

33. Nascent motor unit potentials are short-duration, low-amplitude, polyphasic motor unit potentials seen in severe complete denervation. Similar potentials with an early recruitment pattern are seen in myopathic disorders.

34. In NMJ disorders, the motor unit morphology is mostly normal. In severe cases, short-duration, low-amplitude MUAPs may be seen. MUAPs with varying configuration (unstable MUAPs) are also seen.

35. Decreased CMAP amplitude may be seen with myopathy, NMJ disorders, neuropathies, radiculopathies, and motor neuron diseases.

36. If a patient has sensory loss with normal SNAP in that area, the lesion is likely proximal to the dorsal root ganglia, for example, a radiculopathy.

37. The anterior interosseus nerve (AIN) innervates the flexor pollicis longus, median head of flexor digitorum profundus, and pronator quadratus muscles. Abductor pollicis brevis is not innervated by AIN.

38. Median SNAP changes are the earliest abnormalities seen in patients with carpal tunnel syndrome.

39. Dorsal ulnar cutaneous sensory response can help localize the ulnar nerve lesion in patients with suspected ulnar neuropathy at the elbow.

40. Radial neuropathy at the spiral groove spares the triceps muscle.

41. Posterior interosseous neuropathy presents with wrist and finger extension weakness, but sensation remains normal.

42. Short head of biceps femoris is the only muscle supplied by the peroneal nerve above the level of the fibular neck.

43. Needle EMG of the gluteus medius and tensor fascia lata is abnormal in L5 radiculopathy, but not in peroneal mononeuropathy.

44. In Guillain–Barré syndrome (GBS), the initial nerve conduction study changes include either absent or prolonged F-wave responses.

45. The sural sparing phenomenon (normal sural response with reduced or absent median and ulnar sensory responses) is typically seen in the first few weeks of GBS.

46. In acute inflammatory demyelinating polyneuropathy (AIDP), low CMAP amplitude is the best predictor of poor prognosis.

47. In spinobulbar muscular atrophy (Kennedy's disease), sensory responses are either severely diminished or absent.

48. With medial cord or lower trunk brachial plexopathy, the median sensory responses are preserved, whereas the median motor and ulnar motor and sensory responses are affected.

49. Even in patients with compressive sciatic neuropathies, the peroneal fibers are more affected than tibial fibers.

50. Decrement on slow repetitive stimulation is seen with both presynaptic and postsynaptic NMJ disorders. Significant increment on fast repetitive stimulation or after brief exercise is seen in presynaptic NMJ disorders.

51. After nerve injury, the extent of loss of recruitment correlates with clinical weakness.

52. In demyelinating neuropathies, severely decreased conduction velocity does not correlate with weakness.

53. Fibrillation potentials and positive sharp waves may be absent in hyperacute or chronic denervation.

54. Complex repetitive discharges (CRDs) are usually only seen in chronic neuropathies and myopathies.

55. Myotonic discharges are seen in multiple conditions including acid maltase deficiency (in thoracic paraspinals).

56. Fiber density increases in neurogenic disorders after reinnervation.

57. Nerve conduction studies may be normal in patients with radiculopathy; the pattern of denervation on EMG will help in making the diagnosis.

58. Tibial H-reflex is an electrical correlate of the ankle reflex.

59. Unlike patients with lumbosacral radiculopathies, patients with lumbar canal stenosis have minimal EMG findings.

60. In upper trunk brachial plexopathy, median motor study is normal but the median and radial sensory studies may be abnormal.

61. EMG of deltoid is normal in posterior cord plexopathy, thus differentiating it from radial neuropathy.

62. L4 and L5 fibers in the lumbosacral plexus are commonly affected in postpartum lumbosacral plexopathy.

63. Myokymia is seen with radiation plexopathy but not with plexopathy secondary to infiltration by malignancy.

64. Severe slowing of conduction velocity seen in hereditary demyelinating neuropathies is not a good predictor of weakness.

65. Fibrillations and positive sharp waves may be seen with botulism.

66. Normal single-fiber EMG (SFEMG) in a weak noninflammatory muscle makes a diagnosis of myasthenia gravis (MG) or NMJ disorders unlikely. SFEMG is the most sensitive electrodiagnostic test for MG.

67. When unexpected low CMAP amplitudes are seen in the electrodiagnostic lab, a brief 10-second exercise can help with the diagnosis of LEMS as exercise may result in significant facilitation.

68. Increased spontaneous activity in myopathies does not always indicate "myositis" as these changes can be seen with other noninflammatory myopathies.

69. Sensory responses are preserved in traumatic cervical root avulsion but are abnormal in traumatic brachial plexopathy.

70. In neurogenic thoracic outlet syndrome, the medial antebrachial cutaneous sensory response is almost always abnormal. Median motor fibers are more affected than ulnar motor fibers.

71. Diabetic amyotrophy predominantly affects the anterior and medial thigh muscle groups.

72. Increased jitter on SFEMG is seen even in muscles that are not clinically weak in MG.

73. In patients with length-dependent neuropathy and foot drop, normal EMG of the gluteus medius will help exclude L5 radiculopathy.

74. In patients with axillary neuropathy, denervation may be seen in deltoid and teres minor muscles.

75. Unlike in electrical myotonia, the frequency of discharges remains stable in complex repetitive discharges (CRD).

76. Needle EMG of the extensor indicis proprius muscle can be abnormal in lower trunk brachial plexopathy and helps differentiate it from medial cord brachial plexopathy.

77. Normal EMG of hip adductors suggests femoral neuropathy rather than lumbosacral plexopathy or lumbar radiculopathy.

78. Polymyositis-like picture with motor neuronopathy can be seen with West Nile virus.

79. In L5 radiculopathy, the extensor hallucis longus is weaker than the tibialis anterior muscle.

80. In steroid myopathy, abnormal spontaneous activity is not seen, unlike in patients with polymyositis or dermatomyositis.

81. Lateral antebrachial cutaneous nerve is a branch of the musculocutaneous nerve; side-by-side comparison of this nerve will help in the diagnosis of musculocutaneous neuropathy.

82. The extent of fibrillations or positive sharp waves is not a good indicator of the degree of axonal loss.

83. Unlike myokymia, tremor is characterized by different motor unit potentials firing within each burst of activity.

84. Normal insertional activity lasts less than 300 ms after needle movement.

85. CRDs do not disappear with NMJ blockade as they originate at the muscle fiber level.

86. Fasciculations, doublets, triplets, myokymia, cramps, and neuromyotonia originate at the motor nerve/neuron level and have distinct firing patterns.

87. Monopolar needle has a larger recording area compared to the concentric needle; motor unit potential amplitude with the monopolar needle is larger.

88. Motor unit duration increases with aging. The shortest motor unit duration is seen in the facial muscles.

89. Among the various motor unit potential measures, duration is the most important feature.

90. Before analyzing the motor unit potentials, it is important to make sure that the rise time is short (less than 300–500 ms).

91. In primary central nervous system (CNS) disorders, the motor unit potentials and recruitment remain normal but activation is decreased.

92. Parsonage Turner syndrome is an inflammatory brachial plexopathy, frequently seen after recent viral infections or after surgeries, manifesting with pain and predominant motor nerve involvement.

93. Neuromuscular ultrasound changes in focal neuropathies include increase in nerve cross-sectional area, hypoechogenicity, reduced mobility of the nerve, and increased vascularity of the nerve.

94. Fast and slow repetitive stimulations are performed for NMJ disorders. Slow repetitive stimulation reveals abnormal decrement in both LEMS and MG. Fast repetitive stimulation in LEMS reveals significant increment and no significant changes in MG.

95. Short exercise testing can help with the diagnosis of nondystrophic myotonias.

96. Long exercise testing helps with the diagnosis of periodic paralysis.

97. In contrast to the radiation-induced brachial plexopathy, malignancy or tumor recurrence leading to brachial plexopathy typically cause severe pain and tend to involve the lower trunk.

98. Myelin-associated glycoprotein (MAG) neuropathy is a slowly progressive distal sensory, ataxic neuropathy with distal demyelination changes.

99. In neurogenic thoracic outlet syndrome, the medial antebrachial sensory response is almost always abnormal; the thenar group of muscles are more likely to be affected rather than hypothenar muscles.

100. In myopayhies, short-duration and small amplitude motor unit potentials with early recruitment patterns are typically seen.

101. In neurogenic processes, long-duration and large amplitude motor unit potentials with reduced recruitment are typically seen.

102. Recommended minimal skin temperature is 30°C for lower limbs and 32°C for upper limb nerve conduction studies.

Electroencephalography

1. Alpha wave intrusion occurs in patients with chronic fatigue/pain (e.g., fibromyalgia); it is characterized by the appearance of alpha waves in NREM sleep when delta activity is expected. It is sometimes termed alpha–delta sleep.

2. Paradoxical alpha rhythm represents an alerting response characterized by the appearance of posterior alpha frequencies in the setting of opened eyes and drowsiness.

3. Baclofen and lithium toxicities have been associated with periodic complexes similar to those seen in Creutzfeldt–Jakob disease (CJD).

4. Subacute sclerosing panencephalitis (SSPE) usually presents 5 to 15 years after a primary measles infection with progressive psychoneurological deterioration including personality change and seizures. The EEG is very characteristic, consisting of periodic complexes composed of high-amplitude (300–1,500 microvolts), bisynchronous and symmetrical polyspike- and sharp- and slow-wave complexes occurring every 4 to 15 seconds, which is too long for typical periodic discharges.

5. Generalized periodic discharges (GPDs) can present in a number of clinical scenarios, commonly in anoxia. The period of the discharge, defined as the duration of one cycle in a repeating event (also the reciprocal of frequency), can help with the diagnosis. SSPE has the longest period, typically 4 to 20 seconds, which is longer earlier in the disease and shortens over time. CJD (except the new variant type) and baclofen toxicity also can present with periodic discharges (PDs), but with a shorter period (i.e., higher frequency) on the order of 1 to 2 seconds.

6. EEG patterns evolve over time (typically 6 months) in CJD. Diffuse slowing can be seen initially with periodic complexes appearing and then disappearing; of note, the periodic complexes may subside with drowsiness and recur with stimulation, which is not typical of periodic complexes due to hypoxic–ischemic injury or status epilepticus.

7. Stroke typically results in regional loss of faster frequencies and appearance of slower frequencies; asymmetric normal features (e.g., sleep spindles); and loss of amplitude (in severe stroke).

8. The columnar organization of neurons, along with the sheet-like organization parallel to the scalp, leads to orthogonal dipoles that can be detected by scalp EEG electrodes.

9. Common causes for lateralized PDs (formerly known as periodic lateralized epileptiform discharges [PLEDs]) include herpes simplex virus (HSV) encephalitis, acute or subacute stroke, and seizures.

10. Positive temporal sharp waves can be a normal finding in neonates of 32 to 36 weeks and tend to resolve on subsequent EEGs. However, in pathological groups (e.g., asphyxia, metabolic disorders, and cystic periventricular leukomalacia), this finding tends to be persistent.

11. Trace discontinu may be seen as early as 28 weeks conceptional age (CA), sometimes up to 36 weeks CA; it would not be a marker of severe encephalopathy until beyond 38 weeks CA.

12. Sleep spindles appear at the age of 2 months, when they can be of long duration and be asynchronous but symmetric. After 2 years of age, sleep spindles are normally synchronous and of shorter duration.

13. In a bipolar montage channel G1–G2, the resultant voltage equals the difference between G1 and G2. According to the convention, if the G1 input is more negative than the G2 input, the pen deflection will be upward. It follows that either a more negative event at G1 or a more positive event at G2 would lead to an upward deflection. A more positive event at G1 or a more negative event at G2 leads to a downward deflection. A flat (i.e., an equipotential) deflection occurs if both G1 and G2 have equal inputs.

14. Benign Rolandic epilepsy (BRE) presents with centrotemporal spikes and partial onset seizures, characterized by hemifacial sensorimotor symptoms, oropharyngolaryngeal manifestations, speech arrest, and hypersalivation.

15. Juvenile myoclonic epilepsy (JME) presents with 4 to 6 Hz (fast) spike-wave and polyspike-wave discharges and can present with photoparoxysmal responses.

16. The 14- and 6-Hz positive spikes occur in all age groups but are maximally seen in adolescents. They occur in light sleep, typically last less than 2 seconds, and are usually seen in the posterior temporal region. They are not felt to be clinically significant.

17. Inactivation of sodium channels defines the absolute refractory period.

18. The thalamic reticular nucleus, part of the reticular-activating system (RAS), modulates the thalamocortical pathways and helps to synchronize and desynchronize the EEG.

19. Small sharp spikes (SSS), also known as benign epileptiform transients of sleep (BETS), are brief (less than 50 ms), low-amplitude (less than 50 mV) sharp transients typically seen in the temporal and frontal regions during Stage N1 or N2 sleep.

20. Eye movement causes changes on the EEG due to the dipole nature of the eyeball, with the cornea being relatively positive compared to the retina. Therefore, when looking up or down, the fronto-polar electrodes (Fp1 and Fp2) will be positive or negative, respectively. When looking left or right, the lateral eye electrodes (F7 and F8) will have opposite polarities, with the positive polarity in the direction of the lateral gaze.

21. If only unilateral deflection is noted on the EEG with eye movement, consider enucleation.

22. Slow activity can be better evaluated by viewing a compressed EEG. Sweat artifact presents with slow waves (usually less than 0.5 Hz) with superimposed normal activity. Lateral eye movements would have the homologous anterior channels (i.e., Fp1/Fp2, F7/F8) have opposite polarity due to the dipole effect of the eyeball. Frontal intermittent rhythmic delta activity (FIRDA) would have a frequency between 0.5 and 4 Hz.

23. Looking at the electrocardiogram is helpful because the pulse artifact can be present both on scalp EEGs and intracranial electrocorticography (ECoG); and it typically presents rhythmically, occurring at a frequency equal to but not necessarily synchronous with (may be with a slight lag) the heart rate.

24. Hypsarrhythmia, seen in West syndrome, is an interictal pattern consisting of irregular, high-amplitude (greater than 200 mV), generalized polymorphic slowing in the setting of a chaotic and disorganized background as well as multifocal spikes. It is frequently seen in infants with infantile spasms. Hypsarrhythmia typically disappears or improves during the ictal spasms and/or REM sleep. During NREM sleep, it can become discontinuous and fragmented, resembling a burst-suppression–like pattern. It rarely persists beyond the age of 24 months.

25. Supplementary motor seizures are typically brief, have a nocturnal predilection, and are associated with contralateral head turn, hand elevation and abduction, and possible vocalization.

26. Temporal intermittent rhythmic delta activity (TIRDA) is associated with an increased risk for temporal lobe seizures just like temporal interictal epileptiform discharges.

27. Posterior slow waves of youth are 2 to 4 Hz delta waves, seen bisynchronously with shifting asymmetry in the occipital region. They are considered part of the normal alpha rhythm. They typically form a complex that consists of the slow delta component with superimposed and following alpha rhythm of the waking background, hence the term "fused waves." They are typically seen in preadolescence (6–12 years), but rare before age 2 years or after 21 years. They are best seen with eyes closed in relaxed wakefulness. They attenuate with eye opening, increase with hyperventilation (HV), and disappear in drowsiness. They occur as sporadic single waves or in bursts interspersed by one or several seconds of regular background activity.

28. Cortical blindness can be associated with the presence of occipital spikes.

29. The amplifier sampling frequency, or the frequency at which the amplifier measures the voltage, determines the temporal resolution of the data. Although the screen resolution can impact the resolution of what can be displayed on the screen (e.g., decreasing the number of seconds displayed increases the temporal resolution), it does not impact the resolution of the raw data. The bit rate of the analog-to-digital converter (ADC) and the amplifier input range determine the voltage resolution of the raw data.

30. Note that a channel is comprised of a recording electrode (i.e., G1) and a reference (i.e., G2), which in a bipolar montage is an adjacent electrode. To find the channel voltage, simply subtract G2 from G1 (i.e., G1–G2). A positive voltage will occur if G1 is more positive or less negative than G2, and a negative voltage will occur if G1 is less positive or more negative than G2.

31. EEG sensitivity is equal to the voltage divided by the height of the deflection (typically in mm). For example, a 20 microvolt deflection taking 4 mm to display equals 5 microvolt/mm. Sensitivity goes up if the gain goes down and vice versa.

32. The outside of the cell is by convention defined as zero and the resting membrane potential is, therefore, equal to the voltage inside the cell. In neurons, the usual range of the resting membrane is –60 mV to –70 mV. In muscle, it is typically closer to –90 mV. The typical equilibrium potentials for potassium and sodium are –90 mV and +55 mV, respectively.

33. Sodium contributes the most to neuronal depolarization, and potassium contributes the most to neuronal hyperpolarization. Although potassium helps maintain the resting membrane potential, the resting membrane is most permeable to chloride; hence, the membrane resting potential, typically –60 to –70 mV, is nearest the Nernst potential for chloride (around –65 mV) rather than for potassium (around –90 mV).

34. For a typical posterior dominant rhythm (PDR), the interpeak duration is about 100 ms, which equates to a 10 Hz PDR.

35. As infants grow, the PDR becomes more regular and increases in frequency: 3 Hz at age 3 months; 5 to 6 Hz by age 12 months; 8 Hz by age 3 years; 9 Hz by 9 years. The PDR is abnormal if it is not 8 Hz by 8 years of age. A simplified way of remembering this is 3 (Hz) × 3 (months); 6 × 12 (months); 9 × 9 (years).

36. Hyperventilation (HV) in children can lead to high-amplitude generalized slow activity that can be a normal response. It can also lead to 3 Hz spike-and-wave activity that can be a seizure.

37. When a posterior rhythmic or "spiky" activity is noted on an EEG, a photic-driving response needs to be considered, which can be seen as early as 3 to 4 months. Driving is best seen below 8 Hz flash frequency in children 3 to 5 years of age, and at 6 to 16 Hz in children of 6 to 12 years of age. That said, photic driving can be seen even at 1 Hz.

38. Alpha coma, historically, was felt to be associated with poor outcome; however, the current thinking is that prognosis depends on the underlying etiology. It can be seen after anoxic brain injury (typically unfavorable outcome), although it can also be seen in head trauma, brainstem strokes, and toxic-metabolic dysfunction (typically more favorable outcome). Some reports suggest that it is the most common rhythmic coma pattern in children. It can present with other frequencies, such as theta, resulting in alpha–theta coma, and it can evolve into other coma patterns, including delta or burst-suppression.

39. Spindle coma and beta coma tend to be associated with more favorable outcomes.

40. HV slowing can be exaggerated by hypoglycemia, especially in children. This is one reason for noting the time of the last meal as part of the EEG recording.

41. Photomyogenic effect, felt to be due to a heightened brainstem reflex, results in muscle twitching of the frontalis or eyelids time-locked with the photic stimulus.

42. Subclinical rhythmic epileptiform discharge of adults (SREDA) is typically seen in older adults in the temporoparietal region. It consists of theta range frequencies with a sharply contoured morphology. It usually occurs during rest, drowsiness, or HV. The pattern can evolve into rhythmic activity lasting over 1 minute (average 40–80 seconds). Although the pattern can be misinterpreted as ictal, it is considered nonspecific. Abrupt onset and termination may help distinguish SREDA from an ictal discharge. SREDA pattern is never associated with symptoms or postictal slowing, unlike a seizure pattern.

43. The PDR can occur normally at subharmonic and supraharmonic frequencies, termed "slow alpha variant" (typically half of the PDR) and "fast alpha variant" (typically double the PDR), respectively. These alpha variants are blocked by eye opening, just as the PDR.

44. Positive occipital sharp transients in wakefulness (especially in the setting of scanning the environment) are likely lambda waves. If the transients are seen during sleep, then they are more likely to be positive occipital sharp transients of sleep (POSTS).

45. Inhibitory postsynaptic potential (IPSP) inputs into the cell body and the excitatory postsynaptic potential (EPSP) inputs into the apical dendrites lead to intracellular depolarization and extracellular negativity that can be detected by the scalp EEG.

46. With EPSPs, the synaptic current is carried by the positive ions at the level of the synapse, the ionic current being directed toward the intracellular medium. Therefore, at the level of the synapse, there is an active sink in the case of positive ionic currents (EPSPs) resulting in extracellular negativity and intracellular positivity. The opposite situation occurs with IPSPs, creating a source at the synapse with extracellular positivity and intracellular negativity. Along the cell, away from the synapse, a distributed passive source occurs in the case of EPSPs, whereas a distributed passive sink occurs with IPSPs.

47. The spike-wave complex is not simply an association of a spike and a slow wave. It is believed that the surface negative spike is the result of EPSPs on the apical dendrites of vertically oriented pyramidal type neurons, whereas the surface negative slow wave is the result of IPSPs on or near the soma of similar pyramidal cells. Thus, the slow-wave component is inhibitory, and the spike-wave discharge likely represents alternating excitation and inhibition.

48. The reticular nucleus, part of the reticular activating system (RAS) that modulates the thalamocortical pathways, helps synchronize and desynchronize the EEG. Typically, the EEG is synchronized when the thalamic relay neurons are in the burst mode, and desynchronized when they are in the tonic mode. Stimulation of the RAS suppresses slower activity (e.g., delta) and stimulates faster activity (e.g., gamma). This modulation leads to distinct differences in cerebral electrical activity during wakefulness and sleep.

49. The hippocampus is felt to be a generator for the physiological theta waves.

50. Physiological delta waves (e.g., N3 sleep stage) can originate in the thalamus (in coordination with the reticular formation) or in the cortex (in coordination with the suprachiasmatic nucleus).

51. Dysfunction of white matter typically leads to pathological medium- to high-amplitude polymorphic delta slowing.

52. Thalamic pacemaker cells are felt to mediate the alpha range rhythm, including the PDR, which is generated in the cortex.

53. Sleep spindles are generated within the reticular nucleus of the thalamus (consisting of GABAergic neurons), and persist in the thalamus after decortication and high brainstem transections.

54. Sodium channels are densely populated at the nodes of Ranvier.

55. Active γ-Aminobutyric acid type A (GABAA) receptors increase chloride conductance through a chloride ion-selective pore, driving the membrane potential toward the reversal

potential of the Cl^- ion which is about –65 mV in neurons, in turn inhibiting the firing of new action potentials; this mechanism is responsible for the sedative effects of GABAA allosteric agonists.

56. Baclofen, which acts as a γ-Aminobutyric acid type B (GABAB) receptor agonist, can produce diffuse PDs at toxic levels.

57. Myelin reduces the membrane capacitance and increases the transmembrane resistance, allowing the action potential to jump from node to node, known as saltatory conduction.

58. As established by the Underwriters Laboratories in the United States, the chassis leakage current for medical instruments should be less than 100 microamperes; any higher current applied to the skin can cause ventricular fibrillation in humans.

59. In the ICU, a common ground should be used to prevent electrical injury.

60. In EEG, the ground electrode helps to reduce artifact and electrical injury.

61. Generalized excessive beta activity is usually seen in the setting of benzodiazepine and/or barbiturate administration.

62. In phenytoin toxicity, the EEG tends to show diffuse slow activity (mixture of theta and delta frequencies).

63. POSTS tend to have a positive deflection in a reference montage (e.g., average) when there is usually a negative deflection in the anterior–posterior bipolar montage.

64. Delta brushes are a telltale sign of prematurity; they consist of random 0.3 to 1.5 Hz delta waves with overriding bursts of 18 to 22 Hz beta, giving the illusion of a brush or ripple. They occur asynchronously and symmetrically over homologous areas; at 26 weeks CA, they are infrequent and maximum in the central region; at 29 to 33 weeks CA, they are the prominent feature in active sleep; at about 33 to 38 weeks CA, they are more prominent in quiet sleep with temporal–occipital dominance; they are infrequent at term and disappear by 42 to 43 weeks CA.

65. Mu rhythm is commonly seen in young adults (20% of people younger than 30 years), and represents the resting rhythm of the pre- and post-Rolandic cortex. It is seen in the central region (C3, Cz, C4) with a frequency of 8 to 10 Hz. It may appear asymmetrically during times of relaxation, and is reactive to motor programming. Mu rhythm disappears with movement or the thought of movement of the contralateral arm (e.g., making a fist, wiping nose, etc.). Mu rhythm is a normal variant, not an ictal phenomenon.

66. A salt bridge occurs when the electrolyte in sweat interacts with the electrode gel or paste to produce an isoelectric channel (i.e., the voltage in the two adjacent electrodes appears to be equal).

67. Sturge–Weber syndrome is a rare condition in which there is a "port wine" stain (i.e., birthmark), usually on one side of the face, associated with abnormal blood vessels on the surface of the brain (usually occipital region). This abnormality is associated with focal seizures, with the EEG showing regional or hemispheric amplitude asymmetry.

68. Brain tumors, including gliomas, can present with various changes on the EEG, such as relative voltage suppression in the area of tumor burden, slowing in and around the tumor, spike-wave discharges, lateralized periodic discharges (LPDs; formerly known as PLEDs), and seizures in the surrounding irritative cortex.

69. Sleep features, including vertex waves and POSTS, may occur in runs, especially in children, and should not be misinterpreted as spikes, LPDs, or seizures.

70. Wicket spikes are typically sharp transients with symmetric upslope and downslope but without disruption of the background; they are seen in the temporal region during wakefulness or Stage N1 sleep.

71. Landau–Kleffner syndrome (LKS) is a childhood syndrome characterized by language regression, which typically starts with auditory verbal agnosia. Although they can be associated with clinical seizures, many only present with an electrographic seizure pattern that activates in sleep, referred to as electrographic status epilepticus of sleep (ESES).

72. Although both LKS and continuous spike waves in sleep (CSWS) are epilepsy syndromes with clinical regression and sleep-activated epileptiform EEG patterns in NREM sleep, there are some distinguishing features. The discharges are more bitemporal and/or biparietal in LKS, whereas they are more diffuse in CSWS. The regression in CSWS is more global behavior, whereas in LKS, it is typically limited to language. Both syndromes present with intractable epilepsy and may require multiple antiepileptic agents. Of note, steroids have been noted to be beneficial in both conditions, but carbamazepine has been noted to worsen the EEG patterns in both.

73. Cone waves, also known as O waves, are surface-positive, monophasic or diphasic, high-amplitude, "cone-shaped" delta waves that are seen in the posterior head regions. They are commonly observed during light and deeper stages of sleep. They are interspersed with slow delta waves of sleep. They appear around 6 months of age when sleep patterns evolve from the quiet sleep pattern of neonates to the adult NREM patterns, and persist up to 5 years of age. Although the cone waves are sometimes mistaken for abnormal sharp-wave or slow-wave activity, they do not increase the risk for epileptic seizures.

74. There are many types of occipital sharp transients. In young children, they are likely to be associated with benign epilepsy that may remit in later life; in other words, presence of occipital spikes does not necessarily indicate intractable epilepsy. Lambda waves are occipital sharp transients that occur because of scanning objects, and they disappear with eye closure. Spikes associated with benign occipital epilepsy of childhood attenuate with eye opening. In blind individuals, occipital spikes can be seen without history of seizures.

75. A breach rhythm is due to an underlying skull defect, and can lead to sharper, faster, and higher amplitude EEG activity in the electrodes in and around the skull defect.

76. A burst-suppression EEG pattern consists of high-voltage bursts of mixed activity (slowing, sharp waves, and spikes) alternating with a suppressed background. It can be due to anoxic brain injury, seizures (a late-stage pattern in generalized status epilepticus), and drug effect (e.g., barbiturates, propofol).

77. The semiology of temporal lobe seizures includes motionless staring, oroalimentary automatisms, ipsilateral hand automatisms, contralateral hand dystonic posturing, and ipsilateral postictal nose wiping. Postictal language difficulty is seen with dominant temporal lobe seizures.

78. Increasing the EEG paper speed (i.e., fewer seconds per page) will help detect the faster frequencies better; decreasing the EEG paper speed (i.e., more seconds per page) will help detect the slower frequencies better.

79. The American Clinical Neurophysiology Society (ACNS) "Guideline 3: Minimum Technical Standards for EEG Recording in Suspected Cerebral Death" specifies that electrocerebral inactivity (ECI) recordings need to be at least 30 minutes long; a full set of conventional 10 to 20 scalp electrodes should be used because the study may or may not be ECI; interelectrode impedances should be between 100 and 10K ohms; the integrity of the entire recording system should be tested (i.e., touching each electrode to create an artifact potential on the recording); interelectrode distances should be at least 10 cm; sensitivity must be increased to at least 2 microvolts/mm for at least 30 minutes of the recording with inclusion of appropriate calibrations (i.e., use a 2 or 5 microvolt calibration signal instead of a 50 microvolt signal); filter settings should be set such that the low-frequency filter is no higher than 1 Hz and the high-frequency filter is no lower than 30 Hz; additional signals can be monitored (e.g., EKG); a short-acting neuromuscular blocker is used if muscle artifact is significant; there should be no reactivity to intense stimulation (e.g., auditory, visual, tactile); recordings should be done by a qualified technologist (of note, not mandated to be a registered technologist) working under the supervision of a qualified electroencephalographer; and repeat EEG should be done if there is doubt of ECI.

80. A technically adequate ECI recording with no EEG activity and absent brainstem reflexes would be consistent with (not diagnostic of) brain death; ECI with intact brainstem reflexes is consistent with cortical death; minimally responsive, slow EEG in the setting of some brainstem reflexes with no clear purposeful movements is consistent with a vegetative state (note that in the vegetative state, patients can open their eyelids occasionally and demonstrate sleep–wake cycles but lack cognitive function); minimally responsive slow EEG with some purposeful behavior and intelligible verbalization is consistent with minimally conscious state; clearly reactive normal or mildly slow EEG with limited preserved brainstem reflexes can be seen with locked-in syndrome.

81. Triphasic waves (also known as GPDs with triphasic morphology) are frontally predominant rhythmic activity with triphasic morphology and an anterior–posterior phase gradient. They can be distinguished from rhythmic slowing by the presence of an interval between consecutive waveforms of this type; they occur in the setting of more profound metabolic dysfunction and are classically associated with hepatic and/or uremic encephalopathy. They can also be seen in hypoxic-ischemic insults, other metabolic disorders (e.g., hypercalcemia; hyperthyroidism), status epilepticus, drug toxicity (e.g., baclofen and lithium), and neurodegenerative diseases (e.g., CJD).

82. The electrode pop is the most common electrode artifact caused by abrupt impedance change; it appears in a single electrode as single or multiple sharp waveforms, and characteristically as an abrupt transient without disruption of the background.

83. FIRDA can be interpreted in a variety of ways depending on the situation. It is typically considered normal in children or drowsy elderly individuals. Otherwise, it is considered abnormal (e.g., associated with clinical encephalopathy) and has been associated with metabolic dysfunction, subcortical lesions, or elevated intracranial pressure.

84. Infants with West syndrome (infantile spasms and hypsarrhythmia) can mature into Lennox–Gastaut syndrome, presenting with generalized slow spike-and-wave activity.

85. In Lennox–Gastaut syndrome, the EEG shows generalized slow spike-wave discharges (less than 2.5 Hz) with a slow background in addition to multiple seizure types, including tonic seizures. Clinically, the patients have cognitive impairment.

86. The maximum resolvable frequency within a data set is equal to half of the sampling rate of the ADC.

87. Glossokinetic artifact can be seen in the anterior head electrodes. The tip of the tongue is relatively negative when compared to the base of the tongue.

88. Progressive myoclonic epilepsy can be associated with high-voltage evoked potentials.

89. In term infants, the most common cause of neonatal seizures is hypoxic–ischemic encephalopathy.

90. Absence seizures present with 3 Hz (2.5–4 Hz) generalized spike-and-wave activity.

91. Childhood absence epilepsy (CAE) is associated with occipital intermittent rhythmic delta activity (OIRDA).

92. Paroxysmal fast activity refers to low-amplitude, fast activity (e.g., beta frequencies); when it is generalized, it can be associated with infantile spasms, as well as tonic or atonic seizures, which might be distinguishable by the presence (in tonic seizures) or lack of (in atonic seizures) muscle artifact.

93. Typically, as cerebral blood flow (CBF; milliliters of blood per 100 g of brain tissue per minute) decreases (e.g., during vasovagal syncope or asystole), the EEG changes as follows: normal (above 35 mL/min); loss of beta frequencies (25–35 mL/min); theta slowing (18–25 mL/min); polymorphic delta slowing (12–18 ml/min); suppression of all frequencies (less than 10 mL/min). Of note, ischemia or reversible injury is felt to occur at CBF of 10 to 35 mL/min, whereas infarct or irreversible injury is felt to occur at CBF less than 10 mL/min.

94. The maximum potential (positive or negative) can be assessed by the absolute maximum values on a referential montage or by looking for phase reversals on a bipolar montage. Note that a large field may introduce one or more channels of relative isoelectric potentials (i.e., equal maximums) on a bipolar montage, resulting in a less obvious phase reversal.

95. Negative phase reversals point toward each other (you can imagine that you can fit a minus sign between the phase reversals) while positive phase reversals point away from each other (you can imagine that you can fit a plus sign between the phase reversals).

96. Papez circuit, which is involved in spatial and episodic memory processing, consists of the hippocampus, fornix, mammillary bodies, anterior nucleus of the thalamus, and cingulate cortex. Stimulation of the anterior nucleus of the thalamus, which is part of the Papez circuit, modulates activity in the hippocampus and cortex. This is the basis for deep brain stimulation for epilepsy.

97. Cortical activity gets attenuated by cerebrospinal fluid (CSF), dura, skull, and scalp. It has been shown that approximately 6 cm^2 of the cortical surface needs to be activated for a given activity to be seen at the scalp electrode.

98. Radially oriented dipoles contribute to the EEG activity detected at the scalp, whereas the horizontally oriented diploes, running parallel to the cortical surface, contribute to the magnetoencephalographic (MEG) activity at the scalp.

99. Stereoencephalography (SEEG) has multiple advantages over subdural grid evaluation, including avoidance of large craniotomies, reduced surgical morbidity, and broader coverage area. One limitation SEEG has is poor functional mapping.

100. Encephalopathy can be classified as mild, moderate, severe, and ECI. In general, mild encephalopathy refers to slowing of the PDR (typically less than or equal to 8 Hz), more reactive theta than delta activity, and preservation of some sleep architecture. Moderate encephalopathy has preserved state changes, loss of the PDR, and increased amount of delta slowing. Severe encephalopathy has predominately delta slowing (but can have mixed faster frequencies), diffuse electrodecremental segments or background attenuation, and no reactivity or state changes. ECI has EEG activity less than 2 microvolts.

101. The EEG in Huntington's disease has a characteristic low-voltage background (<10 microvolts), making it hard to appreciate the PDR.

102. EEG patterns in sporadic CJD (sCJD) change with the stage of the disease. Early stages are characterized by diffuse slowing and FIRDA, whereas middle and late stages present with periodic sharp wave complexes (PSWC). Preterminal stages are characterized by a reactive or alpha coma.

Evoked Potentials and Intraoperative Monitoring

1. Pentobarbital decreases amplitudes and prolongs latencies of evoked potentials.

2. The obligate potential for visual evoked potential (VEP) is P100 (generated within the occipital cortex), which can be estimated by the intersection of the slopes of the N75 and N145 waveforms. The N100 is generated in the frontal region, is not obligate, and can help to identify the P100.

3. Full-field stimulation is used to detect lesions anterior to the chiasm and hemifield stimulations are used to detect lesions posterior to the chiasm.

4. Flash frequency VEP is interpreted as either present or absent.

5. Cortical somatosensory evoked potentials (SSEPs) are a combination of the cortical and subcortical signals; the latter are usually subtracted out when the bipolar derivation is used.

6. In a median SSEP, if N13, P14, and N18 (all obligate waveforms) are not recognizable but Erb's potential (N9) and N20 have normal latencies, the study should be considered normal.

7. In a tibial SSEP, if N34 (an obligate waveform) is not recognizable, but LP and P37 have normal latencies, the study should be considered normal.

8. The obligate waveforms for the brainstem auditory evoked potentials (BAEPs) are waves I, III, and V. Wave I is the compound muscle action potential (CMAP) from the cochlear end (distal part) of the eighth nerve (i.e., near field), while the subsequent waves are from multiple generators (i.e., far field). Wave III represents activity in the lower pons and Wave V in the mesencephalon. BAEPs cannot be used to assess pathways rostral to the mesencephalon.

9. Decreasing the click intensity for BAEPs may prolong the absolute latencies and reduce the amplitudes but does not substantially affect the interpeak latencies. To ensure robust testing, the stimulus intensity is typically set for 65 dB above the decibel sensation level (dBSL) or decibel hearing level (dBHL).

10. A more robust Wave I can be elicited by increasing the stimulus intensity if Wave I has a small amplitude or is poorly defined, by decreasing the stimulus intensity if there are too many waves making Wave I not stand out, by changing the click polarity from rarefaction to condensation, by slowing the stimulus rate, by using an external canal electrode (tiptrode), and by administrating sedatives to help patients relax if excessive muscle artifact is present.

11. If a median SSEP is normal and tibial SSEP is abnormal, then the lesion is below the cervical cord and above the most proximal normal tibial SSEP latency.

12. During intraoperative monitoring, nerve manipulation will lead to neurotonic discharges.

13. Conductive hearing loss reduces the effective stimulus reaching the cochlea; on average, a 0.4 ms shift can be expected for each 10 dB of conductive hearing loss.

14. Inhaled anesthetics will increase latencies for cortical potentials.

15. Prolongation of Wave I to III interpeak latency and normal III to V latency is due to a conduction defect between the distal part of CN VIII and the superior olivary nucleus (lower pons) ipsilateral to the stimulated ear.

16. Prolongation of III to V interpeak latency with normal I to III interpeak latency is due to a conduction defect between the superior olivary nucleus (lower pons) and the inferior colliculus (mesencephalon) ipsilateral to the stimulated ear.

17. BAEP tends to be robust in the setting of anesthesia; in particular, Wave I appears to be the least affected by general anesthesia.

18. SSEPs can be used to map the central sulcus by stimulating the median nerve and assessing the negative pseudo-phase reversal of N20 waveform (somatosensory cortex; postcentral gyrus) and the P22 (or P20) waveform (motor cortex; precentral gyrus).

19. Normal N9 and abnormal N13 suggest a lesion proximal to the brachial plexus and distal to the foramen magnum.

20. The loss of N13 can also be seen with a lesion of the lower to mid-cervical cord.

21. If N13 is normal and N20 is abnormal, a lesion proximal to the mid-cervical cord, including the subcortical and cortical pathways, is implicated.

22. Absence of N22 in a tibial SSEP suggests a lesion at or distal to the lumbar region.

23. Normal N22 and delayed N30 potential suggest a lesion between the lumbar and cervical spinal cord.

24. Normal N22 and abnormal P37 suggest a nonlocalizable lesion proximal to the lumbar spinal cord.

25. The yield of abnormal evoked potentials in definite multiple sclerosis (MS) depends on the modality: 70% to 80% for VEPs; 60% to 70% for SSEPs; and 20% to 40% for BAEPs.

26. Bilateral absence of N20 is highly predictive of poor neurological outcome after anoxic or traumatic brain injury but the presence of any response does not necessarily predict a good outcome.

27. Prolongation of bilateral median N20 after cardiac arrest results from a lesion between Erb's point and the cortex.

28. In Huntington's disease, amplitude attenuation rather than latency delay is seen in VEPs and median nerve SSEPs.

29. In neurophysiologic intraoperative monitoring (NIOM), the preservation of wave V of BAEP at the end of a surgical case is a very good indicator that hearing will be preserved.

30. Compared to sensory evoked potential (SEP) monitoring, electromyography (EMG) monitoring has a high sensitivity for detecting mechanical nerve root manipulation but a lower specificity and positive predictive value for postoperative nerve root injury.

31. In general for NIOM, higher sensitivity is preferable to higher specificity.

32. Multifocal VEP (mfVEP) allows for simultaneous recording from multiple visual field regions, leading to an assessment of a much larger cross-sectional area of the optic nerve. This provides a more accurate functional evaluation of the visual pathway, including the periphery, compared to full-field pattern-reversal VEP (PVEP).

Polysomnography and Other Sleep Studies

1. On a polysomnogram (PSG), obstructive sleep apnea (OSA) will typically show frequent arousals, paradoxical chest and abdominal movements, decreased oxygen saturations, and decreased airflow.
2. On a PSG, periodic limb movement disorder will typically show normal breathing with synchronized chest and abdominal movements with good oxygen saturations but with frequent arousals corresponding to leg movements.
3. In neonates, active sleep is equivalent to REM sleep and quiet sleep is equivalent to NREM sleep.
4. Nonrestorative sleep leads to excessive daytime sleepiness, which can be the result of alpha–delta sleep, REM without atonia, OSA, and periodic limb movement disorder.
5. Slow-wave sleep decreases in the elderly.
6. Low hypocretin level is associated with narcolepsy.
7. Sleep spindles (1–3 seconds of 12–16 Hz sinusoidal central activity) are a marker of Stage N2 sleep.
8. Vertex waves, normally seen as single waveforms, can occur in runs or trains of activity, especially in adolescents, and are not considered pathological.
9. REM sleep is characterized by rapid horizontal eye movements, EEG background consisting of low-voltage mixed frequencies (not just theta waves) similar to wakefulness (referred to as paradoxical sleep), and trains of sharply contoured or triangular, 2 to 6 Hz, often serrated waves (sawtooth waves) in the central region.
10. When evaluating for narcolepsy, the patient must undergo an overnight PSG (showing 6 hours of sleep) prior to performing the multiple sleep latency test (MSLT) to ensure that an abnormal MSLT is due to narcolepsy and not due to other causes. Although sleep onset REM periods (SOREMPs) are nonspecific, occurrence of two SOREMPs with a mean sleep latency of less than 8 minutes is consistent with narcolepsy.
11. OSA is worse during REM sleep due in part to the muscle atonia of skeletal muscles of the upper airway and ventilation. Sleeping position also affects OSA, which is typically worsened by sleeping supine.
12. REM sleep behavior disorder (RBD) is a parasomnia, typically occurring in the early morning (due to the predominance of REM later during sleep) in which there is no REM-associated atonia, and thus patients will act out their dreams. Upon waking up, patients are usually able to recall their dreams that match the actions seen by others, yet unaware of their actions. It is most often associated with Parkinson's disease, multiple system atrophy (MSA), and Lewy body dementia.
13. Night terror is another parasomnia, typically occurring in the first few hours of sleep (during NREM sleep), in which the patient feels terror or dread. Nightmares also instill fear but occur as part of REM sleep. Confusional arousal is different from night terror in that it starts with movement and moaning, which can later progress to occasional thrashings or inconsolable crying.

Advanced Topics

1. The term "high-frequency oscillations" (HFOs) refers to EEG activity greater than 70 Hz (30–70 Hz band activity is usually considered as gamma). The 80 to 200 Hz activity is often referred to as ripples, whereas the 250 to 500 Hz activity is referred to as fast ripples. To record HFOs, a sampling rate of 1,000 Hz (preferably 2,000 Hz) is recommended.

2. Although HFOs were recorded using microelectrodes in the initial studies, recent studies have convincingly shown that HFOs can be recorded using clinical depth and subdural electrodes. In patients with epilepsy, HFOs have been recorded from all brain regions including mesial temporal as well as neocortical structures.

3. Recent studies have shown that HFOs are useful in the localization of the epileptogenic zone and are felt to be biomarkers of underlying epileptogenicity.

4. The term "direct current (DC) EEG" refers to a frequency response of the EEG with a minimum at 0 Hz. Although this is typically recorded using dedicated DC-coupled amplifiers, the routine alternating current (AC) amplifiers with long time constants (e.g., 10 seconds) can adequately record the DC shifts as well. They are best seen by decreasing the low-frequency filter (high pass filter) to significantly low values (e.g., 0.016 Hz).

5. Several studies suggest that DC shifts are useful in localizing the seizure onset zone, particularly on intracranial recordings that are relatively artifact-free, unlike scalp recordings.

6. A single electrical stimulus applied to the motor cortex produces multiple volleys within the descending motor tracts, giving rise to D-waves and I-waves. The first volley (called the "D-wave") reflects direct stimulation of the pyramidal axons that comprise the corticobulbar and corticospinal tracts. Subsequent volleys (called "I-waves") reflect activation of the pyramidal neurons via excitatory synaptic input from other cortical neurons that were activated either directly or indirectly by the applied stimulus.

7. M-waves refer to myogenic motor evoked potentials (MEPs) recorded from the muscles (not pyramidal neurons) upon cortical stimulation.

8. Under anesthesia, when I-waves are suppressed and the MEPs consist of D-waves, the myogenic MEPs elicited by transcranial electrical stimulation (TES) are predominantly recorded from muscles contralateral to the anode.

9. Transcranial magnetic stimulation (TMS) does not activate scalp pain fibers as strongly as TES, and is therefore useful for assessing central motor pathways in conscious subjects. However, TMS can also be applied to nonmotor regions in the brain convexity.

10. Repetitive TMS (rTMS)-induced changes in cortical excitability outlast the stimulation, and resemble those of long-term potentiation (LTP) and long-term depression (LTD) that are induced by repetitive electrical stimulation of the cortex or hippocampus. The ability of TMS to produce such lasting and focal changes in cortical excitability forms the basis of its therapeutic effect in major depression, chronic pain, and epilepsy.

11. TMS is not useful for intraoperative monitoring since the MEPs (i.e., I-waves) generated by it are attenuated by anesthesia.

12. The electrical stimuli for TES can consist of a pair of electrodes (anode/cathode) inserted into the scalp. The Fz/Cz electrode pair predominantly stimulates the corticospinal tracts to the legs; C3/C4 preferentially stimulates the corticospinal tracts to the arms; and C1/C2 stimulates corticospinal tracts to both upper and lower extremities. A more laterally placed electrode pair can selectively stimulate the hemisphere ipsilateral to the anode, allowing recording of MEPs in the muscles contralateral to the anode.

13. Magnetoencephalographic (MEG) has better spatial resolution than EEG in localizing the cortical events and is sensitive to activity within the fissural cortex. Currents that are perpendicular to the cortical surface cannot be theoretically detected by MEG. However, current sources that deviate from the radial orientation can be detected.

14. MEG cannot differentiate between ictal and interictal spikes. However, one can position an electrode array over the area of interictal MEG activity, calculate the forward solution, and monitor the ictal activity during EEG to ascertain whether the MEG interictal focus is responsible for the ictal activity as well.

15. In patients with adrenergic failure, Phase II late and Phase IV responses of the Valsalva maneuver are impaired. Generally, Phase IV becomes blunted followed by loss of Phase II Late response.

16. Heart rate deep breathing (HRDB) range is one of the parasympathetic markers of autonomic function. It is the mean change in heart rate over five respiratory cycles.

17. Sudomotor function is typically measured by quantitative sudomotor axon reflex test (QSART) or other forms of sweat testing.

18. Acetylcholine is the neurotransmitter for most parasympathetic postganglionic fibers and norepinephrine is the neurotransmitter for most sympathetic postganglionic fibers. However, sympathetic fibers innervating sweat glands are cholinergic fibers.

19. In postural orthostatic tachycardia syndrome (POTS), there is a profound increase in heart rate without a significant drop in blood pressure.

20. Cardiac sympathetic imaging is the best technique to differentiate Parkinson's disease with autonomic dysfunction from multiple system atrophy (MSA).

21. While performing single-fiber electromyography (SFEMG), the low-frequency filter should be raised to 500 Hz so that distant low-frequency waveforms are not recorded. This allows the SFEMG needle to record only from a few muscle fibers close to the needle tip.

22. A lesion in the right trigeminal nerve or nucleus leads to absent ipsilateral R1, ipsilateral R2, and contralateral R2 responses in a blink reflex study with right trigeminal stimulation.

23. A lesion in the left facial nerve leads to absent contralateral R2 with right trigeminal stimulation and absent ipsilateral R1 and ipsilateral R2 with left trigeminal stimulation.

24. SFEMG is not specific for neuromuscular junction (NMJ) disorders, and can be abnormal in other neurogenic conditions. SFEMG is the most sensitive test for NMJ disorders and a normal SFEMG in a weak muscle is not consistent with myasthenia gravis (MG).

25. Jitter value increases with age.

26. HR varies with deep breathing (decreases with inspiration and increases with expiration), and this variability is measured to calculate HR deep breathing range.

27. HR deep breathing range and other cardiovagal measures decrease with age; therefore, it should always be compared with age-matched controls.

28. HR response to deep breathing and Valsalva ratio are the two commonly measured reflex cardiovagal measures.

29. Pressure recovery time (PRT) is a measure of adrenergic function; it increases with adrenergic failure.

30. QSART evaluates postganglionic, cholinergic, sympathetic sudomotor function.

31. In preganglionic lesions, QSART is normal but thermoregulatory sweat test is abnormal.

32. Phase II Late and Phase IV are the two reflex mediated components of the Valsalva maneuver.

33. Medications such as anticholinergics can have profound effects on autonomic study results, and these should be stopped before autonomic studies.

34. Autonomic dysfunction is seen in both botulism and Lambert–Eaton myasthenic syndrome (LEMS).

35. Quantitative EEG (qEEG) cannot replace expert review of raw EEG.

36. qEEG measures can be used to detect delayed cerebral ischemia (DCI), due to vasospasm.

37. Alpha–delta ratio (ADR) is a measure of the percentage of alpha activity compared to the percentage of delta activity for a given time period. With decreasing cerebral blood flow (CBF), the amount of alpha activity will decrease and the amount of delta activity will increase. Thus, a decreasing ADR would indicate decreasing perfusion, and likely ischemia or infarction.

38. The fast Fourier transform (FFT) spectrogram is a frequency-based qEEG trend that displays a three-dimensional representation of EEG power (which is proportional to the square of the amplitude) over time with respect to the various frequencies. Seizures are typically represented by increasing power that usually evolves from lower to higher frequencies, but the opposite (i.e., higher to lower frequencies) can also occur. Many artifacts (e.g., muscle or electrode) typically present with increased power on the FFT spectrogram as well, but the increase is more abrupt without evolution.

39. Amplitude-integrated EEG (aEEG) is an amplitude-based qEEG trend that displays the minimum and maximum amplitude of the EEG background over a preset time interval (typically 1–2 seconds). On the aEEG, the increase in baseline amplitude and the narrowing of the aEEG band can suggest a seizure discharge. Many other changes on aEEG are nonspecific and often represent artifact.

40. The peak envelope trend is an amplitude-based qEEG trend that displays the median amplitude of the EEG background over a preset time interval (typically 10–20 seconds). On the peak envelope trend, the upward deflection of the tracing represents an increase in median amplitude and can correspond to a seizure.

41. Long leads and ferrous metals can lead to skin heating and burning during acquisition of magnetic resonance (MR) images.

42. Nonferrous metals, such as noble metals (e.g., silver, gold, copper, and platinum) lead to fewer artifacts and are more conducive to being used in MR imaging. Metal electrodes lead to a "starburst" effect on CT images due to deflection, not absorption of x-rays.

43. In about half of all continuous EEG (cEEG) studies, the first seizure is captured within the first hour of recording. Although there may be little benefit of monitoring beyond 24 hours in noncomatose patients, there is some evidence to suggest that extending the monitoring at least another 24 hours in comatose patients may increase the yield by 10%.

44. The American Clinical Neurophysiology Society (ACNS) established standardized critical care EEG terminology to create an objective EEG classification scheme using descriptive terms for frequently encountered EEG patterns in critically ill patients that are not biased about the clinical significance of a given pattern. Standardization allows for comparison of results between readers.

45. Main Term one has four classifications: generalized (G) refers to bilateral activity that is both synchronous and symmetric; if the activity is synchronous and asymmetric, then it falls under the term lateralized (L), which also includes unilateral hemispheric or focal patterns; if the activity is asynchronous, then it falls under the term bilateral independent (BI), and the activity can be hemispheric or more focal; multifocal (Mf) refers to patterns occupying at least three distinct brain regions and involving both hemispheres.

46. Main Term two has three classifications: (a) periodic discharges (PDs) applies only to single discharges with relative uniform morphology lasting less than 0.5 seconds and does not apply to bursts; there is a quantifiable interval between the discharges that have less than 50% variation from one cycle to the next; (b) rhythmic delta activity (RDA) is repetition of a waveform with relatively uniform morphology and duration and can be distinguished from PDs in that RDA does not have an interval between consecutive waveforms; (c) spike wave (SW) consistently follows the pattern of alternating spike or sharp wave followed by a slow wave.

47. Absence of normal sleep architecture, periodic (epileptiform) discharges, nonreactive background, and nonconvulsive status epilepticus are all independent predictors of poor outcome (Modified Ranking Scale (MRS) greater than four) in subarachnoid hemorrhage.

48. The definition of neurogenic orthostatic hypotension is a drop in systolic blood pressure (SBP) of more than 20 mmHg with less than 15beats/min increase in HR during tilt table testing. Nonneurogenic causes of orthostatic hypotension are usually associated with >15beats/min increase in HR along with >20 mmHg drop in BP. If there is no change in BP, but HR increase is more than 30beats/min, it might reflect POTS. Increase in BP during tilt table may be seen with orthostatic hypertension, a rare disorder.

49. Mutation in sodium channel can cause small fiber neuropathy.

50. Chronic inflammatory demyelinating polyneuropathy (CIDP) is not typically associated with significant autonomic neuropathy or failure.

51. Skin biopsy, which assesses epidermal nerve fiber density, has the highest diagnostic yield (sensitivity and specificity) for small fiber neuropathy. QSART testing to assess sudomotor function is the best noninvasive diagnostic test for small fiber neuropathy. Routine nerve conduction and somatosensory evoked potential (SSEP) studies are typically normal in small fiber neuropathy.

52. Excessive beta can also be seen with benzodiazepine and / or barbiturate administration, anesthetics (e.g., nitrous oxide, synthetic opiates), stimulants, (e.g., D-amphetamine, methylphenidate, cocaine), and hallucinogens (e.g., lysergic acid diethylamind (LSD)).

53. At low doses of short-acting synthetic opiates (e.g., fentanyl), slowing of alpha and increase of beta activity occurs. With moderate doses, further higher amplitude predominately theta background slowing occurs. With high doses, further higher amplitude predominately delta background slowing occurs. Of note, burst-suppression or electrocerebral silence (ECS) does not typically occur.

54. Seizures are the most common neurological emergency in abusers of methylenedioxymethamphetamine (MDMA), also known as ecstasy.

55. Epileptogenic zone (EZ) is the presumed area of the brain, removal of which is necessary and sufficient to achieve seizure freedom. It is most commonly defined by the region of the brain that is primarily involved in generating the seizures. In an stereoencephalography (SEEG) evaluation, the EZ is characterized by the presence of rhythmic faster frequency waveforms, repetitive spikes, high-amplitude slow waves with superimposed faster frequency waveforms, or rhythmic synchronous waveforms in multiple electrodes that occur with or without a minor time lag between the electrodes.

Abbreviations

AASM, American Academy of Sleep Medicine
AC, Alternating current
AChR, Acetylcholine receptor
ACNS, American Clinical Neurophysiology Society
ADC, Analog-to-digital converter
ADM, Abductor digiti minimi
ADR, Alpha–delta ratio
AEC, Anatomo-electro-clinical
AEDs, Antiepileptic drugs
aEEG, Amplitude-integrated EEG
AHI, Apnea-hypopnea index
AIDP, Acute inflammatory demyelinating polyradiculoneuropathy
AIN, Anterior interosseus nerve
AIS, Anteriorly predominant intermittent slow
ALS, Amyotrophic lateral sclerosis
ALT, Alanine aminotransferase
AMN, Adrenomyeloneuropathy
AMPA, Alpha-amino-3-hydroxy-5-methyl-4-isoxazolepropionic acid
APB, Abductor pollicis brevis
AS, Active sleep
AST, Aspartate aminotransferase
AVM, Arteriovenous malformation
BAEPs, Brainstem auditory evoked potentials
BECTS, Benign partial epilepsy of childhood with centrotemporal spikes
BETS, Benign epileptiform transients of sleep
BiPAP, Biphasic positive airway pressure
BiPDs, Bilateral periodic discharges
BiPLEDs, Bilateral independent periodic lateralized epileptiform discharges

BP, Blood pressure
BRE, Benign rolandic epilepsy
BSSS, Benign sporadic sleep spikes
CA, Conceptional age
CABG, Coronary artery bypass graft
CAE, Childhood absence epilepsy
CBF, Cerebral blood flow
CCT, Central conduction time
cEEG, Continuous video-EEG
CIDP, Chronic inflammatory demyelinating polyneuropathy
CIRDA, Central intermittent rhythmic delta activity
CISP, Chronic immune sensory polyradiculopathy
CJD, Creutzfeldt–Jakob disease
CMAP, Compound muscle action potential
CMT, Charcot–Marie–Tooth
CNS, Central nervous system
CPA, Cerebellopontine angle
CPAP, Continuous positive airway pressure
CPK, Creatine phosphokinase
CPR, Cardiopulmonary resuscitation
CPSE, Complex partial status epilepticus
CRDs, Complex repetitive discharges
CRRT, Continuous renal replacement therapy
CSA, Central sleep apnea
CSE, Convulsive status epilepticus
CSF, Cerebrospinal fluid
CSWS, Continuous spike waves of sleep
CTS, Carpal tunnel syndrome
dBHL, Decibel hearing level
dBSL, Decibel sensation level
DC, Direct current
DCI, Delayed cerebral ischemia
DNA, Deoxyribonucleic acid
DRG, Dorsal root ganglion
ECI, Electrocerebral inactivity
ECMO, Extracorporeal membrane oxygenation
ECoG, Electrocorticography
EIP, Extensor indices proprius
EMG, Electromyography
EMU, Epilepsy monitoring unit
EOAE, Evoked otoacoustic emission
EOG, Electrooculogram
EP, Evoked potentials
EPSPs, Excitatory postsynaptic potentials
ESES, Electrographic status epilepticus of sleep
EZ, Epileptogenic zone
FDI, First dorsal interosseous

FFT, Fast Fourier transform
FIRDA, Frontal intermittent rhythmic delta activity
FOLD, Female gender, occipital location, low amplitude, drowsiness
GA, Gestational age
GABA, Gamma-aminobutyric acid
GBS, Guillain–Barré syndrome
GIRDA, Generalized intermittent rhythmic delta activity
GPDs, Generalized periodic discharges
GRDA, Generalized rhythmic delta activity
GSD, Glycogen storage disease
GSE, Generalized status epilepticus
GTCs, Generalized tonic-clonic seizures
HFOs, High-frequency oscillations
HFOV, High-frequency oscillatory ventilator
HIHARS, Hyperventilation-induced high-amplitude rhythmic slowing
HLA, Human leukocyte antigen
HMG-CoA, 3-Hydroxy-3-methyl-glutaryl-CoA
HNPP, Hereditary neuropathy with liability to pressure palsy
HR, Heart rate
HSE, Herpes simplex encephalitis
HSV, Herpes simplex virus
HV, Hyperventilation
HVS, High-voltage slow
IBI, Interburst interval
IBM, Inclusion body myositis
ICP, Intracranial pressure
IEDs, Interictal epileptiform discharges
INEM, Isolated neck extensor myopathy
INR, International normalized ratio
IOM, Intraoperative monitoring
IPI, Interpeak interval
IPL, Interpeak latencies
IPS, Intermittent photic stimulation
IPSPs, Inhibitory postsynaptic potentials
IRDA, Intermittent rhythmic delta activity
ISI, Interstimulus intervals
IV, Intravenous
JME, Juvenile myoclonic epilepsy
KA, Kainic acid
LEMS, Lambert–Eaton myasthenic syndrome
LGS, Lennox–Gastaut syndrome
LKS, Landau–Kleffner syndrome
LL, Lateral lemniscus
LPDs, Lateralized periodic discharges
LPs, Lumbar potentials
LSS, Lewis–Sumner syndrome
LTD, Long-term depression

LTP, Long-term potentiation
LTS, Low threshold spike
LVI, Low-voltage irregular
MAC, Minimal alveolar concentration
MAG, Myelin-associated glycoprotein
MCA, Middle cerebral artery
MCN, Modified combinatorial nomenclature
MDMA, Methylenedioxymethamphetamine
MEG, Magnetoencephalography
MELAS, Mitochondrial myopathy, encephalopathy, lactic acidosis, and stroke
MEPs, Motor evoked potentials
MERRF, Myoclonus, epilepsy, ragged red fibers
MFN, Mitofusin
mfVEP, Multifocal visual evoked potentials
MG, Myasthenia gravis
MGA, Martin–Gruber anastomosis
mMEPs, Myogenic motor evoked potentials
MMN, Multifocal motor neuropathy
MR, Magnetic resonance
MRC, Medical Research Council
MRS, Modified Ranking Scale
MS, Multiple sclerosis
MSA, Multiple system atrophy
MSLT, Multiple sleep latency test
MUAP, Motor unit action potential
MUP, Motor unit potentials
MuSK, Muscle-specific kinase antibody
MWT, Maintenance of wakefulness test
NCL, Neuronal ceroid lipofuscinosis
NCS, Nerve conduction studies
NCSE, Nonconvulsive status epilepticus
NIOM, Neurophysiologic intraoperative monitoring
NMDA, N-methyl-D-aspartate
NMJ, Neuromuscular junction
OIRDA, Occipital intermittent rhythmic delta activity
OSA, Obstructive sleep apnea
PAP, Positive airway pressure
PDR, Posterior dominant rhythm
PDS, Paroxysmal depolarization shift
PDs, Periodic discharges
PERG, Pattern electroretinogram
PET, Positron emission tomography
PGO, Ponto-geniculo-occipital
PLEDs, Periodic lateralized epileptiform discharges
PLM, Periodic limb movement
PLMD, Periodic limb movement disorder
PLMS, Periodic limb movement of sleep

PLS, Primary lateral sclerosis
PMEs, Progressive myoclonic epilepsies
PMP, Peripheral myelin protein
PMR, Photomyogenic response
POSTS, Positive occipital sharp transients of sleep
POTS, Postural orthostatic tachycardia syndrome
PPI, Pixels per inch
PPR, Photoparoxysmal response
PRT, Pressure recovery time
PRVEP, Pattern-reversal visual evoked potential
PSE, Partial status epilepticus
PSG, Polysomnogram
PSPs, Postsynaptic potentials
PSWC, Periodic sharp wave complexes
PVEP, Pattern-reversal visual evoked potential
PVS, Persistent vegetative state
QDIRT, Quantitative direct and indirect axonal reflex test
qEEG, Quantitative EEG
QS, Quiet sleep
QSART, Quantitative sudomotor axon reflex test
QST, Quantitative sensory test
RAS, Reticular activating system
RAV, Relative alpha variability
RBD, REM sleep behavior disorder
RC, Resistor–capacitor
RDA, Rhythmic delta activity
RDI, Respiratory disturbance index
RERA, Respiratory effort-related arousal
RINCH, Rhythmic ictal nonclonic hand motions
RLC, Resistor–inductor–capacitor
RLS, Restless leg syndrome
RMP, Resting membrane potential
RMTD, Rhythmic mid-temporal theta bursts of drowsiness
RNS, Responsive neurostimulator
rTMS, Repetitive transcranial magnetic stimulation
SAH, Subarachnoid hemorrhage
SBP, Systolic blood pressure
sCJD, sporadic Creutzfeldt–Jakob disease
SE, Status epilepticus
SEEG, Stereoencephalography
SEP, Sensory evoked potential
SFEMG, Single fiber electromyography
SI, Stimulus induced
SIRPID, Stimulus-induced rhythmic, periodic, or ictal discharges
SMA, Spinal muscular atrophy
SMA, Supplementary motor area
SNAP, Sensory nerve action potential

SOREMPs, Sleep-onset REM periods
SPSE, Simple partial status epilepticus
SREDA, Subclinical rhythmic electrographic discharge in adults
SSEP, Somatosensory evoked potential
SSPE, Subacute sclerosing panencephalitis
SSS, Small sharp spikes
SW, Spike wave
TES, Transcranial electrical stimulation
TIRDA, Temporal intermittent rhythmic delta activity
TMS, Transcranial magnetic stimulation
TSH, Thyroid stimulating hormone
TTR, Transthyretin
VEP, Visual evoked potential
VPL, Ventral posterolateral
WAR, Widespread anteriorly dominant rhythm
WBC, White blood cell
WHAM, Wake, high amplitude, anterior location, male gender
WPS, Widespread persistent slow

Bibliography

Amato A, Russell JA. *Neuromuscular Disorders*. 1st ed. New York, NY: McGraw-Hill Professional; 2008.

American Academy of Sleep Medicine. *AASM Manual for the Scoring of Sleep and Associated Events: Rules, Terminology and Technical Specifications, Version 2*. Westchester, IL: American Academy of Sleep Medicine; 2012.

American Academy of Sleep Medicine. *The International Classification of Sleep Disorders: Diagnostic and Coding Manual*. 2nd ed. Westchester, IL: American Academy of Sleep Medicine; 2005.

American Clinical Neurophysiology Society. *Guideline 3: Minimum Technical Standards for EEG Recording in Suspected Cerebral Death*. Milwaukee, WI: American Clinical Neurophysiology Society; 2006.

American Clinical Neurophysiology Society. *Guideline 14: American Clinical Neurophysiology Society's Standardized Critical Care EEG Terminology: 2012 version*. Milwaukee, WI: American Clinical Neurophysiology Society; 2012.

Bhattacharya, KB. James Wenceslaus Papez, his circuit, and emotion. *Ann Indian Acad Neurol*. 2017;20:207–210.

Blum A, Rutkove S, eds. *The Clinical Neurophysiology Primer*. Totowa, NJ: Humana Press; 2007.

Britton, JW. Electrical stimulation mapping with stereo-EEG electrodes. *J Clin Neurophysiol*. 2018;35:110–114. https://doi.org/10.1097/WNP.0000000000000443

Bulacio. JC, Chauvel. P, McGonigal. A. Stereoelectroencephalography: interpretation. *J Clin Neurophysiol*. 2016;33:503–510. https://doi.org/10.1097/WNP.0000000000000305

Cardinale, F, Casaceli, G, Raneri, F, Miller, J, Lo Russo, G. Implantation of stereoelectroencephalography electrodes: a systematic review. *J Clin Neurophysiol*. 2016;33:490–502. https://doi.org/10.1097/WNP.0000000000000249

Chiappa KH. *Evoked Potentials in Clinical Medicine*. 3rd ed. Baltimore, MD: Lippincott Williams & Wilkins; 1997.

Cossu, M, Cardinale, F, Castana, L, Nobili, L, Sartori, I, Lo Russo, G. Stereo-EEG in children. *Childs Nerv Syst*. 2006;22:766–778. https://doi.org/10.1007/s00381-006-0127-2

Daube JR, Rubin DI, eds. *Clinical Neurophysiology*. 3rd ed. Oxford, England: Oxford University Press; 2009.

Daube JR, Rubin DI. Needle electromyography. *Muscle Nerve*. 2009;39:244–270. https://doi.org/10.1002/mus.21180

Ebersole JS, Pedley TA, eds. *Current Practice of Clinical Electroencephalography*. 3rd ed. Baltimore, MD: Lippincott Williams & Wilkins; 2003.

Fisher R, Salanova V, Witt T, et al. Electrical stimulation of the anterior nucleus of thalamus for treatment of refractory epilepsy. *Epilepsia*. 2010;51:899–908. https://doi.org/10.1111/j.1528-1167.2010.02536.x

Gitter AJ, Stolov WC. AAEM minimonograph #16: instrumentation and measurement in electrodiagnostic medicine—part I. *Muscle Nerve*. 1995;18:799–811. https://doi.org/10.1002/mus.880180803

Gitter AJ, Stolov WC. AAEM minimonograph #16: instrumentation and measurement in electrodiagnostic medicine—part II. *Muscle Nerve*. 1995;18:812–824. https://doi.org/10.1002/mus.880180804

Gutierrez-Hernandez S, Ritzl EK. Motor evoked potentials. In: Husain AM, ed. *A Practical Approach to Neurophysiologic Intraoperative Monitoring*. 2nd ed. New York, NY: Demos Medical Publishing; 2015;33–45.

Hirsch LJ, Brenner RP, eds. *Atlas of EEG in Critical Care*. West Sussex, UK: Wiley-Blackwell; 2010.

Holder, GE. Pattern electroretinography (PERG) and an integrated approach to visual pathway diagnosis. *Prog Retin Eye Res*. 2001;20(4):531–561. doi:10.1016/s1350-9462(00)00030-6

Husain A, ed. *A Practical Approach to Neurophysiologic Intraoperative Monitoring*. New York, NY: Demos Medical Publishing; 2008.

Iber C, Ancoli-Isreal S, Chesson A, Quan SF. *The AASM Manual for the Scoring of Sleep and Associated Events: Rules, Terminology, and Technical Specifications*. Westchester, NY: American Academy of Sleep Medicine; 2007.

Kryger MH, Roth T, Dement WC, eds. *Principles and Practice of Sleep Medicine*. 3rd ed. St. Louis, MO: Elsevier; 2000.

LaRoche S, ed. *Handbook of ICU EEG Monitoring*. New York, NY: Demos Medical Publishing; 2013.

Levin K, Lüders H, eds. *Comprehensive Clinical Neurophysiology*. Philadelphia, PA: W.B. Saunders Company; 2000.

Lüders H, ed. *Textbook of Epilepsy Surgery*. London, UK: Informa Healthcare; 2008.

MacDonald DB. Intraoperative motor evoked potential monitoring: overview and update. *J Clin Monit Comput*. 2006;20(5):347–377. https://doi.org/10.1007/s10877-006-9033-0

Mergos J, Kale EB, Husain AM. Training curriculum for NIOM. In: Husain AM, ed. *A Practical Approach to Neurophysiologic Intraoperative Monitoring*. 2nd ed. New York, NY: Demos Medical Publishing; 2015;334–353.

Miller AE, ed. Autonomic disorders. *Continuum*. 2007;13(6):1–280. https://doi.org/10.1212/01.CON.0000275614.78948.37

Mirandola L, Mai. RF, Francione. S, et al. Stereo-EEG: diagnostic and therapeutic tool for periventricular nodular heterotopia epilepsies. *Epilepsia*. 2017;58:1962–1971. https://doi.org/10.1111/epi.13895

Nuwer MR, ed. *Intraoperative Monitoring of Neural Function: Handbook of Clinical Neurophysiology*. Amsterdam: Elsevier; 2008.

Pellock J, Bourgeois B, Dodson WE, eds. *Pediatric Epilepsy*. 3rd ed. New York, NY: Demos Medical Publishing; 2008.

Preston DC, Schapiro BE. *Electromyography and Neuromuscular Disorders: Clinical-Electrophysiologic Correlations*. 2nd ed. Newton, MA: Butterworth-Heinemann; 2005.

Schomer DL, da Silva FL, eds. *Niedermeyer's Electroencephalography: Basic Principles, Clinical Applications, and Related Fields*. 6th ed. Baltimore, MD: Lippincott Williams & Wilkins; 2010.

Sheybani, A, Brantley, MA, Apte, RS. Pattern electroretinography in age-related macular degeneration. *Arch Ophthalmol*. 2011;129(5):580–584. doi:10.1001/archophthalmol.2011.83

Simon MV. *Intraoperative Neurophysiology: A Comprehensive Guide to Monitoring and Mapping*. New York, NY: Demos Medical Publishing; 2009.

Singh, R, Husain, AM. Electoencephalography. In: Husain, AM, ed. *A Practical Approach to Neurophysiologic Intraoperative Monitoring*. 2nd ed. New York, NY: Demos Medical Publishing; 2015;55–65.

Yamada T, Meng M. *Practical Guide for Clinical Neurophysiologic Testing: EEG*. Philadelphia, PA: Lippincott Williams & Wilkins; 2010.

Yamada T, Meng M. *Practical Guide for Clinical Neurophysiologic Testing: EP, LTM, IOM, PSG, and NCS*. Philadelphia, PA: Lippincott Williams & Wilkins; 2011.

Index